PERINATAL MEDICINE

Management of the High Risk Fetus and Neonate

PERINATAL MEDICINE

Management of the High Risk Fetus and Neonate

RONALD J. BOLOGNESE, M.D.
Associate Professor of Obstetrics and Gynecology,
University of Pennsylvania School of Medicine;
Department of Obstetrics and Gynecology,
Pennsylvania Hospital, Philadelphia;
Board Certified, Maternal and Fetal Medicine

RICHARD H. SCHWARZ, M.D.
Professor of Obstetrics and Gynecology;
Director, The Jerrold R. Golding Division of Fetal Medicine;
University of Pennsylvania, School of Medicine, Philadelphia, Pennsylvania;
Board Certified, Maternal and Fetal Medicine

SANS TACHE

THE WILLIAMS & WILKINS COMPANY/Baltimore

Made in the United States of America

Library of Congress Cataloging in Publication Data

Main entry under title:

Perinatal medicine.

Includes index.
1. Fetus—Diseases. 2. Pregnancy, Complications of. 3. Infants (Newborn)—Diseases. I. Bolognese, Ronald J. II. Schwarz, Richard H. [DNLM: 1. Fetal diseases. 2. Infant, newborn, diseases. W0210 P4415]
RG626.P47 618.9'201 77-1473
ISBN 0-683-00907-9

Composed and printed at the
Waverly Press, Inc.
Mt. Royal and Guilford Aves.
Baltimore, Md. 21202, U.S.A.

Preface

For many years an arbitrary division of responsibility has existed between the obstetrician and the pediatrician. Recognition of perinatal medicine represents a rejection of this separation and an appreciation that the problems of the mother, fetus and newborn are a continuum. Adverse factors affecting the maternal environment can alter significantly fetal development and neonatal morbidity and mortality.

Rapid advances in neonatology have enhanced the survival rate of premature and critically ill term newborn infants. Technologic development of ultrasonic and electronic monitoring equipment and highly sensitive biochemical assays have improved assessment of the fetoplacental unit and have aided in reducing the incidence of stillbirths.

The purpose of this text is to provide the clinician with diagnostic and therapeutic concepts of perinatal medicine. Initially, the high risk gravida must be identified in order to institute genetic, ultrasonic, hormonal and electronic fetal monitoring. Diagnosis of specific complications such as diabetes, Rh sensitization, pregnancy-induced hypertension, dysmaturity and drug addiction require appropriate diagnostic and therapeutic decisions. The neonatal problems associated with prematurity and postmaturity emphasize the importance of intensive care facilities supervised by trained neonatologists. All of these aspects of maternal, fetal and newborn management underscore the role of the perinatal team bridging the traditional disciplines of obstetrics and pediatrics.

Preparation of this information represents the talent and expertise of many authors. Their efforts are most appreciated.

Contributors

Richard H. Aubry, M.D., Associate Professor of Obstetrics and Gynecology, State University of New York, Upstate Medical Center, Syracuse, New York

Tom P. Barden, M.D., Professor of Obstetrics and Gynecology, Associate Professor of Pediatrics, University of Cincinnati, College of Medicine, Cincinnati, Ohio

Richard L. Berkowitz, M.D., Assistant Professor of Obstetrics and Gynecology, Yale University, School of Medicine, New Haven, Connecticut

Samir Beydoun, M.D., Assistant Professor of Obstetrics and Gynecology, State University of New York, Upstate Medical Center, Syracuse, New York

Ronald J. Bolognese, M.D., Associate Professor of Obstetrics and Gynecology, University of Pennsylvania, School of Medicine, Department of Obstetrics and Gynecology, Pennsylvania Hospital, Philadelphia, Pennsylvania

M. Theresa Cabalum, M.D., Fellow in Maternal and Fetal Medicine, State University of New York, Upstate Medical Center, Syracuse, New York

Elsie R. Carrington, M.D., Professor and Chairman, Department of Obstetrics and Gynecology, The Medical College of Pennsylvania, Philadelphia, Pennsylvania

Wayne R. Cohen, M.D., Fellow in Maternal and Fetal Medicine, Beth Israel Hospital, Instructor in Obstetrics and Gynecology, Harvard Medical School, Boston, Massachusetts

James F. Connaughton, Jr., M.D., Assistant Professor of Obstetrics and Gynecology, University of Pennsylvania, School of Medicine, Department of Obstetrics and Gynecology, Pennsylvania Hospital, Philadelphia, Pennsylvania

Stephen L. Corson, M.D., Assistant Professor of Obstetrics and Gynecology, University of Pennsylvania, School of Medicine, Department of Obstetrics and Gynecology, Pennsylvania Hospital, Philadelphia, Pennsylvania

F. Gary Cunningham, M.D., Assistant Professor of Obstetrics and Gynecology, University of Texas Health Sciences Center, Southwestern Medical School, Dallas, Texas

Loretta P. Finnegan, M.D., Associate Professor of Pediatrics, and Associate Director of Nurseries, Thomas Jefferson University, School of Medicine, Philadelphia, Pennsylvania

Roger K. Freeman, M.D., Medical Director of Women's Hospital, Memorial Hospital Medical Center of Long Beach, Long Beach, California; Professor of Obstetrics and Gynecology, University of California at Irvine, Irvine, California

David A. Fuccillo, Ph.D., Director, Advanced Testing and Development Laboratory, Litton Bionetics, Incorporated, Bethesda, Maryland

Norman F. Gant, M.D., Professor and Associate Chairman, Department of Obstetrics and Gynecology, and The Cecil H. and Ida Green Center for Reproductive Biology Sciences, University of Texas, Southwestern Medical School, Dallas, Texas

John C. Hobbins, M.D., Associate Professor, Assistant Chairman, Department of Obstetrics and Gynecology, Assistant Professor, Department of Diagnostic Radiology, Yale University, School of Medicine, New Haven, Connecticut

Calvin J. Hobel, M.D., Chief of Obstetrics, Los Angeles County Harbor General Hospital, Associate Professor, Department of Obstetrics and Gynecology and Pediatrics, University of California, Los Angeles, School of Medicine, Los Angeles, California

John F. Huddleston, M.D., Assistant Professor of Obstetrics and Gynecology, Director, Division of Maternal and Fetal Medicine, University of Alabama, School of Medicine, Birmingham, Alabama

Mhairi G. MacDonald, MBchD, MRCP (UK), FAAP, Neonatologist and Assistant Professor of Pediatrics, Albany Medical Center Hospital, Albany Medical College of Union University, Albany, New York

Michael Mennuti, M.D., Assistant Professor of Obstetrics and Gynecology, University of Pennsylvania, School of Medicine, Philadelphia, Pennsylvania

Uchenna C. Nwosu, M.D., Fellow in Maternal and Fetal Medicine, Pennsylvania Hospital, Instructor in Obstetrics and Gynecology, University of Pennsylvania, School of Medicine, Philadelphia, Pennsylvania

Jack A. Pritchard, M.D., Gillette Professor of Obstetrics and Gynecology, University of Texas Health Sciences Center, Southwestern Medical School, Dallas, Texas

Dian S. Reeser, B.A., Research Assistant, Family Center Program, Thomas Jefferson University, School of Medicine, Philadelphia, Pennsylvania

Herman M. Risemberg, M.D., FAAP, Director of the Capital Regional Neonatal Care Center, Associate Professor of Pediatrics, Obstetrics and Gynecology, Albany Medical Center Hospital, Albany Medical College of Union University, Albany, New York

Barry S. Schifrin, M.D., Director, Maternal and Fetal Medicine, Cedars-Sinai Medical Center, Associate Professor of Obstetrics and Gynecology, University of Southern California, School of Medicine, Los Angeles, California

Richard H. Schwarz, M.D., Professor of Obstetrics and Gynecology, Director, The Jerrold R. Golding Division of Fetal Medicine, University of Pennsylvania, School of Medicine, Philadelphia, Pennsylvania

John L. Sever, M.D., Ph.D., Chief, Infectious Diseases Branch, National Institute of Neurological and Communicative Disorders and Stroke, Bethesda, Maryland; Professor of Pediatrics, Georgetown University Medical School, Washington, D.C.

Margaret L. Williams, M.D., Professor of Pediatrics, State University of New York, Upstate Medical Center, Syracuse, New York

Richard J. Worley, M.D., Assistant Professor of Obstetrics and Gynecology, University of Texas, Southwestern Medical School, Dallas, Texas

Contents

Part IV. NEONATAL

CALVIN J. HOBEL, M.D.

1

Identification of the Patient at Risk

Introduction

To speak of health care for women, neonates and infants as a "continuum" is an apt reminder of the linear nature peculiar to perinatology. Within this branch of medicine, early events flow into and often affect subsequent progress. Ideally, assessment of this continuum should begin well before the antenatal period since the majority of factors which affect reproductive performance are present before a woman becomes pregnant. However, practically speaking, most pregnant patients seeking care already have passed the period of fetal development most greatly affected by adverse factors. Thus, the first prenatal assessment is usually a look back into the continuum; to adolescence, the interconceptional period and gametogenesis and fertilization. Although all these relationships must be seen as a whole, it also is desirable to pinpoint stages of the continuum where important events characteristically take place. The perinatal period is such an area, unique in that later success is vitally reliant upon the early recognition and management of problems during this particular period. The technique of risk assessment used here and intervention can help prevent disabling conditions later during the neonatal period and infancy.

The History of Risk Assessment

The history of risk assessment and why these techniques have not evolved more extensively over the past 15 years has been reviewed recently by Hobel.[21] The inertia centers over two basic problems. Since early studies were retrospective in design and based on an analysis of the medical record, assessment schemes did not clearly identify the high risk patient.[16, 29, 35, 36] Although later studies by Effer[8] and Hebb[19] were prospective, they were incomplete because they limited their assessment only to one time period, usually the antenatal period, which has been shown to be the least predictive.

Risk assessment will attract more perinatologists in the next few years because some of the initial problems have been resolved. More complete prospective assessments recently have been completed by Hobel[21] and Stembera and associates.[41] Changes during the next few years could spark a dramatic change in the way we assess the risks associated with reproduction.

The Team Approach

Perinatal medicine is composed of varied yet interdependent disciplines. To provide effective health care and research, all facets of care must mesh and coordinate smoothly. A team framework allows each individual to make unique contributions in an organized fashion. A perinatal record can reflect a team approach by incorporating all information within a single system to provide a complete patient profile.

As perinatal medicine develops in this

way, we realize more and more that the total need of our patients must be considered. We can no longer address only the medical aspects of care, but we must also address the psychosocial aspects and their effects on health care. Today women are less willing to adopt the role of a sick patient. A recent publication reflects strong contemporary concern regarding health care for women,[1] but physicians have been criticized as early as 1900 for being too scientific and not knowing how to take care of the total needs of patients. Peabody[34] stated in 1927 that "the physician who attempts to take care of a patient while he neglects the emotional life is as unscientific as the investigator who neglects to control all the conditions that may affect his experiment."

The challenge of meeting the total needs of the patient through a spectrum of services provided by a team is incomplete without the participation of the patient. The patient must have a responsible role in helping to achieve and maintain excellent health care. The principle of patient responsibility will become more important as we expand our ambulatory primary care programs to place emphasis on prevention.

How are we to effectuate interdependency and collaboration of our health care team? In order to administrate such a complex program, usually on a regional basis, we must have a means of communication. A problem-oriented perinatal record is the means whereby we can link the components of health care. Each member of the team must play an active role in the development, maintenance and distribution of the data base, problem list and health care plan.

Problem-oriented Perinatal Risk Assessment

The provision of perinatal care is heavily dependent upon the written and spoken word, which generates an array of data elements. Generally speaking there are two systems used to determine the at risk patient from this data. The "clinical impression of risk," whether it be by a nurse or physician, is an individual judgment based on data elements and interpreted as a problem which suggests some degree of risk. An assessment of risk by a "scoring technique" is a refinement of the above described clinical impression. This scoring technique purposely is built into the medical record and its final score gives a precise degree of risk. Both methods identify the patient at risk and both are subject to specific criticisms. On the one hand, many valuable "clinical impressions of risk" are never recorded, buried in the medical record, or forgotten and never passed on to other members of the health team. On the other hand, little of this type of data escapes the higher structured scoring technique. Scoring is sometimes questioned by those who feel that such a system is arbitrary. However, the "clinical impression of risk" is actually more arbitrary in that it is solely dependent upon the individual's personal experience, whereas the "structured scoring technique" is designed and validated on the basis of the experience of hundreds and even thousands of pregnancies. The purpose of this chapter is to acquaint the reader with an existing problem-oriented scoring technique for identification of the high risk patient.

The foundation upon which perinatal medicine is built lies in the system used to collect and analyze our results. This can best be accomplished through the use of an organizational structure, depicted in Figure 1.1, which utilizes a problem-oriented record. In addition to identifying a patient at risk and facilitating a plan of management, the system must provide a mechanism of evaluating medical practice and must support the educational process. Many high risk pregnancies will remain unrecognized until we demand that the record accomplish the above. Only through a well structured system will regionalized perinatal care become effective.

Prenatal Risk Assessment

HISTORIC ASSESSMENT

Assessment for specific *historic problems* is important since many of them are associated with subsequent problems either during the remaining prenatal period, during labor and/or during the neo-

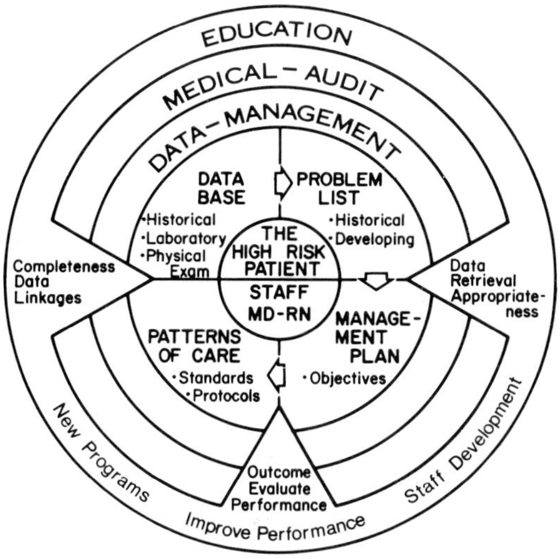

Figure 1.1. The organizational structure of a data collection system for regional perinatal care.

natal period. Because of these associations, cognizance of their presence is necessary to formulate a plan of management.

The development of a data base is the first step in antenatal assessment. To facilitate this process we have found it helpful to have the patient participate in the development of this data base. This is accomplished by providing the patient with a questionnaire which may be completed easily at home or in the doctor's office. The questionnaire which we use has been tested and evaluated for content by our educational staff and has been shown to be an accurate and effective means of facilitating the development of a data base. In the design of this questionnaire we did not want to limit the search to just medical information. We are attempting to incorporate into our assessment an understanding of the psychosocial aspects of illness and patient care. In becoming more involved with these latter two aspects we hope we can shorten the gap between the patient and her physician. The task of designating a patient as low risk or high risk must incorporate a psychosocial as well as a medical assessment. Although pregnancy is not an illness, it can have a profound effect on the behavior of a patient; therefore, to give a patient total care, the physician must also take into consideration the effect of the pregnancy on the patient's emotions and relationships. One additional benefit of the intake questionnaire is that it facilitates communication between the patient and the health care team. Too often, the intake session with a new patient is limited to a question-answer process where the patient is treated only as an information source. The patient must be given sufficient time to reflect on her medical and psychosocial experiences. After this questionnaire is completed, a designated team member completes Form 1 (Prenatal Screening), Figure 1.2, with the aid of the questionnaire. Any positive problem is designated by placing a + sign opposite the listed problem. The time to complete Form 1 varies between 5 and 12 min depending upon the amount of historic information. A high risk patient will require more time, but it is time well spent since an accurate and complete data base will provide more information.

LABORATORY DATA, PHYSICAL EXAM AND DEVELOPING PROBLEMS

The next phase of developing a data base is the collection of *routine laboratory data* and carrying out the initial *physical exam*, Form 2 (Prenatal Screening), Figure 1.3. This begins the formulation of a *developing problem list*. The historic problem list acts as an important background for the patient. Although the historic problems cannot be resolved, many of the developing problems can be resolved. The developing problem list is the active portion of the record used to facilitate continued assessment during pregnancy. This list is divided into five definable categories which are interrelated to special laboratory tests, procedures and follow-up examinations. Habits are included in this section rather than in the historical section because they are potentially soluble.

PRENATAL FLOW RECORD

Form 3 (Prenatal Flow Record), shown in Figure 1.4, is essential for completing the initial assessment. After completing Forms 1 and 2 and entering the initial set of follow-up data (weight, urine test, blood pressure, etc.) on Form 3, the team member (physician or extended role nurse) scans for data which may begin to formu-

AGE	TERM	PREMI	Ab	LIVE	CARRY OVER PROBLEM LIST FROM PATIENT MEDICAL RECORD
LMP	☐ NORMAL ☐ ABNORMAL	CYCLES ☐ Regular ☐ Irregular	EDC		

+	Risk Value	Prob. No.	HISTORICAL PROBLEM LIST — Data Collected ☐ Prospective ☐ Retrospective
	5	1	☐ Age < 17 ☐ AGE > 35 ☐ HEIGHT < 60 inches
	10	2	CHRONIC HYPERTENSION – BP ≥ 140/90 on 2 occasions 1 week apart prior to pregnancy or prior to 26 weeks.
	5	3	PRE-ECLAMPSIA ☐ Required Hospitalization ☐ Required Early Delivery See Problem 16
	10	4	MODERATE TO SEVERE RENAL DISEASE ☐ Chronic pyelonephritis, ☐ Nephrotic Syndrome, ☐ Polycystic Kidney ☐ Other
	5	5	GENITOURINARY INFECTIONS History of ☐ A symptomatic Bacteruria, ☐ Cystitis (Dysuria, Frequency, Treated With Antibiotics), ☐ Pylonephritis (Same as Cystitis but With Temperature Elevation ≥ 100.4°)
	10	6	HEART DISEASE — FUNCTIONAL CLASSIFICATION: ☐ 1 = No limitation of physical activity ☐ 2 = Slight limitation of physical activity ☐ 3 = Marked Limitation of Physical activity ☐ 4 = Inability to Carry On Any Physical Activity w/o Discomfort — CRITERIA FOR DIAGNOSIS (ANY ONE): ☐ A = Diastolic Murmur ☐ B = Cardiac Enlargement ☐ C = Systolic Murmur ≥ Grade III
	10	7	DIABETES White's Classification ☐ B ☐ C ☐ D ☐ E ☐ F (if ☐ Class A evaluate Prob. #28)
	5	8	PULMONARY DYSFUNCTION ☐ Asthma, ☐ Tuberculosis, ☐ Chronic Bronchitis, ☐ Other:
	10	9	HEMOLYTIC DISEASE OF NEWBORN ☐ Rh ☐ ABO ☐ Other:
	5	10	OTHER MEDICAL ☐ EMOTIONAL PROBLEMS ☐ THYROID DISEASE-Type: ☐ Other:
	5	11	HEMORRHAGE DURING PREVIOUS PREGNANCY ☐ 1st ☐ 2nd ☐ 3rd trimester ☐ Post Partum ☐ Transfusion
	5	12	HISTORY OF INFERTILITY ☐ Primary ☐ Secondary ☐ Treated ☐ Untreated
	10	13	UTERINE-CERVICAL ABNORMALITY ☐ Uterine Anomaly ☐ Incompetent Cervix
	5	14	PREVIOUS UTERINE SURGERY ☐ C-Section ☐ Classical ☐ Low Tranverse ☐ Unknown ☐ Hysterotomy ☐ Cerclage ☐ Other
	1	15	PREVIOUS OPERATIONS – Specify:

+	Risk Value	Prob. No.		Preg No.	Delivery Month	Delivery Year	Birth Weight	Gest. Age Weeks	Labor Hours	Alive Yes	Alive No	Age of Death	Abn. Present	Associated Problems (Use Prob. No.)
	10	16	EPILEPSY ☐ ECLAMPSIA											
	5	17	MULTIPARITY (5 or more)	1										
	10	18	PREVIOUS PREMATURE	2										
	10	19	PREVIOUS STILLBIRTH	3										
	10	20	NEONATAL DEATH	4										
	5	21	SUDDEN INFANT DEATH	5										
	5	22	THERAPEUTIC ABORTION	6										
	10	23	HABITUAL ABORTION 3 or MORE CONSECUTIVE	7										
				8										

+	Risk Value	Prob. No.	
	5	24	INFANT GREATER THAN 9 LBS.
	5	25	FAMILY HISTORY OF ☐ Twins ☐ Diabetes ☐ SS Disease ☐ Other:
	5	26	INFANT WITH GENETIC DISEASE ☐ Chromosomal ☐ CNS ☐ Other:
	5	27	FETAL ANOMALY ☐ Extremeties ☐ Trunk ☐ Internal Organs ☐ Other:

DRUGS OR DEVICES USED (WITHIN PAST YEAR)

ITEM	NO	YES	NAME/CODE	DOSE	FROM	TO
BIRTH CONTROL PILLS						
INTRAUTERINE DEVICE						
ASPIRIN						
IRON-VITAMINS						
SEDATIVES-Tranquilizers						
ANTICONVULSANTS						
HORMONES						

SOCIAL STATUS INDEX

PATIENT: FATHER:

EDUCATION
1 - Grad. Prof. Training (17 + yrs)
2 - College or Univ. Grad.
3 - Partial College Training
4 - High School Grad.
5 - Partial High School
6 - Junior High
7 - Less Than 7 yrs of School

INSURANCE COVERAGE
☐ Medical Assistance ______
☐ Other: ☐ None

NUTRITION INDEX

	Excellent	Good	Poor
Protein			
Iron			
Calories			

ALLERGIES

PATIENT ADDRESS			
CITY	MARITAL STATUS	RACE	TELEPHONE
SOCIAL SECURITY NUMBER	BIRTHDATE	CLINIC OR PHYSICIAN - CODE	

1 BR PRENATAL SCREENING

Figure 1.2. This is Form 1, which is the Prenatal Screening form for obtaining the historic data base.

late a developing problem. Identified developing problems are recorded by placing a + sign in the appropriate place on Form 2. The degree of risk next is determined by adding up the risk values for each problem (Forms 1 and 2) and entering the first score in the lower left hand corner on Form 2. A low risk patient is defined as one having a total score of ≤9, whereas high risk patients have total scores of ≥10. This

PRESS HARD — YOU ARE MAKING EXTRA COPIES

ROUTINE LAB		
TYPE ☐ A ☐ B ☐ O ☐ AB		PAP ☐ Neg ☐ Imfl. ☐ Pos
Rh ☐ Pos ☐ Neg ☐ Du+		DYSPLASIA
ANTIBODY SCREEN ☐ Neg ☐ Pos		☐ Mild ☐ Mod
SEROLOGY ☐ Neg ☐ Pos		☐ Severe
FTA ☐ Neg ☐ Pos		PPD ☐ Neg ☐ Pos ______ mm
URINE PROTEIN ☐ Neg ☐ Pos ☐ 1+ ☐ 2+ ☐ 3+		HCT/Hgb
SUGAR ☐ Neg ☐ Pos		GC SCREEN ☐ Neg ☐ Pos
MICRO ☐ Neg ☐ Pos		

PHYSICAL EXAM	NORMAL YES	NO		NORMAL YES	NO	DATE:	NORMAL YES	NO
SKIN			LUNGS			PERINEUM		
HEENT			BREASTS			VULVA		
TEETH			HEART			VAGINA		
GUMS			ABDOMEN			CERVIX		
THYROID			EXTREMITIES			UTERUS		
			NEUROLOGIC			PELVIMETRY		
CLINICAL PELVIMETRY	☐ Adequate		☐ INADEQUATE			☐ Inlet ☐ Mid ☐ Outlet		
X-RAY PELVIMETRY	☐ Adequate		☐ INADEQUATE			☐ Inlet ☐ Mid ☐ Outlet		

DEVELOPING PROBLEMS

COMMENTS

+	DATE POSITIVE	DATE RESOLVED	RISK VALUE	PROB. NO.	POSITIVE LAB
			10	28	DIABETES - Class A
			5	29	POSITIVE PPD
			5	30	POSITIVE SEROLOGY
			5	31	MILD ANEMIA 9-10.9 Gm%
			5	32	SEVERE ANEMIA <9 Gm%
			5	33	Rh NEG. ☐ Not Sent. ☐ Sensitized
			5	34	POSITIVE ROLL OVER TEST
			5	35	SICKLE CELL TRAIT
					ANATOMICAL
			10	36	MULTIPLE PREGNANCY
			10	37	POLYHYDRAMNIOS
			10	38	INCOMPETENT CERVIX
			5	39	WEIGHT ☐ <100 lb. ☐ >200 lb.
			5	40	WEIGHT GAIN ☐ <½ lb./week ☐ >2 lb./week (evaluate at 30 weeks)
			10	41	ABNORMAL FETAL POSITION ☐ Breech ☐ Transverse Lie ☐ Oblique Lie
			5	42	SMALL PELVIS (Any suggestion that the ☐ inlet, ☐ mid-pelvis, or ☐ outlet is small)
					HABITS
			10	43	NARCOTIC USE (Heroin, Cocaine, etc.) Indicate months used and type on Form 1
			5	44	EXCESSIVE USE ☐ Non-Narcotic Drugs ☐ Alcohol
			5	45	SMOKING ☐ 1 pack per day ☐ Less than 1 pack per day
					MEDICAL - SURGICAL - PSYCHOSOCIAL
			5	46	GENITAL-URINARY INFECTION ☐ Vaginitis ☐ Asymptomatic Bacteruria ☐ Cystitis
			10	47	PYELONEPHRITIS - Patient has Bacteruria and Temp. ≥100.4° F.
			5	48	FLU SYNDROME - Any flu like sickness requiring: ☐ 2 days bedrest or ☐ Hospitalization DATE:
			10	49	VIRAL - Other ☐ Toxoplasmosis ☐ Rubella ☐ Cytomegalovirus ☐ Herpes Progenitalis
			10	50	OTHER MEDICAL
			5	51	SURGICAL ☐ Appendectomy ☐ Therapeutic Ab ☐ Cerclage ☐ Other
			5	52	PSYCHOSOCIAL PROBLEMS
					ABNORMALITIES OF FUNCTION
			5	53	MILD PRE-ECLAMPSIA #1 required for the diagnosis ☐ 1 = B.P. ≥140/90 or ↑30 mm Systolic or ↑15 in Diastolic ☐ 2 = Proteinuria 1+ or 2+ ☐ 3 = Persistent edema of hands and/or face
			10	54	SEVERE PRE-ECLAMPSIA ☐ B.P. ≥160/110 or ☐ Proteinuria >2+ both after 26 weeks Gest. Age
			5	55	PERSISTENT HYPOTENSION (Diastolic <65)
			10	56	INTRA UTERINE GROWTH RETARDATION (inadequate uterine growth)
			10	57	POST TERM - Any pregnancy over 42 weeks from LMP or estimated from early physical exam
			10	58	VAGINAL SPOTTING - ☐ Prior to 28 wks ☐ Placenta Previa ☐ Low Lying Placenta
			10	59	ABNORMAL PLACENTAL FUNCTION TEST ☐ E-3 ☐ HPL ☐ OCT

SCORES	DATE	SCORE	SIGNATURES
FIRST SCORE			
REVISED SCORE			
REVISED SCORE			

2 BR PRENATAL SCREENING

Figure 1.3. This is Form 2, which is the Prenatal Screening form for the addition of laboratory data, the physical exam findings and any developing problems.

is referred to as dichotomized scoring.[22] A readjustment of this definition of risk may have to be made after an analysis of more recent data.

Continued assessment during the prenatal period is a requirement since this period is not static. Certain lab tests and procedures are conveniently located on

NOTE ▶ THIS FORM FOR ☐ 0-26 WKS ☐ 27-34 WKS ☐ 35-41 WKS ☐ 42+ WKS

PRE PREG WEIGHT ▶	HEIGHT	> BLOOD PRESSURE < ● FHT ⊗ FUN. HT.	AGE	TERM	PREM	Ab	LIVE	LMP	EDC	CORRECTED EDC

Date	Weight (LBS)	Total Gain	Sug	Albu-min	200	190	180	170	160	150	140	130	120	110	100	90	80	70	60	50	Gest. Age	Fundal Height	Fetal Present	Fetal Heart	Ed-ema	Return Visit - # Weeks	Physician Number
FUNDAL HEIGHT "cm"					42	40	38	36	34	32	30	28	26	24	22	20	18	16	14								

SPECIAL LAB

BLOOD SUGARS					DATE	E-3	HPL	DATE	TITERS	DATE	Hgb ELECT (circle 2)	DATE	REPEAT — LAB
DATE	FAST	1 HR	2 HR	3 HR					Rh:		A_1 A_1 A_2 F		Hct/Hgb =
									Rubella:		S S C		Hct Hgb =
									Serology:		URINE CULTURE		VDRL = ☐ Neg ☐ Pos
													GC SCREEN ☐ Neg ☐ Pos

SPECIAL TESTS

ROLL OVER TEST	LAT /	SUP /	DATE	AMNIO CENTESIS	ULTRA SOUND				
				1. Genetic 3. Optical Density	DATE	PLACENTA	B.P.D.	G.A.	POSITION
OCT	NON STRESS			2. Lung Mat 4. Other					
☐ Neg ☐ Pos	☐ Neg ☐ Pos								
☐ Neg ☐ Pos	☐ Neg ☐ Pos								
☐ Neg ☐ Pos	☐ Neg ☐ Pos								

REFERRAL TO ☐ Social Service ☐ Dietitian ☐ Prep. Child Birth ☐ Med. Ctr. Special OB Clinic ☐ Other:

COUNSEL FOR ☐ Personal Hygiene ☐ Nutrition ☐ Daily Activities ☐ Anesthesia ☐ Other:

CONSULTATION FROM ☐ Medical ☐ Surgical ☐ Psychiatric ☐ Other:

DEVELOPING PROBLEMS CHECK FORM 2 LIST HERE # ______ ______ # ______ ______

DATE	PROB. NO.	PLAN	DATE	PROB. NO.	PLAN

3 BR **PRENATAL FLOW RECORD**

Figure 1.4. This is Form 3 which is the Prenatal Flow Record where serial data is entered and special laboratory tests and procedures are chosen as part of a plan of management.

this form to aid the team member in the search for or resolution of problems. Since each of the problems on Forms 1 and 2 is numbered, the problem number can be recorded on Form 3 in the area designated as "Plan" and a management scheme established. These numbered problems become the baseline reference points which tie the record together and ensure that the record becomes meaningful and manageable.

Once an initial plan is formulated, follow-up information and important interactions should be recorded on separate progress notes. In order to maintain the integration of the record, the number of the problem is included in the entry on the progress notes, and the special "SOAP" editorial device is used; S (subjective data reported by patient), O (objective data), A (assessment status of problem) and P (plan—diagnostic, therapeutic, educational).

ASSESSMENT OBJECTIVES

The purpose of the assessment scheme is to prevent certain problems through the mechanism of early recognition and the implementation of an intervention plan. With the present technique of prenatal assessment using a dichotomized score[22] or the use of a more sophisticated computer analysis, we can expect to predict only approximately 50% of mothers during this time period who later will deliver a neonate with morbidity.[24] The major perinatal problems responsible for this morbidity are listed in Table 1.1. The specific prenatal problems which are related to these major perinatal problems also are listed in Table 1.1. Let us look more carefully at each major problem area and determine what role the assessment of these related problems has in formulating a plan of therapy or prevention.

Risk of Prematurity

Premature labor and the sequel of this complication accounts for 60 to 70% of perinatal morbidity and mortality. Therefore, it is important to be in a position whereby one can predict whether a patient is at risk for premature labor. Unfortunately, utiliz-

Table 1.1. Prenatal assessment objectives*

Major perinatal problems to be identified early	Associated prenatal problems	
	Historic factors	Developing factors
Prematurity <37 weeks	Mother's education† Previous stillbirth Previous premature Previous neonatal death Multiparity ≥5 Uterine malformation Weight <100 lb	Moderate-severe toxemia Incompetent cervix Rh sensitization Smoking Pyelonephritis Narcotic use
Intrauterine growth retardation	Previous stillbirth Previous neonatal death Multiparity ≥5	Moderate-severe toxemia
Toxemia	Chronic hypertension History of renal disease Diabetes Age <17	Weight gain >2 lb/wk Intrauterine growth retardation Positive roll-over test[13] Multiple pregnancy
Diabetes	Age >35 Infant >9 lb Family history Fetal anomaly	Polyhydramnios Pre-eclampsia Genital-urinary infections
Congenital anomalies	Age >35 Diabetes Habitual abortion† Previous fetal anomaly†	

* Five major perinatal problems and the significantly related prenatal problems are listed. The prenatal assessment objective is to identify early the patient at risk for any one of these problems. Prenatal factors except those with references and those marked by daggers (†) were determined by the author to be related to the corresponding major perinatal problem by a prospective analysis of data collected from 1417 pregnancies.

† Those factors with assumed relationship.

ing the criteria listed in Table 1.1, only approximately 50 to 60% of patients with associated factors actually deliver premature infants. This suggests that until the cause of premature labor is determined we can only predict and not yet prevent this complication.

How then is one to use this information? At the present time the medical team and the patient can be informed of the risk of premature labor. If premature labor does occur, proper therapy can be implemented early to halt labor with a well conceived plan rather than treating the event as a catastrophy.

Risk of Intrauterine Growth Retardation

Most of the factors associated with this problem are also historic, yet this condition occasionally is associated with other disease states which affect placental and uterine blood flow, such as severe toxemia and diabetes. Other causes, such as intrauterine infection and genetic defects, are difficult to diagnose clinically. At the present time we must assess carefully the progress of each pregnancy for this risk although we may be unaware of its etiology. Serial fundal measurements to monitor the growth of the fetus is a simple and very useful clinical tool and it may be the first indicator that a problem is developing. Special tests, such as urine or plasma estriol, plasma human placental lactogen levels and procedures like ultrasound measurements, the oxytocin stress test and the nonstress tests, are of value in evaluating fetal and placental growth and function.

Risk for Developing Toxemia

Like the previous problems, most factors can be identified but not resolved. Considerable progress has been made by Gant and associates[13, 14] in the area of predicting the risk of developing pre-eclampsia by utilizing the angiotension infusion test and the supine pressor test (roll-over test). There is recent data to suggest that the roll-over test is not as predictive as the original reports would suggest.[18]

Patients at Risk for Diabetes

O'Sullivan and associates have identified numerous historic factors which are associated with increased risk of glucose intolerance.[32] It is important that the diagnosis of this disease be made as early in pregnancy as possible, so it can be treated in order to reduce the high neonatal morbidity and mortality associated with this problem. Many of the developing factors listed in Table 1.1 are prognostically bad signs, red flags which signal that the management plan has not been optimal. As the adverse factors accumulate, so does the risk of poor outcome. As mentioned above, special tests and procedures are frequently helpful in assessing fetal placental wellbeing.

Risk of Congenital Anomalies

Presently we are very limited in our quest to predict the risk for congenital anomalies. Considerable progress has been made in recent years by focusing on patients with certain risk factors. However, without clear-cut cause and effect relationships we can only speculate what the risks will be. These probabilities are generated only after adequate data collection on large populations. Therefore, if we are to improve our predictions in the future, we must carefully document the potential risks as part of the historic data base today.

Intrapartum Risk Assessment

ANTENATAL RECORD REVIEW

A parturient must be assessed for both the factors which have characterized her prenatal course and those factors which will become apparent during the course of labor. Unfortunately, all too often, important antenatal factors are overlooked either because the team member considers them not important or the information is not available. Prenatal events are important indicators of subsequent risk. Table 1.2 clearly shows that high risk patients during the antenatal period have a greater percentage of high risk neonates and perinatal deaths than do low risk antenatal patients. When prenatal information is not easily available, a quick and thorough assessment should be made. Identified problems are entered in the upper right-

Table 1.2. Prenatal and intrapartum status of patients studied during 1974 divided into four groups*

Group	Risk status			Neonatal outcome	
	Prenatal	Intrapartum	%	Morbidity, %	Mortality, %
I	Low	Low	38	5.0	0.0
II	High	Low	27	5.8	1.4
III	Low	High	17	11.6	2.3
IV	High	High	18	17.4	4.3

* Low risk = score ≤9; high risk = ≥10. Note the differences in percentages of groups when compared with previous published data.[21]

hand portion of Form 4 (Intrapartum Problem List), Figure 1.5. This prenatal information is not only important for the labor and delivery team, but it is of vital importance for the pediatric team. A newborn's data is the mother's prenatal and intrapartum problem list and data sheet.

ASSESSING EARLY PROBLEMS

Our research studies during the intrapartum period have directed our attention toward several time related events.[24] Consequently, our intrapartum record (Form 4) reflects these events. In order to begin an early labor assessment, information regarding the last menstrual period and expected date of confinement, the onset of labor and the time of rupture of the membranes must be obtained. This data sets the stage for identifying whether or not the patient is in premature labor, the first problem on our list, and one of the most serious problems confronting obstetricians and pediatricians today. Each patient must be carefully assessed for each early problem (Problems 101 to 112). If the team member has difficulty with the assessment, consultation is obtained. As soon as a problem can be ruled in or out, a "+" or "−" notation is made opposite the risk factor. At the present time fetal heart rate and uterine motility are not continuously monitored if the patient is defined as low risk (i.e., having a prenatal score of ≤9 or the absence of any early intrapartum problems). We do initiate monitoring of all high risk patients using either external methods or, preferably, internal methods if the membranes have ruptured spontaneously.

ASSESSING INTERIM PROBLEMS

As labor progresses, serial data collection is essential to an ongoing, complete assessment. We have categorized these factors as "interim" because they represent a new series of events which frequently manifest themselves during the active phase of labor. Form 5 (Intrapartum Flow), Figure 1.6, allows for the recording of important data elements. An important component of this approach is to develop a profile of labor based on Friedman's work.[10] Directions for completing Form 5 are located on the back of Form 5 (Figure 1.7).

LATE LABOR ASSESSMENT AND RISK SCORING

We believe that the late stage of labor, beginning with the cervix completely dilated, has not been given sufficient attention. This is most likely true for both previously defined low risk patients and high risk patients. As the interim phase differs from the early phase, so does the late phase differ from previous phases. There is an overlap between these phases, but by reviewing all previous risk items at each of the three assessment periods one is in a better position to recognize developing problems. When the infant is delivered, the delivery data on Form 6 (Intrapartum/Delivery), Figure 1.8, is completed by the nursing team in the delivery room. The late problem list on Form 4 is completed and an intrapartum score is calculated. Copies of Forms 4, 5 and 6 are taken to the nursery as soon as the forms are completed in the delivery room, thus passing on valuable information to the nursery team, who is now responsible for continued care. We are describing an active approach to data collection as compared with the passive approach in the past, where the record was completed after the team left the delivery room. Under these circumstances completion of the record required recall and copies rarely reached the nursery until the newborn was 2 hr old. The prenatal score, intrapartum score and Apgar score should be the first three indicators which alert the

PATIENT WEIGHT	AGE	TERM	PREMI	Ab	LIVE	PRENATAL CARE ☐ NO ☐ YES	CLINIC OR PHYSICIAN	CODE

ADMISSION DATE __/__/__ TIME ____ | LMP | CONDENSED PRENATAL PROBLEM LIST | PROB NO | PROB NO

MEMBRANES RUPTURED __/__/__ TIME ____ | EDC

ONSET LABOR __/__/__ **1** TIME ____

PRENATAL HOSPITALIZATION ☐ No ☐ Yes PRENATAL SCORE ▶

PATIENT TRANSFERRED FROM ANOTHER HOSPITAL ☐ NO ☐ YES - specify:

	+ −	Risk Value	Prob. No.	
EARLY PROBLEMS		10	101	PREMATURE LABOR <37 ▶ Lung Maturity: ☐ Immature ☐ Interm. ☐ Mature Treatment: ☐ Alcohol ☐ B-Mimetic ☐ Other:
		10	102	HYDRAMNIOS – A clinical estimate of excessive amniotic fluid.
		10	103	MULTIPLE PREGNANCY
		10	104	ABN PRESENTATION ☐ Breech ☐ Face ☐ Brow ☐ Compound ☐ Transverse Lie ☐ Other
		10	105	MODERATE SEVERE PRE-ECLAMPSIA - B.P.≥160/110 or Proteinuria>2+ after 26 wks Gest. Age
		5	106	MILD PRE-ECLAMPSIA # 1 required for the Diagnosis ☐ 3 – Persistent edema of Hands or Face ☐ 1 BP≥140/90 or + 30mm in systolic or 15 mm in diastolic ☐ 2 Proteinuria 1 + or 2+
		5	107	INDUCTION ☐ Medical ☐ Elective ☐ Amniotomy ☐ Oxytocin
		5	108	PREMATURE RUPTURE OF MEMBRANES – Rupture 12 hours or more prior to labor onset.
		5	109 *	C-SECTION ☐ Primary ☐ Repeat
		10	110	HEAVY MECONIUM – Dark stained Amniotic Fluid – usually dark green and tenacious
		5	111	LIGHT MECONIUM – Light stained Amniotic Fluid – yellow or greenish
		5	112	PROLONGED LATENT PHASE – Over 13 hours Multipara, over 20 hours Nullipara
INTERIM PROBLEMS		5	113	PRIMARY DYSFUNCTIONAL LABOR - W/O Oxytocin after 4 cm dilatation ☐ 1 - Nullipara - at least 1 cm per hour ☐ 2 - Multipara - 1.5 cm per hour
		1	114	SECONDARY ARREST OF DILATATION – Failure to progress after 5 cm Cervical Dilatation
		5	115	PITOCIN AUGMENTATION OF LABOR – Use of Oxytocin to improve uterine contractions
		10	116	CORD PROLAPSE
		10	117 *	UTERINE BLEEDING ☐ Abruption ☐ Previa ☐ Marginal Separation
		10	118	FETAL TACHYCARDIA > 160 beats per minute lasting more than 30 minutes.
		10	119	AMNIONITIS ☐ Mat. Temp. ≥ 100.4° ☐ Bacteria in Amniotic Fluid
		10	120	FETAL BRADYCARDIA – < 120 Beats/min. or abnormal heart rate patterns (HRP) persisting over 30 min ☐ Mild ☐ Mod ☐ Sev cord comp. or ☐ Mild ☐ Mod ☐ Sev late decel. HRP
		10	121	DECREASE BASE LINE VARIABILITY DUE TO ☐ Medication ☐ Acidosis ☐ Unknown
COMPLETE DILATION DATE __/__/__ **2** TIME ____		5	122	EXCESSIVE MEDICATION ☐ Demerol, greater than 150 mg ☐ Phenobarbitol, greater than 60 mg ☐ Magnesium Sulfate, greater than 25 grams ☐ Other
LATE PROBLEMS		10	123	SEIZURE ☐ Eclampsia ☐ Previous Seizure Disorder ☐ Unknown
		10	124 *	BREECH DELIVERY (VAGINAL) METHOD: ☐ Spontaneous ☐ Assisted ☐ Breech Ext. TYPE: ☐ Single Footling ☐ Double Footling ☐ Frank
		10	125	SHOULDER DYSTOCIA
		5	126 *	☐ OPERATIVE FORCEPS ☐ VACUUM EXTRACTION ☐ FAILED VACUUM
		1	127 *	OUTLET FORCEPS ☐ Simpson ☐ Tucker McLane ☐ Luikart ☐ Other
		5	128	LATE PASSAGE OF MECONIUM - Any stained fluid after previously clear fluid
		10	129	COMPLICATIONS OF ANESTHESIA ☐ Convulsion ☐ Fetal Bradycardia ☐ Hypotension ☐ Other
		5	130	SECOND STAGE > 2.5 HOURS
DELIVERY DATE __/__/__ **3** TIME ____		5	131	PRECIPITOUS LABOR < 3 HOURS TOTAL
		5	132	LABOR > 20 HOURS TOTAL
PLACENTA DATE __/__/__ **4** TIME ____			133	MOTHER-INFANT BONDING ☐ Excellent ☐ Good ☐ Poor
			134	DELIVERED ☐ Home ☐ In Transit ☐ Elsewhere in Hospital
			135	STILLBIRTH ☐ Antepartum ☐ Intra-partum

	HOURS	MIN
STAGE I 1 (-2)	__	__
STAGE II 2 (-3)	__	__
STAGE III 3 (-4)	__	__
TOTAL LABOR TIME		

FINAL SCORE

SIGNATURES

1-

2-

3-

4 B R INTRAPARTUM PROBLEM LIST

Figure 1.5. This is Form 4 (Intrapartum Problem List), which is the initial work sheet for initiating the assessment during the intrapartum period.

nursery team to potential neonatal problems. If the prenatal and intrapartum scores are low and the Apgar score high, the neonate is initially low risk. Subsequent neonatal observations are necessary in order to assure that the neonate remains low risk, or to identify the neonate who becomes high risk for the first time.

When the patient leaves the delivery room, Form 7 (Postpartum/Discharge),

PRESS HARD YOU ARE MAKING EXTRA COPIES

DATE: To Delivery Room – Draw ↓ Arrow Delivery Time – Draw ↓ Arrow

★ Cx DIL	● FHR	× B.P.		▲ STA
		200		–3
9				
		180		–2
8				
		160		
7				–1
		140		
6				
		120		0
5				
		100		
4				+1
		80		
3				
		60		+2
2				
		40		
1				+3
		20		

COMPLETE THE FOLLOWING FOR ALL PATIENTS IN LABOR (See Letter Instructions on Reverse Side)

A	Procedures
B	Temperature
C	Mat. H. Rate
D	Membranes
E	Effacement
F	Position
G	Monitor
H	Frequency
I	Intensity
J	Meds Anal.
K	Anesthesia
L	Oxytocin 0 15 30 45
M	Fetal Distress and Acid Base
N	Initials Physician/Nurse

NURSES INITIALS – SIGNATURE/TIME	PHYSICIANS INITIALS–SIGNATURE/TIME
1 -	1 -
2 -	2 -
3 -	3 -
	PAGE: OF PAGES

5 INTRAPARTUM FLOW

Figure 1.6. This Form 5 which is the Intrapartum Flow record where serial intrapartum data is collected. The data collected on this form is the basis for formulating problems which develop as labor progresses.

Figure 1.9, is initiated and upon arrival in the recovery room postpartum observations are recorded. Problem and procedure lists are included to allow for accurate data collection. This completes the record for the mother when she is discharged.

ASSESSMENT OBJECTIVES

In order to direct our attention toward intrapartum factors which are associated with neonates who are likely to become ill, we will look at the more significant intra-

CERVICAL DILATION every hour during active phase or as necessary to determine progress of labor.

FETAL HEART RATE every 30 minutes (more frequently during the second stage)

BLOOD PRESSURE every hour

A — PROCEDURES — ENTER NUMBER
1 = Prep 2 = Enema 3 = Voided 4 = Shower 5 = I.V. 6 = Catheter
7 = Spec. Exam 8 = Cervical Culture 9 = Amniocentesis 10 = Other

B — TEMPERATURE every 2 hours

C — MATERNAL HEART RATE every (2) hours

D — MEMBRANES — Record Abbreviations 1 - Spontaneous Rupture (SROM) 2 - Artificial Rupture (AROM)

E — EFFACEMENT = 0-25-50-75-100%

F — POSITION — Record Abbreviations
R = Right M = Mentum T = Transverse O = Occiput
L = Left S = Sacrum A = Anterior P = Posterior

G — MONITOR External (EXT) or Internal (INT) and draw line ⟶

H — FREQUENCY = 1 Contraction Every ______ minutes, record as (q^3) etc. (unless patient is being monitored)

I — INTENSITY = 1+ 2+ 3+ if NOT monitored. 1+ (mild), 2+ (ave.), 3+ (mod), 4+ (hypertonus)

J — MEDICINES AND ANALGESIA = Record numbers or abbreviations from Drug Form 6

K — ANESTHESIA
PC = Para Cervical EP = Epidural SP = Spinal Gen = General No = None
PUD = Pudendal CD = Caudal LOC = Local OT = Other - Specify on Form 6 Comments

L — OXYTOCIN — Top space 0-15 minutes, next space 15-30 min., etc. (Enter dose mU /min.)

M — FETAL DISTRESS — Enter Number or Abbreviation
0 = None 4 = Sev. Cord 8 = Tachycardia
1 = Head Comp. 5 = Mild Late Decel 9 = Mild Decrease Base Line Variability
2 = Mild Cord 6 = Mod. Late Decel 10 = Severe Decrease Base Line Variability
3 = Mod. Cord 7 = Sev. Late Decel 11 = Other - Specify on Form 6 Comments

ACID BASE pH Determination F = Fetal M = Maternal

N — ENTER INITIALS OF PHYSICIAN AND NURSE

EXAMPLE:

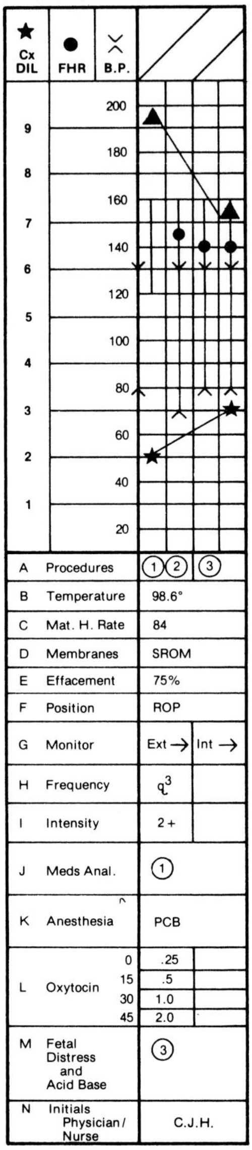

Principles of grading variable and late decelerations

Kubli et. al. Am. J. Obst. & Gynec. 104:1190 1969

CRITERIA OF GRADING	MILD	MODERATE	SEVERE
VARIABLE DECELERATION	Less than 30 sec. duration, irrespective of level	Less than 70 b.p.m. Greater than 30 sec. Less than 60 sec.	Less than 70 b.p.m. Greater than 60 sec.
Level to which FHR drops and duration of deceleration	Greater than 80 b.p.m. irrespective of duration	70-80 b.p.m. Greater than 60 sec.	
	70-80 b.p.m. Less than 60 sec.		
LATE DECELERATION			
Amplitude of drop in FHR	Less than 15 b.p.m.	15-45 b.p.m.	Greater than 45 b.p.m.

Figure 1.7. This is the back of Form 5 and lists definitions and directions for completing Form 5.

partum problems (Table 1.3). This table also lists the prenatal and neonatal or intrapartum problems which are significantly interrelated to those major problems to be prevented. The associated problems were determined by a prospective analysis of the interrelationship between factors in 1417 patients studied between

INTRAPARTUM DATA

HISTORY

PAST — Specify in Comments	YES	NONE
DISEASES		
OPERATIONS		
TRANSFUSIONS		
ALLERGIES		

DATE OF LAST MEAL TIME ☐ Light ☐ Heavy

PHYSICAL EXAM

	NORMAL YES	NORMAL NO		NORMAL YES	NORMAL NO		NORMAL YES	NORMAL NO
HEENT			ABDOMEN			EXT. GENITALS		
LUNGS			EXTREMITIES			VAGINA – CX		
BREASTS			EDEMA			UTERUS		
HEART			DT REFLEXES ☐ 1+ ☐ 2+ ☐ 3+ ☐ Clonus					

CLINICAL PELVIMETRY ☐ Adequate ☐ INADEQUATE: ☐ Inlet ☐ Mid ☐ Outlet

X-RAY PELVIMETRY ☐ Adequate ☐ INADEQUATE: ☐ Inlet ☐ Mid ☐ Outlet

COMMENTS

LAB

BLOOD: TYPE ☐ A ☐ B ☐ O ☐ AB; Rh ☐ Pos ☐ Neg ☐ Du +; HCT; ANTIBODY SCREEN ☐ Neg ☐ Pos — If pos. ident. as:

URINE: PROTEIN ☐ Neg ☐ Trace ☐ 1 + ☐ 2 + ☐ 3 +; SUGAR ☐ Neg ☐ Light ☐ Dark; MICRO ☐ Neg ☐ POS-Result:

AMNIOTIC FLUID

DATE	TIME	1/1	1/1.3	1/2	1/4	L/S

DELIVERY DATA

DATE: TIME:

NEWBORN

APGAR SCORE	0	1	2	1 MIN	5 MIN
HEART RATE	ABSENT	LESS THAN 100	OVER 100		
Resp. Effort	ABSENT	SLOW IRREG	GOOD CRY		
MUSCLE TONE	LIMP	SOME FLEXION	ACTIVE MOTION		
REFLEX Irritability	NO RESPONSE	GRIMACE	CRY		
COLOR	PALE	Body Pink Ext. Blue	ALL PINK		
TOTAL SCORE					

RESUSCITATION
☐ 1 = None
☐ 2 = Oxygen Mask
☐ 3 = Pos. Pressure Mask
☐ 4 = Pos. Pressure Tube
☐ 5 = Umbil. Catheter
☐ 6 = Suction Bulb
☐ 7 = Suction Catheter
☐ 8 = Bicarb cc =
☐ 9 = Cardiac Massage

COMPLICATIONS

MULTIPLE BIRTH ☐ NO ☐ YES = ☐ A ☐ B ☐ C

SEX ☐ Male ☐ Female

CONDITION ☐ Alive ☐ Still-born

CONGENITAL ABNORMALITIES ☐ No ☐ Yes

INFANT PASSED ☐ Urine ☐ Stool

EYE CARE ☐ Yes ☐ No

INFANT'S WEIGHT GMS

LENGTH CM

BREAST FEEDING ☐ YES ☐ NO

BABY HOSPITAL NO.

TAG NUMBER

MOTHER

ANESTHESIA FOR LABOR & DELIVERY
☐ PARA CERVICAL ☐ LOCAL INFILTRATION
☐ EPIDURAL ☐ GENERAL
☐ CAUDAL ☐ NONE
☐ PUDENDAL ☐ * COMPLICATIONS
☐ SADDLE
☐ SPINAL
☐ OTHER:

TYPE OF DELIVERY

VAGINAL VERTEX: ☐ SPONTANEOUS (☐ Del Rm ☐ Bed); ☐ * OUTLET FORCEP; ☐ * MID FORCEP ROTATION; ☐ * VACCUM EXT

* VAGINAL BREECH: ☐ SPONTANEOUS (☐ Del Rm ☐ Bed); ☐ *PIPER (operative forcep)

* C - SECTION: ☐ LOW TRANS; ☐ LOW VERT; ☐ CLASSICAL; ☐ C SEC/HYST

EPISIOTOMY: ☐ NONE; ☐ MID LINE; ☐ MED LAT

LACERATION: ☐ UTERINE; ☐ CERVICAL; ☐ VAGINAL; ☐ PERINEAL; ☐ I° ☐ II° ☐ III° ☐ IV°

PLACENTA

☐ SPONTANEOUS ☐ * PREVIA
☐ EXPRESSED ☐ * ABRUPTION ____ %
☐ MANUAL ☐ * MARGINAL SEPARATION ____ %
☐ OTHER:

WEIGHT: GRAMS

UTERINE EXPLORATION ☐ Yes ☐ No

TOTAL BLOOD LOSS: ML

CORD: ☐ NECK x 1 ☐ NECK x 2 ☐ 2 VESSELS ☐ 3 VESSELS ☐ OTHER:

COMMENTS

DRUG LIST LABOR/DELIVERY

#	MEDICATION	CODE	DOSE	SITE/ROUTE	DATE	TIME	SIGNATURE
1							
2							
3							
4							
5							
6							
7							
8							
9							
10							
11							

DELIVERY PERSONNEL	CODE
Del By:	
Asst.	
Ped.:	
Anesth.	
Nurse:	
Nurse:	

* ENTER INFORMATION ON INTRAPARTUM LIST FORM 4

6 BR INTRAPARTUM/DELIVERY

Figure 1.8. This is Form 6 which contains additional intrapartum information and delivery data.

1969 and 1972.[21] With intervention these intrapartum problems can be modified to reduce the likelihood of poor outcome.

Abnormal Labor

In our study only three of the six types of abnormal labor were found to be associated with subsequent neonatal morbidity (Table 1.3). Prolonged latent phase of labor, secondary arrest of cervical dilatation and precipitious labor were not significantly related to neonatal morbidity or mortality. Secondary arrest of cervical dilatation is not related to either prenatal or

RECOVERY ROOM

Admit Time

OBSERVATIONS EVERY 15 MINUTES X 2, THEN EVERY 30 MINUTES x 3. ADDITIONAL OBSERVATIONS IN NURSES NOTES.

Time	B.P.	Pulse	Resp.	Fundus	BLEEDING MIN	MOD	SEV	MEDS	COMMENTS	SIGNATURE

POSTPARTUM -

	DAY 1	DAY 2	DAY 3
DATE/TIME			
WELL-BEING			
B.P./TEMP.			
HEART			
LUNGS			
BREASTS			
ABDOMEN			
FUNDUS			
PERINEUM			
LOCHIA			
EXTREMITIES			
STOOL			
DYSURIA			
Signatures	M.D.	M.D.	M.D.

	HCT %	PPD ☐ NEG ☐ POS ☐ NOT DONE	VDRL ☐ Neg ☐ Pos ☐ Weak Pos ☐ Pending
		Rh Immune Globulin ☐ NO ☐ YES	FTA ☐ Neg ☐ Pos ☐ Weak Pos ☐ Pending

POSTPARTUM PROBLEMS

- ☐ 151 - Hem. Uterine Atony
- ☐ 152 - Hem. Cx Lac.
- ☐ 153 - Hem. Vag. Lac.
- ☐ 154 - Hem. Ret. Tissue
- ☐ 155 - Endometritis
- ☐ 156 - Cystitis
- ☐ 157 - Pyelonephritis
- ☐ 158 - Pneumonia
- ☐ 159 - Wound Inf.
- ☐ 160 - Fever Unk.
- ☐ 161 - Mastitis
- ☐ 162 - Spinal Headache
- ☐ 163 - Thrombophelebitis
- ☐ 164 - Pulm. Embolus
- ☐ 165 - Mech. Bowel Obst.
- ☐ 166 - Ileus
- ☐ 167 - Coagulopathy
- ☐ 168 - Eclampsia
- ☐ 169 - Anemia
- ☐ 170 - Transfusion
- ☐ 171 - Positive PPD
- ☐ 172 - ________
- ☐ 173 - ________

OPERATIVE PROCEDURES

- ☐ 174 - Tubal Ligation ☐ At C-Sec ☐ P.P.
- ☐ 175 - Repair Laceration ☐ Vag ☐ Cervical ☐ Perineal
- ☐ 176 - Oophorectomy ☐ Right ☐ Left
- ☐ 177 - Salpingectomy ☐ Right ☐ Left
- ☐ 178 - Cystectomy ☐ Right ☐ Left
- ☐ 179 - Cerclage ☐ Shirodkar ☐ McDonald
- ☐ 180 - Appendectomy
- ☐ 181 - Hypogastric Artery Ligation
- ☐ 182 - Curettage
- ☐ 183 - Other

DISCHARGE SUMMARY DATE:

AGE	TERM	PREMI	Ab	LIVE	INFANT ☐ Alive	☐ Still born	☐ Neonatal Death

ADMISSION FOR
- ☐ Labor/Delivery
- ☐ Prenatal Admission without Delivery
- ☐ Prenatal Admission with Delivery
- ☐ Other:

PRIMARY DIAGNOSIS INTRAUTERINE PREGNANCY ______ WEEKS

DIAGNOSTIC PROCEDURES

- ☐ 184 - Placental Function ☐ E-3 ☐ HPL ☐ Other:
- ☐ 185 - Oxytocin Stress Test
- ☐ 186 - Non Stress Test
- ☐ 187 - Amnioscopy
- ☐ 188 - Amniocentesis ☐ Prenatal ☐ Intrapartum
- ☐ 189 - Fetal Monitoring (Labor) ☐ Ext ☐ Int
- ☐ 190 - Screen for Diabetes
- ☐ 191 - Other:

SECONDARY DIAGNOSIS		PROB.NO.		PROB.NO.
	1 -		5 –	
	2 -		6 –	
	3 -		7 –	
	4 -		8 –	

DISCHARGE	☐ HOME	☐ OTHER:	
MEDICATIONS	☐ Fe SO_4	☐ Vitamins	☐ Other:
FOLLOW UP	☐ POSTPARTUM ______ WKS	☐ POSTOP ______ WKS	☐ OTHER ______ WKS
PHYSICIAN'S SIGNATURE			NO.

7 BR POSTPARTUM/DISCHARGE

Figure 1.9. This is Form 7 which contains postpartum information and discharge summary.

neonatal problems. Because abnormal types of labor are also related to other types of intrapartum problems, the recognition of these can be used to predict subsequent events. For example, a prolonged latent phase of labor is significantly related to dysfunctional labor and the latter is associated with prolonged descent and a prolonged second stage of labor. Friedman[10] also has observed little neonatal morbidity associated with secondary arrest of cervical dilatation, whereas pri-

Table 1.3. Intrapartum assessment objectives*

Major problems to be prevented	Associated problems: Prenatal	Associated problems: Neonatal
Abnormal labor		
Prolonged latent phase of labor	Age >35	None
Primary dysfunctional labor	Habitual abortion	Fetal anomalies, low 1-min Apgar scores, meconium aspiration
Prolonged second stage >2.5 hr	None	Hyperbilirubinemia
Precipitous labor	Previous stillbirth Previous premature	None
Prolonged labor >20 hr total	Smoking	Resuscitation at birth Fetal anomalies
Low Apgar scores 1 min <5	Prenatal Moderate-severe pre-eclampsia Maternal cardiac disease Diabetes Previous stillbirth Previous neonatal death Abnormal fetal position Multiple pregnancy	Intrapartum Premature infant Premature rupture of membranes Abnormal presentation Multiple pregnancy Heavy meconium Primary dysfunctional labor Abruptio placenta Fetal acidosis Breech vaginal delivery Operative forceps Shoulder dystocia
5 min <5	Moderate-severe pre-eclampsia Diabetes Previous stillbirth Rh sensitization Abnormal fetal position	Abruptio placenta Heavy meconium Abnormal presentation Premature infant Breech delivery Fetal acidosis Operative forceps
Respiratory distress		
Respiratory distress syndrome	Moderate-severe renal disease Diabetes Previous stillbirth Previous premature Previous neonatal death Multiparity Uterine malformation Rh sensitization Moderate-severe pre-eclampsia Pyelonephritis	Premature labor Moderate-severe toxemia Breech presentation Abruptio placenta Fetal acidosis Breech vaginal delivery
Other respiratory distress (transient tachypnea)	Diabetes Previous neonatal death Previous C section Infant >9 lbs Maternal age >35	Prematurity Premature rupture of membranes C section Heavy meconium

Table 1.3. *Continued*

Table 1.3. Continued

Major problems to be prevented	Associated problems	
	Prenatal	Neonatal
Meconium aspiration	Diabetes Previous stillbirth Multiparity ≥5 Multiple pregnancy Moderate-severe pre-eclampsia	Moderate-severe toxemia Heavy meconium Multiple pregnancy Primary dysfunctional labor Abruptio placenta Fetal acidosis Breech delivery Shoulder dystocia

* Three major perinatal problems and the significantly related prenatal and intrapartum risk factors determined by a prospective analysis of perinatal data collected from 1417 pregnancies are listed. The intrapartum objectives are to identify pregnancies and/or neonates at risk for developing any of these perinatal problems by the recognition of the listed prenatal or intrapartum risk factors.

mary dysfunctional labor is related to morbidity as well as to other intrapartum problems.

Low Apgar Scores

The second objective of intrapartum assessment is to recognize the fetus at risk because of a low Apgar score at birth. It is interesting to note that the prenatal and intrapartum factors related to low 1- and 5-min scores are similar, except for additional items which are more predictive of only low 1-min scores. These are maternal heart disease, multiple pregnancy, premature rupture of the membranes, primary dysfunctional labor and shoulder dystocia. Also, approximately one-half of the items associated with low 1-min scores can be recognized early in labor and three additional items can be recognized during the active phase of labor. We have been interested in why abnormal fetal heart rate patterns (i.e., bradycardia) did not appear in our analysis, although fetal acidosis, as determined by fetal scalp blood sampling, did. We feel that the findings are thus because fetal bradycardia is only a sign of stress and for the fetus to beome ill the pattern must persist until it alters the biochemistry of the fetus. Therefore, fetal bradycardia plus fetal acidosis is a better predictor and determinant of low Apgar scores than is bradycardia alone.

Respiratory Distress

Our next objective is to identify that pregnancy involving a fetus at risk for respiratory distress. A major component of this risk is related to premature labor. For this reason we have listed this problem first on the early intrapartum problem list and have provided a mechanism for recording whether the fetal lungs are immature, mature or of intermediate maturity. If the fetal lungs are immature and in the absence of other obstetric problems which would necessitate delivery, we would inhibit labor with an alcohol infusion (according to the method of Zlatnik and Fuchs[48]) and consider accelerating fetal lung maturity as described by Liggins and Howie.[27] The latter method would be used only if we felt that it was unlikely that labor could be stopped for a reasonable period of time for the fetal lungs to mature naturally. As we mentioned previously, we only can recognize prenatally the patient at risk and attempt to lessen the risk by early intervention, usually during the early intrapartum period. Until we identify the cause of premature labor before its onset, we must continue to function effectively at a less optimal level where we recognize patients at risk by identifying antenatal and intrapartum risk factors.

If premature labor cannot be stopped, attention then must be directed toward other intrapartum factors which may compromise the preterm fetus and increase the likelihood for the development of the respiratory distress syndrome during the neonatal period. Thibeault and associates[43] have demonstrated that factors such as multiple gestation, severe pre-eclampsia, late deceleration fetal heart rate patterns, third trimester bleeding, breech presentation, maternal hypotension and diabetes significantly increase this risk. In addition, Hobel and associates[23] and, more recently, Martin and associates[28] have recognized that abnormal fetal heart rate patterns and fetal acidosis in the preterm fetus also are associated with a greater risk for the development of the respiratory distress syndrome. Therefore, a careful intrapartum assessment and a plan of management for patients with certain risk factors is of vital importance for preventing neonatal morbidity.

There are other types of neonatal respiratory distress, such as the type which does not meet the criteria for the respiratory distress syndrome. The first type, transient tachypnea, is associated with prenatal factors which are related to diabetic pregnancies. In addition, infants delivered by cesarean section frequently develop this type of neonatal respiratory distress which is referred to as the "wet lung." Recent studies by Boddy and associates[2] on fetal gasping suggest that intrapartum events which may promote gasping may initiate intrauterine aspiration of amniotic fluid, which could be an additional cause of this type of respiratory distress. The second additional type of respiratory distress is that which is related to meconium aspiration. This has been a troublesome neonatal problem because it is associated with other neonatal complications such as the development of a pneumothorax, pneumomediastinum and pneumonia.

Our studies indicate that there are events, yet undefined, during the intrapartum period which can significantly increase risk of neonatal morbidity without the patient being at risk as identified by careful risk assessment. At the present time approximately 6% of high risk neonates are delivered from low risk patients.[21] Additional clinical studies are required to identify the remaining risk factors.

Neonatal Risk Assessment

THE INITIAL NEWBORN ASSESSMENT

A prerequisite for early neonatal assessment is having available pertinent delivery data. Form 8 (Newborn Flow Record), Figure 1.10, is initiated in the delivery room where the information located at the top right is collected. This comprises basic information necessary to begin a more complete neonatal assessment. After taking the vital signs, the nurse directs her attention toward the assessment of general problems listed on Form 9 (Newborn Problem List), Figure 1.11. The first problem is hypothermia. If the infant's initial temperature is less than 36°C or 97°F, a + sign is entered in the appropriate box. The prenatal and intrapartum score, the 1- and 5-min Apgar score, presence of asphyxia, the requirement for resuscitation and inadequate lung maturity are obtained from Forms 4 and 6 and positives are recorded as above. The final assessment is to determine the gestational age relationship by plotting the birth weight and calculated gestational age on the appropriate normogram.

DATA COLLECTION AND PROBLEM IDENTIFICATION

The assessment to follow is very similar to the prenatal and intrapartum assessment scheme. In order to identify any new problem, supplementary data must be collected by assessing additional parameters such as activity, tone and color. Information about each of these parameters is conveniently listed on the newborn flow record in a way to clearly illustrate deviations from normal. Abnormal findings frequently require additional assessments. Problems and the tasks to resolve them are summarized in "Progress Notes," where the "SOAP" editorial device is used (see "Prenatal Flow Record"). If a problem begins to emerge with this assessment, then the specific problem is identified on Form 9 with a + sign and the date is entered. The problem number also is recorded in the progress notes under "Assessment," to begin tying together the information system.

THE NEWBORN EXAM

The newborn exam is an important component of the ongoing assessment. The first day exam is completed and recorded on Form 10 (Newborn Physical/Dis-

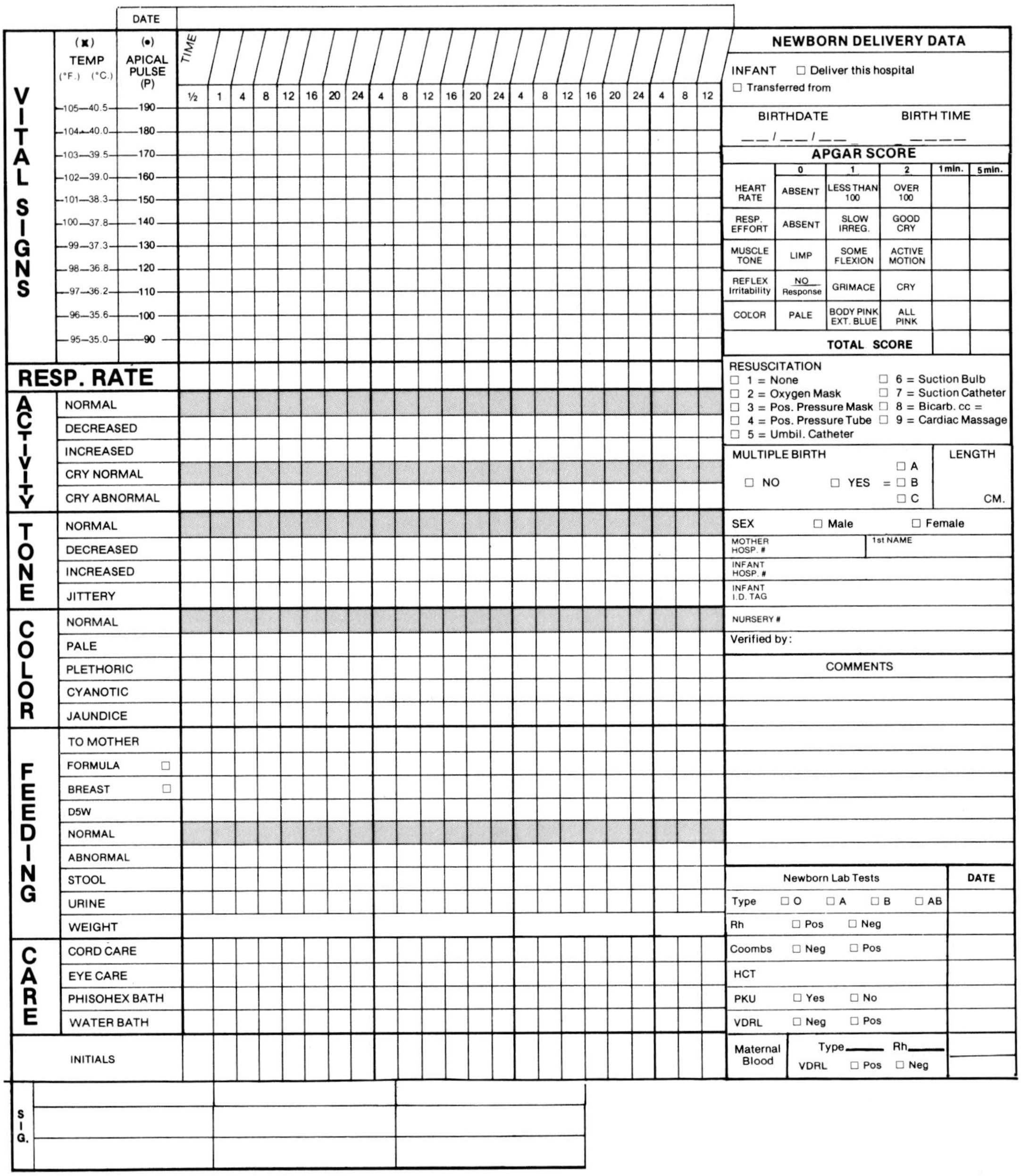

DATE

VITAL SIGNS

(x) TEMP (°F.) (°C.)	(•) APICAL PULSE (P)
105—40.5	190
104—40.0	180
103—39.5	170
102—39.0	160
101—38.3	150
100—37.8	140
99—37.3	130
98—36.8	120
97—36.2	110
96—35.6	100
95—35.0	90

TIME: ½ 1 4 8 12 16 20 24 4 8 12 16 20 24 4 8 12 16 20 24 4 8 12

RESP. RATE

ACTIVITY: NORMAL, DECREASED, INCREASED, CRY NORMAL, CRY ABNORMAL

TONE: NORMAL, DECREASED, INCREASED, JITTERY

COLOR: NORMAL, PALE, PLETHORIC, CYANOTIC, JAUNDICE

FEEDING: TO MOTHER, FORMULA ☐, BREAST ☐, D5W, NORMAL, ABNORMAL, STOOL, URINE, WEIGHT

CARE: CORD CARE, EYE CARE, PHISOHEX BATH, WATER BATH

INITIALS

SIG.

NEWBORN DELIVERY DATA

INFANT ☐ Deliver this hospital
☐ Transferred from

BIRTHDATE __/__/__ BIRTH TIME ____

APGAR SCORE

	0	1	2	1 min.	5 min.
HEART RATE	ABSENT	LESS THAN 100	OVER 100		
RESP. EFFORT	ABSENT	SLOW IRREG.	GOOD CRY		
MUSCLE TONE	LIMP	SOME FLEXION	ACTIVE MOTION		
REFLEX Irritability	NO Response	GRIMACE	CRY		
COLOR	PALE	BODY PINK EXT. BLUE	ALL PINK		
			TOTAL SCORE		

RESUSCITATION
☐ 1 = None ☐ 6 = Suction Bulb
☐ 2 = Oxygen Mask ☐ 7 = Suction Catheter
☐ 3 = Pos. Pressure Mask ☐ 8 = Bicarb. cc =
☐ 4 = Pos. Pressure Tube ☐ 9 = Cardiac Massage
☐ 5 = Umbil. Catheter

MULTIPLE BIRTH ☐ NO ☐ YES = ☐ A ☐ B ☐ C LENGTH CM.

SEX ☐ Male ☐ Female

MOTHER HOSP. # 1st NAME

INFANT HOSP. #

INFANT I.D. TAG

NURSERY #

Verified by:

COMMENTS

Newborn Lab Tests					DATE
Type	☐ O	☐ A	☐ B	☐ AB	
Rh	☐ Pos	☐ Neg			
Coombs	☐ Neg	☐ Pos			
HCT					
PKU	☐ Yes	☐ No			
VDRL	☐ Neg	☐ Pos			
Maternal Blood	Type__ Rh__ VDRL	☐ Pos	☐ Neg		

8 BR NEWBORN FLOW RECORD

Figure 1.10. This is Form 8 (Newborn Flow Record), which is initiated in the delivery room. This record is for data collection based on serial observations.

charge), Figure 1.12. Positive findings again direct the physician or nurse practitioner to the Newborn Problem List (Form 9), Figure 1.11, to record any problems. If further assessment is required, a problem-oriented "SOAP" note is completed in the progress notes. Laboratory results are recorded as objective data in the progress notes, and only the appropriate high or low values are recorded on Form 9 (Figure 1.11) for problems which require certain criteria to establish a particular diagnosis.

CODE = SHADED AREAS
A = Date Active R = Date Resolved

+	Val	GENERAL
	5	1) Hypothermia ≤ 97°F. or 36.2°C. ®
	10	2) Prenatal Score ≥10
	10	3) Intrapartum Score ≥10
	5	4) Apgar 1 min ≤5
	10	5) Apgar 5 min ≤5
	10	6) Asphyxia
	10	7) Resuscitation
	5	8) Neg Foam Test or L/S < 1.5
	1	9) Intermed. F.T. or L/S 1.5-2.0
	10	10) Preterm ≤37 wks.
	1	11) Term 38-42 wks.
	5	12) Post Term > 42 wks.
	10	13) SGA <10% ile
	1	14) AGA
	5	15) LGA >90% ile
		SKIN
	1	16) Positive Finding
		Type Code
		A R
		HEAD-NECK
	5	17) Low set ears
	10	18) Cleft Palate
	10	19) Choanal Atresia
	10	20) Retrolental Fibroplasia
		A R
	10	21) Retinoblastoma
		22) Other
		RESPIRATORY
	10	23) Meconium Aspiration
		A R
	5	24) Aspiration (other)
		☐ Am. Fl. ☐ Blood ☐ Formula
		A R
	5	25) Mild respiratory distress (T.T.N.)
		A R
	5	26) Mild RDS (Syndrome)
		A R
	10	27) Severe RDS (Syndrome)
		A R
	10	28) Congenital Pneumonia
		A R
	10	29) Apnea
		A R
	10	30) Pneumothorax
		A R
	10	31) Pneumomediastinum
		A R
	10	32) Interstitial Emphysema
		A R
	10	33) Broncho-pulm. dysplasia
		A R
	10	34) Anomaly
		Type
		35) Other

	Val	CARDIOVASCULAR
	10	36) Congenital Heart Disease
		A R
		Type
	10	37) Patent Ductus Arteriosus
		A R
	10	38) Persistent Fetal Circulation
		A R
	10	39) Congestive Heart Failure
		A R
	5	40) Heart Murmur
		A R
		Type
		41) Persistent Cyanosis
		42) Other
		GASTRO-INTESTINAL
	5	43) Distended Abdomen
		A R
	5	44) Vomiting
		A R
	10	45) Diarrhea/Gastroenteritis
		A R
	5	46) Blood in stool
		A R
	10	47) Bowel obstruction
		A R
	10	48) Pyloric Obstruction
		A R
	5	49) Meconium Plug
		A R
	10	50) Necrotizing Enterocolitis
		A R
	10	51) Tracheo-Esophageal Fistula
		52) Other
		METABOLIC
	10	53) Hypoglycemia
		A R
		Lowest Value
	10	54) Hypocalcemia
		A R
		Lowest Value
	5	55) ☐ Hypo ☐ Hypermagnesemia
		A R
		Low/High Value
	10	56) ☐ Hypo ☐ Hyperthyroidism
		A R
		Low/High Value
	10	57) ☐ Hypo ☐ Hypernatremia
		A R
		Low/High Value
	10	58) Inappropriate ADH
		A R
	10	59) Persistent Metabolic Acidosis
		A R
	5	60) Failure to Gain
		A R
		61) Other

+	Val	GENITO-URINARY
	10	62) Renal Failure
		A R
		63) Anomaly
		Type
		64) Other
		HEMATOLOGICAL
	5	65) Isoimmunization
		A R
		☐ Rh ☐ ABO ☐ Other
	10	66) Hyperbilirubinemia
	5	☐ Indirect
		☐ Direct
		Highest value ____ mg %
	10	67) Hemorrhagic Diathesis
		A R
		Type
	5	68) Anemia
		A R
		Type
	5	69) Polycythemia
		A R
		Highest Hct
		70) Other
		INFECTION
	1	71) Scalp Abscess
		A R
	5	72) Eye Infection
		A R
	1	73) Monilia
		A R
	5	74) Omphalitis
		A R
	10	75) Sepsis
		A R
	10	76) Meningitis
		A R
	10	77) ☐ T ☐ O ☐ R ☐ C ☐ H
		A R
	5	78) Urinary Tract Infection
		A R
	10	79) Syphilis
		A R
	5	80) Elevated IgM
		81) Other
	Code	82) List Organisms
		1 -
		2 -
		3 -
		FINAL NEWBORN SCORE ►

Val	NEUROLOGICAL	
	83) Abnormal Head	
	☐ Micro ☐ Hydro ☐ Anen.	
5	84) CNS Depression <24 hrs.	
	A R	
10	85) CNS Depression >24 hrs.	
	A R	
10	86) Seizure	
	A R	
	Type	
10	87) Jittery-Hyperactive	
	A R	
10	88) Withdrawal Symptoms	
	A R	
	Type	
10	89) Paralysis	
	A R	
	Type	
	90) Other	
	ORTHOPEDIC	
10	91) Fracture	
	Type	
10	92) Hip Dislocation R L	
	93) Other	
	GENETIC/ENDOCR.	
10	94) Downs Syndrome	
10	95) Other	
	SPECIAL TREATMENT	
	Pulmonary	
	1. ☐ O_2 >1 day	5. ☐ Chest Tube
	2. ☐ Ambu Bag	6. ☐ Chest X-Ray
	3. ☐ C-PAP	7. ☐ Other
	4. ☐ Respirator	8. ☐
	HEMATOLOGIC	
	9. ☐ Phototherapy	11. ☐ Transfusion
	10. ☐ Exch. Trans.	12. ☐
	SPECIAL TESTS	
	13. ☐ Biopsy - Type	16. ☐ Spinal Tap
	14. ☐ Cardiac Cath	17. ☐ Other
	15. ☐ EKG	18. ☐
	OPERATIONS — PROCEDURES	
	19. ☐ PDA Ligation	22. ☐ UV Cath.
	20. ☐ UA Cath.	23. ☐
	21. ☐ Circumcision	24. ☐
	DRUGS	
	25. ☐ Antibiotics	29. ☐ Digitalis
	26. ☐ Bicarb	30. ☐
	27. ☐ Calcium	31. ☐
	28. ☐ Glucose	32. ☐

9 B R **NEWBORN PROBLEM LIST**

Figure 1.11. This is Form 9 (Newborn Problem List), which is used as a code sheet as well as a reference guide for assessing neonatal risk.

DISCHARGE EVALUATION

On the day of discharge a final physical examination is carried out and Form 9 is reviewed to update the discharge problem list and record whether or not any problems have been resolved. To establish the risk status of the patient for problems present during this period, all values (scores) are added and a final newborn

F = First Day Exam D = Discharge Exam

F	D	GENERAL CONDITION	F	D	EYES	F	D	ABDOMEN	F	D	NEUROLOGIC
		Normal			Cataracts R L			Distended			Decreased Activity
		Abnormal			Abnormal Retina R L			Palpable Mass			Increased Activity
F	D	**SKIN**			Conjunctivitis R L			Probably = Code			Asymmetric Movement
		Cyanosis ☐ Body ☐ Extrem.			Scleral Hemorrhage R L			Hepatomegaly			Hypotonia
		Pallor			Other:			Umbilical Cord Abnormal			Hypertonia
		Plethora			Normal Eyes			Other:			Abnormal Cry
		Jaundice ☐ Face ☐ Chest ☐ Abd						Normal Abdomen			Moro Abnormal
		Bruising	F	D	**LUNGS/THORAX**						Clin. Est. Gestational Age
		Petechiae			↑ A-P Diameter	F	D	**GENITAL-ANAL**			Weeks
		Meconium Staining			Respirations ↑ > 60/min			Ambiguous			Other
		Edema			Respirations ↓ < 25/min			Hypospadius			Normal Neurologic
		Other:			Grunting			Abnormal Female Genitalia	F	D	**MUSCULOSKELETAL**
		Normal Skin			Retractions			Testes Undescended R L			Abnormal Back - Spine
					Stridor			Imperforate Anus			Hip Dislocation ☐ R ☐ L
F	D	**HEAD-NECK**			Breath Sounds ↓ R L			Other:			Fracture ☐ R ☐ L
		Microcephaly			Rales R L			Normal Genital-Anal Area			Type Code
		Macrocephaly			Breasts (abnormal) R L						Paralysis
		Abnormal Facies			Other:						Malformation
		Cephalohematoma			Normal Chest						Other:
		Caput due to Vac. Ext.	F	D	**CARDIOVASCULAR**						Normal Musculoskeletal
		Abnormal Sutures			Precordial Thrill						
		Abnormal Fontanelle			Precordial Activity ↑						
		Scalp Electrode Mark			Perfusion ↓						
		Scalp Abscess			Perfusion ↑						
		Nasal Flaring			Bradycardia < 100/min						
		Abnormal Oral Cavity			Tachycardia > 200/min						
		Other:			Arrhythmias						
		Normal Head-Neck			Abnormal Sounds						
					Murmur						
F	D	**EARS**			Displaced Apical Beat						
		Abnormal Location R L			Cardiomegaly						
		Abnormal Form R L			Femoral Pulses ☐ ↓ ☐ ↑						
		Other:			Brachial Pulse ☐ ↓ ☐ ↑						
		Normal Ears			Other:						
					Normal Heart						

FIRST EXAM	DATE	TIME	DISCHARGE EXAM	DATE	TIME
Length	cm	%	Length	cm	%
Weight	gms	%	Weight	gms	%
Head Circ.	cm	%	Head Circ.	cm	%
Sig:			Sig:		

COMMENTS:

CONSULTATION	Dr.	Date
	Dr.	Date
	Dr.	Date
TRANSPORT	To	
	Date	

DISCHARGE SUMMARY DATE SEX ☐ M ☐ F ☐ Unk

NEONATAL CONDITION ☐ Healthy No Disease ☐ Multiple Birth ☐ A ☐ B ☐ C ☐ Neonatal Disease Active ☐ Neonatal Death → AUTOPSY ☐ No ☐ Yes

DIAGNOSIS CODE A = Active R = Resolved		Code	A	R		Code	A	R
	1 -				5 -			
	2 -				6 -			
	3 -				7 -			
	4 -				8 -			

DISCHARGE ☐ Home with mother ☐ Home after mother ☐ Other

FEEDING ☐ Breast ☐ Enfamil ☐ Similac ☐ SMA ☐ Evaporated Milk ☐ Other:

CLINIC ☐ Community Health ______ ______ wks. ☐ PMD ______ ______ wks. ☐ Hosp. Follow-Up Clinic ______ wks. ☐ Specialty Clinic ______ wks.

SCREEN ☐ PKU - ☐ Yes ☐ No ☐ T-4 - ☐ Yes ☐ No

MEDS ☐ Vitamins ☐ Iron ☐ Other 1.) ______
2.) ______ 3.) ______ 4.) ______
5.) ______ 6.) ______ 7.) ______

PHYSICIAN CODE

10 BR NEWBORN PHYSICAL/DISCHARGE

Figure 1.12. This is Form 10 (Newborn Physical/Discharge). A physical exam is carried out on day 1 and again at discharge. The structured "Discharge Summary" facilitates discharge procedures.

score is calculated on Form 9. We are presently using a dichotomized score to designate the level of risk. A low risk neonate is one with a total score of ≤9 and a high risk infant is one who has a total score of ≥10. The level at which risk is defined many have to be readjusted as more follow-up data is collected. The exact value of this score may not be as important as a specific problem, or cluster of problems; however,

CODE = SHADED AREAS
A = Date Active R = Date Resolved

+	Val	GENERAL
	5	1) Hypothermia ≤ 97°F. or 36.2°C. ®
	10	2) Prenatal Score ≥10
	10	3) Intrapartum Score ≥10
	5	4) Apgar 1 min ≤5
	10	5) Apgar 5 min ≤5
	10	6) Asphyxia
	10	7) Resuscitation
	5	8) Neg Foam Test or L/S < 1.5
	1	9) Intermed. F.T. or L/S 1.5-2.0
	10	10) Preterm ≤37 wks.
	1	11) Term 38-42 wks.
	5	12) Post Term >42 wks.
	10	13) SGA <10% ile
	1	14) AGA
	5	15) LGA >90% ile

+	Val	SKIN
	1	16) Positive Finding
		Type Code
		A R

+	Val	HEAD-NECK
	5	17) Low set ears
	10	18) Cleft Palate
	10	19) Choanal Atresia
	10	20) Retrolental Fibroplasia
		A R
	10	21) Retinoblastoma
		22) Other

+	Val	RESPIRATORY
	10	23) Meconium Aspiration
		A R
	5	24) Aspiration (other)
		☐ Am. Fl. ☐ Blood ☐ Formula
		A R
	5	25) Mild respiratory distress (T.T.N.)
		A R
	5	26) Mild RDS (Syndrome)
		A R
	10	27) Severe RDS (Syndrome)
		A R
	10	28) Congenital Pneumonia
		A R
	10	29) Apnea
		A R
	10	30) Pneumothorax
		A R
	10	31) Pneumomediastinum
		A R
	10	32) Interstitial Emphysema
		A R
	10	33) Broncho-pulm. dysplasia
		A R
	10	34) Anomaly
		Type
		35) Other

Val	CARDIOVASCULAR
10	36) Congenital Heart Disease
	A R
	Type
10	37) Patent Ductus Arteriosus
	A R
10	38) Persistent Fetal Circulation
	A R
10	39) Congestive Heart Failure
	A R
5	40) Heart Murmur
	A R
	Type
	41) Persistent Cyanosis
	42) Other

Val	GASTRO-INTESTINAL
5	43) Distended Abdomen
	A R
5	44) Vomiting
	A R
10	45) Diarrhea/Gastroenteritis
	A R
5	46) Blood in stool
	A R
10	47) Bowel obstruction
	A R
10	48) Pyloric Obstruction
	A R
5	49) Meconium Plug
	A R
10	50) Necrotizing Enterocolitis
	A R
10	51) Tracheo-Esophageal Fistula
	52) Other

Val	METABOLIC
10	53) Hypoglycemia
	A R
	Lowest Value
10	54) Hypocalcemia
	A R
	Lowest Value
5	55) ☐ Hypo ☐ Hypermagnesemia
	A R
	Low/High Value
10	56) ☐ Hypo ☐ Hyperthyroidism
	A R
	Low/High Value
10	57) ☐ Hypo ☐ Hypernatremia
	A R
	Low/High Value
10	58) Inappropriate ADH
	A R
10	59) Persistent Metabolic Acidosis
	A R
5	60) Failure to Gain
	A R
	61) Other

+	Val	GENITO-URINARY
	10	62) Renal Failure
		A R
		63) Anomaly
		Type
		64) Other

+	Val	HEMATOLOGICAL
	5	65) Isoimmunization
		A R
		☐ Rh ☐ ABO ☐ Other
	10	66) Hyperbilirubinemia
	5	☐ Indirect
		☐ Direct
		Highest value ____ mg %
	10	67) Hemorrhagic Diathesis
		A R
		Type
	5	68) Anemia
		A R
		Type
	5	69) Polycythemia
		A R
		Highest Hct
		70) Other

+	Val	INFECTION
	1	71) Scalp Abscess
		A R
	5	72) Eye Infection
		A R
	1	73) Monilia
		A R
	5	74) Omphalitis
		A R
	10	75) Sepsis
		A R
	10	76) Meningitis
		A R
	10	77) ☐ T ☐ O ☐ R ☐ C ☐ H
		A R
	5	78) Urinary Tract Infection
		A R
	10	79) Syphilis
		A R
	5	80) Elevated IgM
		81) Other
	Code	82) List Organisms
		1 -
		2 -
		3 -

FINAL NEWBORN SCORE ▶

Val	NEUROLOGICAL
	83) Abnormal Head
	☐ Micro ☐ Hydro ☐ Anen.
5	84) CNS Depression < 24 hrs.
	A R
10	85) CNS Depression >24 hrs.
	A R
10	86) Seizure
	A R
	Type
10	87) Jittery-Hyperactive
	A R
10	88) Withdrawal Symptoms
	A R
	Type
10	89) Paralysis
	A R
	Type
	90) Other

Val	ORTHOPEDIC
10	91) Fracture
	Type
10	92) Hip Dislocation R L
	93) Other

Val	GENETIC/ENDOCR.
10	94) Downs Syndrome
10	95) Other

SPECIAL TREATMENT	
Pulmonary	
1. ☐ O_2 >1 day	5. ☐ Chest Tube
2. ☐ Ambu Bag	6. ☐ Chest X-Ray
3. ☐ C-PAP	7. ☐ Other
4. ☐ Respirator	8. ☐
HEMATOLOGIC	
9. ☐ Phototherapy	11. ☐ Transfusion
10. ☐ Exch. Trans.	12. ☐
SPECIAL TESTS	
13. ☐ Biopsy - Type	16. ☐ Spinal Tap
14. ☐ Cardiac Cath	17. ☐ Other
15. ☐ EKG	18. ☐
OPERATIONS — PROCEDURES	
19. ☐ PDA Ligation	22. ☐ UV Cath.
20. ☐ UA Cath.	23. ☐
21. ☐ Circumcision	24. ☐
DRUGS	
25. ☐ Antibiotics	29. ☐ Digitalis
26. ☐ Bicarb	30. ☐
27. ☐ Calcium	31. ☐
28. ☐ Glucose	32. ☐

9 B R NEWBORN PROBLEM LIST

Figure 1.11. This is Form 9 (Newborn Problem List), which is used as a code sheet as well as a reference guide for assessing neonatal risk.

DISCHARGE EVALUATION

On the day of discharge a final physical examination is carried out and Form 9 is reviewed to update the discharge problem list and record whether or not any problems have been resolved. To establish the risk status of the patient for problems present during this period, all values (scores) are added and a final newborn

F = First Day Exam D = Discharge Exam

F	D	GENERAL CONDITION
		Normal
		Abnormal

F	D	SKIN
		Cyanosis □ Body □ Extrem.
		Pallor
		Plethora
		Jaundice □ Face □ Chest □ Abd
		Bruising
		Petechiae
		Meconium Staining
		Edema
		Other:
		Normal Skin

F	D	HEAD-NECK
		Microcephaly
		Macrocephaly
		Abnormal Facies
		Cephalohematoma
		Caput due to Vac. Ext.
		Abnormal Sutures
		Abnormal Fontanelle
		Scalp Electrode Mark
		Scalp Abscess
		Nasal Flaring
		Abnormal Oral Cavity
		Other:
		Normal Head-Neck

F	D	EARS
		Abnormal Location R L
		Abnormal Form R L
		Other:
		Normal Ears

F	D	EYES
		Cataracts R L
		Abnormal Retina R L
		Conjunctivitis R L
		Scleral Hemorrhage R L
		Other:
		Normal Eyes

F	D	LUNGS/THORAX
		↑ A-P Diameter
		Respirations ↑ > 60/min
		Respirations ↓ < 25/min
		Grunting
		Retractions
		Stridor
		Breath Sounds ↓ R L
		Rales R L
		Breasts (abnormal) R L
		Other:
		Normal Chest

F	D	CARDIOVASCULAR
		Precordial Thrill
		Precordial Activity ↑
		Perfusion ↓
		Perfusion ↑
		Bradycardia < 100/min
		Tachycardia > 200/min
		Arrhythmias
		Abnormal Sounds
		Murmur
		Displaced Apical Beat
		Cardiomegaly
		Femoral Pulses □ ↓ □ ↑
		Brachial Pulse □ ↓ □ ↑
		Other:
		Normal Heart

F	D	ABDOMEN
		Distended
		Palpable Mass
		Probably = Code
		Hepatomegaly
		Umbilical Cord Abnormal
		Other:
		Normal Abdomen

F	D	GENITAL-ANAL
		Ambiguous
		Hypospadius
		Abnormal Female Genitalia
		Testes Undescended R L
		Imperforate Anus
		Other:
		Normal Genital-Anal Area

F	D	NEUROLOGIC
		Decreased Activity
		Increased Activity
		Asymmetric Movement
		Hypotonia
		Hypertonia
		Abnormal Cry
		Moro Abnormal
		Clin. Est. Gestational Age Weeks
		Other
		Normal Neurologic

F	D	MUSCULOSKELETAL
		Abnormal Back - Spine
		Hip Dislocation □ R □ L
		Fracture □ R □ L
		Type Code
		Paralysis
		Malformation
		Other:
		Normal Musculoskeletal

FIRST EXAM	DATE	TIME	DISCHARGE EXAM	DATE	TIME
Length	cm	%	Length	cm	%
Weight	gms	%	Weight	gms	%
Head Circ.	cm	%	Head Circ.	cm	%
Sig:			Sig:		

COMMENTS:

CONSULTATION	Dr.	Date
	Dr.	Date
	Dr.	Date
TRANSPORT	To	
	Date	

DISCHARGE SUMMARY DATE SEX □ M □ F □ Unk

NEONATAL CONDITION □ Healthy No Disease □ Multiple Birth □ A □ B □ C □ Neonatal Disease Active □ Neonatal Death → AUTOPSY □ No □ Yes

DIAGNOSIS / CODE A = Active R = Resolved		Code	A	R		Code	A	R
	1 -				5 -			
	2 -				6 -			
	3 -				7 -			
	4 -				8 -			

DISCHARGE □ Home with mother □ Home after mother □ Other

FEEDING □ Breast □ Enfamil □ Similac □ SMA □ Evaporated Milk □ Other:

CLINIC □ Community Health ______ ______ wks. □ PMD ______ ______ wks. Hosp. Follow-Up □ Clinic ______ wks. Specialty □ Clinic ______ wks.

SCREEN □ PKU - □ Yes □ No □ T-4 - □ Yes □ No

MEDS □ Vitamins □ Iron □ Other 1.) ______
2.) ______ 3.) ______ 4.) ______
5.) ______ 6.) ______ 7.) ______

PHYSICIAN CODE

10 BR **NEWBORN PHYSICAL/DISCHARGE**

Figure 1.12. This is Form 10 (Newborn Physical/Discharge). A physical exam is carried out on day 1 and again at discharge. The structured "Discharge Summary" facilitates discharge procedures.

score is calculated on Form 9. We are presently using a dichotomized score to designate the level of risk. A low risk neonate is one with a total score of ≤9 and a high risk infant is one who has a total score of ≥10. The level at which risk is defined many have to be readjusted as more follow-up data is collected. The exact value of this score may not be as important as a specific problem, or cluster of problems; however, it facilitates the division of neonates into certain risk categories for follow-up assessments.

NEONATAL ASSESSMENT OBJECTIVES

In the nursery the purpose of problem-oriented risk assessment is to identify the high risk neonate and develop a plan of management. Because certain perinatal conditions are related to problems during infancy, the prenatal, intrapartum and neonatal risk score is the basis for planning longitudinal care, whether it be medical or nursing. This approach is similar to the "Risk Register" concept developed in England during the late 1950's.[36] Certain high risk infants were selected by a retrospective analysis of single perinatal events and placed on "the register" and their developmental program followed carefully. Our present approach differs in two respects. First, it utilizes our neonatal score which takes into account multiple factors to identify which infant requires follow-up. The second difference is that the decision to provide careful follow-up is based on prospectively collected data at the time the neonate is discharged.

From the above discussion it can be determined that our approach to neonatal assessment is to focus on a cluster of problems represented by a total score rather than to focus on single factors to define morbidity. This approach is in agreement with our prenatal and intrapartum risk assessment. As shown, high risk patients (score ≥ 10) during the prenatal and/or intrapartum period are more likely to deliver high risk infants than low risk patients (Table 1.2). The majority of studies, including the "Risk Register" concept, have not been successful in relating single prenatal problems to later developments. Several more recent studies have suggested that combinations of perinatal problems are more predictive of outcome. Table 1.4 lists those studies and the combination of problems which are most predictive. However, one must be cognizant of the fact that all high risk neonates do not experience later difficulty. Besides single or multiple perinatal problems, there are socioeconomic and environmental factors during infancy which can also influence outcome whether the infant is initially high or low risk. Developmental disabilities are most likely the result of a specific constellation of interrelated perinatal events occurring at critical periods throughout the continuum.

The Advantages of Problem-oriented Risk Assessment

The problem-oriented perinatal record described in this chapter has been designed to effectuate the collaboration of the team members providing perinatal care. Its configuration facilitates the following.

IDENTIFICATION OF HIGH RISK PATIENT

The structure of the record allows for a systematic recording of data from which problems are identified. The uniformity of recording this information makes it possible for any member to quickly identify data elements without getting lost, the usual case with unstructured records. In order to determine the degree of risk, we have incorporated risk scoring to separate out those items considered to be most predictive of outcome. As a result, any member of the team can quickly grasp the degree of risk as well as specific items which characterize that level of risk. Identification of the specific high risk factors and the quantification of risk are the essential elements of an effective problem-oriented record.

DEVELOPMENT OF PLAN OF MANAGEMENT

The problem-oriented record is the stimulus to begin synthesizing protocols of management in the development of standard operating procedures for nursing as well as medical tasks. It also is beneficial for integrating the system as well as for becoming the basis for a medical audit.

FACILITATION OF AUDIT

The medical record must be audited in order to maintain a certain standard of medical care. The high risk patient is identified in terms of certain factors and the performance of the team and the care

Table 1.4. Relationship of multiple perinatal variables to poor outcome*

Author	Prenatal variables	Intrapartum variables	Neonatal variables	Infant and/or childhood outcome
Drage and Berendes[6]	0	0	2	Abnormal Bayley at 8 months. Abnormal neurologic exam at 1 year
Drorbaugh et al[7]	0	1	3	Central nervous system dysfunction at 7 years
Graham et al[17]	7	17	3	Less optimal behavioral measures and Binet IQ at 3 years
Honzik et al[25]	4†, ‡	13	7	Abnormal Bayley's mental and motor scales at 8 months
Niswander et al[30]	0	1	3	Abnormal Bayley's and neurologic exam at 8 months
Prechtl[35]	←42‡→		1	Less optimal behavioral intelligence at age 2–4 years
Smith et al[39]	4	1†, ‡	4	Less optimal developmental outcome at 7 years
Stembera et al[41]	16	9	9	Cerebral palsy and neurologic, psychic and social development at 18 months
Stevenson[42]	5†, ‡	4	3	Poorly adjusted child at 5–8 years
Werner et al[47]	17	18	17	Below normal physical status and intellectual and social development
Weiner et al[46]	3	3	3	Impaired mental development in 8–10-year-old children

* This table lists eleven authors who found more than one perinatal variable to be related to poor developmental outcome during infancy and childhood.

† More than the indicated variables were probably used to predict outcome.

‡ Authors who did not list the variable used in their analysis.

given can be measured in terms of the plan of management and the actions taken to resolve problems. If certain standards are not met, improved levels at least can be attained through the educational process, whether it be the training of new staff members, in-service education or the development of new programs. Weed[45] has outlined four conditions which the medical record must meet to facilitate auditing medical practice and care. (a) The data in the record must be linked with a problem to determine whether the data was necessary in solving that problem. (b) All data for any particular problem must be easily retrieved and must be immediately available to the staff. This refers to the pattern and the types of data needed to resolve certain problems. In the future, as the data bank grows, these patterns of care will be more clearly formulated and new standards can be developed. (c) The development of standards becomes complex when patients have more than one problem, all of which may or may not be interrelated. The complex array of data elements must be sorted in the record. This leads us to Weed's final premise. (d) The above problem cannot be met easily without computerization of the data. We are in complete agreement with the above condition as outlined by Weed. Computerization of our perinatal record has allowed us to more carefully define and organize our problems and data elements. It already has improved our performance and it will continue to facilitate the development of our regional perinatal program.

INTERDISCIPLINARY EDUCATION

Education must encompass the whole patient care system. The problem-oriented record can bring about a change in perinatal education by replacing fragmented assessment with a logical and integrated approach to patient care. The record incorporates a sequence of activities from various sources and when accomplished it is considered an educational experience. With established objectives and management protocols the record is a self-contained learning unit. The medical audit discussed above is an important step toward developing a continuing education program because there is a link between audit and the educational process (Figure 1.1).

PREVENTION OF IATROGENIC PROBLEMS

Why should we be addressing the problem of iatrogenic perinatal problems? The subject of problems induced by the physician is not new. For the past century medicine has become more mechanical and with this we have seen varied problems as a result of intervention. Since the progress of medicine is often based on prevention through intervention, the incidence of iatrogenic problems could increase and we must now consider how these could be prevented. Through the use of a structured problem-oriented perinatal record, we believe that these types of problems could be more easily identified, because the record focuses on the identification of risk factors and the performance of the team providing care. Table 1.5 lists the proven iatrogenic perinatal problems as well as a few which are presently speculative. With the wider use of management protocols and/or standard operating procedures, fewer numbers of management errors will be made. When iatrogenic problems are recognized through the audit mechanism, the educational process should provide the feedback mechanism to alter behavior. The above discussion on the advantages of a problem-oriented perinatal record is important because the structured medical record has far-reaching implications for improving health care and the management of complex interactions of our specialty.

Table 1.5. Iatrogenic perinatal problems*

Problems	Cause
Proven iatrogenic	
Respiratory distress syndrome	Elective induction of labor
	Elective repeat cesarean (C) section[15]
Rh sensitization	Complications of amniocentesis[3, 4]
Fetal trauma	
Fetal anemia	
Premature labor	Induced abortion[26]
Vaginal adenosis	In utero exposure to diethylstilbestrol[20]
Vaginal clear cell adenocarcinoma	
Masculinization of the female fetus	Use of ^{18}C and ^{19}C agents during pregnancy[5]
Fetal and neonatal hypothyroidism	Treatment of maternal hyperthyroidism[9]
Increased incidence of variable heart rate patterns	Elective inductions[38]
Neonatal lung disease	Oxygen and respiratory therapy[44]
Retrolental fibroplasia	Oxygen therapy[33]
Neonatal jaundice	Operative delivery[11]
Increased neonatal insensible water loss	Phototherapy[31]
Protracted labor	Conduction anesthesia[12]
Alteration of neonatal behavior	Anesthesia[37, 40]
Speculative iatrogenic	
Low 1-min Apgar scores	Maternal transfer from labor room to delivery room
Neonatal neurologic sequelae	Elective induction[38]

* Those iatrogenic problems and causes which have been clearly identified as well as those about which there has been considerable recent speculation are listed.

Conclusion

The only way in which we can understand the future potential of the neonate is to follow the clinical course of pregnancy and attempt to understand the complex interactions that occur before, during and after pregnancy. A method by which the physician and members of his health team can accomplish this task readily has been described in this chapter. We utilize this approach of assessment to identify the high risk patient in order to plan intervention programs with the goal of preventing perinatal problems which have been shown to be related to neonatal and infant mortality and morbidity. The prenatal, intrapartum and neonatal assessment is the analytic assessment profile or mechanism whereby we can begin to predict future events. If we are interested in quality then let us know what can assure it; likewise, let us understand those events which are responsible for developmental delay.

REFERENCES

1. Arms, S.: *Immaculate Deception: A New Look at Women and Childbirth in America, 1975.*
2. Boddy, K., Dawes, G. S.: Fetal Breathing. Br Med Bull 31: 3, 1975.
3. Creasman, W. T., Lawrence, R. A., Thiede, H. A.: Fetal complications of amniocentesis. JAMA 204: 949, 1968.
4. Curtis, J. D., Cohen, W. N., Richerson, H. B., White, C. A.: The importance of placental localization preceding amniocentesis. Obstet Gynecol 40: 194, 1972.
5. Dmowski, W. P., Greenblatt, R. B.: Ambiguous external genitalia in the newborn and prepubescent child. JAMA 212: 308, 1970.
6. Drage, J. B., Berendes, H. W.: Apgar scores and outcome of the newborn. Pediatr Clin North Am 13: 635, 1966.
7. Drorbaugh, E. D., Moore, D. M., Warram, J. H.: Association between gestational and environmental events and central nervous system function in 7-year-old children. Pediatrics 56: 529, 1975.
8. Effer, S. B.: Management of high risk pregnancy: Report of a combined obstetrical and neonatal intensive care unit. Can Med Assoc J 101: 55, 1969.
9. Fisher, D. A., Burrow, G. N., Editors, *Perinatal Thyroid Physiology and Disease*. New York, Raven Press, Publishers, 1975.
10. Friedman, E. A.: *Labor: Clinical Evaluation and Mangement*. New York, Appleton-Century-Crofts, 1967.
11. Friedman, E. A., Sachtleben, M. R.: Neonatal jaundice in association with oxytocin stimulation of labor and operative delivery. Br Med J 24: 198, 1976.
12. Friedman, E. A., Sachtleben, M. R.: Station of the fetal presenting. V. Protracted descent patterns. Obstet Gynecol 36: 558, 1970.
13. Gant, N. F., Chand, S., Warley, R. J., Whalley, P. J., Crosby, V. D., MacDonald, P. C.: Clinical test useful for predicting the development of acute hypertension in pregnancy. Am J Obstet Gynecol 120: 1, 1974.
14. Gant, N. F., Daley, G. L., Chand, S., Whalley, P. J., MacDonald, P. C.: A study of angiotensin II pressor response throughout primigravid pregnancy. J Clin Invest 52: 2682, 1973.
15. Goldenberg, R. L., Nelson, K.: Iatrogenic respiratory distress syndrome. Am J Obstet Gynecol 123: 617, 1975.
16. Goodwin, J. W., Dunne, J. T., Thomas, B. W.: Antepartum identification of the fetus at risk. Can Med Assoc 109: 458, 1969.
17. Graham, F. K., Emhard, C. B., Thurston, D., Craft, M.: Development three years after perinatal anoxia and other potentially damaging newborn experiences. Psychol Mongr 76: Whole No. 522.
18. Gusdon, J. P.: A clinical evaluation of the "Roll-over test" for pregnancy induced hypertension (Abstract). Gynecol Invest 7: 9, 1976.
19. Hebb, M.: Nova Scotia Fetal Risk Project. Annual Progress Report, 1974.
20. Herbst, A. L., Kurman, R. J., Scully, R. E.: Vaginal and cervical abnormalities after exposure to stilbestrol in utero. Obstet Gynecol 40: 287, 1972.
21. Hobel, C. J.: Recognition of the high risk pregnant woman. *Management of the High Risk Pregnancy,* Chapter 1. Edited by W. N. Spellacy, Baltimore, University Park Press, 1976.
22. Hobel, C. J., Hyvarinen, M. A., Okada, D. M., Oh, W.: Prenatal and intrapartum high risk screening. 1. Prediction of the high risk neonate. Am J Obstet Gynecol 117: 1, 1973.
23. Hobel, C. J., Hyvarinen, M. A., Oh, W.: Abnormal fetal heart rate patterns and fetal acid-base balance in low birth weight infants in relation to respiratory distress syndrome. Obstet Gynecol 39: 85, 1972.
24. Hobel, C. J., Youkeles, L., Forsythe, A.: A multiple logistic regression analysis of prenatal and intrapartum events. Identification of optimal factors for assessing risk. (In preparation)
25. Honzik, M. P., Hutchings, J. J., Burnip, S. R.: Birth record assessments and test performances at eight months. Am J Dis Child 109: 416, 1965.
26. Klinger, A.: Demographic consequences of the legalization of induced abortion in Eastern Europe. Int J Gynaecol Obstet 8: 680, 1970.
27. Liggins, G. C., Howie, R. N.: A controlled trial of antepartum glucocorticoid treatment for the prevention of the respiratory distress syndrome in premature infants. Pediatrics 50: 515, 1972.
28. Martin, C. B., Siassi, B., Hon, E. H.: Fetal heart rate patterns and neonatal death in low birth weight infants. Obstet Gynecol 44: 503, 1974.
29. Nesbitt, R. E. L., Aubry, R. H.: High risk obstetrics. II. Value of semiobjective grading system in identifying the vulnerable group. Am J Obstet Gynecol 103: 972, 1969.
30. Niswander, K. R., Friedman, E. A., Hoover, D. B., Pietrowski, H., Westphal, M. C.: Fetal morbidity following potentially anoxigenic obstetrical conditions. I. Abruptio placenta. II. Placenta previa. III. Prolapse of the umbilical cord. Am J Obstet Gynecol 95: 838, 1966.
31. Oh, W., Karecki, H.: Phototherapy and insensible water loss in the newborn infant. Am J Dis Child 124: 230, 1972.

32. O'Sullivan, J. B., Mahan, C. M., Charles, D., Dandrow, R. V.: Screening criteria for high risk gestational diabetic patients. Am J Obstet Gynecol 116: 895, 1973.
33. Patz, A.: Retrolental fibroplasia. Surv Ophthalmol 14: 1, 1969.
34. Peabody, F. W.: The care of the patient. J Am Med Assoc 88: 877, 1927.
35. Prechtl, H. F. R.: Neurological sequelae of prenatal and perinatal complications. Br Med J 4: 763, 1967.
36. Rogers, M. G. H.: The Risk Register: A critical assessment. Med Officer 118: 253, 1967.
37. Scanlon, J. W., Brown, W. V., Weiss, J. B., Alper, M. H.: Neurobehavioral responses of newborn infants after maternal epidural anesthesia. Anesthesiology 40: 121, 1974.
38. Schwarcz, R. L., Belizan, J. M., Cifuentes, J. R., Cuadro, J. C., Marques, M. B., Caldeyvo-Barcia, R.: Fetal and maternal monitoring in spontaneous labors and in elective inductions. Am J Obstet Gynecol 120: 356, 1974.
39. Smith, A. C., Flick, G. L., Ferriss, G. S., Sellmann, A. H.: Prediction of developmental outcome of seven years from prenatal, perinatal and postnatal events. Child Dev 43: 495, 1973.
40. Standley, K., Soule III, A. B., Copans, S. A., Duchowny, M. S.: Local regional anesthesia during childbirth: Effect on newborn behaviors. Science 186: 634, 1974.
41. Stembera, Z. K., Zezulokova, J., Dittrichova, J., Znamenacek, K.: Identification and quantification of high risk factors affecting fetus and newborn. Proceedings of the 4th European Congress of Perinatal Medicine. Prague, August 28–31, 1974.
42. Stevenson, S. S.: Paranatal factors affecting adjustment in childhood. Pediatrics 2: 154, 1948.
43. Thibeault, D. W., Hobel, C. J.: The relationship of the foam stability test, in maturity, and intrapartum complications in the respiratory distress syndrome. Am J Obstet Gynecol 118: 56, 1974.
44. Thibeault, D. W., Lachman, R. S., Laul, V. R., Kwong, M. S.: Pulmonary interstitial emphysema, pneumomediastinum and pneumothorax. Am J Dis Child 126: 611, 1973.
45. Weed, L.: Medical records that guide and teach. N Engl J Med 278: 652, 1968.
46. Weiner, G., Rider, R. V., Oppel, W. C., Harper, P. A.: Correlates of low birth weight: Psychological status at eight to ten years of age. Pediatr Res 2: 110, 1968.
47. Werner, E., Simonion, K., Bierman, J. M., French, F. E.: Cumulative effect of perinatal complications and deprived environment on physical intellectual and social development of preschool children. Pediatrics 39: 490, 1967.
48. Zlatnik, F. J., Fuchs, F. A.: A controlled study of ethanol in threatened premature labor. Am J Obstet Gynecol 112: 610, 1972.

Part I

ANTEPARTUM EVALUATION

MICHAEL T. MENNUTI, M.D.

2

Genetic Counseling and Diagnosis during Pregnancy*

Introduction

The rapidly expanding knowledge of human genetics has made clinical medical genetics an important aspect of comprehensive health care. Optimally, genetic counseling should be offered before conception. During the past decade, however, methods for the diagnosis of a number of birth defects during the second trimester of pregnancy have been developed. These advances, coupled with the liberalization of attitudes and laws regarding termination of pregnancy, have made genetic counseling practical during early pregnancy in certain situations. Experience with the application of these techniques has served to document the safety and accuracy of prenatal genetic diagnosis, as well as the problems and pitfalls associated with it.

Medical centers and physicians who offer care to the high risk mother and her fetus have experienced a continuing increase in the number of requests for these studies. The broad body of scientific knowledge and medical resources required for this have necessitated establishing multidisciplinary programs to provide these services. It would be impossible to discuss here all of the aspects of medical knowledge which are offered by such a team. Rather, it is the purpose of this chapter to review principles and problems of genetic counseling and diagnosis during pregnancy which are most relevant for the obstetrician.

Genetic Counseling during Pregnancy

Genetic counseling is a process whereby individuals or families are given information which is needed for the understanding of a hereditary disorder. One purpose of this process is to enable the patients to make important personal decisions regarding a particular genetic disease, either in themselves or their families. During pregnancy, this most often deals with reproductive decisions. Although the basic approach and principles are the same as those used at other times, certain situations, such as critical time limitations for the decision-making aspect, occur more frequently during pregnancy.

IDENTIFICATION OF FAMILIES AT RISK

The identification of patients at risk for bearing a child with a genetic disorder or birth defect has become an important responsibility in primary obstetric care. A careful medical history, as well as a family pedigree of the father and mother of the pregnancy, should be obtained at the initial prenatal visit. Attention should be directed to specific areas which might iden-

* This research was supported in part by United States Public Health Service Training Grant GM 005303.

tify an increased risk for certain birth defects, such as age or geographic or ethnic background. Family members with suspected genetic disorders, birth defects or mental retardation, as well as viral illnesses and drug use during pregnancy, should be reviewed in detail.

INITIATION OF COUNSELING DURING PREGNANCY

As previously stated, it is optimal to offer genetic counseling before conception. Once a pregnancy has been established, there is often a great deal more anxiety associated with the discussion of genetic disorders. In addition, the options available to the patient may be more limited. Unfortunately, however, many patients deny a genetic risk until they are pregnant. Increasing anxiety results in the not infrequent occurrence of these patients seeking genetic counseling for the first time during pregnancy. It is also important for obstetricians to recognize that by a denial mechanism, some patients may presume that a risk is not significant by the failure of their physician to call attention to it. Once genetic counseling has been requested by a pregnant patient or it has been suggested for her, it is important that it be made available rapidly. Some patients may be reassured by counseling because they have presumed a risk that is not present, or perhaps a higher risk than is actually the case. Often, however, genetic counseling during pregnancy is only of value when more than one option is available for the patient. In many cases where patients are at increased risk, the only potential option, other than continuation of the pregnancy and assuming that risk, is termination of the pregnancy. Because of this, one must be aware of the gestational age of the fetus, the availability of pregnancy termination and the patient's attitude regarding this option very early in the course of genetic referral or counseling.

Correct Diagnosis

This is a prerequisite for all genetic counseling. Through the process of genetic counseling, patients may make important decisions regarding choices in their life patterns, especially in terms of reproduction. The impact of how genetic counseling and testing may alter their views of themselves and family members in terms of health or disease is significant. For these reasons, it is absolutely essential that the most accurate diagnosis and information be given to the patient. In many cases which the obstetrician encounters, the correct diagnosis for counseling may be made relatively simply. For example, in patients who are of advanced maternal age, the recognition of their age-related risk permits counseling without further diagnostic studies. In many other instances, couples have a previous child with a specific genetic disorder or birth defect which can be readily ascertained by review of the medical records. Occasionally, however, there may be previously lost pregnancies, children or other family members with abnormalities which may arouse suspicion. In these cases, it is important to review all of the available medical information regarding these individuals. This may require reevaluation and testing of various family members. Detailed autopsy reports, x-rays, and photographs of previously lost pregnancies may be of invaluable assistance. Because of the multidisciplinary approach to the diagnosis of many of these problems, and the time required for obtaining records or studies of family members, employing a nonphysician coordinator has proven to be useful in many centers.

Appropriate Gestational Age

Appropriate gestational age is important in regard to the availability of options, and also from the point of view of the technical aspects of the diagnostic procedures. Because pregnancy termination may be an important option for the patient, the limitation of the gestational age at which this is available is critical. The time required to arrive at an accurate diagnosis of family members, or the length of time necessary for the completion of a genetic study on a pregnancy frequently constitutes an emergency.

COUNSELING PROCESS

There are three aspects of a genetic disorder which are discussed during the counseling process. These include the medical aspects (the burden), an explanation of the mode of inheritance (the risk) and a presentation of the options available (the decision).

Medical Aspects

Counseling regarding the medical aspects of the disease essentially presents the concept of burden. Through the counseling, the patient should have an understanding and an appreciation of the burden of the disease on the affected person, as well as the family. Pregnant patients frequently present two extremes of medical knowledge regarding a disease for which their pregnancy is at risk. In some cases, a previous child or a close family member may have had the disease. In these instances, patients may have had personal experience with the disease and its burden. When this occurs, it is often unnecessary to engage in detailed medical counseling. If the expression of the disease, or the burden of the disease, is variable, this should be explained in detail. It may also be important to discuss new or anticipated developments in therapy when these are relevant. When a patient has little or no knowledge regarding the disorder for which their pregnancy is at risk, the necessary time should be spent in discussing the medical aspects of the disease. For example, in the case of advanced maternal age, it is important that the patient understand not only the risks of having a child with Down's syndrome, but also the burden of the disease, in order to make an informed decision regarding prenatal diagnosis. Studies performed in genetic counseling clinics have shown that burden often plays a major role in the patient's decision-making process following counseling.[1]

Risk

In defining risk, it is important that patients have an understanding of the mode of inheritance of the disorder. The genetic mechanisms involved and the derivation of the risk figure should be explained to the patients in a way that they are able to understand them. It may be necessary to review and summarize the information several times. Having the patient relate the information back to the counselor or another individual present is useful in assessing the effectiveness of this aspect of the counseling. In dealing with numerical risk figures, the parents should obtain a proper perspective on their particular situation. It is useful to compare the patient's risk to that of the general population for a specific birth defect, and also the population risk for all birth defects. Pointing out the converse of a risk, for example, a 1% risk means a 99% chance that a given disorder will not occur, is helpful.

Options

The counselor must be aware of and present all of the available options to the patient using a nondirective approach.[2] He or she should be well versed in discussing the options and the potential implications of each of these. Those most frequently available during pregnancy are: (a) assumption of a risk with continuation of the pregnancy; (b) termination of the pregnancy, with a subsequent review of the options available for future reproduction (e.g., adoption, donor insemination, etc.); (c) prenatal diagnosis and selective abortion. It is most important that the counselor not predetermine which course of action is most appropriate for any particular patient. Through counseling, the patients should be able to reach their own decisions. Many patients who are not familiar with the process of counseling seek specific recommendations either directly or indirectly by asking the counselor what he or she would do in their situation. When this occurs, it should be pointed out that because of the variability of each family situation, only the patients can make the best decision for themselves.

When prenatal diagnosis and selective abortion are considered, the patients should understand the important aspects of the diagnostic procedure. This requires an explanation of the method of diagnosis, the attendant risks involved, both to the mother and the fetus, and the anticipated accuracy of the test procedure. Limitations of the test procedure which may result in error or failure to complete the study should be explained, as well as any other relevant problems or pitfalls.

After counseling, the patients are given the time necessary for reaching a decision. Because of the critical time restrictions imposed by pregnancy, this may be difficult, but specific time limitations should be set when necessary. It is valuable to have at least two sessions so that questions which arise from the initial counseling can be answered, or areas which have not been understood can be reviewed. Many genetic counselors give patients written information to use in the interval between the two visits. This can be in the form of a letter from the counselor, or a booklet. Although the number of disorders amenable to prenatal diagnosis has rapidly increased, certain indications (e.g., advanced maternal age, previous trisomic child, etc.) constitute the majority of the cases in prenatal diagnosis clinics. Nevertheless, the unique aspects of each family make counseling for repetitive indications a continuing challenge.

METHODS

Radiography

Plain x-ray has been utilized during late pregnancy for estimation of pelvic size, and on occasion, for fetal evaluation. A number of genetic disorders have been diagnosed by these studies either purposely, fortuitously or retrospectively. These include fetal anencephaly, hydrocephaly, osteogenesis imperfecta, etc., as well as chromosomal abnormalities.[3–5] Nevertheless, fetal skeletal visualization during the first half of pregnancy generally is not adequate for a diagnosis of genetic disorders. In isolated instances, early radiologic diagnosis may be made when there are diagnostic changes of major skeletal areas. The diagnosis of infantile osteopetrosis has been made late in the second trimester.[6] Omenn et al[7] reported the exclusion of the diagnosis of TAR syndrome (thrombocytopenia, absent radii) by visualization of a fetal radius at 16 weeks of gestation. Optimal visualization of the fetal skeleton is obtained when there has been mechanical emptying of the maternal large bowel, and with the use of maternally administered sedation, in an attempt to diminish fetal movement.[8] It seems likely that the diagnosis of certain skeletal disorders such as achondrogenesis, osteogenesis imperfecta, etc., may be possible at 20 weeks of pregnancy or shortly after, if there is careful attention to detail.

Amniography

The injection of water-soluble contrast material intra-amniotically has been safely performed during the second and third trimester. Its use for the late pregnancy diagnosis of birth defects has been evaluated.[9] It has been suggested as a tool for the early diagnosis of soft tissue defects, especially meningomyelocele. Frigoletto and Griscom[10] reported a series of six cases in which they felt the procedure was able to adequately exclude these defects. No positive diagnosis of open neural tube defects has been reported using this technique. Amniography, performed in two cases reported by Allan et al[11] and three cases reported by Mennuti et al,[12] failed to delineate neural tube defects which were present in the fetuses. On the basis of this experience, it seems likely that the procedure is of limited value in this regard. Notably, amniography frequently provides an outline of the fetal head, trunk, and often one or more limbs (see Figure 2.1). It is quite possible that this procedure may prove to be a useful adjunct to plain x-ray in the early diagnosis of certain skeletal abnormalities such as short-limbed dwarfism. The initiation of uterine contractility by the use of hypertonic dye is a concern that has not been borne out, although the number of cases reported is small. Labor inhibitors, such as intravenous alcohol have been used in a limited number of cases. The value of this has not been determined, although its use is probably not necessary.

Fetography

Fetography was first described by Erbsloh.[13] A lipid-soluble radiopaque dye is instilled into the amniotic cavity, either sep-

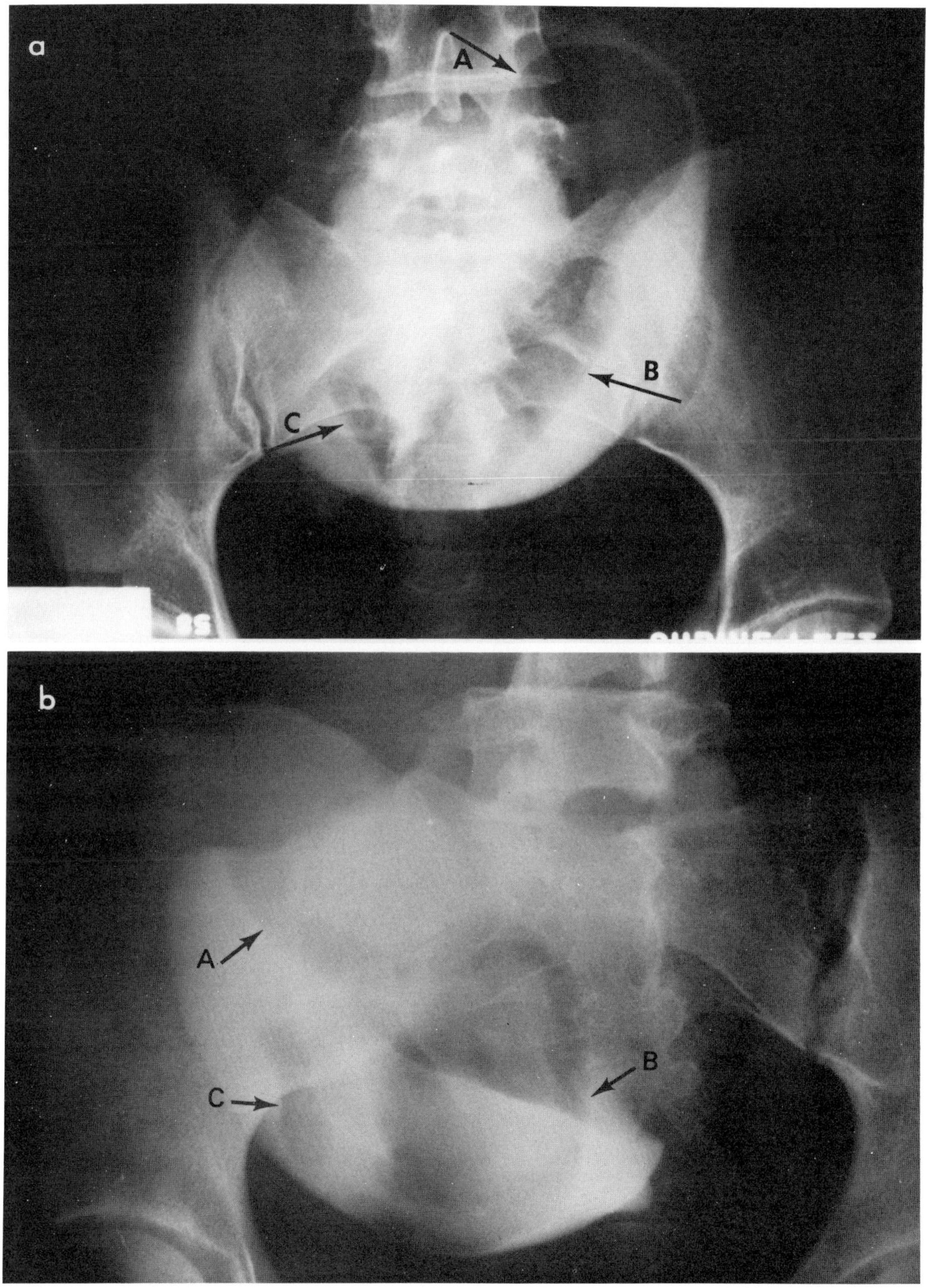

Figure 2.1. Amniograms performed at 18 weeks of gestation. A points to fetal head, B points to dorsal thorax, C points to fetal thigh.

arately or in conjunction with amniography. The dye provides a positive outline of the fetal skin surfaces by its adherence to the vernix caseosa. The fetal visualization obtained is very dramatic. It has been suggested that this procedure be utilized for the study of pregnancies when there is polyhydramnios, rhesus sensitization, multiple gestation or suspected congenital abnormality.[14–16] A number of birth defects diagnosed in late pregnancy have been reported, including trisomy 18.[17] Studies specifically evaluating the safety of the procedure are not available. The isolated report of fetal aspiration of the oil base dye is a cause for concern.[18] The use of this technique during the early second trimester has not been of value because of the absence of vernix caseosa.

These radiologic procedures which require amniocentesis (i.e., amniography and fetography) have been recommended in late gestation when fetal abnormalities are suspected by virtue of the presence of unexplained polyhydramnios or by ultrasonic findings. The simultaneous initiation of amniotic fluid studies such as cell culture and karyotyping or viral studies may be useful if subsequent fetal demise compromises the ability to successfully diagnose these abnormalities.

Ultrasound

Ultrasound examination for early prenatal diagnosis of birth defects is most useful as an adjunct to amniocentesis (see "Amniocentesis," below). A number of congenital defects have been diagnosed with this tool.[19, 20] As with radiographic procedures, this has been largely restricted to the late pregnancy investigation of clinical abnormalities such as polyhydramnios. The successful diagnosis or exclusion of anencephaly during midtrimester has become well accepted.[21, 22] More recently, the early delineation of a spina bifida by ultrasound has been reported.[23] Refinements in equipment and further experience hold the promise of more accurate diagnosis of this disorder, as well as the ability to evaluate other areas of the fetal anatomy. It is anticipated that a number of single organ defects may be detectable with this tool. Perhaps more importantly, the evaluation of a single involved organ, when normal, may permit the exclusion or reduction of a risk for a particular multiple malformation syndrome.

Placental Aspiration

Aspiration of placental blood is probably performed inadvertently during amniocentesis quite frequently. Often mixed samples of maternal and fetal blood of varying proportions are obtained. Recently, investigators have reported the successful use of these samples for rapid analysis of fetal chromosomes by standard lymphocyte culture techniques.[24] The successful prenatal diagnosis of hemoglobinopathies has been reported, utilizing blood obtained by this approach.[25, 26] Placental aspiration should be ultrasonically directed. Aspiration of fetal blood cells is often best achieved when the placenta is implanted anteriorly in the uterus. The safety of this procedure in regard to pregnancy wastage, fetal-maternal transfusion, etc., has not been evaluated, and for that reason, the risks of the procedure cannot be well defined for the patient.

Fetoscopy

The development of an endoscope for the direct visualization of the fetus, with the ability to obtain fetal tissue biopsy, including blood samples, is perhaps the most dramatic and exciting recent development in prenatal diagnosis.[27] Relatively few instances of its use for diagnosis have been reported. It is anticipated that studies requiring small samples of fetal blood, such as those for hemoglobin synthesis disorders, will be the prominent indication for its use. A limited number of cases have been reported in which this procedure has been applied clinically for this purpose.[28] In addition, there is the potential for visualization of a number of fetal abnormalities not detectable by other means. Benzie et al[29] have recently reported the use of fetal visualization to exclude the diagnosis of arthrogryposis multiplex congenita. Reports regarding the evaluation of its potential in pregnancies about to be terminated are impressive, but also point out limitations of the instrument, especially in terms of fetal visualization.[30, 31] Continued investigation to improve the technical aspects of the instrument promises to enhance the usefulness.[32] As with placental aspiration, the diagnostic potential and safety of this procedure for general clinical use need further clarification.

Amniocentesis

Amniocentesis has become an important and frequently used tool for fetal evaluation during the third trimester. Anticipation of its widespread application for genetic diagnosis generated concerns regarding the safety of the procedure during the early second trimester. Over a relatively short period of time, studies have established its status as a safe and accurate clinical tool. The availability of amniotic fluid during the second trimester of pregnancy has permitted the diagnosis of a large number of birth defects. The cell-free supernatant may be utilized for biochemical determinations, such as for alphafetoprotein, as well as studies for viral diseases.[33] Studies of the cellular fraction of fresh amniotic fluid samples have generally not proven useful because of the variable sources and viability of the cellular element. Nevertheless, the high rate of success with tissue culture of amniotic fluid cells which reflect the fetal genotype has made possible diagnosis of cytogenetic, as well as many single gene disorders.

Ultrasound Guidance

The value of ultrasound examination before midtrimester amniocentesis continues to be a controversial area. It was initially anticipated that this procedure, by virtue of placental localization, might have a direct impact on the safety of second trimester amniocentesis with regard to fetal wastage. Large studies have not shown this to be the case.[34] Nevertheless, it would seem advisable, if only on theoretic grounds, to avoid placental puncture whenever possible. Ultrasound has proven useful in determining needle placement when the placental implantation only partially covers the anterior wall of the uterus. If the placenta covers the entire anterior wall of the uterus, avoidance of the central area of the placenta, where cord insertion is most frequent, can be attempted. Direct ultrasound guidance of amniocentesis may be useful when there is failure to obtain fluid after repeated attempts. A reduction in the incidence of amniotic fluid samples contaminated by blood, as well as fetomaternal microtransfusion, has been noted when preliminary placental localization is available.[35–37] The issue of blood group sensitization due to midtrimester amniocentesis will be discussed subsequently. Some investigators have experienced less successful cell culture with bloody samples.[38, 39] A reduction in the incidence of bloody samples, if important in increasing the frequency of successful tissue culture or, perhaps, shortening the time required to complete a study, certainly justifies the use of preliminary ultrasound.

Anticipation of fetal blood contamination of the amniotic fluid specimen is an important aspect of counseling for certain diagnostic procedures such as alphafetoprotein determination for neural tube defects (see "Neural Tube Defects"). Ultrasound examination is also useful in detecting multiple gestation and abnormalities of amniotic fluid volume, such as polyhydramnios or olighydramnios, as well as confirming the gestational age. This latter aspect is most important for biochemical studies which vary with the length of gestation (e.g., amniotic fluid alphafetoprotein levels). An additional benefit is the exclusion of anencephaly by the detection of a well defined, normal appearing fetal vertex. For these reasons, the continued use of this examination prior to midtrimester amniocentesis is recommended by a number of authorities.[40]

The technique of amniocentesis during the midtrimester of pregnancy is not unlike that used during later pregnancy, with the exception that determination of fetal position is not possible. The patient is asked to empty her urinary bladder immediately before the procedure. A pelvic examination may be useful in determining placement of the needle, especially when gestational age is relatively early. After mechanical antiseptic skin preparation, a sterile field is established. The use of local anesthesia for the skin, subcutaneous tissue and peritoneum is advisable to avoid movement of the patient during placement of the needle into the uterine cavity. A standard 18- to 20-gauge spinal needle is used for withdrawal of fluid. A stylet is kept in place until the uterine cavity has been entered, in an attempt to avoid contamination of the bore of the needle with maternal tissues or blood from the uterine wall. After withdrawal of the stylet, a small amount (approximately 1 cc) of amniotic fluid is aspirated or allowed to run out of the open needle for the same reason. If blood-tinged fluid is obtained, frequently it will clear with this technique. Fluid specimens are collected in sterile plastic syringes. Duplicate aliquots are usually withdrawn as a precaution against microbial contamination as well as laboratory error. The amount of fluid withdrawn is contingent upon the duration of gestation, as well as that necessary to complete the diagnostic study. Most often, 20 to 30 cc of fluid is sufficient. After withdrawal of the specimen, the stylet is replaced in the needle, and the needle withdrawn from the uterine cavity. The patient may resume normal activities immediately after the procedure, and the fluid samples are delivered to the laboratory for immediate processing.

Risks of Amniocentesis

A number of investigators have reported their individual experience with the safety and accuracy of amniocentesis in midtrimester. In an attempt to further define these aspects of midtrimester amniocentesis for prenatal diagnosis, prospective controlled studies of a large number of patients have been performed. The results of these studies have recently been made available.

Pregnancy Wastage. Data has been analyzed from 1040 women undergoing the procedure, and 929 appropriate control subjects in a study in the United States, and a comparable study of 1020 pregnancies monitored by amniocentesis performed in Canada.[34–41] The age-adjusted fetal loss rate in the United States study was 3.3% for amniocentesis cases and 3.4% for the control subjects, there being no significant difference between the two groups in this regard. The incidence of fetal loss between the amniocentesis group and selected control subjects in the Canadian study confirms this finding. These two studies attest to the safety of the procedure. It would appear that the incidence of fetal loss directly related to amniocentesis is exceedingly low.

Maternal Complications. A number of immediate maternal complications were experienced by a small percentage of patients. Minor discomfort at the site of the needle insertion was not uncommon. Vaginal bleeding was reported in approximately 1% of cases. This is often self-limited. Likewise, leakage of amniotic fluid was reported in a comparable portion of cases, and once again, was usually transient. Amnionitis occurred in two cases in the Canadian study.

Fetal Injury. Injury of the fetus during the third trimester with an amniocentesis needle has been well documented.[42–50] These injuries range from minor cosmetic scars to fatal fetal exsanguination. It has generally been anticipated that the possibility of fetal injury during the second trimester would be less, because of the relatively larger volume of amniotic fluid in relationship to fetal size. Newborn evaluation and a 1-year follow-up of patients in the United States controlled study failed to reveal evidence of physical injuries resulting from amniocentesis, or significant differences in physical, neurologic or developmental status. Nevertheless, there have been recent reports of skin scars attributed to second trimester amniocentesis.[51] In view of the large number of early second trimester amniocenteses performed with careful newborn examination and follow-up, it would appear that the risk of fetal injury, either cosmetic or otherwise, is present, although very low.

Technical Failure. The necessity for repeated amniocentesis occurs in approximately 10% of cases. In about half of the instances, this is due to failure to obtain fluid at the initial attempt. Although the fetal loss rate for women requiring more than one amniocentesis was not statistically significantly different in the studies, there was a suggestion of an increasing incidence of fetal loss with increasing number of needle insertions during the tap. In the author's experience, multiple needle insertions in rapid succession are often unrewarding, and may represent an increased risk, whereas a single repeat amniocentesis at a 7- to 10-day interval, when time permits, usually meets with success in obtaining amniotic fluid. In approximately one-half of the cases which require repeat amniocentesis, the indication is failure of cell culture. Successful culture in more than 95% of cases has been achieved by a number of laboratories. Careful attention to the early growth of amniotic cells should permit an early decision for repeat amniocentesis in almost all cases when necessary. This becomes clinically important in view of the time limitations for completion of these studies.

Accuracy. The accuracy of midtrimester amniocentesis for prenatal genetic diagnosis is also of critical importance. In instances in which amniotic tissue culture is to be performed, it is generally advisable that samples be processed in duplicate. It is beneficial to have this processing performed in laboratories which have independent equipment and supplies. This potentially prevents loss of samples because of contamination, equipment failure or energy failure, as well as human error in labeling of samples, etc. The accuracy of the procedure is often contingent upon the accuracy of specific test procedures involved. One important source of error, that of maternal cell contamination, has been recognized through cytogenetic studies. In the series of 1040 cases evaluated in the United States, six erroneous diagnoses occurred, resulting in an overall accuracy rate of 99.4%. In some instances, recognition of the error was made by the birth of a normal male fetus when karyotype of the cultured amniotic cells was consistent with that of a normal female. Presumably, comparable instances in which maternal cells were cultured and a normal female fetus was born, would have been unrecognized. On this basis, the rate for maternal cell contamination may be in the range of 0.05–1%. Potential methods for elimination of the source of error are an important avenue for investigation. Identification of specific paternal marker chromosomes is useful in individual cases. Likewise, determination of sex steroids in amniotic fluid supernatant is also of value in instances where a female karyotype is obtained from a pregnancy with a male fetus (see "X-linked Recessive" under "Mendelian Patterns of Inheritance").

A second important source of potential error exists when there is a multiple gestation. Because of the increasing frequency of dizygotic twin gestation with advanced maternal age, it is anticipated that this will be encountered in patients undergoing midtrimester amniocentesis more often than in the general population.[52] As previously mentioned, it is felt that the exclusion of the diagnosis of multiple gestation constitutes one of the important indications for ultrasound prior to amniocentesis for genetis diagnosis. A technique for the successful genetic study of a twin gestation has been described. Ultrasound guidance and the injection of a dye (Congo red or methylene blue) after the initial entry into the amniotic cavity permitted the assessment of fluid from each amniotic sac in the reported cases.[53, 54] Use of chromosome markers may be of value in an individual case of dizygotic twins to determine the success of this technique.

Other Risks. The possibility of blood group sensitization due to fetomaternal microtransfusion as a result of amniocentesis is an area of concern. Uncontrolled studies of the effect of late pregnancy amniocentesis on antibody titers have shown conflicting results.[55–57] Thus far, no documented cases of primary sensitization attributable to second trimester amniocentesis have been reported. Because of the natural history of this disease, this is not entirely unexpected. Detection of this phenomenon would require follow-up through subsequent pregnancies in a large number of Rh-negative women. The incidence of blood contamination of amniotic fluid during second trimester amniocentesis has been reported in a range of 6 to 22%.[54, 58–60] It is well accepted that the incidence of microscopic blood contamination is a good deal higher than recognized by gross examination of the fluid specimen. The presence of fetal blood in a significant portion of these specimens has been documented by hemoglobin identity, as well as the Kleihauer technique.[61, 62] The incidence of fetomaternal microtransfusion after second trimester amniocentesis has been found to be as high as 10 to 15%.[62, 63] For this reason, the administration of Rh immunoglobulin has been recommended after amniocentesis in Rh-negative women whose spouses are Rh positive.[54, 58, 64] The safety of this therapy has not been evaluated in a large number of patients. The administration of Rh immunoglobulin produces a very low passive antibody titer, and because placental immunoglobulin transfer may not be well developed at this time,[65] it seems likely that the effects of this prophylaxis would not be any greater than those seen in patients with mild (low titer) sensitization in early pregnancy. It is appropriate to inform Rh-negative patients of this information before amniocentesis, especially when the placental implantation is on the anterior wall of the uterus. Administration of Rh immunoglobulin probably should be reserved for patients who demonstrate a fetomaternal microtransfusion when the father is Rh positive. This is perhaps most essential for those patients being studied for high risk situations who anticipate repeated pregnancies utilizing prenatal diagnosis, e.g., a Tay-Sachs carrier couple. The large group of patients who have amniocentesis undergo the procedure on the basis of advanced maternal age. This is often their final pregnancy. Because of the natural history of Rh sensitization and the absence of reports of problems during the pregnancy studied by amniocentesis, it does not seem unreasonable to withhold Rh immunoglobulin therapy in these cases if there is any question regarding the necessity for its use.

Chromosomal Disorders

During the past two decades there have been rapid advances in the field of human cytogenetics. Methodology developed during the 1960's allowed for the standardization of the conventional human karyotype. In addition to the description of a number of "chromosomal syndromes," a great deal of information has been gained regarding the frequency of chromosomal abnormalities in human populations, and the relationship of these to reproductive failure. During the early 1970's, specialized chromosome staining techniques were developed and standardized.[66] Patterns demonstrated by these methods provide discrimination of each chromosome in the human karyotype, as well as a higher resolution of specific chromosomal segments and rearrangements. These staining techniques have become collectively known as "banding." The "G-banding" pattern of the normal human karyotype illustrated in Figure 2.2 has become the standard tool for cytogenetic diagnosis. With the use of banding, chromosomal syndromes associated with imbalance of small segments of human chromosomes are being reported with increasing frequency.[67]

The successful culture and cytogenetic study of human amniotic fluid cells was first reported in 1966 by Steele and Breg.[68] Since that time, cytogenetic investigation of human pregnancies has been the most frequently applied tool for prenatal diagnosis. The proper application of prenatal cytogenetic diagnosis is contingent upon an understanding of the frequency of chromosomal abnormalities and the mechanisms involved in their occurrence.

FREQUENCY OF CHROMOSOME ABNORMALITIES

Extensive cytogenetic surveys of consecutive newborn infants have been performed. Hamerton[69] has compiled a number of these studies comprising a total of 46,150 newborn infants. The results indicate that major chromosome abnormalities occur in between 1:150 and 1:200 liveborn babies.[69] In a study of approximately 14,000 newborns, he found 20 with sex chromosome aneuploidy, 18 autosomal trisomies, and 24 infants with balanced structural rearrangements (11 reciprocal and 13 Robertsonian translocations). One infant had an unbalanced structural rearrangement and two others had additional identified fragments.

Studies of pregnancy wastage have documented a high frequency of chromosome

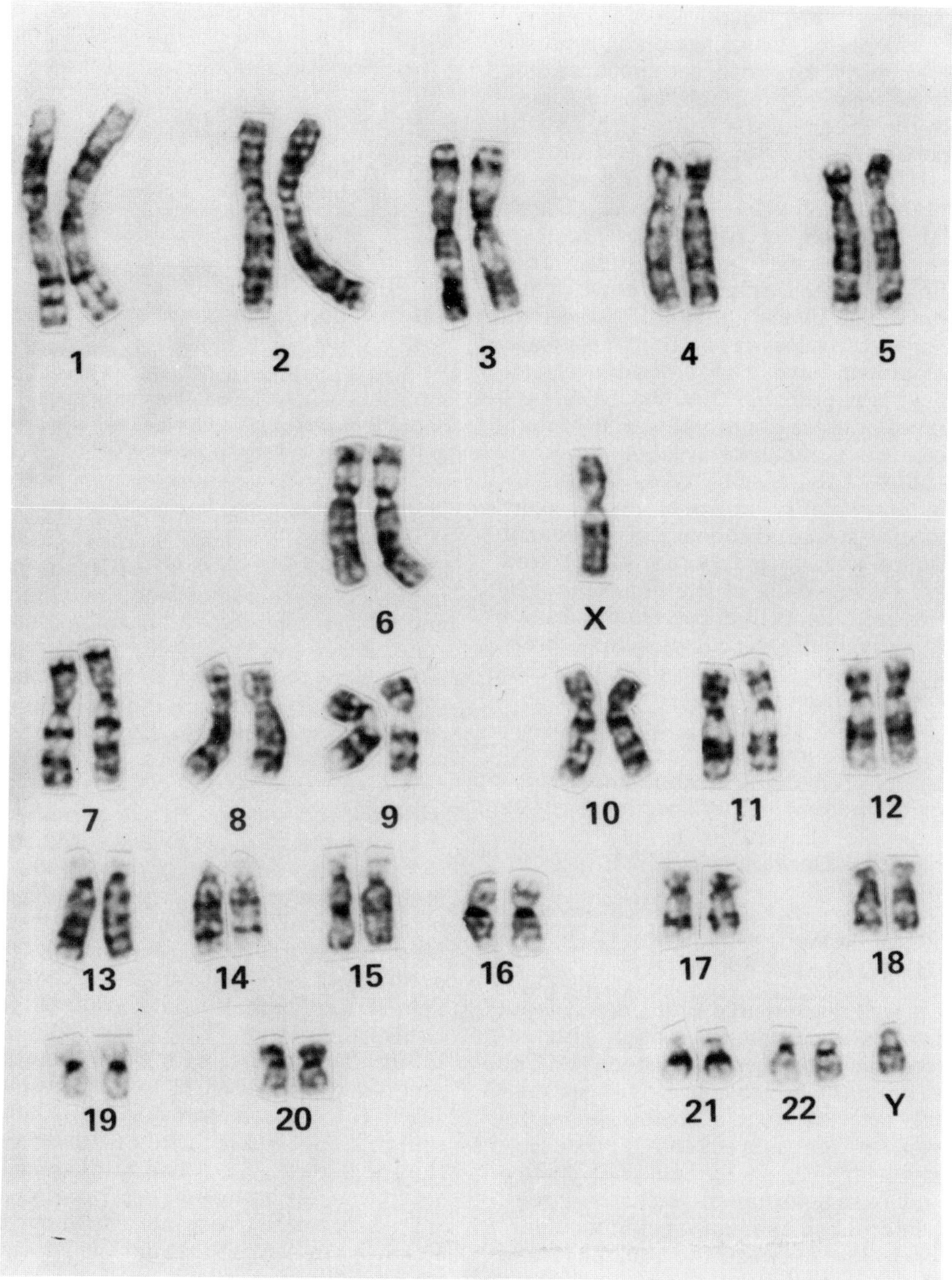

Figure 2.2. Normal G-banded human karyotype.

abnormalities in lost conceptions. Investigations of late pregnancy loss, including stillbirth and neonatal deaths in two studies, have shown frequencies of chromosome abnormalities of 5.6% and 7.2%.[70, 71] Also notable was the frequency of 10.2% and 13% of these abnormalities when there were congenital malformations, as opposed to 4.4% and 2.5% when they were not present. When the malformations were not limited to the central nervous system, the incidence of chromosome abnormality was 18.9%. It has also become apparent that the frequency of chromosome abnormality in pregnancy wastage is inversely proportional to the duration of gestation at the time of fetal loss.[72–75] In a review of spontaneous abortion material, Carr[72] found that 36% of aborted pregnancies have chromosome abnormalities. This finding has been confirmed by other investigators. The Boues[76] have estimated that 70% of embryos lost at less than 6 weeks of development have a chromosome abnormality. It is probable that the overall occurrence of these abnormalities in human conceptions is remarkably high.

Studies of the specific types of chromosome abnormality in spontaneous abortions show a high frequency of autosomal trisomies (45%), polyploidy (25%) and 45,XO (20%). Many of the autosomal trisomies seen, as well as polyploidy, are almost universally lethal in early pregnancy. Nevertheless, this data has confirmed that even the majority of Turner's syndrome and Down's syndrome conceptions result in pregnancy loss.[72, 77] The application of banding techniques to the study of this problem will further identify the specific abnormalities, and perhaps clarify the mechanisms which are involved.[78]

CHROMOSOME ABNORMALITIES RELATED TO MATERNAL AGE

It is well documented that the incidence of Down's syndrome increases with advanced maternal age (see Table 2.1). The most dramatic increase begins at approximately age 35, with a steep rise in frequency in the subsequent reproductive years.[79, 80] The cause for this phenomenon has not been determined. Recently, Hook[81] has determined the age-specific incidence for each year between the ages of 34 and 41. An increased frequency of nondisjunction related to advanced maternal age, leading to other autosomal trisomies (13 and 18), has also been shown.[82, 83] New prospective data regarding the frequency of chromosomal abnormalities in pregnancies of older women have been gained from prenatal cytogenetic studies. These have uniformly indicated a higher incidence than seen in newborn studies. Chromosome abnormalities detected in the pregnancies of mothers between the ages of 35 and 40 are reported to be approximately 1.5%. After the age of 40, positive diagnoses have been found in approximately 5% of cases.[84] The marked discrepancy between the retrospective and the prospective data for chromosome errors due to advanced maternal age is a source of controversy and concern.[85–87] It is important that patients be made aware of the potential frequency for positive diagnosis in the midtrimester of pregnancy, and the possible diagnosis of trisomies other than Down's syndrome. The actual risk, however, which is significant in terms of burden, still remains the data available from liveborn surveys. The discrepancy certainly lies, in part, with the frequency of pregnancy loss after 16 weeks' gestation, when the fetus is chromosomally abnormal.[70, 71, 75, 85] Other factors, such as selection of patients for prenatal diagnosis or correction for maternal age at the estimated date of delivery, may be important. Further analysis of this data is necessary to clarify the age-specific incidence of chromosomal abnormalities for prenatal counseling.

Table 2.1. Incidence of Down's syndrome births related to maternal age*

Retrospective data		Age by year		Prospective data	
Age, yr	Ratio	Age, yr	Ratio	Age, yr	%
<20	1:2300	34	1:527	35	0.5
20–25	1:1600	35	1:413	35–40	1.5
25–30	1:1200	36	1:333	40	5.2
		37	1:266		
30–35	1:880	38	1:183		
35–40	1:290	39	1:135		
		40	1:106		
40–45	1:100	41	1:83		
>45	1:46				

* Retrospective data for maternal age-related risk of Down's syndrome from Collman and Stoller[79] and Hook.[81] Prospective data based on age of mother at amniocentesis from Ferguson-Smith.[84]

PREVIOUS TRISOMIC OFFSPRING

With the current availability of cytogenetic studies, all children who have a clinical diagnosis of Down's syndrome should have a karyotype performed. In approximately 95% of cases, a primary trisomy (47,XX or XY,+21) is found. A number of instances of siblings with primary trisomies are reported. In some cases, this has been found to be due to parental mosaicism, with a low percentage cell line, having a 47,XX or XY,+21 karyotype.[88] In other cases, no explanation is found. The higher than expected frequency of double trisomies (48 XXY,+21) and cases of familial mosaicism support the concept of predisposition to nondisjunction in certain individuals or families.[89, 90]

A recurrence risk for Down's syndrome due to a primary trisomy has been given as approximately 1%. Data concerning the recurrence risk for other autosomal trisomies is not available. Prospective data from amniocentesis studies regarding the risk in these situations should be forthcoming. In the data from Canada,[41] 238 pregnancies of mothers less than 35 years of age were studied because of a previous child or other family member with Down's syndrome. The diagnosis of Down's syndrome was made in a single case in which the mother was subsequently shown to be mosaic for a trisomy 21 cell line. Other investigators have found a 1 to 1.5% incidence of positive findings in this group of patients, but have not specifically defined the recurrence risk for trisomy 21. The general experience of the author has been that many couples who have had a child with an autosomal trisomy elect prenatal diagnosis based more on burden than risk. It will be important, however, to further clarify the actual risk for counseling.

ROBERTSONIAN TRANSLOCATION

Centric fusion translocations occur between the D group and G group chromosomes in man (D/D, D/G, G/G). The frequency of these in population studies is approximately 1:1000.[91, 92] DqDq translocations most frequently involve the nos. 13 and 14 chromosomes. An imbalance caused by these translocations infrequently accounts for a child born with trisomy 13. The risk of bearing a child with a chromosome abnormality, when a parent is a carrier for a D/D translocation, is very low. Translocations between a D and G group chromosome (D/G) most often involve chromosomes 14 and 21.[93] The risk for bearing a child with Down's syndrome, when a parent carries a D/G translocation, is less than the theoretically expected value, based on random segregation of the chromosomes at meiosis. This may be accounted for by nonrandom segregation, prezygotic selection of gametes or early loss of imbalanced conceptions. Hamerton[91] has calculated that the risk to a heterozygous mother with a balanced D/G translocation is 10.9%, whereas for a similarly heterozygous father, it is 2.4%. The risk for specific D/G translocations (i.e., 13/21 vs. 14/21 vs. 15/21) has not been determined, but might be of importance for counseling. With G/G translocations involving chromosomes 21 and 22, the risk to a heterozygous parent is approximately 6 to 7%. When Robertsonian translocations involve the same chromosome (e.g., 13/13, 21/21, etc.), all conceptions will be either monosomic (presumably lethal) or trisomic for that chromosome. In these cases, prenatal diagnosis would not be of value.

RECIPROCAL TRANSLOCATIONS

Children with unbalanced chromosome material due to parental reciprocal translocations are being reported with increasing frequency, utilizing chromosome banding methods. The actual risk of bearing a chromosomally abnormal child when a parent is a balanced carrier for any specific reciprocal translocation cannot be precisely determined.[94] In most instances, because of current limitation of family size, information from the pedigree cannot be considered reliable to determine risk figures. When ascertainment has been on the basis of a liveborn child with a chromosome abnormality, it would seem that the risk is probably significant.

Increasingly, couples in which one member carries a structural rearrangement are being ascertained by chromosome banding studies of patients with recurrent reproductive wastage (Figure 2.3). The incidence of translocation in one member of a couple with this history is approximately 1 in 15.[95–97] When the reproductive loss has been first trimester abortion, the risk of a

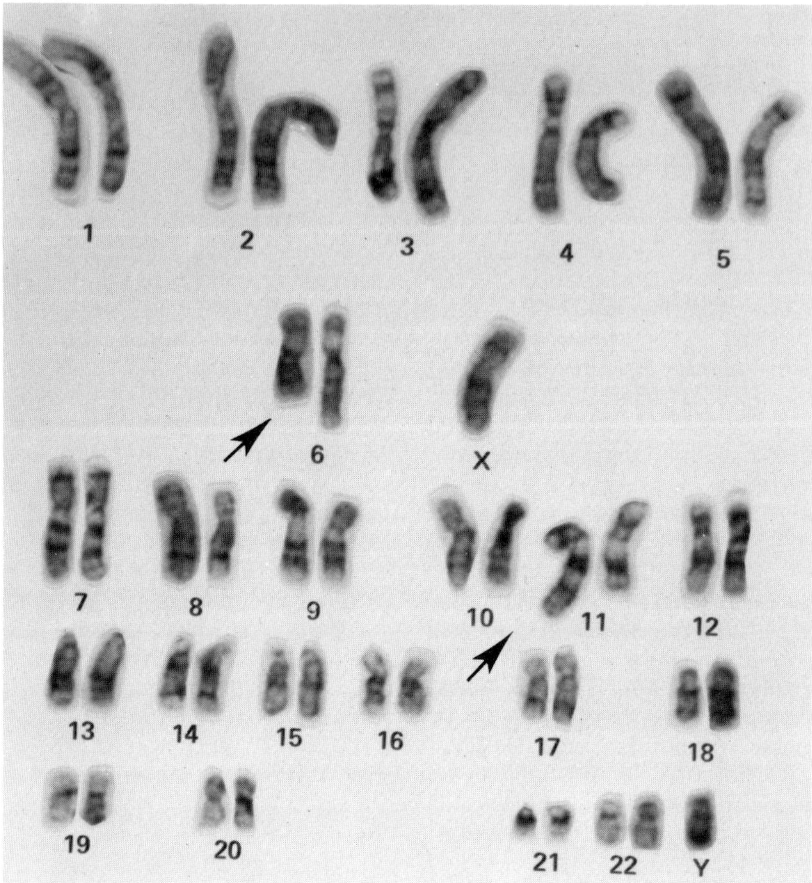

Figure 2.3. G-banded karyotype. Male partner of couple with history of habitual abortion. Balanced reciprocal translocation between chromosomes 6 and 11 (arrows point to involved chromosomes).

chromosome abnormality in a pregnancy maintained into the second trimester cannot be predicted. After appropriate counseling, the couple may elect prenatal diagnosis for reassurance. When the husband is a balanced carrier of this type of rearrangement and there is a history of habitual early abortion, donor insemination is an option which should be discussed. In view of this information, it is also important that parental chromosome studies be performed when there is a history of recurrent pregnancy wastage in patients undergoing prenatal diagnosis for other indications, in order that a chromosome imbalance due to a structural rearrangement does not go undetected in an amniotic fluid study.

PROBLEMS IN PRENATAL DIAGNOSIS OF CHROMOSOME ABNORMALITY

A number of problems and pitfalls with prenatal cytogenetic diagnosis have been recognized. Increasing experience with several of these findings has permitted more accurate interpretation of the results of the studies. On the other hand, certain problems, such as mosaicism, continue to be a dilemma.

Since very early experience with amniotic cell culture, a high and quite variable frequency of polyploidy has been noted. Although tetraploidy occurs in human fibroblast cultures, it is usually present in a low percentage of cells. It has been suggested that this finding in amniotic cell culture may represent an in vitro occurrence, or may arise from cells originating in the amnion.[98–101] Neither explanation has been felt to be entirely satisfactory. Since this varies both within one laboratory and from one laboratory to another, it would be difficult to explain on the basis of certain aspects of culture technique. Tegenkamp and Hux[102] have shown an increase in the percentage of tetraploidy in fibroblast-like cultures, as opposed to epithelial-like cultures. The finding of a high percentage of polyploidy with an otherwise normal cytogenetic study has not been clinically significant.[103] A relationship between polyploidy and aneuploidy in amniotic cell culture has not been noted or suggested.

The finding of an autosomal trisomy of a chromosome other than the no. 21 should not be unexpected in samples studied for the indication of advanced maternal age. Because of the poor prognosis for development and survival with trisomy 13 and 18, this does not usually present a clinical dilemma. The incidental finding of sex chromosome aneuploidy should be anticipated, based on its known frequency and the large number of these studies being performed. When this occurs, the chromosomal error and its clinical implications should be explained to the parents. In these situations, the decision-making process may be quite difficult.

Chromosomal variants or markers usually cause concern in prenatal diagnosis because the phenotype of the patient cannot be ascertained. When these occur, the problem can usually be resolved by parental chromosome studies to identify the variant in one of the phenotypically normal parents. For example, variations in the short arms of the acrocentric chromosomes (e.g., Dp−, Dp+, Gp−, Gp+) may lead to this type of study. The frequency of these and other variants in populations has been studied.[104] Their occurrence in phenotypically normal individuals is well documented. In order to avoid undue patient anxiety, it is useful to explain the possible necessity for comparing parental chromosomes with those obtained from amniotic cell culture in a portion of cases at the initial counseling session. By taking this approach, patients have not been alarmed when this becomes necessary. On occasion, when these marker chromosomes are of paternal origin in amniotic cell cultures, they have been useful to exclude the possibility of maternal cell contamination.

Mosaicism in amniotic cell culture continues to be a troublesome finding. Many laboratories with large prenatal diagnosis experience have encountered this problem. The concern of course arises because of the possibility that mosaicism may truly reflect the fetal genotype. It is known that the incidence of mosaicism varies with the tissue studied and number of cells analyzed, as well as the laboratory methods and experience.[105] Nevertheless, the occurrence of mosaicism in phenotypically abnormal individuals and in spontaneously aborted second trimester pregnancies causes concern when seen in studies of cultured amniotic fluid cells.[75, 105] In most instances in which mosaicism has been detected, this finding has not been confirmed in repeat amniotic fluid studies, fetal tissues at abortion or in the newborns from these pregnancies. Based on these findings, mosaicism is generally felt to most often represent a culture phenomenon.[106–111] Other important possibilities include an aneuploid cell focus in the amnion, misdivision of a free amniotic cell in vivo or true fetal mosaicism. Trisomy C mosaicism has been found in repeated amniotic fluid samples from the same patient in one case in which fetal tissues failed to grow after induced abortion. In this instance, the fetus appeared phenotypically normal.[112] Importantly, Bloom et al[113] have made the prenatal diagnosis of trisomy D mosaicism, which was confirmed by fetal tissue studies following abortion. When mosaicism occurs in an amniotic cell culture, the patient should be informed of this finding, and the most current experience with it. At times, the absence of this finding in a second amniotic fluid sample may reassure the patient and the physician. Because complete reassurance cannot be given regarding the initial results, the option of pregnancy termination should be made available when the informed patient requests it.

Another source of problems occurs when

chromosome translocations or other complex structural rearrangements (inversions, etc.) are detected. In these instances, the concept of "aneusomie de recombinaison" may apply.[114, 115] This phenomenon could result in a chromosome imbalance in a fetus from a parent with a balanced rearrangement although the chromosomes of the two may appear morphologically identical. The use of appropriate banding techniques in selected cases should reduce this risk. The occurrence of a de novo structural rearrangement detected by amniocentesis presents a similar problem regarding assurance of a balanced state. An additional concern arises because spontaneous chromosome rearrangements in cell culture have been observed.[116] If this phenomenon were to occur in an amniotic fluid cell culture, the difficulty of interpretation would be similar to that which occurs when mosaicism has been found.

SINGLE GENE DISORDERS

The prenatal diagnosis of a number of disorders due to single mutant genes has been accomplished. In addition, a number of other disorders are deemed potentially diagnosable (see Table 2.2). Most of the biochemical disorders which are amenable to prenatal diagnosis are autosomal recessive in their inheritance. Only a few disorders inherited in the other Mendelian patterns are able to be studied. It is not the purpose of this discussion to enumerate the specific metabolic basis of each disorder and the method of diagnosis, but rather to point out general principles which apply in many of these situations. The use of amniotic fluid supernatant is of very limited value except for a few disorders. Problems with assays of the cellular element arise because of the variable sources of cells in the amniotic fluid, and more importantly, the variation in their viability. For these reasons, most of the studies are performed using cultured amniotic fluid cells. Biochemical assays which measure the deficient enzyme, its substrate or the end products of its metabolic reaction are the basis for many of these assays. The number of cells necessary for these tests is often greater than that needed for chromosome analysis. This frequently causes a more extended delay from amniocentesis to the final test results (4 to 6 weeks as opposed to 2 to 3 weeks).

It is important to consider certain aspects of amniotic fluid cell culture which are relevant to biochemical diagnosis. Early investigators noted the presence of morphologically distinct clones in amniotic cell culture. Two dominant cell types, epithelial-like and fibroblast, have usually been observed. One group of investigators evaluating clonal morphology and growth potential have described a third type of clone, designated amniotic fluid cells (AF).[117] Enzymatic differences between the fibroblast and epithelial cells have been described in regard to histidase and cystathionine synthase.[118, 119] Nadler has appropriately called attention to the need for recognition of other factors in amniotic cell culture which may alter the biochemical properties of the cells. In general, enzyme activity in cultured skin fibroblasts cannot be extrapolated directly to amniotic fluid cell cultures. Preliminary studies on control amniotic cultures have preceded clinical application of these assays by necessity. With regard to certain enzymes, it has also been important to evaluate control of a gestational age comparable to that anticipated for clinical use in order that qualitative or quantitative enzymatic changes related to gestational length be detected. When studies are performed for biochemical disorders, it is appropriate that several simultaneous control cultures be initiated in order to avoid any influence of the particular culture techniques on the result, as well as to serve as a source of presumably normal material. Many investigators cooperate by providing a "back-up" assay, as well as cell cultures from known affected pregnancies, for comparison. Because of the rarity of most of these disorders, referral of samples to centers actively involved with the specific biochemical assay has become commonplace, and is to be recommended.

MENDELIAN PATTERNS OF INHERITANCE

The different Mendelian patterns of inheritance relevant to prenatal diagnosis

Table. 2.2. Inborn errors of metabolism diagnosable before birth*

Lipidoses	
Cholesterol-ester storage disease†	Juvenile GM_2 gangliosidosis (GM_2 gangliosidosis type 3)†
Fabry disease‡	GM_3 sphingolipodystrophy†
Farber disease†	Krabbe's disease (globoid cell leukodystrophy)‡
Gaucher disease‡	Metachromatic leukodystrophy‡
Generalized gangliosidosis (GM_1 gangliosidosis type 1)‡	Niemann-Pick disease type A‡
Juvenile GM_1 gangliosidosis (GM_1 gangliosidosis type 2)‡	Niemann-Pick disease type B†
Tay-Sachs disease (GM_2 gangliosidosis type 1)‡	Niemann-Pick disease type C†
Sandhoff's disease (GM_2 gangliosidosis type 2)‡	Refsum disease†
	Wolman disease‡
Mucopolysaccharidoses (MPS)	
MPS I (Hurler)‡	MPS IV (Morquio's syndrome)†
MPS I (Scheie)†	MPS VIA (Maroteaux-Lamy syndrome)†
MPS (Hurler/Scheie)†	MPS VIB (Maroteaux-Lamy syndrome)†
MPS IIA (Hunter)‡	MPS VII (β-glucuronidase deficiency)†
MPS IIB (Hunter)‡	
MPS III (Sanfilippo A)‡	
MPS III (Sanfilippo B)†	
Amino acid and related disorders	
Argininosuccinic aciduria‡	Cystathionine synthase deficiency (homocystinuria)†
Aspartylglucosaminuria†	Cystathioninuria†
Citrullinemia‡	Cystinuria‡
Congenital hyperammonemia†	Hartnup disease†
Histidinemia†	Methylenetetrahydrofolate reductase deficiency†
Hypervalinemia†	Ornithine-α-ketoacid transaminase deficiency†
Iminoglycinuria†	Propionyl coenzyme A (CoA) carboxylase deficiency (ketotic hyperglycinemia)†
Isovaleric acidemia†	Succinyl-CoA: 3-ketoacid CoA-transferase deficiency†
Maple syrup urine disease	Vitamin B_{12} metabolic defect†
Severe infantile‡	
Intermittent†	
Methylmalonic aciduria	
Unresponsive to vitamin B_{12}†	
Responsive to vitamin B_{12}‡	
Isoleucine catabolism disorder†	
Disorders of carbohydrate metabolism	
Fucosidosis†	Glycogen-storage disease (type IV)‡
Galactokinase deficiency†	Mannosidosis†
Galactosemia‡	Phosphohexose isomerase deficiency†
Glucose-6-phosphate dehydrogenase deficiency†	Pyruvate decarboxylase deficiency†
Glycogen-storage disease (type II)‡	Pyruvate dehydrogenase deficiency†
Glycogen-storage disease (type III)†	
Miscellaneous hereditary disorders	
Acatalasemia†	Familial hypercholesterolemia†
Acute intermittent prophyria†	Glutathionuria†
Adenosine deaminase deficiency‡	Hypophosphatasia‡
Chediak-Higashi syndrome†	I-cell disease‡
Congenital erythropoietic porphyria†	Leigh's encephalopathy†
Congenital nephrosis‡	Lesch-Nyhan syndrome‡
Lysosomal acid phosphatase deficiency‡	Protoporphyria†
Lysyl-protocollagen hydroxylase deficiency†	Saccharopinuria†
Myotonic muscular dystrophy†	Sickle cell anemia†
Nail-patella syndrome†	Testicular feminization†
Orotic aciduria†	Thalassemia‡
Cystinosis‡	Xeroderma pigmentosum‡

* Data courtesy of Dr. Aubrey Milunsky, Massachusetts Medical Society, and *The New England Journal of Medicine*.[40]

† Prenatal diagnosis potentially possible.

‡ Prenatal diagnosis made.

will be discussed in regard to general principles of counseling.

Autosomal Dominant Disorders

Disorders are classified as autosomal dominant when an individual who is heterozygous for the gene may be expected to express it. An affected child may be born by transmission of the gene from a parent (50% risk), or by virtue of a new mutation. Of interest is the association between this latter phenomenon and advanced paternal age, described for a number of disorders.[120] Importantly, the specific risk for this phenomenon is not known, but is presumably quite low. Optimally, counseling regarding the occurrence of a dominant mutation in a child of unaffected parents is conducted shortly after the birth of that child. The situation which lends itself to prenatal counseling regarding a dominant trait is most often when the gene is familial. It is important that the counselor be familiar with the frequency of penetrance and the variability of expression of the gene for a disease when discussing the risk and the burden with the family. The development of biochemical assays for prenatal diagnosis of many of the more common familial autosomal dominant disorders in the very near future is not promising. Improved methods of fetal evaluation through the use of ultrasound or fetoscopy may allow detection of some of the structural defects present in certain of these disorders. The detection of a genetic marker in amniotic fluid closely linked to a gene for a specific autosomal dominant disorder would be able to substantially alter the projected 50% risk. This approach, of course, requires close linkage and an informative mating in regard to the particular loci. An example of this which has been well defined is the linkage of the loci for myotonic dystrophy and ABH secretion.[121, 122] This latter marker can be determined by amniocentesis.[123] Perhaps with the rapid advances in genetic knowledge and gene localization, this type of approach may prove useful for other autosomal dominant or X-linked disorders.

Autosomal Recessive Disorders

Disorders are classified as autosomal recessive when the gene for the disorder is located on an autosome and is expressed when present in the homozygous state. Subtle expression, measurable by laboratory studies, allows for detection of the heterozygous or carrier state. In this situation, unaffected parents may have one or more children affected. The risk for each conception is 25%. Because of the rarity of many of these genes, a negative family history is not unusual. An increased likelihood that parents are both heterozygous for the same gene is seen in consanguinous marriages. The frequency of the heterozygous state for certain genes is higher in particular groups by virtue of ethinic, racial or geographic background. The increased frequency of heterozygosity for the Tay-Sachs disease in Jews of Eastern European origin is an example of this. Availability of carrier testing, as well as accurate prenatal diagnosis, has allowed pilot programs to examine the feasibility of screening a high risk population. These couples are able to be identified before the birth of an affected child, and prenatal diagnosis may be offered to them.[124] The analysis of the benefits of this type of program, in addition to the difficulties associated with it, should be of importance to those interested in prenatal diagnosis, as well as those persons concerned with population genetics and screening.

For prenatal diagnosis of a recessive disorder, it is essential that the discrimination between the heterozygous and homozygous states for the gene be highly accurate. Since 50% of the offspring would be expected to be heterozygous, one can see that failure to make the distinction of these fetuses from those that are homozygous, would incur a 75% incidence of a positive study (of which two-thirds would be normal carriers). This concept is perhaps more acutely appreciated when one is aware that we are all normal carriers for several mutant genes.

When a couple is at risk for bearing children who may have a specific autosomal recessive disorder not amenable to prenatal diagnosis, the only available options during pregnancy are assumption of that 25% risk or pregnancy termination. Donor insemination for future pregnancies should be included in the discussion of options. This is perhaps most satisfactory when reliable testing is available, to exclude heterozygosity of the semen donor. When this is not available, the use of a low risk donor by virtue of geographic, racial or ethnic background may be preferable to a random donor. Nevertheless, because of the relatively low frequency of heterozygosity for many of these genes, the risk with a random donor insemination is often quite low.

X-linked Recessive

Disorders which are inherited by an X-linked recessive pattern almost universally affect only male offspring of a female carrier. When a woman carries an X-linked recessive gene, the risk of the disease to her male children is 50%. Only a few of these disorders are specifically diagnosable during the midtrimester of pregnancy (e.g., Fabray's disease, Lesch-Nyhan syndrome and Hunter's syndrome). As with dominant disorders, the birth of a child with an X-linked recessive disorder may occur because of familial transmission of the gene or new mutation. Because of this, and the difficulties with carrier detection for most of these disorders, the determination of the precise risk to future male offspring may be quite complex when the family history is negative. The reader is referred to sources which demonstrate the approaches used in determining this risk.[125]

For patients at risk of bearing sons with X-linked recessive disorders, other than those specifically diagnosable by amniocentesis, the options available during pregnancy are assumption of the risk, or sex determination followed by termination of pregnancies in which the fetus is male. A number of methods of fetal sex determination have been investigated. They have included examination for Y chromosome fluorescence in maternal peripheral lymphocyte culture, endocervical smears and amniotic fluid cells.[126–129] These procedures, as well as the Barr body analysis of amniotic fluid cells, have not been generally recommended because of the reliability required for prenatal genetic diagnosis. For this reason, karyotype of cultured amniotic fluid cells continues to be used for this purpose. Because of the possibility of maternal cell contamination of amniotic fluid cell culture (see "Accuracy" under "Risks of Amniocentesis"), a reliable confirmatory method would be of value. Young and associates[130] reported testosterone levels of greater than 90 pg per ml in pregnancies with male fetuses, and less than 90 pg per ml in pregnancies with female fetuses. In 100 cases studied in our laboratory, amniotic fluid values of 100 pg per ml or greater were found in all but two pregnancies in which the fetus was male, and were less than 100 pg per ml in all pregnancies in which the fetus was female.[131]

Neural Tube Defects

A large portion of birth defects are attributed to multifactorial inheritance. These malformations are due to the additive effects of several genes and environmental influences. The risk to future siblings of an affected child is based on empiric data, and is often in a range of 2 to 7%.[132] The prenatal diagnosis of some of these defects may be possible with the advances in technology which are anticipated (e.g., ultrasound, fetoscopy, etc.).

Of the disorders due to multifactorial inheritance, only the neural tube defects (anencephaly, spina bifida, etc.) are able to be reliably diagnosed by currently available methods. The recurrence risk to siblings of a child with a neural tube defect is 3 to 5%.[133, 134] A recurrence within a family may be any type of neural tube defect, rather than the specific one seen in the index case. When there have been two affected children, the risk for subsequent pregnancies is approximately 10 to 12%.[135] The risk to children of adult survivors with spina bifida is 3%.[136] Neural tube defects are also seen with other syndromes. In some situations, these may be sporadic, or chromosomal. In other cases, the disorder is due to a single mutant gene (e.g., Meckel's syndrome, which is autosomal recessive). Because of the genetic heterogeneity of these defects, accurate diagnosis before counseling is essential.[137]

The prenatal diagnosis of anencephaly may be suspected by the absence of a well defined fetal vertex on ultrasound examination.[21, 22] Although ultrasound diagnosis of certain neural tube defects is possible in late pregnancy, only a single case of spina bifida has been demonstrated in the early second trimester with this tool.[19, 23] Early amniography for the visualization of these malformations (other than anencephaly) has thus far been disappointing.[11, 12] Since the demonstration of the reliability of amniotic fluid alphafetoprotein assay for the diagnosis of open neural tube defects, patients seeking this test constitute an increasing percentage of the caseload for prenatal diagnosis centers.[138] This protein is present in fetal serum very early in gestation, reaching peak values up to 4 mg per ml, at about the 13th week of gestation. After this, levels decrease sharply until delivery. The concentration of alphafetoprotein in amniotic fluid parallels that in fetal serum, however the ratio between the two is 1:150. Weiss et al[139] have demonstrated that alphafetoprotein normally enters the amniotic fluid compartment via the fetal urine. As opposed to fetal serum and amniotic fluid levels, the maternal serum concentration is low during the early pregnancy (the ratio with fetal serum being 1:10,000), rising sharply during the second trimester and peaking at approximately 34 to 36 weeks of pregnancy.

Elevations of amniotic fluid or maternal serum alphafetoprotein levels have been demonstrated with a number of disorders. The common denominator of this phenomenon appears to be some breakdown of the normal barriers between the compartments of the pregnancy, i.e., the fetal circulation-amniotic fluid-maternal circulation. Brock and Sutcliffe[140] first demonstrated raised amniotic fluid alphafetoprotein in which neural tube defects were present in the fetus. Elevation of the amniotic fluid alphafetoprotein is the most reliable market at present for the prenatal diagnosis of open neural tube defects. The reliability of this assay, when used before 20 weeks of gestation, has become well accepted. In an analysis of 2495 cases, Milunsky and Alpert found all 49 cases of open neural tube defects to be diagnosed by amniotic fluid alphafetoprotein levels greater than 3 SD.[61, 141]

As with the other methods of prenatal diagnosis of birth defects, a number of important problems and pitfalls have been encountered. Elevated values have also been found with intrauterine fetal death, as well as a number of other fetal disorders, including omphalocele, congenital nephrosis, duodenal atresia, esophageal atresia, Turner's syndrome and sacrococcygeal teratoma.[142, 147] False positive values may be obtained due to fetal blood contamination of the amniotic fluid during amniocentesis. Because of the marked difference in concentration of alphafetoprotein between fetal blood and amniotic fluid, very small quantities of fetal blood may markedly alter the results of this testing.[148, 149] Patients electing this procedure who have an anterior placenta should be counseled regarding this possibility. Bloody amniotic fluid samples should be studied for the presence of fetal red cells or fetal hemoglobin in these cases. Because of the change in normal levels of amniotic fluid alphafetoprotein with gestational age, errors in "dating" may cause false positive as well as false negative results. The use of preliminary ultrasound to assess gestational age as well as reduce the incidence of fetal blood contamination of the fluid, is necessary. Nevertheless, Milunsky and Alpert[61] have encountered a true false positive rate of 1.2%. It is likely that fetal problems as yet not determined may account for this, as well as elevated values found in normal pregnancy. An important cause of false negative results occurs when the neural tube defect is covered by skin. It has been estimated that as many as 10% of these defects fall into this group.[150] Because of these problems associated with alphafetoprotein assay for open neural tube defects, a number of other amniotic fluid components have been investigated for the diagnosis of these disorders, including beta-trace spinal fluid protein, macrophage counts, fibrin split products and macroglobulin in amniotic fluid.[151–155] Although these methods may be confirmatory, none has yet proven to be reliable for the exclusion of the false positives and false negatives encountered with the alphafetoprotein assay.

Since the large majority of children with neural tube defects are born to parents with negative family histories, the detection of high risk pregnancies through maternal serum screening has been proposed. Brock and associates[156] first reported the prenatal diagnosis of anencephaly by maternal serum alphafetoprotein measurement. Since that time, a number of investigators have found detection rates with this method varying from only 40 to 80%.[157–161] As with amniotic fluid alphafetoprotein, errors may occur because of fetal-maternal bleeding secondary to amniocentesis, inappropriate gestational age (less than 13 weeks or greater than 22 weeks) at the time of testing, errors in gestational dating, closed neural tube defects or other fetal abnormalities, as well as true false positives and false negatives. Because maternal AFP is elevated with multiple gestation or maternal liver disease, these conditions are additional sources of false positive results. As with amniotic fluid measurement, certain of these discrepancies may be overcome with the preliminary use of ultrasound and studies to detect fetal-maternal bleeding. Because of the high frequency of errors in gestational dating, or nonspecific last menstrual period, it would appear that this will be the greatest problem encountered by maternal serum alphafetoprotein screening projects.[162] In spite of this, it would seem that continued investigation of the clinical application of this test may be rewarding.

An additional comment is now necessary regarding the diagnosis of anencephaly by ultrasound. Recently the absence of a fetal vertex on ultrasound examination in the presence of normal amniotic fluid alphafetoprotein has been encountered in the diagnosis of fetal hypophosphatasia. This has occurred in pregnancies when the parents were known to be heterozygous for that gene.[163, 164] The data regarding amniotic fluid alkaline phosphatase levels is conflicting, but this disorder should be suspected in a pregnancy when these combinations of findings are obtained. Alkaline phosphatase determinations on parental serum in a carrier range might serve as further evidence of the diagnosis.

Goals of Prenatal Genetic Counseling and Diagnosis

PATIENT REASSURANCE

Much important effort has been spent discussing the goals and impact of prenatal diagnosis and selective abortion in terms of society. The monetary cost-benefit ratio is obvious. Ultimately, however, persons involved with these services must establish their goals in terms of the individual patients who consult with them. Since the majority of the pregnancies studied are normal, the final result is most often one of parental reassurance. The ability to obtain this reassurance may foster reproduction in patients who might not have otherwise considered it. Couples with a great deal of anxiety during pregnancy are able to be more comfortable after prenatal diagnosis. Although they must recognize that these tests do not "guarantee a normal baby," the reliable exclusion of a diagnosis for which they are at increased risk is often of immeasurable value to them. Thus, a primary goal of prenatal counseling and diagnosis is patient reassurance.

PREVENTION OF BIRTH DEFECTS

In almost all cases in which there is prenatal diagnosis of a genetic disorder, selective abortion of affected pregnancies is the option elected. The issue of obtaining a commitment to abort from patients before performing a diagnostic procedure is controversial, but probably a moot point. Through appropriate counseling, the patients should recognize this possibility, and it should be discussed early in the course of the counseling. Because patients seeking prenatal diagnosis have "wanted pregnancies," the issue of abortion may be difficult to consider. Not infrequently, patients who have negative feelings regarding pregnancy termination in general wish to postpone a commitment for abortion until the result of a study indicates it. Acceptance of this situation by the counselor is reasonable in that insistence on pregnancy termination for a positive diagnosis might only generate anxiety in a setting which is primarily designed to reassure patients. When a patient feels that she would not terminate a pregnancy under any circumstances, the risk-benefit ratio must be rediscussed. It is conceivable that some couples may find appropriate benefits to justify the risks of prenatal diagnosis exclusive of selective abortion. It is anticipated that this situation will be quite rare. On occasion, patients have elected not to terminate a pregnancy after a positive diagnosis has been made.

Only limited information is available regarding the effects of selective abortion on families. Blumberg and associates[165] conducted testing and interviews on 13 of these families. A very high frequency of depression was found in both partners of the marriages, as well as marital separation. The results of this study indicate a need for further analysis of the impact of prenatal diagnosis, and especially of selective abortion, on the families who elect these procedures. Inclusion of psychiatric or marriage counseling services in the scope of the services offered by a prenatal diagnosis team seems advisable. Before informing patients of positive results, all studies should be completed and verified. In the author's experience, these patients often desire termination as rapidly as possible. Arrangements for this should be made in a way that will conform to the patient's wishes, whenever possible. The method of termination is selected with the maternal safety as the greatest priority. The value of confirmation of the diagnosis for scientific purposes, as well as the frequent desire of patients to have this information in the future, should be secondary.

Plans for careful evaluation of the fetus should be made in advance. Detailed gross examination, photographs, histopathology and other special studies should be performed when necessary. Standards for the morphologic assessment of fetuses are largely restricted to evaluation of "normal" populations.[166] Information from individual cases after selective abortion for specific diagnoses is accumulating in the medical literature. Operative pregnancy termination by hysterotomy offers the best method for confirmation of the diagnosis. The maternal interest, however, rarely justifies this approach. As an alternative, the diagnosis is most reliably confirmed by the study of amniotic fluid samples obtained at the time of abortion. The intra-amniotic instillation of hypertonic solutions or prostaglandins is the most frequently used method. The culturability of fetal tissue after these techniques is not highly reliable. Park and associates[167, 168] have reported greater success of fetal skin culture following prostaglandin-induced abortion (68% and 73%) over those in which either hypertonic saline (0%) or urea (8%) was used. Successful placental cultures have been obtained from pregnancies aborted using hypertonic saline.[169] The frequency of maternal tissue growth requires detailed analysis of culture results with banding to identify maternal markers. This method is obviously less satisfactory from the laboratory point of view. Nevertheless, the value of confirming the prenatal diagnosis justifies its use when other fetal tissues fail to grow.

THERAPY

Optimally, the goal of any diagnostic procedure should be that of appropriate therapy. The prospects for genetic manipulation are as exciting scientifically as they are controversial in terms of human society. Specific therapy for the genetic disorders amenable to prenatal diagnosis is relatively limited. The repeated demonstration of histopathologic changes in fetuses aborted after genetic diagnosis has confirmed the need for investigation of intrauterine, rather than extrauterine, therapy for certain disorders. Ampola and associates[170] have reported the first prenatal diagnosis and therapy for a fetus with vitamin B_{12}-responsive methylmalonic acidemia.

PROSPECTS FOR OBSTETRIC CARE

In spite of the limitations of specific genetic therapy, advances in medical care have permitted prolonged survival of individuals with certain birth defects or genetic disorders. Many of these individuals lead productive lives and reproduce. Perhaps the most dramatic example of this is the changing pattern of heart disease in pregnancy from a predominance of acquired disorders, such as rheumatic heart disease, to a higher frequency of patients with congenital heart defects. Increasingly, obstetricians who deal with high risk pregnancy are called upon to care for women with genetic disorders such as sickle cell disease, acute intermittent porphyria, cystic fibrosis, von Willebrand's disease, dwarfism, myotonic dystrophy, and many others. The medical-obstetric complications in these patients presents a challenge to their skills.

The fetal effects of maternal metabolic disorders, which are genetic, is an important area for investigation. Adverse effects due to a maternal genetic disorder may be noted only when the fetus has inherited the gene. An example of this is the speculation that myotonic dystrophy in a woman may alter the course of the disease in her children who inherited the gene by virtue of some intrauterine environmental influence.[171] With other disorders, the maternal metabolic disturbance influences fetal development, although the child will not have the disease. Although the genetics of diabetes mellitus is not entirely clear, this represents the most common example of this problem.[172] The effect of maternal phenylketonuria on the heterozygous fetus is well recognized, and also illustrates this problem. The description of women with unrecognized phenylketonuria and the high frequency of mental retardation in their offspring has prompted some to recommend maternal prenatal screening for this disorder.[173–175] The value of maternal dietary control for the prevention of mental retardation of the offspring must be studied further.[176]

It is also possible that other inborn errors of metabolism, perhaps as yet undescribed, may not cause clinical disease in the mother, but may influence fetal development. Histidinemia is probably a benign metabolic disorder which does not require therapy.[177] Defects in offspring of female mice with a disorder which appears to be a homolog of human histidinemia have been demonstrated.[178, 179] The intellectual development of children born to histidinemic women has been evaluated in a limited number of cases.[188, 181] Impairment of intellectual ability attributed to maternal histidinemia has been considered and needs evaluation.

REFERENCES

1. Leonard, C. D., Chase, G. A., Childs, B.: Genetic counseling: A consumer's view. N Engl J Med 287: 433, 1972.
2. World Health Organization Expert Committee: Genetic counseling. WHO Tech Rep Ser 416: 1, 1969.
3. Russell, J. G. B.: Radiology in the diagnosis of fetal abnormalities. J Obstet Gynecol B Commonw 76: 345, 1969.
4. Birmbaum, S. J.: Prenatal diagnosis of mongolism by X-ray. Obstet Gynecol 37: 394, 1971.
5. Bishop, E. H.: *Radiographic Studies of the Gravid Uterus*. New York, Harper & Row, 1965.
6. Jenkinson, E. L., Pfisterer, W. N., Latteier, K. K., et al: A prenatal diagnosis of osteopetrosis. Am J Roentgenol 49: 455–462, 1943.
7. Omenn, G. S., Figley, M. M., Graham, C. B., et al: Prospects for radiographic intrauterine diagnosis: The syndrome of thrombocytopenia with absent radii. N Engl J Med 288: 777, 1973.
8. Hall, J.: Personal communication.
9. Queenan, J. T., Gadow, E. C.: Amniography for detection of congenital malformations. Obstet Gynecol 35: 648, 1970.
10. Frigoletto, F. D., Griscom, N. T.: Amniography for the detection of fetal myelomeningocele. Obstet Gynecol 44: 286, 1974.
11. Allan, L. D., Ferguson-Smith, M. A., Donald, I., et al: Amniotic alpha fetoprotein in the antenatal diagnosis of spina bifida. Lancet 2: 522, 1973.
12. Mennuti, M. T., Moranz, J. G., Schwarz, R. H., et al: Amniography for the early detection of neural tube defects. Obstet Gynecol 49: 25, 1977.
13. Erbsloh, S.: Das intrauterine fetogram. Arch Gynaecol 14: 28, 1942.
14. Wisenhaan, P. F.: Fetography. Am J Obstet Gynecol 113: 818, 1973.
15. Aguero, O., Zighelboim, I.: Fetography and molegraphy. Surg Gynecol Obstet 130: 649, 1970.
16. Daw, E.: Fetography. Am J Obstet Gynecol 115: 718, 1973.
17. Ogita, S., Hasegawa, H., Matsumoto, M., et al: Prenatal dagnosis of E trisomy syndrome by fetography. Obstet Gynecol 43: 887, 1974.
18. Crosby, W.: Fetal respiratory distress following fetography. Am J Obstet Gynecol 121: 958, 1975.
19. Santo-Ramos, R. Duenholter, J. H.: Diagnosis of congenital fetal abnormalities by sonography. Obstet Gynecol 45: 279, 1975.
20. Garrett, W. J., Greenwald, G., Robinson, D. E.: Prenatal diagnosis of fetal polycystic kidney by ultrasound. Aust NZ J Obstet Gynecol 10: 7, 1970.
21. Campbell, S., Johnstone, F. D., Holt, E. M., et al: Anencephaly: Early ultrasonic diagnosis and active management. Lancet 2: 1126, 1972.
22. Thiery, M., Van Kets, H., YoLe Sian, A., et al: Early diagnosis of anencephaly. Lancet 1: 599, 1973.
23. Campbell, S., Pryse-Davies, J., Coltart, T. M., et al: Ultrasound in the early diagnosis of spina bifida. Lancet 1: 1065, 1975.
24. Ogita, S., Hasegawa, H., Matsumato, M., et al: Prenatal diagnosis of genetic anomalies by placental puncture. Obstet Gynecol 43: 709, 1974.

25. Kan, Y. W., Valenti, C., Guidotti, R., et al: Fetal blood-sampling in utero. Lancet 1: 79–80, 1974.
26. Kan, Y. W., Golbus, M. S., Trecartin, R.: Prenatal diagnosis of sickle cell anemia. N Engl J Med 294: 1039, 1976.
27. Valenti, C.: Endoamnioscopy and fetal biopsy: A new technique. Am J Obstet Gynecol 114: 561, 1972.
28. Alter, B. P., Friedman, S., Hobbins, J. C., et al: Prenatal diagnosis of sickle cell anemia and alpha G Phila. N Engl J Med 294: 1040, 1976.
29. Benzie, R. J., Malone, R. M., Miskin, M., et al: Prenatal diagnosis by fetoscopy with subsequent normal delivery: Report of a case. Am Obstet Gynecol 126: 287, 1976.
30. Levine, M. D., McNeil, D. E., Kaback, M. M., et al: Second trimester fetoscopy and fetal blood sampling: Current limitations and problems. Am J Obstet Gynecol 120: 937, 1974.
31. Hobbins, J. D., Mahoney, M. J.: In utero diagnosis of hemoglobinopathies: technic for obtaining fetal blood. N Engl J Med 290: 1065, 1974.
32. Kaback, M. M., Valenti, C., Editors, *Intrauterine Fetal Visualization: A Multidisciplinary Approach*. New York, American Elsevier Publishing Co., 1976.
33. Levin, M. J., Oxman, M. N., Moore, M. G., et al: Diagnosis of congenital rubella in-utero. N Engl J Med 290: 1187, 1974.
34. NICHD National Registry for Amniocentesis Study Group. JAMA (In press.)
35. Mishkin, M., Doran, T. A., Rudd, N., et al: Use of ultrasound for placental localization in genetic amniocentesis. Obstet Gynecol 43: 872, 1974.
36. Harrison, R., Campbell, S., Craft, I.: Risks of fetomaternal hemorrhage resulting from amniocentesis with and without ultrasound placental localization. Obstet Gynecol 46: 389, 1975.
37. Curtis, J. D., Cohen, W. N., Richerson, H. B., et al: The importance of placental localization preceding amniocentsis. Obstet Gynecol 40: 194, 1972.
38. Milunsky, A., Editor, *The Prevention of Genetic Disease and Mental Retardation*. Philadelphia, W. B. Saunders Co., 1975.
39. Young, P. E., Matson, M. R., Jones, O. W.: Amniocentesis for antenatal diagnosis: A review of problems and outcomes in a large series. Am J Obstet Gynecol 125: 495, 1976.
40. Milunsky, A.: Current concepts: Prenatal diagnosis of genetic disorders. N Engl J Med 295: 377, 1976.
41. The Canadian Registry for Prenatal Diagnosis of Genetic Diseases: Preliminary report. MRC (Canada) Prenatal Diagnosis Newsletter, Vol. 5, p. 1, 1976.
42. Creasman, W. T., Lawrence, R. A., Thiede, H. N.: Fetal complications of amniocentesis. JAMA 204: 949, 1968.
43. Grove, C. S., Trombetta, G. C., Amstey, M. S.: Fetal complications of amniocentesis. Am J Obstet Gynecol. 115: 1154, 1973.
44. Hyman, C. J., Depp, R., Pakravan, P., et al: Pneumothorax complicating amniocentesis. Obstet Gynecol 41: 43, 1973.
45. Leake, R. D. Hobel, C. J., Lachman, R. D.: Neonatal pneumothorax and subcutaneous emphysema secondary to diagnostic amniocentesis. Obstet Gynecol 43: 884, 1974.
46. Egley, C. C.: Laceration of fetal spleen during amniocentesis. Am J Obstet Gynecol 116: 582, 1973.
47. Gottdiener, J. S., Ellison, R. C., Lorenzo, R. L.: Arteriovenous fistula after fetal penetration at amniocentesis. N Engl J Med 293: 1302, 1975.
48. Berner, H. W., Seisler, E. P., Barlow, J., et al: Fetal cardiac tamponade, a complication of amniocentesis. Obstet Gynecol 40: 702, 1972.
49. Ryan, G. T, Ivy, R., Peason, J. W., et al: Fetal bleeding, a major hazard of amniocentesis. Obstet Gynecol 40: 702, 1972.
50. Goodlin, R. D., Clewell, W. H.: Sudden fetal death following diagnostic amniocentesis. Am J Obstet Gynecol 118: 285, 1974.
51. Broome, D. L., Wilson, M. G., Weiss, B., et al: Needle puncture of fetus: A complication of second trimester amniocentesis. Am J Obstet Gynecol 126: 247, 1976.
52. Benirschke, K., Kim, C. K.: Multiple pregnancy. N Engl J Med 288: 1276, 1973.
53. Bang, J., Nielsen, H., Philip, J.: Prenatal karyotyping of twins by ultrasonically guided amniocentesis. Am J Obstet Gynecol 123: 695, 1975.
54. Young, P. E., Carson, K., Jones, O. W.: A technique for managing amniotic fluid studies in twin pregnancies. J Reprod Med 13: 163, 1974.
55. Fairweather, D. V. I., Parkin, D., Murray, S., Walker, W.: Possible immunological implications of amniocentesis. Lancet 2: 1190, 1963.
56. Cassady, G., Cailleteau, J., Lockard, D., Milstead, R.: The hazard of fetal-maternal transfusion after transabdominal amniocentesis. Am J Obstet Gynecol 99: 284, 1967.
57. Aickin, D. R.: The significance of rises in rhesus antibody titer following amniocentesis. J Obstet Gynecol Br Commonw 78: 149, 1971.
58. Robinson, A., Bowes, W., Droegmueller, W., et al: Intrauterine diagnosis: Potential complications. Am J Obstet Gynecol 116: 937, 1973.
59. Doran, T. A., Rudd, N. C., Gardner, H. A., et al: The antenatal diagnosis of genetic disease. Am J Obstet Gynecol 118: 314, 1974.
60. Milunsky, A., Atkins, L., Littlefield, J. W.: Amniocentesis for prenatal genetic studies. Obstet Gynecol 40: 104, 1972.
61. Milunsky, A., Alpert, E.: Prenatal diagnosis of neural tube defects. II. Analysis of false positive and false negative alpha-fetoprotein results. Obstet Gynecol 48: 6, 1976.
62. Blajchman, M. A., Maudsley, R. F., Uchida, I., et al: Diagnostic amniocentesis and fetal-maternal bleeding. Lancet 1: 993, 1974.
63. Mennuti, M. T., Brummond, W.: Unpublished data.
64. Antenatal diagnosis of genetic disorders. ACOG Tech Bull 39, 1976.

65. Scott, J. R., Beer, A. E.: Reproductive immunology. *Obstetrics and Gyencology Annual*, Vol. 3. Edited by R. M. Wynn, New York, Appleton-Century-Crofts, 1974.
66. Paris Conference (1971): Standardization in human cytogenetics. Birth Defects, Original Article Series, Vol. VIII, No. 7, 1972.
67. Lewandowski, R. C., Yunis, J. J.: New chromosomal syndromes. Am J Dis Child 129: 515, 1975.
68. Steele, M. W., Breg, W. R., jr.: Chromosome analysis of human amniotici-fluid cells. Lancet 1: 383, 1966.
69. Hamerton, J. L., Canning, N., Ray, M., et al.: A cytogenetic survey of 14,069 newborn infants. 1. Incidence of chromosome abnormalities. Clin Genet 8: 223, 1975.
70. Bauld, R., Sutherland, G. R., Bain, A. D.: Chromosome studies in investigation of stillbirths and neonatal deaths. Arch Dis Child 49: 782, 1974.
71. Machin, G. A.: Chromosome abnormality and perinatal death. Lancet 1: 549, 1974.
72. Carr, D. H.: Chromosomes and abortion. *Advances in Human Genetics*, Vol. 2. Edited by H. Harris, K. Hirschorn. New York, Plenum Press, 1971.
73. Kajii, T., Omaha, K., Niikawa, N., et al: Banding analysis of abnormal karyotypes in spontaneous abortion. Am J Hum Genet 25: 539, 1973.
74. Dhadial, R. K., Machin, A. M., Tait, S. M.: Chromosome anomalies in spontaneously aborted human fetuses. Lancet 2: 20, 1970.
75. Ruzicska, P., Czeizel, A.: Cytogenetic studies on mid-trimester abortions. Humangenetik 10: 273, 1970.
76. Boue, J. G., Boue, A.: Frequence des aberrations chromosomiques dans les avortements spontanes humains. C R Acad Sci (D) Paris 269: 283, 1969.
77. Creasy, M. R., Crolla, J. A.: Prenatal mortality of trisomy 21, Down's syndrome. Lancet 1: 473, 1974.
78. McConnell, H. D., Carr, D. H.: Recent advances in the cytogenetic study of human spontaneous abortions. Obstet Gynecol 45: 547, 1975.
79. Collman, R. D., Stoller, A.: A survey of mongoloid births in Victoria, Australia, 1942–1957. Am J Pub Health 52: 813, 1962.
80. Penrose, L. S., Smith, G. F.: *Down's Anomaly*, London, Churchill, 1966.
81. Hook, E. B.: Estimates of maternal age-specific risks of a Down-syndrome birth in women aged 34–41. Lancet 2: 33, 1976.
82. Magenis, R. E., Hecht, F., Milham, S.: Trisomy 13 (D1) syndrome: Studies on parental age, sex ratio and survival. J Pediatr 73: 222, 1968.
83. Taylor, A. I.: Autosomal trisomy syndromes: A detailed study of 27 cases of Edwards' syndrome and 27 cases of Patau's syndrome. J Med Gent 5: 117, 1968.
84. Ferguson-Smith, M. A.: Prospective data on risk of Down syndrome in relation to maternal age. Lancet 2: 252, 1976.
85. Bain, A. D., Smith, I. I., Bauld, R., et al: Prenatal diagnosis, stillbirths and the macerated fetus. Lancet 2: 375, 1976.
86. Hook, E. B.: Risk of Down syndrome in relation to maternal age. Lancet 2: 465, 1976.
87. Poland, P. E., Alberman, E., Berry, A. C., et al: Chromosome abnormalities and maternal age. Lancet 2: 516, 1976.
88. Hsu, L. Y. F., Gertner, M., Leiter, E., et al: Paternal trisomy 21 mosaicism and Down's syndrome. Am J Hum Genet 23: 592, 1971.
89. Drets, M. E., Cardoso, J. H., Deffino, J. H., et al: Familial normal-partial trisomy 16 with selective endoreduplication in malformed proband. Cytogenetics (Basel) 9: 333, 1970.
90. Green, J. R., Krovetz, L. J., Taylor, W. J.: Two generations of 13–15 mosaicism: Possible evidence for a genetic defect in the control of chromosomal replication. Cytogenetics (Basel) 7: 286, 1968.
91. Hamerton, J. L.: Robertsonian translocations in man: Evidence of prezygotic selection. Cytogenetics 7: 260, 1968.
92. Friedrich, U., Nielsen, J.: D/D translocations in newborn children. Ann Human Genet 38: 97, 1974.
93. Hecht, F., Case, M. P., Lovrien, E. W., et al: Nonrandomness of translocations in man: Preferential entry of chromosomes into 13–15/21 translocations. Science 161: 371, 1968.
94. Nielsen, J., Rasmussen, K.: Autosomal reciprocal translocations and 13/14 translocations: A population study. Clin Genet 10: 161, 1976.
95. Kim, H. Y., Hsu, L. Y. F., Pacine, S., et al: Cytogenetics of fetal wastage. N Engl J Med 293: 844, 1975.
96. Tsengi, C., Metaxotou-Stavridaki, C., Strataki-Benetou, M., et al: Chromosome studies in couples with repeated spontaneous abortions. Obstet Gynecol 47: 463, 1976.
97. Schmidt, R., Nitowsky, H. M., Dar, H.: Cytogenetic studies in reproductive loss. JAMA 236: 369, 1976.
98. Walker, S., Lee, C. L. Y, Gregson N. M.: Polyploidy in cells cultured from amniotic fluid. Lancet 2: 1137, 1970.
99. Milunsky, A., Atkins, L., Littlefield, J. W.: Polyploidy in prenatal genetic diagnosis. Pediatr 79: 303, 1971.
100. Klinger, H. P., Schwarzacher, H. G.: The sex chromatin and heterochromatic bodies in human diploid and polypoid nuclei. J Biophys Biochem Cytol 8: 345, 1960.
110. Book, J. A., Kjessler, B., Santesson, B.: Karyotypes of cultured cells from fetal membranes of normal newborns. J Med Genet 5: 224, 1968.
102. Tegenkamp, T. R., Hux, C. H.: Incidence of tetraploidy as related to cell type. Am J Obstet Gynecol 120: 1066, 1974.
103. Kohn, G., Robinson, A.: Tetraploidy in cells cultured from amniotic fluid. Lancet 2: 778, 1970.
104. Nielsen, J., Friedrich, N., Hreidarsson, A. B.: Frequency of deletion of short arm satellites in acrocentric chromosomes. J Med Genet 11: 177,

1974.
105. Nielsen, J.: Chromosome mosaicism in a population sample. Humangenetik 29: 155, 1975.
106. Cox, D. M., Niewczas-Late, V., Riffell, M. E., et al: Chromosomal mosaicism in diagnostic amniotic fluid cell cultures. Pediatr Res 8: 679, 1974.
107. Kajii, T.: Pseudomosaicism in cultured amniotic fluid cells. Lancet 2: 1037, 1971.
108. Kardon, N. B., Chernay, P. R., Hsu, L. Y. F., et al: Problems in prenatal diagnosis resulting from chromosome mosaicism. Clin Genet 3: 83, 1972.
109. Mannanalal, G. S.: The issue of chromosomal mosaicism in prenatal diagnosis. J Pediatr 81: 422, 1971.
110. Katayama, K. P., Park, I. J., Heller, R. H.: Errors of prenatal cytogenetic diagnosis. Obstet Gynecol 44: 693, 1974.
111. Pernoll, M. L., Prescott, G. H., Hecht, F., et al: Prenatal diagnosis: Practice, pitfalls, progress. Obstet Gynecol 44: 773, 1974.
112. Kohn, G., Mennuti, M. T., Kaback, M., et al: Chromosomal mosaicism in amniotic cell culture: A diagnostic dilemma. Israel J Med Sci 5: 476, 1975.
113. Bloom, A. D., Schmickel, R., Barr, M., et al: Prenatal detection of autosomal mosaicism. J Pediatr 84: 732, 1974.
114. Lejune, J., Berger, R.: Sur deux observations familiales de translocations complexes. Ann Genet 8: 21, 1965.
115. DeGrouchy, J., Aussannaire, M., Brissaud, H. E., et al: Aneusomie de recombinasion: Three further examples. Am J Human Genet 18: 467, 1966.
116. Kohn, G., Aronson, M., Mellman, W. J.: Spontaneous D/G translocation in fibroblasts derived from a patient with trisomy 21 mosaicism. Clin Genet 5: 113, 1974.
117. Hoehn, H., Bryant, E. M., Karp, L. E., et al: Cultured cells from diagnostic amniocentesis in second trimester pregnancies. I. Clonal morphology and growth potential. Pediatr Res 8: 746, 1974.
118. Melancon, S. B, Lee, S., Nadler, H. L.: Histidase activity in cultivated human amniotic fluid cells. Science 173: 627, 1971.
119. Burton, B. K., Gerbie, A. B., Nadler, H. L.: Intrauterine diagnosis of genetic defects. Am J Obstet Gynecol 118: 718, 1974.
120. Jones, K. L., Smith, D. W., Harvey, M. A., et al: Older paternal age and fresh gene mutation: Data on additional disorders. J Pediatr 86: 84, 1975.
121. Renwick, J. H., Bolling, D. R.: An analysis procedure illustrated on a triple linkage of use for prenatal diagnosis of mystonic dystrophy. J Med Genet 8: 399, 1971.
122. Scrott, H. G., Karp, L., Omenn, G. S.: Prenatal prediction in myotonic dystrophy: Guidelines for genetic counselling. Clin Genet 4: 34, 1973.
123. Harper, P., Bias, W. B., Hutchinson, J. R., et al: ABH secretor status of the fetus: A genetic marker identifiable by amniocentesis. J Med Genet 8: 438, 1971.
124. Kabach, M. M.: Heterozygote screening for the control of recessive genetic disease. *The Prevention of Genetic Disease and Mental Retardation*. Edited by A. Milunsky, Philadelphia, W. B. Saunders Co., 1975.
125. Murphy, E. A, Chase, G. A.: *Principles of Genetic Counselling*. Chicago, Year Book Medical Publishers, Inc., 1975.
126. Grosset, L., Barrelet, V., Odartchenko, N.: Antenatal fetal sex determination from maternal blood during early pregnancy. Am J Obstet Gynecol 120: 60, 1974.
127. Rhine, S. A., Cain, J. L., Cleary, R. E., et al: Prenatal sex detection with endocervical smears: Successful results utilizing Y-body fluorescence. Am J Obstet Gynecol 122: 115, 1975.
128. Manuel, M., Park, I. J., Jones, H. W.: Prenatal sex determination by fluorescent staining of cells for the presence of Y-chromatin. Am J Obstet Gynecol 119: 853, 1974.
129. Khudr, G., Benirschke, K.: Fluorescence of the Y chromosome: A rapid test to determine fetal sex. Am J Obstet Gynecol 110: 1091, 1971.
130. Young, P. E., Judd, H. L., Robinson, J. D., et al: Sex differences of amniotic fluid androgens and estrogens at mid-gestation. Philadelphia, Society for Gynecologic Investigation, March 25, 1976.
131. Mennuti, M. T., Wu, C. H.: Unpublished data.
132. Holmes, L. B.: Current concepts in genetics: Congenital malformations. N Engl J Med 295: 204, 1976.
133. Yen, S., MacMahon, B.: Genetics of anencephaly and spina bifida. Lancet 2: 623, 1968.
134. Carter, C. O., David, P. A., Lawrence, K. M.: A family study of major central nervous system malformations in South Wales. J Med Genet 5: 81, 1968.
135. Carter, C. O., Roberts, J. A. F.: The risk of recurrence after two children with central nervous system malformations. Lancet 1: 306, 1967.
136. Carter, C. O., Evans, K.: Children of adult survivors with spina bifida cystica. Lancet 2: 924, 1973.
137. Holmes, L. B., Driscoll, S. G., Atkins, L.: Etiologic heterogeneity of neural tube defects. N Engl J Med 294: 365, 1976.
138. Brock, D. J. H.: The prenatal diagnosis of neural tube defects. Obstet Gynecol Surv 31: 32, 1976.
139. Weiss, R. R., Macri, J. N., Elligers, K. W.: Origin of amniotic fluid alpha-fetoprotein in normal and defective pregnancies. Obstet Gynecol 47: 697, 1976.
140. Brock, D. J. H., Sutcliffe, R. G.: Alpha fetoprotein in the antenatal diagnosis of anencephaly and spina bifida. Lancet 2: 197, 1972.
141. Milunsky, A., Flyate, E.: Prenatal diagnosis of neural tube defects. 1. Problems and pitfalls: Analysis of 2495 cases using the alpha-fetoprotein assay. Obstet Gynecol 48: 1, 1976.
142. DeBruijn, H. W., Huisjes, H.: Omphalocole and raised alpha fetoprotein in amniotic fluid. Lancet 1: 525, 1975.
143. Igessler, B., Johansson, S. G., Sherman, M., et al: Alpha feto proteins in antenatal diagnosis of congenital nephrosis. Lancet 1: 432, 1975.

144. Weinberg, A. G., Milunsky, A., Harrod, M. J.: Elevated amniotic fluid alpha-feto protein and duodenal atresia. Lancet 2: 496, 1975.
145. Seppala, M., Laes, E., Harvo-Noponen, M.: Elevated amniotic fluid alpha-feto protein in congenital esophageal atresia. J Obstet Gynecol Br Commonw 81: 827, 1974.
146. Seller, M. J., Creasy, M. R., Alberman, E. D.: Alpha feto protein levels in amniotic fluids from spontaneous abortions. Br Med J 1: 524, 1974.
147. Schmid, W., Muhlethaler, J. P.: High amniotic fluid alpha-1-fetoprotein in a case of sacrococcygealteratoma. Humangenetik 26: 353, 1975.
148. Milford, W. A., Stewart, C. R.: False positive results in antenatal diagnosis of neural tube disorders. Lancet 2: 345, 1974.
149. Brock, D. J. H.: Antenatal misdiagnosis of neural-tube defects. Lancet 2: 495, 1975.
150. Laurence, K. M., Tew, B. J.: Natural history of spina bifida cystica and cranium bifidum cysticium. Arch Dis Child 46: 127, 1971.
151. Milunsky, A., Macri, J. N., Weiss, R. R., et al: Prenatal detection of neural tube defects: Comparison between alpha-fetoprotein and beta-trace protein assay. Adv J Obstet Gynecol 122: 313, 1975.
152. Olsson, J. E., Sherman, M. S., Kjessler, B.: Beta-trace protein and neural tube defects. Lancet 2: 347, 1974.
153. Macri, J. N., Weiss, R. R., Joshi, M. S., et al: Antenatal diagnosis of neural-tube defects using cerebrospinal fluid proteins. Lancet 1: 14, 1974.
154. Purdie, D. W., Howie, P. W., Edgar, W., et al: Raised amniotic fluid FDP in fetal neural-tube anomalies. Lancet 1: 1013, 1975.
155. Sutherland, G. R., Brock, D. J. H., Scrimgeour, J. B.: Amniotic fluid macrophages and the antenatal diagnosis of anencephaly and spina bifida. J Med Genet 12: 135, 1975.
156. Brock, D. J. H., Bolton, A. E., Monaghan, J. M.: Prenatal diagnosis of anencephaly through maternal serum-alpha fetoprotein measurement. Lancet 2: 923, 1973.
157. Seller, M. J., Singer, J. D., Coltart, T. M., et al: Maternal serum-alpha-fetoprotein levels and prenatal diagnosis of neural-tube defects. Lancet 1: 428, 1974.
158. Harris, R., Jennison, R. G., Barson, A. J., et al: Comprison of amniotic-fluid and maternal serum alpha-fetoprotein levels in the early antenatal diagnosis of spina bifida and anencephaly. Lancet 1: 429, 1974.
159. Macri, J. N, Weiss, R. R., Starkovsky, N. A., et al: Maternal serum alpha-fetoprotein and prospective screening. Lancet 2:719, 1975.
160. Leighton, P. C., Gordon, Y. B., Kitau, M. J., et al: Levels of alpha-fetoprotein in maternal blood as a screening test for fetal neural-tube defect. Lancet 2: 1012, 1975.
161. Brock, D. J. H., Scrimegeout, J. B., Bolton, A. E., et al: Effect of gestational age on screening for neural-tube defects by maternal plasma AFP measurement. Lancet 2: 719, 1975.
162. Werner, W. H., Young, E. B.: Nonspecific date of last menstrual period. Am J Obstet Gynecol 120: 1071, 1974.
163. Rudd, N. L., Miskin, M., Hoar, D. I., et al: Prenatal diagnosis of hypophosphatasia. N Engl J Med 295: 146, 1976.
164. Mennuti, M. T., Mullivor, R.: Unpublished case.
165. Blumberg, B. D., Golbus, M. S., Hanson, K. H.: The psychological sequelae of abortion performed for a genetic indication. Am J Obstet Gynecol 122: 799, 1975.
166. Tanimura, T., Nelson, T., Hollingsworth, R. R., et al: Weight standards for organs from early human fetuses. Anat Record 171: 227, 1971.
167. Park, I. J., Wentz, A. C., Jones, H. W., Jr.: The viability of fetal skin of abortuses induced by saline or prostaglandin. Am J Obstet Gynecol 115: 274, 1973.
168. Ju, K. S., Park, I. J., Jones, H. W., Jr.: The culturability of fibroblasts from the skin of abortuses after intra-amniotic instillation of urea or prostaglandin. Am J Obstet Gynecol 125: 1155, 1976.
169. Gardner, H. A., Wood, E. M., Stecker, E.: Placental cultures for cytogenetic assessment in saline aborted fetuses. Am J Obstet Gynecol 126: 350, 1976.
170. Ampola, M. G., Mahoney, M. J., Nakamura, E., et al: Prenatal therapy of a patient with vitamin B-12-responsive methylmalonic acidemia. N Engl J Med 293: 313, 1975.
171. Harper, P. S., Dyken, P. R.: Early onset dystrophia myotonica: Evidence supporting a maternal environmental factor. Lancet 2: 53, 1972.
172. Zonana, J., Rimoin, D. L.: Inheritance of diabetes mellitus. N Engl J Med 295: 603, 1976.
173. Maternal phenylketonuria. ACOG Tech Bull No. 25, December, 1973.
174. Cockburn, F., Farquhar, J. W., Forfar, J. O., et al: Maternal hyperphenylalaninaemia in the normal and phenylketonuric mother and its influence on maternal plasma and fetal fluid amino acid concentrations. J Obstet Gynecol Br Commonw 79: 698, 1972.
175. Perry, T. L., Hansen, S., Tischler, B., et al: Unrecognized adult phenylketonuria: Implications for obstetrics and psychiatry. N Engl J Med 289: 395, 1973.
176. Farquhar, J. W.: Baby of a phenylketonuric mother: Inferences drawn from a single case. Arch Dis Child 49: 205, 1974.
177. Levy, H. L., Shih, V. E., Madigan, P. M.: Routine newborn screening for histidinemia: clinical and biochemical results. N Engl J Med 291: 1214, 1974.
178. Bulfield, G., Kacser, H.: Histidinaemia in mouse and man. Arch Dis Child 49: 545, 1974.
179. Kacser, H., Bulfield, G., Wallace, M. E.: Histidinaemic mutant in mouse. Nature 244: 77, 1973.
180. Lyon, I. C. T., Gardner, R. J. M., Veale, A. M. O.: Maternal histidinaemia. Arch Dis Child 49: 581, 1974.
181. Neville, B. G. R., Harris, R. F., Stern, D. J., et al: Maternal histidinaemia. Arch Dis Child 46: 119, 1971.

ELSIE R. CARRINGTON, M.D.

3

Biochemical Monitoring of the Fetus

Perinatal mortality and physical and mental handicaps in the newborn are always tragic and sometimes unexpected events. Disaster strikes often enough in apparently normal pregnancies for the inadequacy of clinical methods alone in predicting certain cases of impending fetal death to be recognized. The practicality of applying objective laboratory methods to the task of fetal diagnosis on the one hand, and fetal therapeutics on the other, was demonstrated beyond question in the classic works of Bevis[7] in 1952 and Liley[38] in 1963, respectively, in Rh-sensitized patients. These successes served as a driving force for acquisition of new knowledge of the developing fetus and its environment and the search for new methods of fetal evaluation.

In the past decade or two, many direct and indirect methods using cytogenetic, biochemical and biophysical methods have appeared. In many cases, more than one modality is required for an individual fetal health survey. The biochemical tests employed for antenatal monitoring of the fetus measure substances, generally hormones or enzymes, produced uniquely by the fetus, the placenta or both. Each test reflects a different dynamic function or combinations of functions. Clearly, no one test is capable of detecting all types of disorders that affect the fetus. Each should be considered in terms of the source of the substance measured, its reliability in clinical use and its limitations.

Estrogen Assays

Laboratory tests using one of the many available methods for measuring estrogenic substances have proven applicable in a wider variety of conditions that pose risks for the fetus than most other fetal health survey tests. The striking increase in production of hormones, particularly estriol, during pregnancy, and the fact that a fetal component as well as placental component are essential for synthesis of estriol are major advantages.

METABOLIC PATHWAYS

Clarification of the biosynthetic steps in the production and excretion of estrogen during pregnancy [17, 19] has led to identification of factors that may alter estriol values and has greatly enhanced the clinical usefulness of estriol assays.

Estriol precursors are produced by the fetal adrenal cortex. At least 90% of the precursors are produced in the large fetal zone of the adrenals, mainly as sulfates of dehydroepiandrosterone (DHEAS) and 16-α-hydroxy dehydroepiandrosterone (16-αOH DHEAS). Much of the DHEAS is converted to 16-OH DHEAS in the fetal liver. Conversion of the precursors to estriol is entirely a placental function. This step involves enzymatic separation of the sulfates and aromatization of the 16-OH DHEA to estriol. Estriol is conjugated, mainly with glucuronic acid and, to a lesser extent, with sulfate in the maternal liver and then is excreted, mainly in the conjugated form, by the maternal kidney. A portion of the estriol conjugate passes from maternal liver via the enterohepatic circulation into the gut. Hydrolysis of the conjugate by bacterial flora is essential for reabsorption of estriol and its return to the liver for reconjugation.[1, 58]

Estriol excretion increases approximately 1000-fold during pregnancy. Of the total estrogen, 90% is excreted in the form of sodium estriol glucosiduronate. Normally, estriol values reach approximately 2 to 3 mg per 24 hr at 18 to 20 weeks of gestation and increase to 12 to 50 mg per 24 hr at term. The need for a rapid, reproducible and accurate means of determining estriol concentration has resulted in the development of a wide variety of methods. Those most commonly used involve acid or enzyme hydrolysis, extraction, purification and measurement by spectrophotometry or fluorometry.[6, 9, 21] The method used in our laboratory is that of Greene and Touchstone[22] modified by substituting the extraction procedure of Hobkirk and Metcalfe-Gibson,[29] which is intended for quantitation of low titer estrogens. Recovery rates average 77% with a standard deviation of less than 10%. Gas chromatographic[61, 62] and radioimmunoassay methods[24] are also available. Campbell and Gardner[10] developed a simple automated fluorometric method capable of analyzing 150 samples per day. The test measures total urinary estrogens rather than estriol. The authors report a correlation coefficient of 0.91 between the automated method for total estrogens and their manual method for urinary estriol. Further proof of the reliability of the automated test is apparently necessary since no such method is yet available for general use.

CLINICAL CONSIDERATIONS

Day to day fluctuations in estriol excretion rate are seen in normal gestations, but a fall of 40% below a previous peak or values below 4 mg after the 34th week of pregnancy is cause for serious concern. Although the range of normal values for gestational age is wide, the gradual increase in excretion rate to term is quite consistent. These facts emphasize the importance of serial estriol determinations in the individual patient and the necessity for correct dating of gestational age for each determination.

The estriol/creatinine ratio (E/C) is sufficiently useful in assessing the accuracy of the 24-hr urine collection to warrant its use routinely. Aubrey and coworkers[2] and others[16] utilized the E/C ratio of random urine samples to predict the 24-hr E/C ratio and considered it satisfactory as a screening procedure in an ambulatory prenatal high risk clinic. However, one should be cautioned regarding the use of random samples, particularly in patients with any reduction in renal function. In our hands, short collection periods of 4 to 8 hr provided only an approximation of the true 24-hr E/C ratio. Short collection periods therefore are used only to estimate the state of affairs in unusual situations.

VALIDITY OF URINARY ESTRIOL LEVELS

High or normal urinary estriol values which in general follow the mean for gestational age are reassuring, even in high risk pregnancies. Avoidance of untimely premature delivery has proven to be one of the most important and practical uses of the test. This is not to imply that all complicated pregnancies can proceed until spontaneous labor ensues if the estriol levels are normal. With maternal complications such as severe diabetes, hypertension or pre-eclampsia, in which the risk of sudden events including abruptio placentae or deterioration are ever present, delay in delivery beyond the period of good fetal viability because the estriol value is normal can be regretable. Nevertheless, the addition of serial 24-hr urinary estriol determinations to clinical methods has resulted in better management of high risk pregnancies complicated by hypertension, intrauterine growth retardation, preeclamptic toxemia, diabetes, prolonged pregnancy, a history of previous stillbirth and a number of other conditions in which fetoplacental function may be compromised. The estriol test will not predict early fetal distress in cases of erythroblastosis since neither the fetal adrenal nor the placenta is primarily involved. Consequently, in some cases with Rh sensitization, the urinary estriol value may be surprisingly high before fetal decompensation, possibly as a result of stress initiated by the hemolytic process (Figure 3.1).

Low urinary estriol values are more difficult to evaluate because technical, chemical or physiologic factors may be reflected in the sample despite adequate estriol production. Fortunately, most of these can be identified. When these factors are kept in mind, correct interpretation of the test is possible in a very high percentage of cases with low estriol values, making the test the mainstay so far as laboratory assessment of fetal jeopardy is concerned. Other causes for low estriol values may be summarized as follows.

Lack of Estriol Precursors

This is a major factor responsible for the exceedingly low values noted after fetal death or in the absence of the fetus (hydatidiform mole and choriocarcinoma) and with certain types of congenital anomalies, particularly anencephaly.[19] Absence of fetal pituitary ACTH is reflected in marked hypoplasia of the fetal adrenal cortex. Low estriol values also are found in other types of major malformations, many of which are also associated with fetal growth retardation. Severe congenital heart disease and Down's syndrome[31] are well documented examples. Figure 3.2 illustrates the low estriol values in an infant with trisomy 18 and multiple major anomalies who expired at 12 hr after birth. Applying estriol determinations to the study of an obstetric population, Beischer and Brown[4] reported a total of 115 newborns with congenital anomalies in 10,000 pregnancies. Eighty of these were major malformations and estriol excretion was subnormal in 61% of this group. The authors calculated that a major fetal anomaly will be encountered once in every 30 pregnancies in which maternal urinary estriol values are very low. These findings underscore the importance of considering major malformation when exceptionally low estriol levels consistently are present. Ultrasound or x-ray examination may be capable of discovering some of these deformities before interference or cesarean section is carried out.

Impairment of Maternal Renal Function

When renal function is impaired to a degree sufficient to reduce consistently the

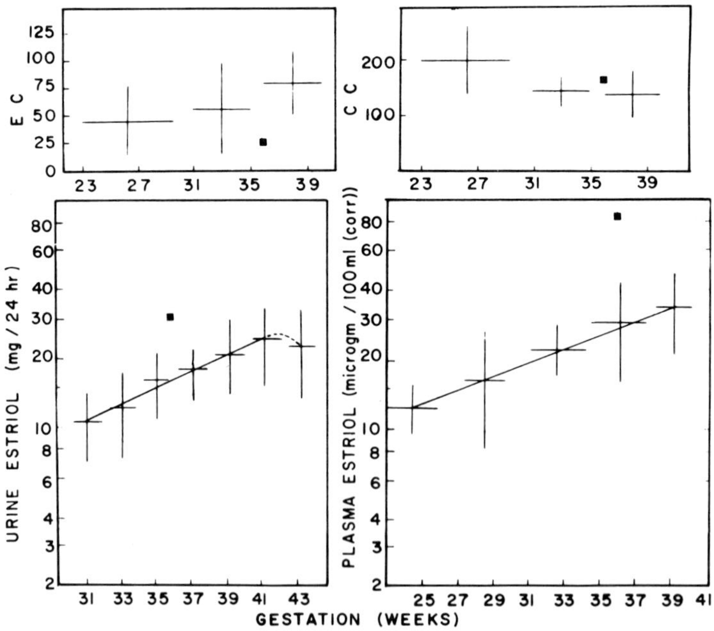

Figure 3.1. Patient R. C. Rh-negative sensitized gestational diabetic. Estriol clearance (EC) 25.8; creatinine clearance (CC) 170 ml per min. Estriol: urine 31.6 mg per 24 hr; plasma 85 μg per 100 ml. Cesarean section at 36 weeks of gestation. Living, but clearly affected newborn required three exchange transfusions, although estriol production and excretion were above normal.

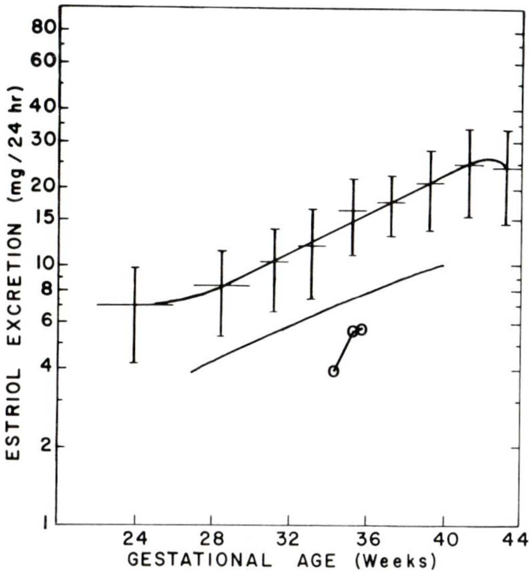

Figure 3.2. Patient G. B. Estriol excretion rate consistently below the normal range is graphed on logarithmic scale. Horizontal lines represent mean values for 168 normal pregnant subjects; vertical bars extend one standard deviation above and below the means. Infant had multiple anomalies (trisomy 18, hypoplastic adrenals, ovarian agenesis, esophageal atresia) and died at 12 hr.

clearance of endogenous creatinine, estriol clearance also is reduced.[13] Conditions in which this situation exists, which include primary renal disease, severe pre-eclampsia, eclampsia and advanced stages of diabetes or hypertension, are serious problems for both the mother and her baby. Thus, low urinary values may be valid indicators of fetal distress, but this cannot be ascertained without determining the plasma estriol level and renal clearance rates. If renal function is reduced but the fetus is not yet affected, the urinary estriol level may be misleadingly low and the plasma estriol misleadingly high. An exceptional example of this phenomenon is seen in Figure 3.3, *A* and *B*. This patient had severe chronic pyelonephritis with superimposed severe pre-eclamptic toxemia which required dialysis before and after cesarean section was performed at 34 weeks. The urinary estriol value was only 2 mg per 24 hr, but the plasma estriol at 55 μg per 100 ml was high for gestational age. Both creatinine and estriol clearances were reduced consistently. The newborn weighed 3 pounds 3 ounces. The Apgar score was 8 at 1 min, 9 at 5 min; the infant survived. It should be noted in this case that the superimposed severe pre-eclampsia undoubtedly played a major role in renal impairment. Erroneously low estriol values usually are not associated with pyelonephritis unless there is sufficient renal damage to diminish renal clearance. Neither bacteriuria nor proteinuria per se interfere with the yield of urinary estriol.[13]

Estriol Conjugation

Placental sulfatase deficiency is an infrequent cause for low estriol excretion. France and Liggins[18] demonstrated the lack of placental sulfatase activity in a patient whose urinary estriol values never exceeded 1.5 mg per 24 hr. The fetus produced ample quantities of estrogen precursors in the form of DHEAS and 16-OH DHEAS, but the ability of the placenta to hydrolyze sulfoconjugates was limited. The newborn infant delivered by cesarean section was normal. Beischer and Brown[4] reported a case in which estriol values did not exceed 2.1 mg per 24 hr, whereas pregnanediol values reached 67 mg per 24 hr. This infant also was delivered by cesarean section at 42 weeks when induction of labor failed. Reduction of the conjugating capacity of the maternal liver may account in part for the low urinary estriol values inconsistent with the fetal status observed in some cases of severe pre-eclampsia/eclampsia.

Chemicals

Certain drugs interfere with the estriol test and give spuriously low results.[8] *Methenamine mandelate* (Mandelamine), which liberates formaldahyde during acid hydrolysis, causes almost complete destruction of the estriol present. *Corticosteroids* suppress maternal and, to a lesser extent, the fetal adrenals and can reduce estriol excretion, particularly when relatively large doses in excess of 75 mg of cortisone or its equivalent are administered.[43] *Glucose* in the urine causes partial destruction of estriol in acid hydrolysis. This can be overcome without altering recovery rate significantly by dilution of the sample.[13, 28] *Ampicillin* causes a reduction

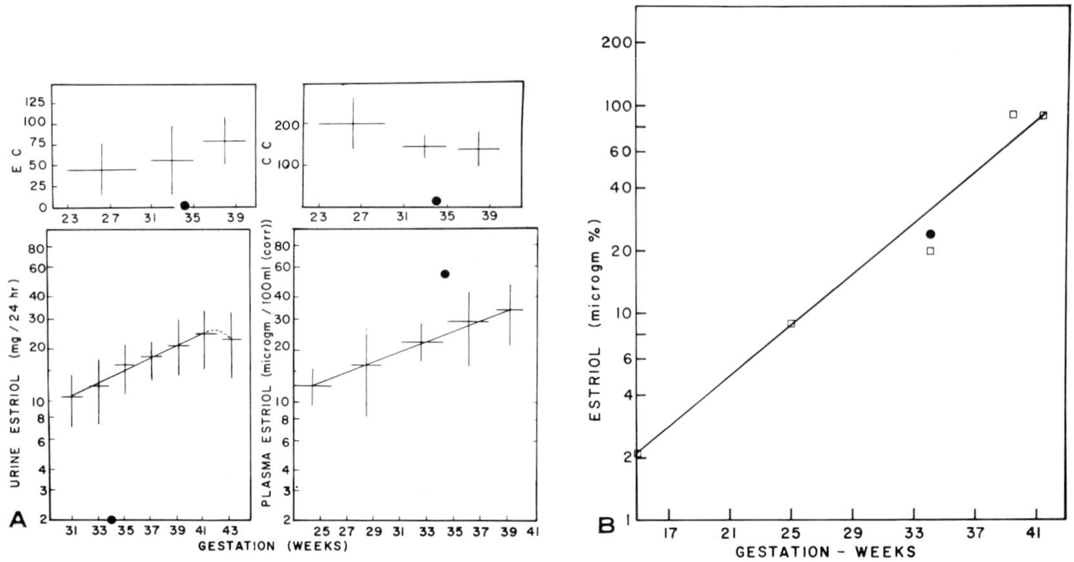

Figure 3.3. Patient B. M. *A*, chronic pyelonephritis and severe pre-eclampsia with blood pressure 140/100 to 170/120; urine protein +4; blood-urea nitrogen 84 mg per 100 ml; uric acid 12.2 mg per 100 ml. Estriol clearance (EC): 3.4 ml/min, creatinine clearance (CC): 14.1 ml per min. Estriol: urine 2.7 mg per 24 hr; plasma 55 μg per 100 ml. Cesarean section at 34 weeks of gestation. Weight: 3 pounds 3 ounces; Apgar: 8 to 9. Samples obtained courtesy of Richard Schmidt, Cincinnati, Ohio. *B*, amniotic fluid estriol. In contrast to the exceptionally low urinary E_3 value, the amniotic fluid E_3 is within normal limits and proved to be consistent with the clinical condition of the newborn in this case.

in hydrolysis of estriol conjugates by bacterial flora in the intestinal tract.[58] This hydrolysis is essential for reabsorption of estriol and its return to the liver for reconjugation. There is an increase in fecal estrogen excretion and a reduction in estrogens excreted in the maternal urine early in the course of ampicillin therapy. This effect is blunted if ampicillin is continued for several days.

PLASMA ESTRIOL ASSAY

Plasma estriol determinations obviate the 24-hr delay and possible errors in collection of the specimen. The test is technically more difficult than the urinary estriol test, but when mastered is comparable in accuracy to the simpler test in a high percentage of cases.[41, 42] In normal and in many high risk pregnancies the increases in estriol values with gestational age are correlated consistently in the two tests. In a small but important group of patients with significant impairment of renal function, correlation is poor and inconsistencies are observed between both plasma and urinary estriol values and the clinical results.[13] The inconsistencies are in the opposite direction if the fetoplacental function of estriol is adequate (Figure 3.3*A*). Nachtigall, Levitz and coworkers,[37, 41] who pioneered the use of plasma estriols in this country, found puzzlingly elevated values for plasma estriol inconsistent with the condition of the fetus in patients with class D diabetes and chronic renal disease. Under these circumstances reliance upon high plasma values will result in some unnecessary fetal losses. Renal clearance studies have helped to explain these findings.[13]

We continue to use urinary estriol determinations as the primary guide and resort to plasma estriol determination and clearance studies only if the urinary levels are low. If both urine and plasma values are low, fetoplacental function clearly is failing. Figure 3.4 is an example. Patient A. B. had marked hypertension and moderate reduction in creatinine clearance. Both urinary and plasma estriol values

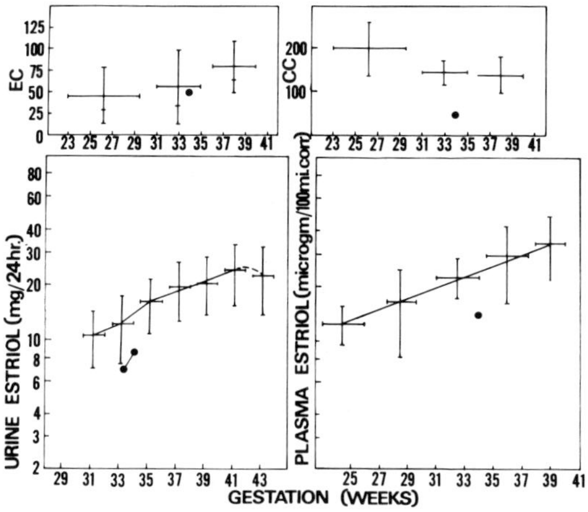

Figure 3.4. Patient A. B., 23 years of age, para 1, gravida 3. Hypertensive plasma creatinine: 2.02 mg per 100 ml. Previous stillbirth. Amniocentesis performed at 34 weeks was green stained/cesarean section delivery of male infant, 4 pounds, 2 ounces; Apgar 6 in at 1 min; 8 at 5 min.

were extremely low and gestational age was in doubt. Since the lecithin to sphingomyelin ratio may be accelerated in the fetus subjected to chronic stress, an amniocentesis was performed. Dark green amniotic fluid was obtained and cesarean section was performed immediately. A living infant weighing 4 pounds 2 ounces was delivered. The Apgar score was 6 at 1 min and 8 at 5 min.

AMNIOTIC FLUID ESTRIOL

Amniotic fluid estriol levels increase progressively to term.[40] From the practical point of view the clinical use of amniotic fluid estriol determination is limited to very special problems. The regulatory mechanism determining the concentration of estriol in the amniotic fluid compartment is different from that in the urine or plasma. The conjugation of estriol to a sulfate is performed by many fetal tissues, such as skin and lung, but glucosiduronate conjugation is performed mainly by the fetal liver. The sulfate portion excreted into the amniotic fluid is readily hydrolyzed by the amniotic membrane and transferred to the maternal circulation. Estriol glucosiduronate is hydrolyzed slowly and its accumulation accounts for most of the estriol in the amniotic fluid. Schindler and coworkers[50] used amniotic fluid estriol determinations before and after intrauterine transfusion in Rh isoimmunization to determine the effect of the procedure in improving hepatic function as an objective guide to fetal prognosis.

15-α-HYDROXY ESTRIOL (ESTETROL) ASSAYS

This form of estrogen is produced from precursors, mainly from placental estradiol and estrone and apparently some from the fetal adrenal, but the fetal liver is presumably the exclusive site of final hydroxylation steps in its synthesis.[35] Both urinary and plasma assays have been used in clinical practice. The information provided is similar to that obtained from estriol determination.[26, 59] Estetrol did not predict the grave fetal condition in patients with severe Rh isoimmune disease, although one would expect the fetal liver to be significantly involved in such cases. The ability of estriol and estetrol assays to predict fetal distress is not significantly different. This includes the finding of low values in each test in patients with a living anencephalic fetus.

Human Placental Lactogen

Human placental lactogen (HPL), also known as human chorionic somatomammotrophin or chorionic growth hormone-prolactin,[34] was first isolated from placental tissue and retroplacental blood by Josimovich and MacLaren in 1962.[33] During pregnancy the hormone is synthesized solely by syncytiotrophoblast of the placenta, but it also is found in the tissues of hydatidiform mole or choriocarcinoma and in the serum of patients with these disorders.[23, 47] HPL shows immunologic cross reaction, although incomplete, with human pituitary growth hormone.

HPL is readily detectable in the maternal circulation by the 6th week of gestation and increases progressively until about the 36th week when levels reach a plateau. After delivery it disappears rapidly from the circulation. Small but increasing amounts are transferred to the amniotic fluid, but negligible amounts appear in the fetal circulation. Placental production rate of HPL is very high, on the order of 1 g or more per day near term. This is greatly in excess of that produced by any other known peptide hormone.[14] It is metabolized rapidly in the maternal liver and kidneys. The short half-life of HPL of approximately 20 min is a potential advantage in that impairment of placental synthesis should be reflected rapidly by a fall in the level of HPL in the maternal circulation.

Maternal plasma levels of HPL are measured by radioimmunoassay.[33, 34] Various modifications have been developed to shorten the procedure,[49] including semiautomation.[14, 36] Values differ slightly in individual laboratories because of the lack of a universally recognized reference standard. Those obtained by Josimovich[32] and his colleagues for normal single fetus pregnancies and for multiple pregnancies are shown in Figure 3.5. The mean value of 7.5 μg per ml found at 32 to 36 weeks in this study is typical and provides assurance of HPL standard purity.

Other immunotechniques have been

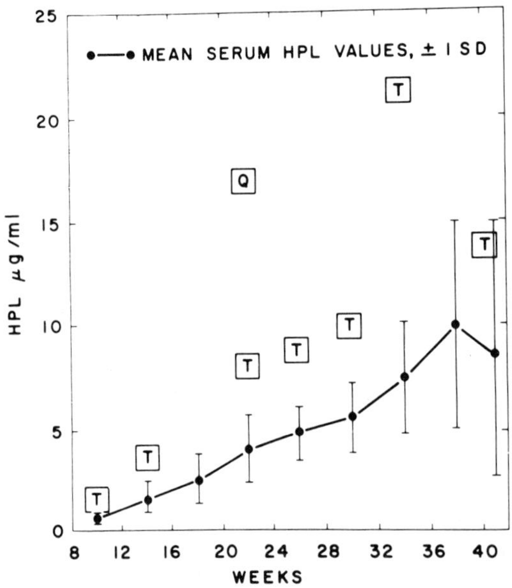

Figure 3.5. Mean maternal serum HPL concentration in normal single-fetus pregnancies during each 4-week period of gestation. Individual symbols represent twin (T) or quintuplet (Q) pregnancies. From Josimovich et al[32] by permission of *Obstetrics and Gynecology.*

tested. Gusdon[25] used a modified hemagglutination inhibition assay and found mean values of HPL compatible with those obtained by radioimmunoassay. Spellacy et al.[55] compared a simple radioactive immunodiffusion kit system with a standard solid phase radioimmunoassay test for HPL. The sensitivity of the simpler test was satisfactory in the upper normal levels but less so in the critical levels below 4 μg per ml.

CLINICAL APPLICATION

Serial HPL determinations have been studied extensively as a fetal monitoring method, both in this country and abroad. Reports regarding its merits have been conflicting.[15, 32, 39, 46, 48, 49, 52, 54, 56] Sufficient clinical and experimental data are now available to indicate its usefulness as an adjunct in fetal monitoring and at the same time to define specific limitations. Conditions that compromise placental function to jeopardize the fetus sufficiently cause falling HPL values approaching the fetal danger zone, defined by Spellacy[54, 56] as any value below 4 μg per ml after 30 weeks of gestation. Thus, obstetric complications in which serial HPL values have proved useful in predicting fetal distress include hypertensive disorders of pregnancy, placental insufficiency associated with intrauterine growth retardation, postmature pregnancies or maternal disease in which hypertension is a significant factor. The test has not proved capable of predicting fetal compromise in certain fetal disorders in which placental function remains adequate, i.e., in maternal diabetes, class A or B, unassociated with hypertension, fetal congenital anomalies or erythroblastosis.

Belanger and coworkers[5] used the primate as an experimental model to study the factors that influence HPL synthesis and secretion in more detail. After surgical removal of the primate fetus with retention of the placenta at various stages of pregnancy, the fall in placental lactogen concentration was only modest, ranging from 10 to 20%. A drastic fall in placental lactogen concentration was seen only when experimental abruptio placentae was induced, suggesting that a major compromise in placental function is required before a significant change in the hormone concentration is observed. There is reason to believe that the regulatory mechanism for HPL secretion in human pregnancy is similar to that in the primate.

The most extensive, well controlled human study was conducted by Spellacy[54] prospectively over a 3-year period. Serial HPL determinations were performed throughout 2733 pregnancies. In one-half of this group HPL values were made available to the obstetric team. The other half served as controls. Although the frequency of low HPL values falling within the fetal danger zone area was similar in the two groups (8.6% and 8.2%, respectively), intrauterine fetal death rate was 2.6% in the treated group and 14.2% in the control group. However, in the 71 cases of eventual fetal death, HPL values fell in the fetal zone in 72.5% of the cases of toxemia but in only 55% of the cases of fetal death in patients with diabetes. Overall HPL values falling within the fetal danger zone area predicted fetal death in 50.7% of the total group of 71 stillbirths. In summarizing their wide experience with the test, the authors concluded the HPL test is not an end point but is clearly an adjunct to fetal monitoring.

Heat-stable Alkaline Phosphatase

The heat-stable isoenzyme of alkaline phosphatase (HSAP) originates in the placenta.[20] Production of HSAP by chorionic tissue has been demonstrated by histochemical electrophoretic and immunologic techniques.[51] The progressive rise in maternal serum alkaline phosphatase throughout the course of pregnancy is due almost entirely to this heat-stable fraction. Alkaline phosphatases from sources other than the placenta are heat labile and largely, but not entirely, inactivated at 56°C within 30 min. Hunter[30] demonstrated that the critical temperature for removal of all nonplacental alkaline phosphatase actually requires a temperature of 65°C. He attributes the lack of success experienced by some investigators to incomplete heat inactivation.

Although the range of normal HSAP values is fairly wide, serial determinations for normal pregnancy quite consistently follow a rising mean value. Elevation of maternal serum HSAP above the upper limits of normal is highly suggestive of placental damage. Hunter postulates that cellular enzymes are liberated from the compromised placenta as from infarcted heart muscle. The sudden and rapid additional increase of previously elevated levels often precedes impending or actual fetal death by 2 to 3 weeks. An example of this is shown in Figure 3.6. This patient had essential hypertension and subclinical diabetes. An extremely high HSAP value was observed at 28 weeks of gestation. An additional sharp rise was seen approximately 2 weeks before the drop in urinary estriol value was observed and intrauterine fetal death occurred.

HSAP is a relatively simple, inexpensive test and has proven to be a valuable adjunct to estriol monitoring, particularly in patients in whom placental dysfunction is suspected. High HSAP values in such patients may be seen at 28 to 30 weeks, and when this occurs, estriol determinations are performed more frequently, even if the pregnancy at that time appears normal.

Plasma Diamine Oxidase

Diamine oxidase (DAO) increases significantly and in a characteristic fashion in the maternal plasma during pregnancy. Swanberg,[57] using a biologic method, demonstrated that the major site of origin of DAO is in the retroplacental maternal decidua. This was confirmed by Southern and coworkers,[53] who used a sensitive, highly specific radioassay procedure, a modification of the method of Okuyama and Kobayashi.[44] The physiologic significance of this enzyme in the maternal circulation may well represent an adaptive response designed to protect the pregnant woman against histamine and possibly other amines formed in the fetus.[60] Histamine is present in increased amount in rapidly growing tissues such as healing wounds and in certain tumors. It is present in high concentration in fetal tissues. Within the decidua, and to a lesser extent within the placenta, it acts as both the inducer and the substrate for the enzyme.

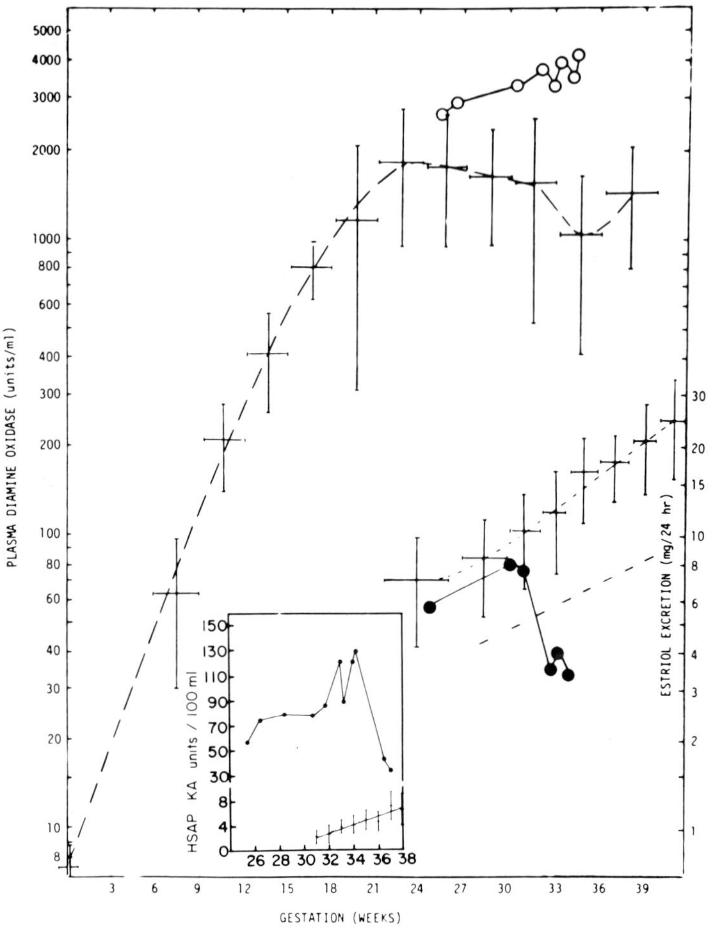

Figure 3.6. Patient C. L., gravida 5, para 4, 41 years of age. Essential hypertension. HSAP elevated during second and early third trimesters with additional sharp rise, approximately 1 to 2 weeks before intrauterine fetal death occurred and estriol levels fell. DAO values fail to predict or to detect fetal demise.

The early rise in plasma DAO is rapid and consistent. When mean values for normal pregnant subjects are plotted on a logarithmic scale against weeks of gestation, the rise is essentially linear until about the 20th week of pregnancy (Figure 3.6). Values are doubled or tripled above nonpregnant levels by the 6th week of gestation, reaching at least 100 units by the 11th week and 500 units by the 21st week.

Throughout this period, the test has proved useful, but by no means the only diagnostic procedure available for dealing with problems related to threatened or missed abortion, some types of ectopic pregnancy and hydatidiform mole or choriocarcinoma. In all of these conditions DAO levels are abnormally low. During the more critical last half of gestation, values tend to plateau within a wide range of normal and frequently fail to predict the fetal status during the third trimester period, when the information is most important.[11, 12] DAO levels may not only fail to drop precipitously in the presence of fetal distress and falling urinary estriol values, but in some patients the DAO level may actually rise during the interval between fetal demise and delivery of the dead fetus (Figure 3.6).

Oxytocinase

Oxytocinase is the main cystine aminopeptidase enzyme capable of inactivating oxytocin during pregnancy. Page and coworkers[45] presented evidence for its origin in the syncytiotrophoblast. Considering its placental source, Babuna and Yemen[3] developed a rapid, inexpensive colorimetric method for measurement of maternal serum oxytocinase and studied its clinical use as an index of placental function. Enzyme activity increases sharply and steadily after the 16th week of gestation to term. Falling levels of oxytocinase were found in cases of pre-eclamptic toxemia and postmaturity in which fetal distress was due specifically to placental dysfunction. In contrast, the test proved incapable of predicting fetal distress of fetal origin as long as the placenta remained functional.[27] In cases of therapeutic abortion oxytocinase levels did not fall after ligation of the umbilical cord until 5 days after the procedure, when placental function finally diminished. On the other hand, when intraamniotic hypertonic saline was injected for interruption of pregnancy, chemical damage to the placenta was reflected promptly by a precipitous drop in serum oxytocinase activity.

Oxytocinase assays have been used less frequently in clinical practice than either HPL or HSAP measurements. All reflect specific placental function. The relative sensitivity of these tests in terms of the amount of placental compromise that will cause fetal distress in a given case is unknown. All three are relatively simple, rapid and inexpensive tests. Serial tests can be performed frequently and serve as practical screening procedures for placental disorders or as an adjunct to one of the estriol tests measuring fetal as well as placental function.

REFERENCES

1. Aldercrentz, H., Luukainen, T.: Identification and determination of oestrogens in various biological materials in pregnancy. Ann Clin Res 2: 365, 1970.
2. Aubrey, R. H., Rouke, J. E., Cuenca, V. G., Marshall, L. D.: The random urine estrogen/creatinine ratio: A practical and reliable index of fetal welfare. Obstet Gynecol 46: 64, 1975.
3. Babuna, C., Yemen, E.: Enzymatic determination of placental function. Am J Obstet Gynecol 95: 925, 1966.
4. Beischer, N. A., Brown, J. B.: Current status of estrogen assays in obstetrics and gynecology: A review. Part 2. Estrogen assays in late pregnancy. Obstet Gynecol Surv 27: 303, 1972.
5. Belanger, C., Shome, B., Friesen, H., Myers, R.: Studies of the secretion of monkey placental lactogen. J Clin Invest 50: 2660, 1971.
6. Beling, C. G.: Estrogen assays. *Endocrinology of Pregnancy*. Edited by A. Klopper, New York, Harper & Row, 1971, p 50.
7. Bevis, D. C. A.: Antenatal prediction of haemolytic disease of the newborn. Lancet 1: 395, 1952.
8. Bolognese, R. J., Corson, S. L., Touchstone, J. C.: Factors affecting the yield of urinary estriol. Obstet Gynecol 39: 683, 1972.
9. Brown, J. B., Coyle, M. G.: Urinary excretion of oestriol during pregnancy. J Obstet Gynecol Br Commonw 70: 219, 1963.
10. Campbell, D. G., Gardner, G.: The automated analysis of urinary oestrogens during pregnancy. Clin Chem Acta 32: 153, 1971.
11. Carrington, E. R.: Diabetes in pregnancy. Clin Obstet Gynecol 16: 28, 1973.
12. Carrington, E. R., Frishmuth, G. J., Oesterling, M. J., Adams, F. M., Cox, S. E.: Gestational and postpartum plasma diamine oxidase values. Obstet Gynecol 39: 426, 1972.
13. Carrington, E. R., Oesterling, M. J., Adams, F. A.: Renal clearance of estriol in complicated pregnancies. Am J Obstet Gynecol 106: 1131, 1970.
14. Chard, T.: The hormonal assessment of foetal and placental function. Clin Obstet Gynaecol 1: 85, 1974.
15. Cohen, M., Haour, F., Dumont, M., Bertrand, J.: Prognostic value of human chorionic somatomammotrophin plasma levels in diabetic patients. Am J Obstet Gynecol 115: 202, 1973.
16. Dickey, R. P., Grannis, G. F., Hanson, F. W.: The use of estrogen/creatinine ratio and the "estrogen index" for screening of normal and "high risk" pregnancy. Am J Obstet Gynecol 113: 880, 1972.
17. Diczfalusy, E.: Endocrine functions of the human placental unit. Fed Proc 23: 791, 1964.
18. France, J. T., Liggins, G. C.: Placental sulfatase deficiency. J Clin Endocrinol 29: 138, 1969.
19. Frandsen, V. A., Stakemann, G.: Site of production of estrogenic hormones in human pregnancy: Hormone excretion in pregnancy with anencephalic fetus. Acta Endocrinol 38: 383, 1961.
20. Ghosh, N. K., Fishman, W. H.: Characterization of placental isoenzyme of alkaline phosphatase in human pregnancy serum. Can J Biochem 47: 147, 1969.
21. Greene, J. W., Jr., Duhring, J. L., Smith, K.: Placental function tests: A review of methods available for assessment of the fetoplacental complex. Am J Obstet Gynecol 92: 1030, 1965.
22. Greene, J. W., Jr., Touchstone, J. C.: Urinary estriol as an index of placental function. Am J Obstet Gynecol 85: 1, 1963.
23. Grumbach, M. M., Kaplan, S. L., Sciarra, J. J., Burr, I. M.: Chorionic growth hormone–prolactin (CGP): Secretion, disposition, biologic activity in man, and postulated function as the "growth hormone" of the second half of pregnancy. Ann N Y Acad Sci 148: 501, 1968.
24. Gurpide, E., Giebenhain, M. E., Tsing, L.,

Kelly, W. G.: Radioimmunoassay for oestrogens in human pregnancy urine, plasma and amniotic fluid. Am J Obstet Gynecol 109: 897, 1971.
25. Gusdon, J. P., Jr.: Improved hemagglutination-inhibition assay: Clinical application to measurement of human placental lactogen. Obstet Gynecol 33: 397, 1969.
26. Heikkila, J., Luukkainen, T.: Urinary excretion of estriol and 15α-hydroxyestriol in complicated pregnancies. Am J Obstet Gynecol 110: 509, 1971.
27. Hensleigh, P. A., Krantz, K. E.: Oxytocinase and placental function. Am J Obstet Gynecol 107: 1233, 1970.
28. Hobkirk, R.: Hydrolysis of estrogen conjugates in diabetic pregnancy urine. J Clin Endocrinol Metabol 19: 1352, 1959.
29. Hobkirk, R., Metcalfe-Gibson, A.: Urinary estrogens. Stand Methods Clin Chem 4: 65, 1963.
30. Hunter, R. J.: Serum, heat stable alkaline phosphatase: An index of placental function. J Obstet Gynecol Br Commonw 77: 987, 1970.
31. Jorgensen, P. I., Trolle, D.: Low urinary œstriol excretion during pregnancy in women giving birth to infants with Down's syndrome. Lancet 2: 782, 1972.
32. Josimovich, J. B., Koser, B., Boccella, L., Mintz, D. H., Hutchinson, D. L.: Placental lactogen in maternal serum as an index of fetal health. Obstet Gynecol 36: 244, 1970.
33. Josimovich, J. B., MacLaren, J. A.: Presence in human placenta and term serum of a highly lactogenic substance immunologically related to pituitary growth hormone. Endocrinology 71: 209, 1962.
34. Kaplan, S. L., Grumbach, M. M.: Immunoassay for human chorionic "growth hormone prolactin" in serum and urine. Science 147: 751, 1965.
35. Korda, A. R., Challis, J. J., Anderson, A. B. M., Turnbull, A. C.: Plasma unconjugated 15α-hydroxyoestriol (oestetrol) levels in normal human pregnancy. Br J Obstet Gynecol 82: 882, 1975.
36. Letchworth, A. T., Boardman, R., Bristow, C., Landon, J., Chard, T.: A rapid semi-automated method for the measurement of HCS. J Obstet Gynecol Br Commonw 78: 542, 1971.
37. Levitz, M., Salinger, M.: Plasma estriol levels in Class D diabetes of pregnancy. Am J Obstet Gynecol 108: 82, 1970.
38. Liley, A. W.: Intrauterine transfusion of the foetus in haemolytic disease. Br Med J 2: 1107, 1963.
39. Lindberg, B. S., Nilsson, B. A.: Human placental lactogen (HPL) levels in abnormal pregnancies. J Obstet Gynecol Br Commonw 80: 1046, 1973.
40. Michie, A. E., Livingstone, J. R. B.: Oestriol concentration in amniotic fluid. Acta Endocrinol 61: 329, 1969.
41. Nachtigall, L., Bassett, M., Hogsander, U., Levitz, M.: Plasma estriol levels in normal and abnormal pregnancies: An index of fetal welfare. Am J Obstet Gynecol 101: 638, 1968.
42. Nachtigall, L., Bassett, M., Hogsander, U., Slagle, S., Levitz, M.: A rapid method for assay of plasma estriol in pregnancy. J Clin Endocrinol 26: 941, 1966.
43. Oakey, R. E.: The interpretation of urinary oestrogen and pregnanediol excretion in pregnant women receiving corticosteroids. J Obstet Gynecol Br Commonw 77: 922, 1970.
44. Okuyama, T., Kobayashi, Y.: Determination of diamine oxidase activity by scintillation counting. Arch Biochem Biophys 95: 242, 1961.
45. Page, E. W., Titus, M. A., Mohun, G., Glendening, M. B.: The origin and distribution of oxytocinase. Am J Obstet Gynecol 82: 1090, 1961.
46. Samaan, N. A., Bradbury, J. T., Gopelrud, C. P.: Serial hormonal studies in normal and abnormal pregnancy. Am J Obstet Gynecol 104: 781, 1969.
47. Samaan, N., Yen, S. C. C., Friesen, H., Pearson, O. H.: Serum placental lactogen levels during pregnancy and in trophoblastic disease. J Clin Endocrinol 26: 1303, 1966.
48. Saxena, B. N., Emerson, K., Jr., Selenkow, H. A.: Serum HPL levels as an index of placental function. N Engl J Med 281: 225, 1969.
49. Saxena, B. N., Refetoff, S., Smerson, K. J., Selenkow, H. A.: Rapid radioimmunoassay for human placental lactogen: Application to normal and abnormal pregnancies. Am J Obstet Gynecol 101: 874, 1968.
50. Schindler, A. E., Ratanasopa, V., Lee, T. Y., Herrmann, W. L.: Estriol and Rh isoimmunization: A new approach to the management of severely affected pregnancies. Obstet Gynecol 29: 625, 1967.
51. Shane, J. M., Suzuki, K.: Placental alkaline phosphatase: A review and re-evaluation of its applicability in monitoring fetoplacental function. Obstet Gynecol Surv 29: 97, 1974.
52. Singer, W., Desjardins, P., Friesen, H. G.: Human placental lactogen: An index of placental function. Obstet Gynecol 36: 222, 1970.
53. Southern, A. L., Kobayashi, Y., Brenner, P., Weingold, A. B.: Diamine oxidase activity in human maternal and fetal plasma and tissues at parturition. J Appl Physiol 30: 1048, 1965.
54. Spellacy, W. N., Buhi, W. C., Birk, S. A.: The effectiveness of HPL measurements as an adjunct in decreasing perinatal deaths. Am J Obstet Gynecol 121: 835, 1975.
55. Spellacy, W. N., Buhi, W. C., McCreary, S. A.: Measurement of human placental lactogen with a simple immunodiffusion kit (Plac-Gest). Obstet Gynecol 43: 306, 1974.
56. Spellacy, W. N., Teoh, E. S., Buhi, W. C.: Human chorionic somatomammotrophin (HCS) levels prior to fetal death in high risk pregnancies. Obstet Gynecol 35: 635, 1970.
57. Swanberg, H.: Histaminase in pregnancy with special reference to its origin and formation. Acta Physiol Scand 23, Suppl 79: 1–69, 1951.
58. Tikkanen, M. J., Aldercreutz, H.: Effect of antibiotics on oestrogen metabolism in pregnancy. Br Med J 2: 369, 1973.
59. Tulchinsky, D., Frigoletto, F. D., Ryan, K. J., Fishman, J.: Plasma estetrol as an index of fetal well-being. J Clin Endocrinol Metab 40: 560,

1975.
60. Weingold, A. B., Southern, A. L.: Diamone oxidase as an index of the fetoplacental unit: Clinical applications. Obstet Gynecol 32: 593, 1968.
61. Wotis, W. H., Martin, H. F.: Studies in steroid metabolism. XI. Gas chromatographic determination of estrogens in human pregnancy urine. Anal Biochem 3: 97, 1962.
62. Yousem, H. L.: Simple gas chromatographic method for estimation of urinary estriol in pregnant women. Am J Obstet Gynecol 88: 375, 1964.

JOHN F. HUDDLESTON, M.D.
ROGER K. FREEMAN, M.D.

4

The Use of the Oxytocin Challenge Test for the Management of Pregnancies at Risk for Uteroplacental Insufficiency

It would be of inestimable value to the practicing obstetrician and pediatrician if it were possible to prospectively and precisely identify that minority of pregnancies which, without special prophylactic and therapeutic efforts, would eventuate in significant maternal and/or perinatal morbidity or mortality. Safe in the conviction that the pregnancies not so identified would enjoy favorable outcomes, obstetricians could confidently entrust most of their care to associates with less medical training, but with more time to deal with the physical and emotional needs of normal pregnancy and impending motherhood. Obstetricians could then devote most of their time and energy to the identified minority who require and deserve the benefits of their special training. Unfortunately, such an ability to identify all serious obstetric problems early in pregnancy does not exist at this time. Indeed, considering the unpredictable emergencies inherent in current obstetric practice, this ability is unlikely to become a reality in the near future. Problems such as premature rupture of the membranes, abnormal presentation and intrapartum cord occlusion will prove very difficult to predict during the early prenatal course. However, although they are imperfect at the present time, useful methods do currently exist for prospectively identifying many actual and potential obstetric problems.

This chapter will address the issue of separating from the identified high risk pregnancies those at risk for uteroplacental insufficiency (UPI). Within the subset of high risk pregnancies at risk for UPI exist at least two further subsets: (a) those pregnancies which will eventuate in normal perinatal outcome without obstetric intervention and (b) those pregnancies for which intervention should be considered because of a high liklihood of adverse perinatal outcome. The oxytocin challenge test (OCT) is one of the clinical tools which can be of value in making this latter discrimination, more commonly to support a plan of nonintervention but at times strongly to suggest delivery. The physiologic principles, methods of performance and interpretation, clinical usefulness and clinical limitations of the OCT will be considered.

Defining Uteroplacental Respiratory Insufficiency

SCREENING FOR HIGH RISK PREGNANCY

During the past several years, much interest has been focused on identification of the so-called high risk pregnancy. Although most of the conditions associated with adverse maternal or fetal outcome generally have been recognized for some time, only recently have methods been published which allow the clinician to quantitate the risks of unfavorable outcome for an individual pregnancy.[2, 22, 28, 38] These methods, which take into consideration numerous historic, physical and laboratory factors, will identify prospectively about one-fourth to one-third of pregnancies as high risk: those from which will arise the majority of the eventual perinatal morbidity and mortality. By such identification and subsequent careful survillance and treatment, it is anticipated that the frequency of these adverse outcomes will be reduced.[28]

UTEROPLACENTAL INSUFFICIENCY

Many of the identifiable high risk factors are associated with conditions known or presumed to interfere with uterine blood flow, intervillous space (IVS) perfusion and placental exchange.[39] For example, the pregnant woman with rheumatic mitral stenosis is at risk for developing cardiorespiratory distress because of volume load across the stenotic valve. Her fetus, however, is not at greatly increased risk, since uterine blood flow and placental exchange are relatively normal. On the other hand, a maternal condition such as chronic hypertension may be associated with diminished vascular caliber, hypovolemia and decreased uterine blood flow. The consequent inadequate exchange of nutrients and/or blood gases across the placenta, defined as UPI[14, 29, 39] (Figure 4.1), is at times clearly detrimental to the developing fetus. In other instances, placental transfer is impeded because of fetal

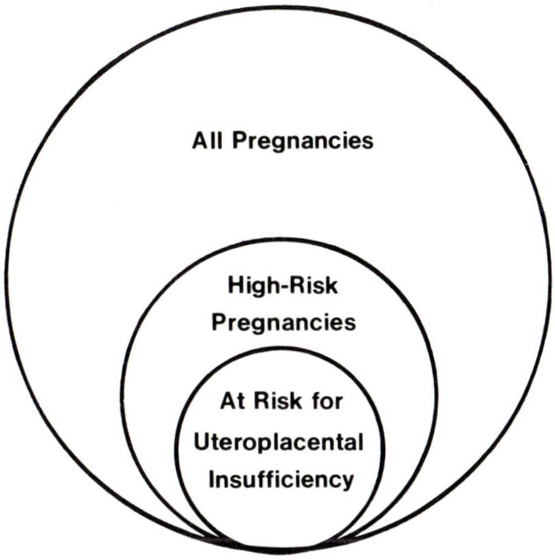

Figure 4.1. Diagram representing the total population of all pregnancies, a smaller population of high risk pregnancies and a subset of high risk pregnancies representing those at risk for uteroplacental insufficiency.

or maternal conditions other than inadequate placental perfusion.[39] In its worst forms, UPI is associated with intrauterine growth retardation (IUGR), chronic fetal hypoxemia and intrauterine fetal demise (IUFD). It is with these high risk pregnancies which are additionally at risk for UPI that modern methods of fetal surveillance find their greatest usefulness.

Kubli and associates[34] have for operational purposes separated the nutritive and the respiratory functions of the placenta. They considered the serial measurements of fetal biparietal diameter by ultrasound[52] and the serial measurement of urinary estriol (E_3)[23] to reflect the nutritive function. The OCT was considered to reflect the respiratory function.[25] More recently, Parer[39] has suggested that as uteroplacental function deteriorates, nutritive function decline precedes impairment in respiratory function. The very useful surveillance methods involving ultrasonography and hormonal monitoring are dealt with elsewhere in this volume. In order to better understand how the OCT might be related to uteroplacental respiratory function, a brief review of uteroplacental respiratory physiology is appropriate.

UTEROPLACENTAL RESPIRATORY PHYSIOLOGY

The developing fetus requires a rather constant supply of nutrients and oxygen for survival and growth. Because storage depots in the forms of glycogen and proteins exist for energy-producing nutrients, the fetus is able to survive brief reductions or interruptions in the supply of these nutrients. On the other hand, no such storage mechanism exists for oxygen, the gas which is so essential for minute-by-minute energy production and prevention of lactic acidosis. Fetal blood oxygen is consumed at a rate which effectively exhausts its concentration within one circulation through the fetal vascular system. Perhaps surprisingly, the normal partial pressure of oxygen in the umbilical vein averages only 25 to 30 mm Hg, which may seem low by usual clinical standards.[7, 37] However, the oxygen dissociation curve, the Bohr effect and the high hematocrit of fetal blood all function to compensate for this normally low partial pressure and thus to provide the fetus with adequate oxygen.[39]

Data from both animal[24, 43] and human[41, 42] experiments have established clearly that uterine blood flow, including the vital flow to the IVS, normally slows or ceases during uterine contractions of normal intensity. It follows that such periodic interruptions of IVS perfusion necessarily subject the fetus during labor to repetitive hypoxic stresses. The normally oxygenated fetus presumably tolerates these stresses without difficulty and recoups its oxygen debt during the periods of uterine diastole. However, the fetus existing under conditions of basal hypoxia may respond adversely to these additional hypoxic stresses.

Hon and Quilligan[30] and Caldeyro-Barcia and colleagues[8] described various patterns of the fetal heart rate (FHR) relative to uterine contractions (UC). The pattern designated as late deceleration[30] (type II dip[8]), for which the nadir of the FHR deceleration occurs late in time relative to the peak of the UC, was claimed to be due to hypoxic myocardial depression and was shown to be associated with fetal hypoxemia, acidosis and poor perinatal outcome.[7, 8, 29, 30] Myers and associates,[37] using direct fetal blood sampling in pregnant rhesus monkey experiments, have demonstrated that late decelerations accompany only those UC's which occur during fetal hypoxia. Even the acidotic fetus apparently will not exhibit late decelerations if oxygenation is normal. Myers[36] has also demonstrated that hypoxic brain damage and hypoxic fetal death are predictable from the measurement of oxygenation in the hypoxic monkey fetus. Using a tissue electrode implanted transabdominally into the muscle of the human fetal buttock, Pose and colleagues[41] also showed that late decelerations occur only with basal fetal hypoxia. They described a threshold partial pressure of oxygen below which the hypoxic stresses of uterine contractions regularly cause late decelerations by further depressing fetal oxygenation (Figure 4.2). Myers and associates[37] have noted a similar threshold phenomenon in fetal monkeys. It thus seems well established that repetitive late decelerations of the FHR represent a reliable reflection of intrauterine hypoxia. This interpretation does not imply that all perinates will be depressed if delivered immediately after such a pattern is noted. Indeed, such is not the case.[29] Hypoxia alone would be ex-

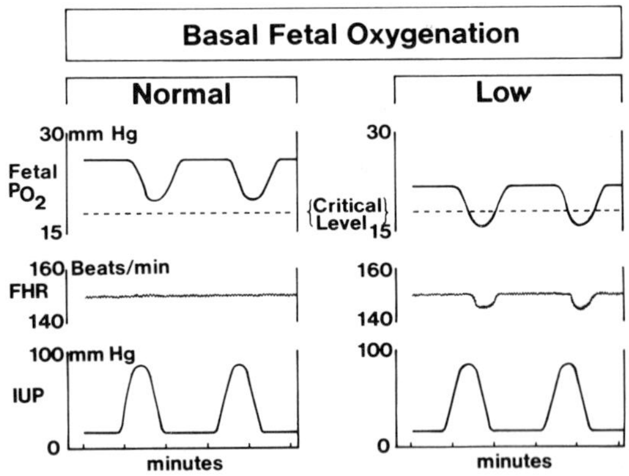

Figure 4.2. Schematic representation of the decrease in fetal pO_2 which normally accompanies uterine contractions. In the fetus with low basal oxygenation, this decrease falls below a critical pO_2 level. Below this critical level the fetal myocardium is depressed and the heart rate slows, resulting in the pattern of late deceleration. Modified from Pose and colleagues.[41]

pected to clear rapidly during the first few breaths after delivery. However, prolonged intrauterine hypoxia will lead to lactic acidosis, which clears more slowly and is more frequently associated with depression in the newborn. Thus, it would be reasonable to interpret late decelerations occurring for a short time in response to normal contractions as representing a very early sign of fetal distress, one which, if acted upon, should preclude significant fetal acidosis and neonatal depression.

Development of Interest in OCT

EARLY STUDIES UTILIZING OCT

Several investigators, armed with the physiologic data presented above, then reasoned that it might be possible to identify basal fetal hypoxia by studying, during the last several weeks of pregnancy, the FHR response to spontaneous or induced UC's.

Hammacher, in 1966,[25] was the first to propose that this procedure be used as an indicator of fetal well being. Hammacher and coworkers[26] reported using the OCT in a study of 207 pregnancies, most of which were high risk. They found the presence of late decelerations to be associated frequently with low Apgar scores. Moreover, this abnormal FHR pattern was associated with 17 of the 23 stillbirths in their study. No information was given relating the time of testing to either delivery or to fetal death.

Pose and colleagues[40] conducted a study of 33 OCT's in 20 high risk patients during late pregnancy. Tests were repeated at weekly intervals in 10 patients, and clinical management was not influenced by test results. These investigators also noted that for all 12 cases in which the last test was negative (late decelerations absent), the 5-min Apgar score was high. For the eight cases in which one test was positive (late decelerations present), three had low 5-min Apgar scores and three others were stillborn. Two of the stillbirths occurred before labor, 3 and 7 days after the positive test. Thus, although their frequency of positive results was quite high, the outcome was unfavorable in fully 75% of the fetuses who manifested a positive test. Perhaps more importantly, the outcome was uniformly good when the OCT, repeated at weekly intervals, was negative.

Kubli and associates[34] studied the OCT in an investigation of several parameters of fetal surveillance. They likewise found the OCT predictive of fetal outcome. Those perinates with negative tests had good Apgar scores; those with a positive test frequently had IUFD or low Apgar scores.

Sánchez-Ramos and coworkers[46] reported a study of 191 tests in 132 patients. In the 98 fetuses exhibiting only normal FHR responses, there were no stillbirths; there were only 2 infants with 5-min Apgar scores below 6. There were 34 patients with abnormal tests: 2 infants were stillborn and 5 had low Apgar scores.

Spurrett[48] performed a total of 181 OCT's on 164 patients at risk for UPI. He was able to show clearly higher rates of low Apgar scores, IUGR and IUFD in these perinates exhibiting abnormal FHR responses compared with those for whom the OCT's were negative. He suggested prompt delivery for patients with a positive test, an interpretation given to at least one test from 23 patients.

The first published OCT report from the United States was that of Ray and coworkers[44] in 1972. Their study included 113 tests in 66 patients at risk for UPI. Weekly testing was employed and neonatal follow-up was complete. The OCT results were not made available to the clinicians rendering patient care. These investigators again suggested that the negative test, if repeated weekly, was reassuring in the diagnosis of fetal well-being. Of the 15 fetuses with positive tests, there were three intrauterine deaths (20%); all occurred within 72 hr of the positive OCT. The overall incidence of low 5-min Apgar scores in the positive group was a very significant 53%. The convention of weekly testing, the criteria for performance of the test and the definitions of test interpretation defined in their report have been those generally followed in most subsequent studies.

MORE RECENT STUDIES

Since early 1974, a number of OCT series, collectively representing a very large clinical experience, have been presented and form the basis for a realistic appraisal of the clinical value of the OCT (Table 4.1).[4, 5, 9–12, 14, 19, 27, 32, 47, 51] The above publications, which exclude those papers which are only case reports,[17, 33, 50] and those for which data are included in other studies,[16] represent a total experience of 4920 tests in 2307 patients. Within this experience there are only five cases of IUFD within a week of a negative test, a rate of 3.9 per 1000 tested patients. Among these five stillbirths, there were four with possible explanations: one total placental abruption[4]; one with a triple nuchal cord[14]; one for which the OCT, in retrospect, was probably not negative[12]; and one which revealed thrombosis of the chorionic vessels.[5] The latter two cases[5, 12] occurred at the temporal limit of the time interval now recommended: 7 days after a negative test. Klapholz and Burke[33] reported a single case of unexplained IUFD 6 hr after a negative OCT and 9 hr after a diagnostic amniocentesis. No needle trauma was defined at autopsy.

Performance of OCT

INDICATIONS AND CONTRAINDICATIONS

Patients to be managed using the OCT are those which would ordinarily be identified as at risk for UPI. Table 4.2 lists the more common of these indications used at our institutions and in most other studies. Since, at both of our centers, the perinatal mortality rate in uncomplicated class A diabetes mellitus is no higher than in our low risk patients, the class A diabetics are not followed with OCT's (or E_3 determinations) unless (a) the fasting blood sugar becomes elevated, (b) there has been a previous unexplained stillbirth, or (c) insulin has been required in a previous pregnancy.[13, 31] Although meconium in the amniotic fluid is listed as an indication, its presence is not ordinarily sought by amnioscopy or amniocentesis unless one of the other listed indications exists. Indeed, there is some disagreement between us as to the actual importance of antepartal meconium in determining fetal well-being.[15]

The listed contraindications (Table 4.2) include those conditions for which the risks of premature labor or contraction-associated morbidity usually outweigh the possible benefits of defining uteroplacental respiratory status. Thus, after thoughtful consideration of the risk-benefit ratio, the OCT may be performed on some of these patients. In fact, several twin pregnancies have been knowingly tested without precipitating labor, and several patients with placenta previa have been inadvertently but uneventfully tested before recognition of that abnormality.

INSTRUMENTATION

The type of fetal monitoring equipment used for the OCT varies somewhat among

Table 4.1. Test series reported since 1974

Senior author	Reference no.	No. of OCT's	No. of patients	Patients with positive OCT, %	Instances of IUFD*	Patients with recurrent LD's in labor, %†
Boehm	4	266	152	9.9	2	0.0
Boyd	5	46	41	12.2	1	13.3
Christie	9	60	50	18.0	0	2.9
Cooper	10	116	89	14.6	0	0.0
Ewing	11	86	58	13.8	0	0.0
Farahani	12	767	333	7.2	1	0.3
Freeman	14,16	1500	600	16.9‡	1‡	§
Gaziano	19	81	72	9.7	0	0.0
Hayden	27	225	105	7.6	0	5.1
Huddleston	32	1209	533	12.9	0	2.6
Schifrin	47	189	120	7.5	0	3.0
Weingold	51	375	154	9.1	0	2.8

* Intrauterine fetal demise within 7 days of negative OCT.

† LD: late decelerations (% of patients laboring within 7 days of negative OCT).

‡ Data based only upon first 390 patients studied.

§ Data not presented.

Table 4.2. Choice of patients for oxytocin challenge testing

Indications	Contraindications
Diabetes mellitus (see text)	Rupture of chorioamnion
Chronic hypertension	Multiple pregnancy
Acute hypertension	Previous premature labor
Chronic renal disease	Hydramnios
Homozygous hemoglobinopathies	Previous classical cesarean section
Prolonged pregnancy (≥42 weeks)	Placentae previa
Intrauterine growth retardation	
Elderly gravida (≥40)	
Previous unexplained stillbirth	
Rhesus sensitization	
Cyanotic maternal heart disease	
Maternal hyperthyroidism	
Meconium-stained amniotic fluid	

various institutions. In general, noninvasive transducers for FHR and UC must be utilized. Since the test is not conducted as a prelude to labor, the integrity of the fetal membranes must be preserved. However, both Pose and colleagues[40] and Cooper and associates[10] have used transabdominal catheters for intra-amniotic pressure recording during the OCT. Although this method allows the precise quantitation of uterine activity, and thus allows a standardization of the hypoxic stress or challenge, we consider it too cumbersome and potentially morbid (uterine hypertonus,[10] infection) to be of widespread practical value.

The most widely available noninvasive techniques employ an ultrasonic transducer for the detection of fetal cardiac activity and a strain gauge contraction detector. This "standard" combination is usually quite satisfactory and has been used in most studies to date. However, certain limitations to the ultrasound-strain gauge system should be appreciated.

The first limitation is that the strain gauge does not quantitate intrauterine pressure and therefore can be used only for simple detection and timing of uterine contractions. Unfortunately then, standardization of fetal challenge is not possible. Since the strain gauge method of contraction detection is common to all noninvasive methods, this limitation applies to them all.

The second limitation of the "standard" combination concerns the ultrasound system and its inherently "noisy" signal output. Artifical FHR variability is introduced, which usually renders unreliable any conclusion that the beat-to-beat variability of the FHR is normal.[14, 26, 29] This artificial variability becomes more pronounced as the distance from the transducer to the fetal heart increases. Therefore, this effect may be more pronounced with obese or hydramic patients. Uncommonly, the "noisy" ultrasound FHR recording is unsatisfactory for interpretation. However, there is occasionally an OCT tracing in which the FHR obtained from an ultrasound transducer has very little variability. In this latter case, one is probably safe in concluding that the actual variability is decreased, since the ultrasound system will not obscure actual beat-to-beat fluctuations unless there is electronic "smoothing" of the FHR output.

The same type strain gauge has been used in combination with a sensitive abdominal microphone equipped with a manual gain control We both have experience with this combination, and the results have been quite satisfactory. The FHR output of this system correlates much better with the actual fetal-scalp electrocardiogram (ECG) than does that obtained with ultrasound.[14] Therefore, more valid comments can be made concerning the FHR beat-to-beat variability and more accurate interpretation of the FHR recording can be made because of the less "noisy" signal. Most experience with the microphone system has been with equipment not available commercially.[14] However, we anticipate that most companies producing fetal monitoring equipment will soon be offering this feature, at least as an option.

The fetal ECG obtained from electrodes applied to the maternal abdomen can be utilized by some equipment to record the FHR. Of the noninvasive methods, the abdominal fetal ECG theoretically should provide the best input signal. Some technical problems have been encountered in separating the fetal ECG from the much stronger maternal ECG signal, especially when the two signals are coincident. Although imperfect at the present time, the external fetal ECG and strain gauge combination is most likely to become the standard method of noninvasive antepartum fetal monitoring.

Suffice it to say that there exist and are under development various means of determining FHR and UC signals adequate for OCT interpretation. The currently "standard" ultrasound-strain gauge transducers will generally produce the most consistently readable tracings.[47] Some of the more sophisticated techniques, although offering more accurate determination of beat-to-beat variability and a less "noisy" FHR signal, will, in general, not offer significant advantage over standard methods in the detection of late decelerations.

SPECIAL FACILITY AND PERSONNEL

In our centers the OCT is conducted in a special facility, located separately from the actual labor and delivery area, but close enough to deal swiftly with any problems which might arise. The facility is staffed by a specially trained nurse whose only job is preforming the test. Immediate physician backup must always be available. Since she is free from the interruptions inherent in the unpredictable exigencies of the labor and delivery area, the OCT nurse is free to devote her entire attention to obtaining a high quality OCT recording. This diligent attention not only adds to the safety of the procedure, but also results in a greater percentage of recordings of a quality acceptable for interpretation. We realize that the demand for performing this test on smaller, nonindigent obstetric services may not justify the employment of one nurse just to perform OCT's. This objection can be overcome by having a single OCT facility perform the tests for all hospitals in a given area.

CONDUCTION OF OCT

The test is conducted as previously described.[14, 44] The test procedure is explained carefully by the requesting physician to the patient, who then is asked to sign a consent form (Figure 4.3). She is given an appointment and asked to arrive at the OCT facility within a few hours of a meal. This timing is chosen because the fetus appears to be less active after the mother eats, and because bowel sounds are usually less frequent and intense. Both of these considerations are in the interest of a more interpretable recording. The consideration of bowel sounds assumes importance only when the phonocardiographic transducer is used.

The patient is positioned either in the semi-Fowler[44] or lateral tilt[32, 51] position, in an effort to prevent aortocaval compression[42] and its consequent reduction in cardiac output, uterine blood flow and IVS perfusion. It is possible that even the normally oxygenated fetus might develop basal hypoxia and late decelerations secondary to this positioned effect. In order to detect any systemic arterial hypotension, the blood pressure is taken initially and thereafter at least every 10 min until the test is completed. Since many of these

I, ______________________, give permission to ______________________, M.D. and his associates to perform upon me an Oxytocin Challenge Test. I understand that (1) this is a test to check on the well-being of my baby, (2) the test information will be obtained from painless and harmless devices placed upon my abdomen to record the contractions and the baby's heartbeat, (3) oxytocin (the drug ordinarily given in larger doses to induce labor) will be given me by vein in small doses to cause a few contractions, (4) the test may need to be repeated on several occasions, (5) although my doctor(s) feel(s) the test is reasonably safe, there is a small chance that I will go into labor as a result of the test or that the baby may respond abnormally to the test, and (6) that the results of the test may cause my doctor(s) to advise immediate hospitalization with or without immediate delivery. I recognize and accept all of the above-stated risks in order that my doctor(s) may better determine the correct management for my complicated pregnancy.

Witnesses:__________________ Signed:__________________

__________________ Date: __________________

Figure 4.3. Informed consent for the oxytocin challenge test.

Table 4.3. Interpretation of oxytocin challenge test

Result	Interpretation
Negative	Uterine activity (UA) adequate*; no late deceleration(s) (LD) present.
Positive	LD occur with most (≥50%) contractions, even if UA less than that defined as adequate.
Suspicious	UA adequate; definite LD present, but only with some (<50%) contractions.
Hyperstimulation	LD present, but occur with or following period of excessive† UA; excessive UA without LD is considered negative.
Unsatisfactory	Adequate UA not achieved *or* tracing quality too poor to exclude LD.

* Three contractions of 40-sec duration within 10 min.

† Contraction(s) lasting >90 sec or occurring more frequently than every 2 min.

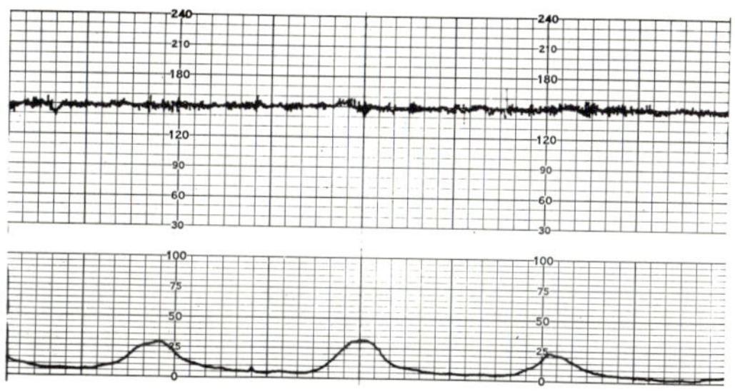

Figure 4.4. Negative oxytocin challenge test: upper channel (beats per min); lower channel, uterine contractions (arbitrary units).

gravidas are hypertensive, one must consider this diagnosis in interpreting the brachial arterial pressure readings.

The monitoring equipment is applied to the maternal abdomen. The strain guage generally functions best when placed over the fundus; the FHR transducer is positioned so as to obtain the highest quality fetal signal. Since the fetus is often quite active, it is frequently necessary to reposition the FHR transducer many times during the test in order to obtain a readable tracing. A 15- to 20-min observation period is then routinely undertaken. A significant percentage of these gravidas will be having spontaneous uterine activity sufficient for what is arbitrarily considered an adequate challenge: three contractions of 40 to 60 sec duration within a 10-min period.[14, 44] If an amniocentesis is performed within a few hours before the test, spontaneous uterine activity is even more frequently adequate. What is considered adequate uterine activity for the OCT may or may not be considered uncomfortable or even noticed by the gravida.

If, on careful observation, spontaneous uterine activity is inadequate and no late decelerations are present, dilute intravenous oxytocin is begun via infusion pump at a low rate: 0.5 milliunits per min. This rate is doubled only every 10 to 15 min until uterine activity is adequate or until repetitive late decelerations appear. The dosage of oxytocin necessary to produce adequate uterine activity is not great, a dosage in excess of 8.0 milliunits per min rarely being required. The OCT generally takes 1 to 2 hr. If there is adequate spontaneous uterine activity noted during the observation period and oxytocin is unnecessary, much less time is needed. The nurse specialist is able to complete about four or five tests per day. When the test is over, the monitoring is continued until the contractions become less frequent than every 10 min.

Interpretation of OCT (Table 4.3)[14]

NEGATIVE

When three adequate contractions have been achieved within a 10-min period, and no late decelerations are noted (Figure 4.4) the test is concluded, interpreted as negative, and repeated only every 7 days. A strict policy of assigning a negative interpretation only if late decelerations can definitely be excluded is fundamentally important in relying upon the negative test result for 7 subsequent days. Accelerations of the fetal heart rate coincident with fetal movements (AFM) are noted when present (Figure 4.5).[26] The significance of AFM will be considered subsequently.

POSITIVE

An OCT is interpreted as positive when persistent and consistent late decelerations are noted in association with most

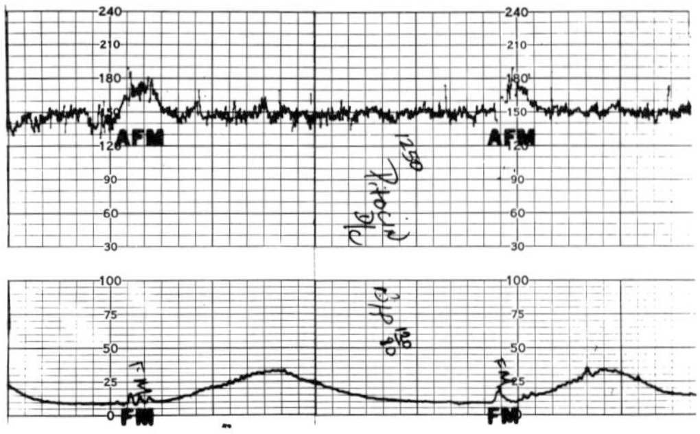

Figure 4.5. Negative oxytocin challenge test demonstrating accelerations (AFM) of the fetal heart rate in response to fetal movements (FM). Upper and lower channels as in Figure 4.4.

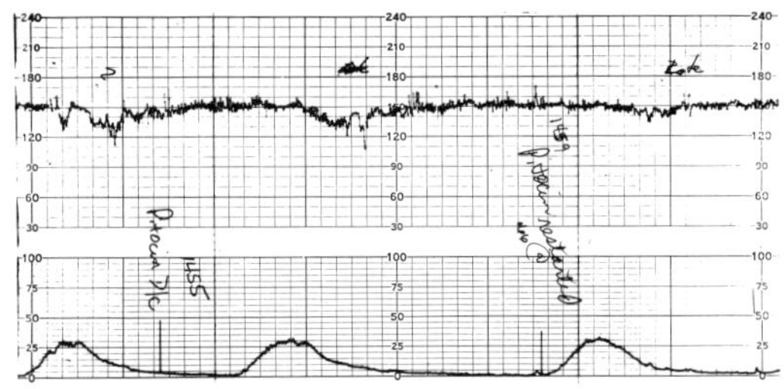

Figure 4.6. Positive oxytocin challenge test. Late decelerations occur with each uterine contraction. Upper and lower channels as in Figure 4.4.

(more than half) of the adequate contractions (Figure 4.6). It is to be emphasized that definite, repetitive late decelerations, no matter how shallow the amplitude, probably reflect fetal myocardial hypoxia and should be considered significant. It is likewise important to state that if repetitive late decelerations (either spontaneus or oxytocin-induced) occur with less than the level of uterine activity defined as adequate, further uterine stimulation is unnecessary and is contraindicated.

SUSPICIOUS, HYPERSTIMULATION AND UNSATISFACTORY

The definitions for these interpretations are also given in Table 4.3. In general, these interpretations should be considered inconclusive, giving no information useful in clinical management. The patients should be retested 24 hr later. Together, these three interpretations constitute less than one-fourth of the OCT's; therefore, in more than three-fourths a definite negative or positive answer is available.[32]

Considerations Concerning Clinical Use of OCT Results

CONCEPT OF INTACT SURVIVAL

In the management of pregnancies at risk for UPI, our philosophy is based upon the concepts not only of perinatal survival, but of survival without damage. If the placenta is functioning sufficiently well to normally oxygenate the fetus (as determined by a negative OCT), the chances are extremely small (3.9 per 1000 fetuses) that IUFD will occur during the 7 subsequent days (Table 4.1). This information is of tremendous value in supporting a policy of nonintervention in cases where fetal jeopardy is of great concern but where the fetus is not yet sufficiently mature for extrauterine survival. However, survival alone is a rather crude index of perinatal success. Schifrin and coworkers[47] have pointed out that a negative OCT is also valuable in predicting whether the fetus will tolerate labor occurring within 1 week of the test. They noted that only 3.0% of such fetuses developed recurrent late decelerations during labor. Analysis of the recent series (Table 4.1) lends some support to their contention; labor was tolerated without distress in the great majority of patients who had a negative OCT within 7 days of labor. However, the primary value of the negative OCT is to support a policy of nonintervention in pregnancies at risk for UPI. Other clinical tests, such as serial 24-hr urinary E_3 determinations, also can be very reassuring if they remain normal.[21, 23]

MEANING OF POSITIVE OCT

On the other hand, a positive OCT is far less reassuring. The early clinical reports support the contention that a positive OCT is ominous.[26, 34, 40, 44, 46, 48] In most of the recent reports, clinicians have considered the positive OCT as indicating fetal jeopardy and have acted accordingly to hasten delivery. More recently, Freeman and associates[16] reported on an analysis of 390 patients, 66 of whom had at least one positive OCT, the remaining 324 having no OCT positive. They showed significantly more adverse results for the positive OCT perinates with respect to low E_3 values, stillbirths, 5-min Apgar scores, IUGR and neonatal morbidity. These differences were all significant at a probability of less than 0.001. The recent blinded study of Schifrin and coworkers[47] also suggests that the positive test identifies the fetus in jeopardy.

It seems reasonable to conclude from these data that the great majority of perinatal morbidity and mortality derives from perinates who will manifest a positive OCT. The average fraction of patients eventually exhibiting a positive result in the recent studies is 11.6% (Table 4.1). It is with this small fraction of those patients at risk for UPI that we believe intervention should be considered in most cases.

The threshold for intervention should always be tempered with all clinical information. This information includes other tests of fetal well being, fetal maturity studies and an assessment of the neonatal support facilities.

ESTRIOL DETERMINATIONS

For more than a decade, 24-hr urinary E_3 measurements[23] have been the standard test for fetal well-being. Although frought with difficulties of inadequate urine collections, interfering medical conditions and medications, unreliability in certain high risk situations and need for frequent determinations, this test, when normal, is still considered highly reliable for following most pregnancies at risk for UPI.[21] This and other hormonal studies are covered in detail in another chapter.

FETAL MATURITY STUDIES

A frequent problem when considering delivery of one of these high risk fetuses is that of functional maturity. Although many tests have been described which correlate with fetal age, in reality the greatest threat to the survival of the premature infant is that of pulmonary immaturity, the cause of idiopathic respiratory distress syndrome (IRDS). The tests which correlate most closely with the functional pulmonary maturity of the fetus are those which measure some aspect of amniotic fluid surfactant. At this time, the most widely used and best studied of these is the lecithin to sphingomyelin (L/S) ratio, first described by Gluck and associates.[20] If their technique is followed precisely, a qualification which because of its complexity does not always occur, an L/S ratio of 2.0 or greater correlates nearly always with an infant who will not succumb to IRDS in the nursery. Ratios less than 2.0 do not always mean that IRDS will develop, but the chances of its development rise as the L/S ratio decreases below this value. We utilize this test in judging functional pulmonary maturity and consider it to be reliable, even in diabetes mellitus, where the L/S ratio frequently matures later than in nondiabetic pregnancies. It is to be noted that even a fetus at term occasionally has an immature L/S ratio and thus is at risk for developing IRDS. Therefore, those tests (such as ultrasonic cephalometry) which correlate well with fetal age do not necessarily correlate with lung maturity. Perinatal asphyxia for any reason occasionally can cause depression of surfactant production and respiratory distress, even when the prior L/S ratio is 2.0 or greater.

NEONATAL SUPPORT FACILITIES

Oxytocin challenge testing is begun at such time as a pathologic result would cause the clinician to act positively upon this result. In general, weekly testing is begun at 34 weeks of gestation. In those cases where serious problems are manifest before 34 weeks (such as severe chronic hypertension or IUGR), we occasionally began testing as early as 28 weeks. In these cases where early intervention may be considered, the adequacy of the neonatal support unit must carefully be considered. In the highly sophisticated neonatal units staffed by our pediatric colleagues, 28 weeks is currently the approximate gestational age limit at which consideration may be given to pregnancy intervention for fetal indications. An attempt to improve the chances of a 1000-g perinate by delivery in a center with 24-hr neonatal physician coverage and the capacity for infant ventilation and blood gases may be much more realistic than delivery of this infant in a hospital without these sophisticated facilities and personnel.

INSUFFICIENCY OF PLACENTAL NUTRITIVE FUNCTION

The OCT is considered to be an evaluation of basal fetal oxygenation only and to give no information regarding the nutritive or other placental functions.[14, 34] Although the various functions of the placenta obviously are interrelated, one function may be deranged more than another.[39] An example might be the fetus with clinically and ultrasound-confirmed IUGR whose weekly OCT's remain negative. Certainly, many such fetuses will exhibit positive OCT's, but all will not.[16, 17, 35, 47] Although with a negative OCT anoxic fetal death is unlikely, the advisability of allowing such a fetus to persist in a nutritionally deficient environment is unknown at this time. One must also consider the possibility of chronic intrauterine infection or genetic abnormality in deciding upon management in such cases of IUGR in which the OCT is negative.

CHOICE OF PATIENTS FOR DELIVERY

A schematic of our recommendations for high risk pregnancy management based upon the OCT is presented in Figure 4.7. As noted, we consider the negative test to be very reassuring and repeat it only every 7 days. In many cases, spontaneous labor may safely be awaited. However, if other clinical considerations suggest earlier delivery, this can be effected without fear of IRDS at such time as the L/S ratio is mature (≥ 2.0). Even with L/S maturity documented, one should consider waiting until about 38 weeks in order to diminish the chances of other potential problems of prematurity in the neonate, such as hyperbilirubinemia, poor feeding and apnea. Moreover, unless clinical factors demand earlier delivery, a cervix favorable for induction can be awaited in those patients with weekly negative OCT's. Obviously, all of these factors must be weighed in the management decisions for each patient.

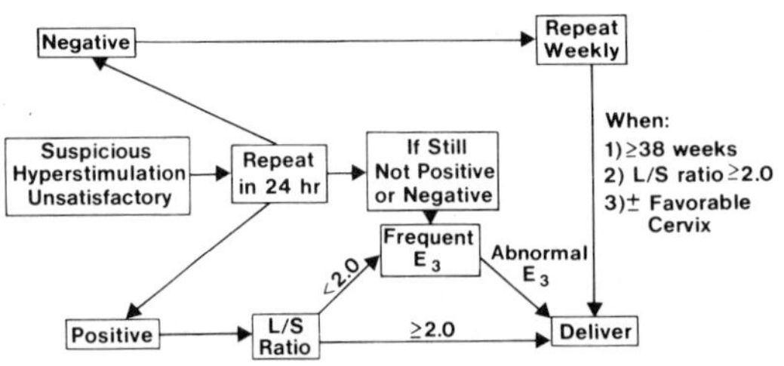

Figure 4.7. Clinical use of the oxytocin challenge test. L/S, lecithin/sphingomyelin; E_3, estriol.

For the three inconclusive OCT interpretations (suspicious, hyperstimulation and unsatisfactory), the test is repeated the next day; if still no definite positive or negative interpretation is possible, then 24-hr urinary E_3 levels are utilized, the frequency of their collection depending upon the clinical disorder (daily for insulin-dependent diabetes mellitus,[21] two or three times weekly for other indications). Attempts to obtain a positive or negative OCT result are continued.

The management of the positive test depends primarily upon the L/S ratio. If it is mature the perinate is delivered. If the L/S ratio is immature, a significant risk exists for either intervention or nonintervention: a risk of neonatal death from IRDS for early delivery; a risk of IUFD for inaction. Under these circumstances of a positive OCT and immature L/S ratio, we advise hospitalization, persistent lateral positioning and daily urinary (or more recently plasma) E_3 measurements. If the E_3 levels are normal and rising, then L/S maturation is awaited. If the E_3 measurements are abnormal, the infant is delivered regardless of the L/S ratio. We consider that on finding two abnormal tests (OCT, E_3) indicative of UPI, the perinate has a better chance of survival in the nursery than in the uterus. Fortunately, the delivery of a low L/S infant for these reasons is an infrequent event: only two infants have died from IRDS among those positive OCT perinates so managed in our combined experience.[16, 32]

Of course, in order to effectively interpret urinary E_3 values, a backlog of several previous values is necessary. In order to have such a backlog of serial E_3 measurements when a critical need arises for their availability (positive or inconclusive OCT), these data must have been collected previously.

ROUTE OF DELIVERY

When a decision to deliver is made, the delivery route is predicated upon the standard obstetric indications and the Bishop score[3] of the cervix (Figure 4.8). We believe that, in the presence of a somewhat favorable cervix and if no other obstetric conditions contraindicate, a trial of carefully monitored labor is justified. Preparations are made for possible cesarean section. Before rupturing fetal membranes and connecting internal monitoring equipment, the mother is turned to and kept in the lateral position; oxygen is administered by mask.[1] Freeman and associates[16] found that under these conditions 24% of patients with a positive test showed no late decelerations during labor. In the study of Huddleston and coworkers,[32] labor was tolerated without late decelerations by 38% of the positive OCT patients allowed to labor. These so-called false positive tests may have several possible explanations.

FALSE POSITIVE OCT

First, the patients with positive OCT's are given standard treatment for UPI (persistent lateral positioning; mask oxygen) on admission to the labor floor and before membrane rupture and internal monitor placement. Such treatment likely allows some fetuses with borderline oxygenation to overcome marginal deficiencies and to tolerate a controlled labor. Second, the uterine hemodynamics after membrane rupture may be subtly changed so as to improve IVS profusion. Third, with external monitoring during the OCT, the intensity and duration of contractions and/or the level of the baseline intrauterine pressure may be greater than appreciated. Such unappreciated abnormalities may at times decrease transplacental oxygen transfer below the critical level, even in some normal patients. Fourth, although a strong attempt is made to prevent poor IVS perfusion due to aortocaval compression during the OCT, subtle changes in this perfusion may occur and not be reflected in the brachial artery pressure. Which, if any, of these possibilities is involved is uncertain.

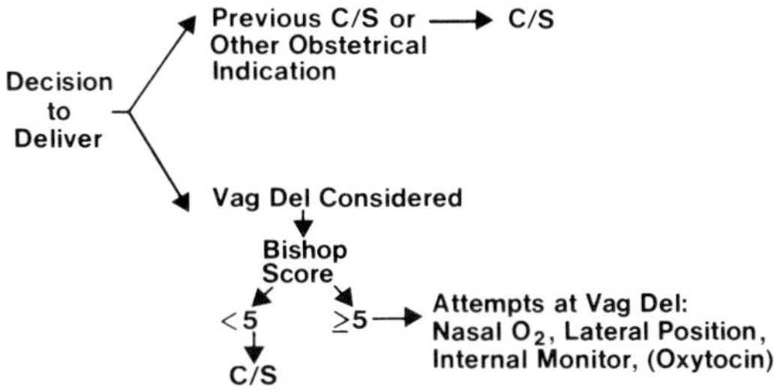

Figure 4.8. Choice of delivery route for patients with a positive oxytocin challenge test. C/S, cesarean section; Vag Del, vaginal delivery.

ACCELERATION WITH FETAL MOVEMENT

In an attempt to clarify which patients with positive OCT's will tolerate labor, attention has been directed toward the use of AFM noted before or during the OCT as a possible discriminator. AFM was earlier described by Hammacher and coworkers[26] and by Kubli et al.[34] Schifrin and associates[47] noted that AFM during the OCT accurately predicted tolerance of labor. Rochard and colleagues[45] claimed that fetuses demonstrating AFM during baseline observation uniformly tolerated labor well. It was suggested on this basis that such nonstressed FHR monitoring be the primary test for fetal respiratory function and that only those fetuses not demonstrating AFM on nonstressed monitoring be subjected to an oxytocin challenge.[47] This concept was supported by a retrospective study by Trierweiler and coworkers,[49] who noted no positive OCT's in those cases where AFM was noted during baseline observation.

Subsequently, we have become concerned about this approach by finding that some fetuses with AFM during a baseline recording will develop a positive OCT after oxytocin is added.[6, 32] Braly and Freeman[6] noted that AFM seen during a positive OCT was not a reliable indicator of subsequent tolerance of labor. They did, however, find that a positive OCT without AFM uniformly identified those fetuses which would not tolerate labor. We also have heard of a recent case of IUFD in a diabetic patient who had a normal nonstressed test (AFM) but was not given an oxytocin challenge.[18] It is probably fair to state that a question remains as to whether simple observation of the baseline FHR for AFM, although valuable in terms of time savings to patients and personnel, will be as accurate as the OCT or E_3 levels in defining fetal well-being. This concept deserves further study.

VAGINAL OR ABDOMINAL DELIVERY

Several investigators have recommended immediate cesarean section for positive OCT patients who have mature L/S ratios.[11, 12, 27] We strongly feel that safe vaginal delivery is possible for many of these patients under the conditions alluded to above. A possible exception to this is that group of patients in whom no AFM is demonstrable during a positive OCT.[6] In those who develop distress, cesarean section can be performed expediently with the expectation of good neonatal outcome. Once the decision to deliver is made, however, efforts toward that end should begin promptly. Freeman and associates[16] reported three positive OCT patients in whom IUFD occurred while plans were being made for cesarean section.

CONCERN OVER SUSPICIOUS OCT

Although positive tests often are preceded by suspicious tests, the great majority of suspicious tests are not positive when retested.[32] Thus, the suspicious test should not be used to influence clinical management. It should be ascertained that a test which appears suspicious is associated with adequate uterine activity. If not, then the oxytocin infusion rate should be increased until three adequate contractions occur within 10 min. Only if the late decelerations remain intermittent under these conditions should the suspicious interpretation be given.

OTHER DEFINITIONS OF POSITIVE TEST

Although most OCT reports define recurrent late decelerations as constituting a positive test, some reports note that variable decelerations, baseline tachycardia, baseline bradycardia and/or diminished beat-to-beat variability are used for defining a positive test.[26, 46, 48] Using the management plan based upon the late deceleration concept (Figure 4.7), we have seen little reason to change. Three cases of unusual deceleration patterns, all eventuating in perinatal mortality, have been reviewed.[17] In two of these, a variant deceleration pattern defined as "atypical variable deceleration" was noted. In this probably ominous pattern, the deceleration is followed by acceleration. Variable decelerations themselves are seen uncommonly in OCT tracings. When seen, they should raise the suspicion of oligohydramnios and associated cord entrapment. Primarily because of artifactual FHR variability inherent in most external monitoring techniques, the evaluation of baseline variability is of little clinical usefulness.[6] Baseline FHR variability may assume more significance for OCT interpretation as more experience is gained with external fetal ECG techniques.

SAFETY OF OCT

Justifiable concern exists over whether the administration of oxytocin for the OCT may induce premature labor in some of these patients. However, experience in three large series has shown that only one of those patients with a fetus less than 38 weeks of gestational age commenced labor and delivered within 48 hr of an OCT.[14, 32, 51] Another three patients delivered prematurely within this time period but had demonstrated adequate spontaneous uterine activity without oxytocin, so the drug was not administered.[32] Thus, they were probably in early subclinical labor at the time the FHR-UC recording was made. This safety record emphasizes the importance of a 15- to 20-min observation period before beginning oxytocin. It is possible that if this protocol is not rigidly followed, oxytocin might augment the spontaneous uterine activity to such a degree that more premature labors might occur.

TEST WHEN OXYTOCIN IS CONTRAINDICATED

In those pregnancies where a relative contraindication to the OCT exists and where amniocentesis is indicated, one can take advantage of the significant chance of being able to interpret the FHR-UC recording from adequate spontaneous uterine activity, provided the test is performed within a few hours of the amniocentesis. Less frequently, spontaneous uterine activity is adequate without prior amniocentesis.

CORRELATION WITH OTHER MEASURES OF FETAL DISTRESS

In the previously cited studies in which OCT results were not used to influence clinical management, other commonly accepted measures of fetal distress, such as repetitive late or severe variable FHR decelerations in labor, Apgar scores and perinatal mortality correlated highly with these OCT results.[44, 47] Urinary E_3 measurements have correlated well with OCT results in some studies,[16, 44] but not in others.[8, 12, 51] In the larger series where the OCT was used to influence intervention, the results were also correlated with FHR patterns of distress during labor.[16, 51] However, since constant vigilance was afforded those positive OCT patients allowed to labor, any ominous FHR pattern was quite promptly acted upon and the 5-min Apgar scores were generally very good. Indeed, in a large clinical study in which the OCT was used to influence clinical management of high risk pregnancies, the outcome was uniformly good for positive OCT patients.[32] None of the four perinatal deaths in the study could be related to possible flaws in the concept of nonintervention for weekly, negative OCT's. This is not to apologize for what some might consider "unnecessary" intervention, since we believe in the early monitor diagnosis of distress as an early indicator of fetal hypoxia, before significant hypoxia-induced metabolic acidosis. The delivery of a depressed infant, even after a positive OCT, is not necessary or even desirable to "prove" that active intervention is appropriate. The fact that high risk perinates, many of whom are expected to do poorly, do well under such management should be reasonable justification of its appropriateness.[2, 44, 47] Farahani and coworkers[12] have related this philosophy reasonably to the liberalized use of cesarean section for breech presentation, a much more common occurrence than that of the high risk patient with a positive OCT.

Pitfalls in Test Conduction and Interpretation and in Patient Management

HYPERSTIMULATION

As noted previously, a baseline observation period is most important. Also important in preventing hyperstimulation of the sensitive uterus is a low (0.5 milliunits per min) initial dose of oxytocin.[10, 47] This rate can be achieved accurately only by a mechanical flow-regulating device. Subsequent upward adjustments of this dosage should be at intervals (10 to 15 min) infrequent enough to allow adequate observation of the effects of the previous dosage increase. In some studies, higher initial doses were used, and these studies may have been responsible for some of the unfavorable results obtained.[5, 9] In our experience, very rarely is it necessary to use a dosage higher than 8.0 milliunits per min to achieve the desired three contractions within a 10-min period.

CERTAINTY OF NEGATIVE INTERPRETATION

Since such reliance is placed upon a negative OCT, one must be absolutely critical in interpreting the test. Because recurrent late decelerations may be of very low amplitude, it is important to have a recording without artifactual variability of a degree which might obscure these subtle changes. If the absence of late decelerations cannot be determined with certainty, the test must be called unsatisfactory and repeated. It is again for this reason that a nurse specialist with no other distractions should be available to devote full attention to obtaining a high quality recording. There is at times a reluctance to interpret a test honestly which is not clearly negative, since that patient must be retested the next day. This reluctance must be avoided, lest errors be made.

ADHERENCE TO 7-DAY TEST INTERVAL

As noted previously, there have been several reports of fetal deaths within a week of a negative OCT.[4, 5, 12, 14, 33] Most of these possibly were explainable on some other basis than chronic uteroplacental respiratory insufficiency. Two occurred on the seventh day after the negative test; in another study, an unexplained IUFD occurred 10 days after a negative test.[32] It is obvious that certain complications, such as abruptio placenta, cord accidents and diabetic ketoacidosis may rather suddenly cause death in some fetuses, irrespective of the adequacy of uteroplacental respiratory function at the time of a recent OCT. Although the 7-day time interval was originally chosen arbitrarily, generally it has proved very reliable. It is possible that as more experience is gained, slightly less time between tests may prove more appropriate.

Advantages and Disadvantages of OCT

ADVANTAGES

The OCT exhibits certain advantages and disadvantages compared with other tests of fetal well-being. Among the advantages is that the only technical expertise necessary is that of understanding and adequately performing external fetal monitoring. Although most of these tests should be done on a scheduled basis by a specialist and in a separate facility as noted previously, the OCT can be performed by the concerned clinician at any hour, including late nights and weekends. The result is then immediately available, and the negative test permits a policy of nonintervention for one subsequent week. In contradistinction to urinary E_3 analyses, no background data are necessary for adequate OCT interpretation. In the outpatient who is prescribed bedrest, a once-weekly test perhaps will serve her better than having to travel more frequently to her clinic for urine (or serum) studies.

DISADVANTAGES

The disadvantages include a substantial investment of time, the test frequently taking 1 to 2 hr. This leads to considerable expense, although (because only weekly tests are required if negative) probably less than that of more frequently measured urinary (or serum) hormone values. A physician comfortable in interpreting the OCT records must be available at all times. Although very rare in our experience, a small chance of initiating premature labor or precipitating fetal distress by uterine hyperstimulation must be acknowledged. There is a significant incidence of equivocal recordings which must be repeated within 24 hr.

Perhaps the greatest disadvantage is that, because intrauterine pressure is not recorded, the fetal challenge cannot be exactly standardized. With external recording methods, this problem seems insoluble at this time.

Summary

The oxytocin challenge test is an evaluation of uteroplacental respiratory status. The test is performed on those high risk pregnancies which are also at risk for UPI. The test interpretation is based upon the physiologic principle that the response of the FHR to the hypoxic stress of uterine contractions is a reflection of basal fetal oxygenation. Those fetuses exhibiting a normal response (negative OCT) can, with a high degree of assurance, be expected to survive in utero for 7 subsequent days. Thus, the principal value of the OCT is that it can allow the physician caring for patients at risk for chronic UPI to avoid unnecessary, premature intervention. Within the smaller group of fetuses exhibiting repetitive late decelerations in response to uterine contractions (positive OCT) are most of those destined for IUFD, distress in labor and low Apgar scores. We advocate an aggressive approach in the management of these latter pregnancies for which the OCT is positive. We have found that if the cervix is favorable a significant proportion of those fetuses with positive tests are able to tolerate, under certain conditions, carefully monitored labor. These conditions include prophylactic administration of oxygen by mask and persistent lateral positioning of the mother. With the OCT we can probably better identify that small group of pregnancies in which many of the fetuses are in great jeopardy. There is need to define more exactly which fetuses with positive OCT's must be rescued from their hostile intrauterine environments, especially if fetal pulmonary maturity cannot be assured.

REFERENCES

1. Althabe, O., Jr., Schwarcz, R. L., Pose, S. V., Escarcena, L., Caldeyro-Barcia, R.: Effects on fetal heart rate and fetal Po_2 of oxygen administration to the mother. Am J Obstet Gynecol 98: 858, 1967.
2. Aubrey, R. A., Pennington, J. C.: Identification and evaluation of high-risk pregnancy: The perinatal concept. Clin Obstet Gynecol 16: 3, 1973.
3. Bisho, E. H.: Pelvic scoring for elective induction. Obstet Gynecol 24: 266, 1964.
4. Boehm, F. H., Braun, R. D., Growdon, J. H., Jr., Sherrell, J. W.: The oxytocin challenge test. South Med J 69: 884, 1976.
5. Boyd, I. E., Chamberlain, G. V. P., Fergusson, I. L. C.: The oxytocin stress test and the isoxsuprine placental transfer test in the management of suspected placental insufficiency. J Obstet Gynaecol Br Commonw 81: 120, 1974.
6. Braly, P., Freeman, R. K.: Fetal heart rate reactivity assessment for discrimination between a true and false positive OCT. Contemp Ob/Gyn (In press.)
7. Caldeyro-Barcia, R., Cusacuberta, C., Bustos, R., Giussi, G., Gulin, L., Escarcena, L., Méndez-Bauer, C.: Correlation of intrapartum changes in fetal heart rate with fetal blood oxygen and acid base balance. *Diagnosis and Treatment of Fetal Disorders*. Edited by K. Adamssons, New York, Springer-Verlag, 1968, p. 205.
8. Caldeyro-Barcia, R., Méndez-Bauer, C., Poseiro, J. J., Escarcena, L. A., Pose, S. V., Bieniarz, J., Arnt, I., Gulin, L., Althabe, O.: Control of the human fetal heart rate during labor. *The Heart and Circulation in the Newborn and Infant*. Edited by D. E. Cassels, New York, Grune and Stratton, 1966, p.7.
9. Christie, G. B., Cudmore, D. W.: The oxytocin challenge test. Am J Obstet Gynecol 118: 327, 1974.
10. Cooper, J. M., Soffronoff, E. C., Bolognese, R. J.: Oxytocin challenge test in monitoring high-risk pregnancies. Obstet Gynecol 45: 27, 1975.
11. Ewing, D. E., Farina, J. R., Otterson, W. N.: Clinical application of the oxytocin challenge test. Obstet Gynecol 43: 563, 1974.
12. Farahani, G., Vasudeva, K., Petrie, R., Fenton, A. N.: Oxytocin challenge test in high-risk pregnancy. Obstet Gynecol 47: 159, 1976.
13. Freeman, R. K.: Obstetric management of the diabetic patient. Contemp Ob/Gyn 1(1): 58, 1973.
14. Freeman, R. K.: The use of the oxytocin test for antepartum clinical evaluation of uteroplacental respiratory function. Am J Obstet Gynecol 121: 481, 1975.
15. Freeman, R. K., Depp, R., Huddleston, J. F., Spellacy, W. N.: The enigma of prolonged pregnancy. Contemp Ob/Gyn 7(3): 116, 1976.
16. Freeman, R. K., Goebelsmann, U., Nochimson, D., Cetrulo, C.: An evaluation of the significance of a positive oxytocin challenge test. Obstet Gynecol 47: 8, 1976.
17. Freeman, R. K., James, J.: Clinical experience with the oxytocin challenge test. II. An ominous atypical pattern. Obstet Gynecol 46: 255, 1975.
18. Gabbe, S. G.: Personal communication.
19. Gaziano, E. P., Hill, D. L., Freeman, D. W.: The oxytocin challenge test in the management of high-risk pregnancies. Am J Obstet Gynecol 121: 947, 1975.
20. Gluck, L., Kulovich, M. V., Borer, R. C., Brenner, P. H., Anderson, G. G., Spellacy, W. N.: Diagnosis of respiratory distress syndrome by amniocentesis. Am J Obstet Gynecol 109: 440, 1971.
21. Goebelsmann, U., Freeman, R. K., Mestman, J. H., Nakamura, R. M., Woodling, B. A.: Daily urinary estriol assays in the management of the pregnant diabetic woman. Am J Obstet Gynecol 115: 795, 1973.
22. Goodwin, J. W., Dunne, J. T., Thomas, B. W.: Antepartum identification of the fetus at risk. Can Med Assoc J. 101: 458, 1969.
23. Green, J. W., Jr., Touchstone, J. C.: Urinary estriol as an index of placental function. Am J Obstet Gynecol 85: 1, 1963.
24. Greiss, F. G., Anderson, S. G.: Uterine blood flow during labor. Clin Obstet Gynecol 11: 96, 1968.
25. Hammacher, K.: Früherkennung intrauteriner gefahrenzustände durch electrophonokardiographie und fokographie. *Prophylaxe Frühkindlicher Hirnshäden*. Edited by R. Elert, K. A. Hüter, Stuttgart, Georg Theime Verlag, 1966, p. 120.
26. Hammacher, K., Hüter, K. A., Bokelmann, J., Werners, P. H.: Foetal heart frequency and perinatal condition of the foetus and newborn. Gynaecologia 166: 349, 1968.
27. Hayden, B. L., Simpson, J. L., Ewing, D. E., Otterson, W. N.: Can the oxytocin challenge test serve as the primary method for managing high-risk pregnancies? Obstet Gynecol 46: 251, 1975.
28. Hoebel, C. J., Hyvarinen, M. A., Okada, D. M., Oh, W.: Prenatal and intrapartum high-risk screening. I. Prediction of the high-risk neonate. Am J Obstet Gynecol 117: 1, 1973.
29. Hon, E. H.: Additional observations on "patho-

logic" bradycardia. Am J Obstet Gynecol 118: 428, 1974.
30. Hon, E. H., Quilligan, E. J.: Classification of fetal heart rate. II. A revised working classification. Conn Med 31: 779, 1967.
31. Huddleston, J. F., Hurst, J. M.: Modern management of the pregnant diabetic. J Med Assoc State Ala 44: 614, 1975.
32. Huddleston J. F., Sutliff, G., Carney, F. E., Jr., Flowers, C. E. Jr.: Oxytocin challenge test for antepartum fetal assessment. Am J Obstet Gynecol (In press.)
33. Klapholz, H., Burke, L: Intrauterine fetal demise with a negative oxytocin challenge test. J Reprod Med 15: 169, 1975.
34. Kubli, F. W., Kaeser, O., Hinselmann, M.: Diagnostic management of chronic placental insufficiency. *The Foeto-Placental Unit.* Edited by A. Pecile, C. Finzi, Amsterdam, Excerpta Medica Foundation, 1969, p. 323.
35. Low, J. A., Pancham, S. R., Worthington, D.: Fetal heart deceleration patterns in relation to asphyxia and weight-gestational age percentile of the fetus. Obstet Gynecol 47: 14, 1976.
36. Myers, R. E.: Threshold values of oxygen deficiency leading to cardiovascular and brain pathological changes in term monkey fetuses. *Oxygen Transport to Tissue,* Edited by D. F. Bruley, H. I. Bicher, New York, Plenum, 1973, p. 1047.
37. Myers, R. E., Mueller-Heubach, E., Adamsons, K.: Predictability of the state of fetal oxygenation from the quantitative analysis of the components of late deceleration. Am J Obstet Gynecol 115: 1083, 1973.
38. Nesbitt, R. E., Jr., Aubrey, R. H.: High-risk obstetrics. II. Value of semiobjective grading system in identifying the vulnerable group. Am J Obstet Gynecol 103: 972, 1969.
39. Parer J. T.: Normal and impaired placental exchange. Contemp Ob/Gyn 7(2): 117, 1976.
40. Pose, S. V., Castillo, J. B., Mora-Rojas, E. O., Soto-Yances, A., Caldeyro-Barcia, R.: Test of fetal tolerance to induced uterine contractions for the diagnosis of chronic distress. *Perinatal Factors Affecting Human Development.* Washington, D. C., Pan American Health Organization, 1969, p. 96.
41. Pose, S. V., Escarcena, L., Althabe, O., Schwarcz, R. L., Ibarra-Polo, A. A., Quintanilla, R., Caldeyro-Barcia, R.: The influence of uterine contractions on the partial pressure of oxygen of the human fetus. *Effects of Labour on the Foetus and Newborn.* Oxford, Pergamon Press, 1967, p. 48.
42. Poseiro, J. J., Méndez-Bauer, C., Pose, S. V., Caldeyro-Barcia, R.: Effect of uterine contractions on maternal blood flow through the placenta. *Perinatal Factors Affecting Human Development.* Washington, D. C., Pan American Health Organization, 1969, p. 161.
43. Ramsey, E. M.: Uteroplacental circulation during labor. Clin Obstet Gynecol 11: 78, 1968.
44. Ray, M., Freeman, R., Pine, S., Hesselgesser, R.: Clinical experience with the oxytocin challenge test. Am J Obstet Gynecol 114: 1, 1972.
45. Rochard, F., Schifrin, B. S, Goupil, F., Legrand, H., Blottiere, J., Sureau, C.: Non-stressed fetal heart cardiotachometry in the antepartum period. Am J Obstet Gynecol 126: 699, 1976.
46. Sánchez-Ramos, J., Santísimo, J. L., Pemán, F. C.: La prueba de la oxitocina en el diagnóstico del estado fetal anteparto. Acto Ginecol (Madrid) 22: 679, 1971.
47. Schifrin, B. S., Lapidus, M., Doctor, G. S., Leviton, A.: Contraction stress test for antepartum fetal evaluation. Obstet Gynecol 45: 433, 1975.
48. Spurrett, B.: Stressed cardiotocography in late pregnancy. J Obstet Gynaecol Br Commonw 78: 894, 1971.
49. Trierweiler, M. W., Freeman, R. K., James, J.: Baseline fetal heart rate characteristics as an indicator of fetal status during the antepartum period. Am J Obstet Gynecol 125: 618, 1976.
50. Tushuizen, P. B. T., Stoot, J. E. G. M., Ubachs, J. M. H.: Abnormal antepartum cardiotocograms in patients with placental insufficiency. Am J Obstet Gynecol 119: 638, 1974.
51. Weingold, A. B., De Jesus, T. P. S., O'Keiffe, J.: Oxytocin challenge test. Am J Obstet Gynecol 123: 466, 1975.
52. Willocks, J., Donald, J., Campbell, S., Dunsmore, I. R.: Intrauterine growth assessed by ultrasonic foetal cephalometry. J Obstet Gynaecol Br Commonw 74: 639, 1967.

RICHARD L. BERKOWITZ, M.D.
JOHN C. HOBBINS, M.D.

5

Ultrasonography in the Antepartum Patient

Introduction

Because ultrasound is a noninvasive diagnostic tool, it has been used in a variety of medical subspecialties. As technical experience increases and manufacturers produce more sophisticated machinery, the practical applications of this modality grow. Nowhere is this more true than in the field of obstetrics where ultrasound provides an opportunity to safely and accurately study the human fetus in utero. In addition to static data, we can now obtain dynamic information on single or serial examinations without exposing the mother or fetus to the risks associated with radiologic studies. Furthermore, the ultrasonic evaluation of an ongoing gestation has become an extremely useful adjunct to a number of special procedures. This chapter will review the ways in which ultrasound can be utilized to assist the obstetrician in his care of the fetus at risk.

Basic Principles of Ultrasound Scanning

Ultrasound in clinical practice is sound limited to frequencies in the range from 1 to 10 million cps (i.e., 1 to 10 MHz). Obstetric ultrasound examination is performed in the range of 2 to 5 MHz. Current methods employ the detection and analysis of reflected echoes of this high frequency sound. As it traverses the body, some of the sound is reflected back to its source by various tissue interfaces. The amount of energy reflected is a function of the orientation of the interface and the difference in acoustic impedance of the tissues involved. The sound pulses are transmitted and received by the same transducer, which is possible because of the relatively long pauses between transmissions. Most systems utilize pulses of 1 μsec fired 1000 times per sec, which means that sound is emitted only 1% of the time. There are several methods of displaying the reflected echoes. The first is A Mode (amplitude modulation), in which echoes are displayed as vertical spikes along the baseline of a cathode ray tube. The amplitude of the spike is proportional to the intensity of the reflected echo. The second method is B Mode (brightness modulation), in which echoes are displayed as a spot of light on the cathode ray tube, the brightness of which reflects the intensity of the reflected echoes. A two-dimensional picture of a given slice of the subject being studied is displayed, i.e., an echotomogram. The last is M Mode, a variation of B Mode in which information is provided for time-motion studies. This is used primarily for echocardiography.

A Mode scanning rarely is used alone in obstetric ultrasound because the anatomic information provided by a series of spikes is often difficult to interpret. When used in conjunction with B Mode scanning to provide the anatomic orientation, however, the A Mode can be used to measure amplitude and distance accurately.

There is a variety of ways to produce B scans. The most commonly used technique in obstetric work is the compound contact B scan. In this method the transducer is moved over the surface of the maternal abdomen, and the echo is displayed as a static picture on a cathode ray tube. Sine-cosine potentiometers in the transducer arm provide positional and directional orientation for the scan.

When conventional compound contact scanners are used and no storage of the image is maintained on the cathode ray tube, intensity modulation is obtained (i.e., the brightness of the points of light correspond to the intensity of the reflected echo.). When a storage tube is used, however, an arbitrary cut-off level is made, below which no echoes are represented and above which all echoes are of the same brightness. Because the storage tube is capable of representing only these two levels (i.e., on and off) its display is referred to as being bistable.

With the development of the scan converter in 1974, a major technologic advance was achieved. This device contains a matrix of elements, each of which is capable of exhibiting several levels of intensity. By coupling the scan converter to the cathode ray tube, it became possible to use compound contact scanning and produce a stored display with a wide range of intensity modulation. These various levels of intensity are displayed as different shades of gray in a black and white picture; therefore, this is referred to as "gray scale."

Real-time ultrasound has opened up a new dimension in diagnostic scanning. The principle of real-time is that multiple different echograms are taken in rapid succession and viewed on the same screen. If the transducer is held in a steady position, the "picture" that one observes shows motion of the object being studied. A commercially available real-time scanner made by the ADR company utilizes 64 transducers which are fired four at a time in a sequence which produces 40 images per sec. Since the images are not stored, the machine has gray scale potential. The advantage of real-time scanning is that a dynamic view of intrauterine life is instantaneously obtained. The disadvantages are that resolution is somewhat inferior to that of the compound scanners, and measurements are more difficult to obtain accurately. In centers using ultrasound for obstetric diagnosis, gray scale compound contact scanners and real-time are frequently employed in a complementary fashion.

Estimation of Gestational Age

The most frequent request made to an obstetric ultrasonographer is to determine the gestational age of a fetus. The importance of dating a pregnancy is obvious, especially in a high risk situation when intervention is being considered. Uterine fundal height and the date of the patient's last menstrual period frequently are misleading. Ultrasound has given us the means to assess gestational age with a high degree of accuracy.

The ultrasonic diagnosis of pregnancy can be made as early as 5 to 6 weeks after the last menstrual period when the gestational sac can be noted clearly within the uterine cavity. By 8 weeks, the fetus consistently can be discerned within the sac, and at 10 weeks fetal activity and heart beat can be observed with real-time equipment.

Robinson[46] has studied the crown-rump length of early gestations and has shown that this increases from 10 mm at 7 weeks to 85 mm at 14 weeks (Figure 5.1). Because of the mobility of the very young fetus, this measurement can be technically difficult to obtain. By using multiple sections to locate the correct obliquity for a true determination of the longest fetal axis, however, Robinson has demonstrated an impressive accuracy of plus or minus 3 days in dating these early pregnancies.

A somewhat less accurate but much easier way to assess first trimester gestational age is to divide the period from 6 to 12 weeks into 2-week intervals. At 6 weeks the sac will be about 2 cm in diameter and occupy one-third of the uterine cavity. At 8 weeks it occupies two-thirds of the space and at 10 weeks measures about 5 cm and fills the cavity. At 12 weeks the fetal head is detectable, and a biparietal diameter can be measured.

Measurement of the biparietal diameter (BPD) has become the accepted method of ultrasonically determining fetal age in the second and third trimester (Figure 5.2). A number of nomograms for biparietal diameters plotted against weeks of gestation have been published (Figure 5.3). These vary according to the population being studied, the method of measuring the scans (i.e., leading edge to leading edge vs. outer table to outer table) and the type of ultrasound machinery being used.

Since the fetal skull grows more rapidly in the second trimester than in the third, a

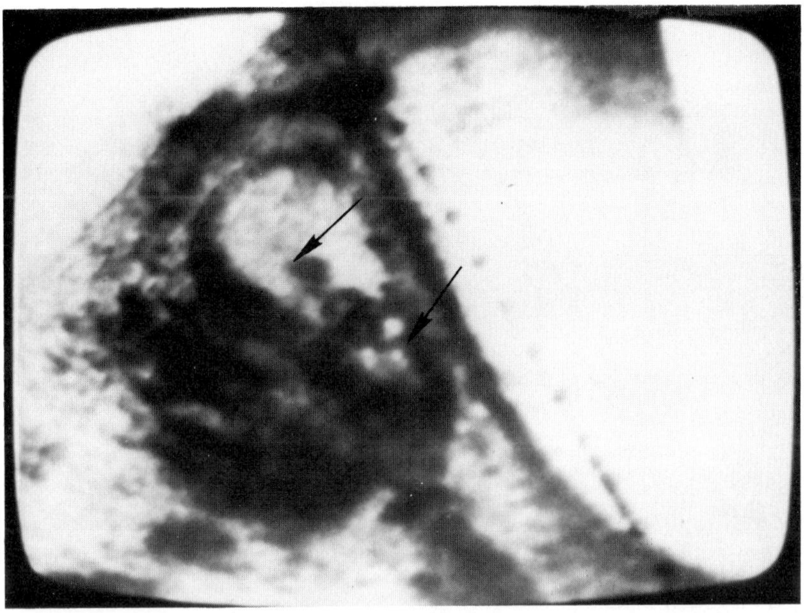

Figure 5.1. Crown-rump measurement of 25 mm, corresponding to a gestation of 9 weeks and 3 days.

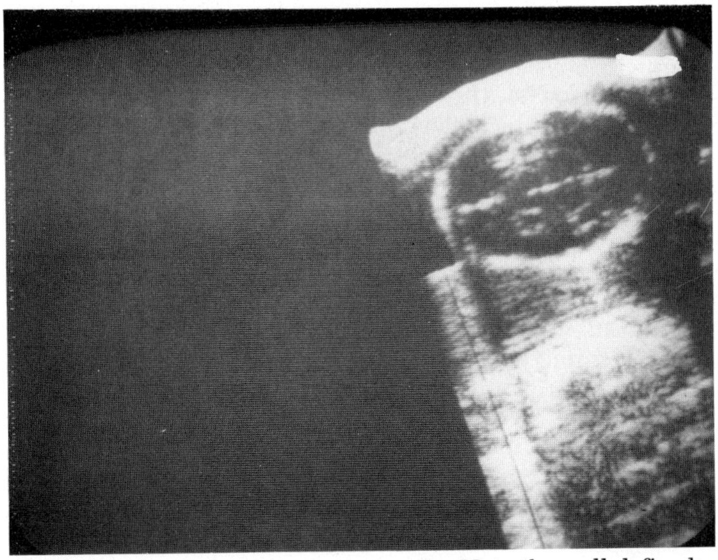

Figure 5.2. A biparietal diameter on gray scale. Note the well defined midline echo.

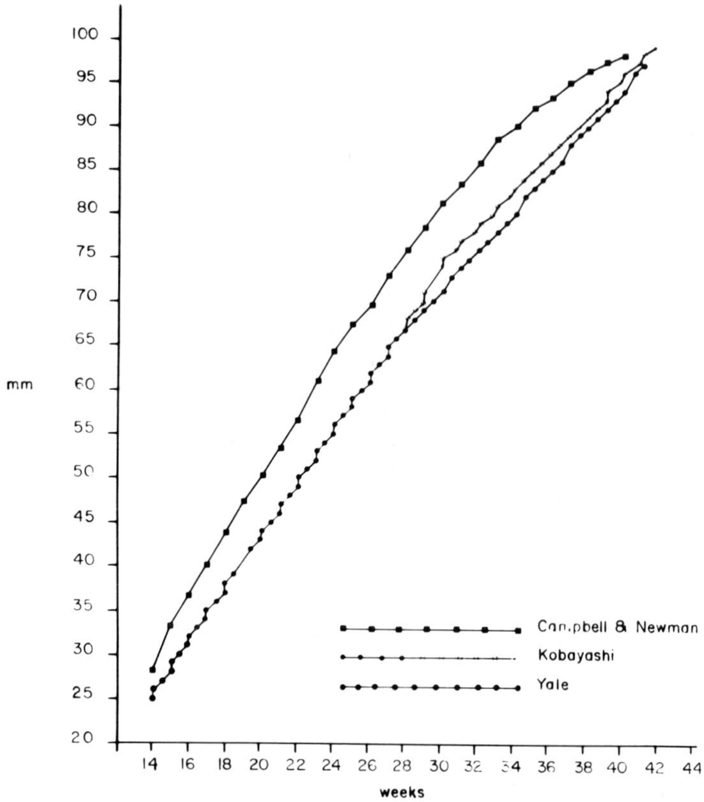

Figure 5.3. The relationship between BPD and gestational age (three different curves). Reprinted with permission from Anderson, G. G., Hobbins, J. C., Speroff, L.: Obstetrical management of the high risk patient. *Medical Complications of Pregnancy*. Edited by G. N. Burrow, T. F. Ferris, Philadelphia, W. B. Saunders Co., 1975.

given measuring error will have less significance during the former. For example, a 4-mm error corresponds to approximately 1 week of growth before 20 weeks and almost 4 weeks of growth after 34 weeks. Furthermore, although the biologic variation in biparietal diameter for a particular week of gestation is confined within relatively narrow limits up to 30 weeks, the splay increases after that time. It therefore follows that the most reliable predictions of gestational age can be made up to 30 weeks. Because the cranial growth is still relatively rapid between 30 and 34 weeks, assessments made during this period still can be useful. After 34 weeks, however, variation in skull size for each week, as well as the delayed rate of growth, make gestational age predictions considerably less accurate. This is also true of serial third trimester measurements to ascertain appropriate cranial growth. The ultrasonic evaluation of the potentially growth-retarded infant will be discussed in a separate section. The reader is referred to the article by Davison et al[12] for a detailed discussion of the statistic problems involved in assessing fetal age and growth by means of the biparietal diameter.

An excellent trend in most hospitals has been the attempt to document fetal maturity before elective inductions or repeat cesarean sections. The biparietal diameter can be a misleading index of maturity in gestational diabetics or in very large but otherwise normal babies. Therefore, if possible, in our institution we like to document pulmonic maturity with an amniotic fluid lecithin to sphingomyelin (L/S) ratio before elective deliveries. If there is no evidence of growth retardation and the biparietal diameter is less than 8.6 cm (our mean BPD for 37 weeks), the amniocentesis is postponed for 1 week. We have felt in the past that a BPD greater than 9.0 in a nondiabetic was compatible with fetal maturity. A recent retrospective study in our institution, however, has shown that 29% of the fetuses with BPD's of 9.0 or greater who underwent amniocenteses had L/S ratios less than 2.0. Furthermore, 40% of the fetuses with BPD's between 8.7 and 9.0 had L/S ratios less than 2.0. Because of the immature L/S ratios, none of these babies were delivered, and so we have no idea how many of them would have developed the respiratory distress syndrome (RDS). Recent work by Gluck et al[25] suggests that if phosphatidyl glycerol is present in the amniotic fluid of patients with immature L/S ratios, they will not develop RDS. Perhaps that is the situation in those patients with BPD's greater than 9.0 and L/S ratios less than 2.0. A study currently is being conducted to investigate this possibility.

In summary, the BPD is an accurate means of dating second and early third trimester pregnancies. Measurements greater than 8.5 cm do not correlate well with gestational age. It is, therefore, recommended that biparietal diameter measurements be made in the mid-second trimester for accurate gestational dating. A series of BPD's is better than a single determination since it provides a further check on the accuracy of a single reading and gives useful information about the rate of growth of the fetus.

Placenta

A great deal of information can be obtained by the ultrasonic study of the placenta. In addition to determining its location and size, an appreciation of subtle textural changes can be a useful tool in assessing some high risk pregnancies.

LOCATION

Various radioactive tracers and radiopaque dyes have been used to locate the placenta, but these techniques are invasive and potentially dangerous. The Doppler method can identify the area of placental implantation in most cases, but cannot accurately define its borders. This information is of no use in determining whether a low lying placenta is a previa and cannot indicate the best site for an amniocentesis. Ultrasonic scanning, on the other hand, permits accurate location of the placenta and in most cases clearly delineates its margins. Furthermore, it frequently permits identification of the site of cord insertion (Figure 5.4).

The placenta is easily identified by its juxtaposition with the amniotic fluid as well as by its appearance. The chorionic plate is visualized as a strong echo because of the fibrous tissue just beneath its surface. The characteristic placental texture will be discussed in more detail in a separate section.

Anterior placentas are very easy to identify. Reverberations from the abdominal wall can mimic an anterior placenta, but they exactly parallel the contour of the abdomen and often can be traced forward into the bladder. Posterior placentas do not differ acoustically from their anterior counterparts but can look different because of interference with the sonic beam by intervening fetal parts. This produces a phenomenon called shadowing. Frequently, different densities within a fetal part will cast shadows of varying intensity (i.e., bones within the soft tissue of a limb) (Figure 5.5). With real-time equipment where fetal movement can be appreciated, the shadowing will be seen to change in correspondence to fetal motion.

PLACENTA PREVIA

Although in all cases placental location can be determined by ultrasonic scanning, it is not always possible to be certain of the diagnosis of placenta previa. This is because of the difficulty of precisely locating the cervical internal os. When the bladder is full, the cervix usually lies at the point where the bladder-uterus interface intersects the posterior vaginal wall. As Sanders[49] has demonstrated, however, the internal os may lie somewhat above this point. Situations can arise, therefore, where a marginal previa is suspected but cannot be diagnosed with assuredness.

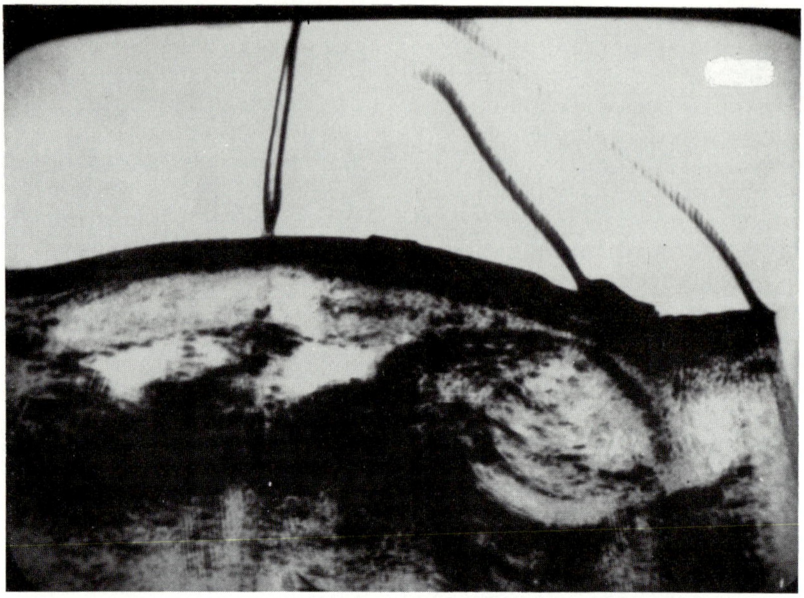

Figure 5.4. Anterior placenta with cord insertion.

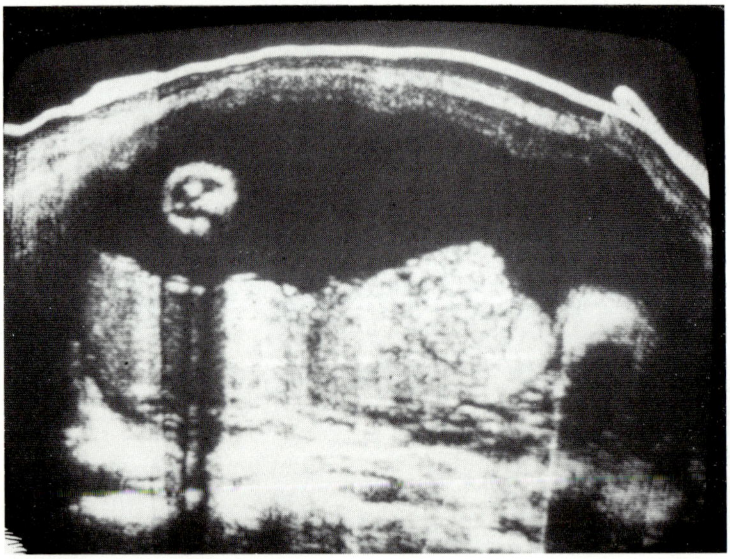

Figure 5.5. Shadowing of a posterior placenta. Note the differential effects of bone and soft tissue within the fetal limb.

When anterior placentas cross the cervix, interpretation of the scans is straightforward. Posterior placental margins are more difficult to appreciate, however, because of the shadowing described above. With a vertex presentation, one may observe a clear space between the fetal head and posterior uterine wall rather than seeing the placenta itself. If the distance to the uterine wall does not decrease when the fetal head is manually depressed, this space must be occupied by placental tissue. Another maneuver which can be attempted is to place the patient in Trendelenberg position and displace the head out of the pelvis. Rescanning will then clarify the issue (Figure 5.6, *A* and *B*). With transverse lies or breech presentations, movement of the fetal small parts immediately above the internal os can be observed with the real-time scanner. The space-occupying placenta will prevent the movement of limbs into this area if it is a previa.

It is now well established that the location of the placenta relative to the cervix changes as pregnancy progresses. This is probably related to the development of the lower uterine segment. Even some previas which completely cover the cervix have been demonstrated to "migrate" away and permit subsequent vaginal delivery. For this reason, it is recommended that asymptomatic previas which are discovered on routine scans be followed with repeat examinations at 2-week intervals. Under no circumstances should a diagnosis of placenta previa made more than 2 weeks before the time of delivery be used as the basis for an elective cesarean section.

TEXTURE

Early work with obstetric ultrasound contains very few references to placental texture. This is primarily because bistable scanning does not provide enough detail to appreciate subtle changes within the complex parenchymal structure of the placenta. The advent of gray scale scanning has permitted the ultrasonographer to observe these subtleties.

The homogeneous placental texture of the first trimester is replaced by a uniform speckled appearance in the second trimester. The chorionic plate becomes visible at approximately 18 to 22 weeks. In the second trimester there may be an apparent separation of the placenta from the uterine wall, making it appear as if it were detached and floating freely in the cavity (Figure 5.7). The explanation for this phenomenon is unclear, but it has no prognostic significance. Many of these pregnancies have been followed closely and have been demonstrated to progress uneventfully. Around 28 weeks of gestation, a number of echo-free spaces begin to appear within the placental tissue which persist and grow in diameter until term. These represent villous-free spaces which are probably the sites where maternal blood is being forced into the placental substance under significant pressure. As the needs of the growing fetus increase, these spaces may represent a physiologic increase in the amount of maternal blood made available to meet those demands. At 35 to 36 weeks, dense echoes begin to appear which represent the fibrous intervillous septas with some reticular calcification (Figure 5.8, *A* and *B*).

States of intrauterine stress can accelerate placental maturation prematurely. Some patients with severe pre-eclampsia have been demonstrated at 32 weeks to have placentas with the textural appearance one would expect at term (Figure 5.9). In addition, large placental infarctions can be appreciated ultrasonically by the demonstration of areas of concentrated echoes which are devoid of the normal patterns of healthy placental parenchyma. The reader is referred to the excellent review by Fisher et al[13] for a more detailed description of the ultrasonic study of the placenta.

VOLUME

Placental volume can be calculated by utilizing the formula for a planoconvex object. This is somewhat tedious, however; accurate longitudinal and horizontal measurements can be difficult to obtain because the placenta often extends from one uterine surface to another. Nonetheless, a visual estimation of placental volume can provide useful information. In fetal hydrops from Rh disease or other causes there will be an increase in placental volume because of edema (Figure 5.10). Enlarged placentas also can be observed with macrosomic infants of diabetic mothers and congenital syphilis. Decreased placental volume is noted in some patients with intrauterine growth retardation.

ABRUPTIO PLACENTA

Patients are frequently referred to the obstetric ultrasonographer to rule out the presence of an abruptio placenta. This diagnosis is rarely clear-cut unless the abruption is severe. The placenta will not

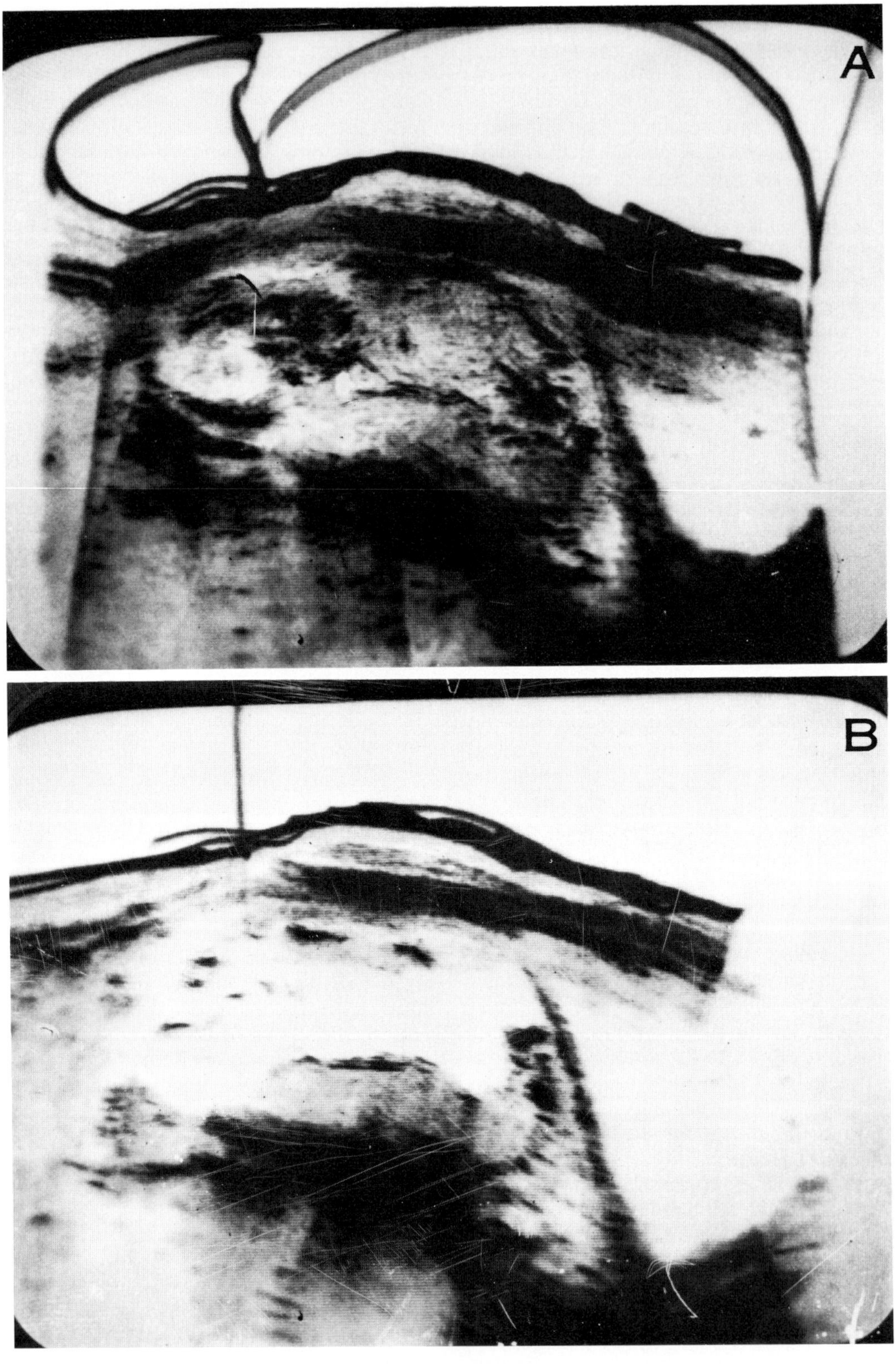

Figure 5.6. *A* posterior placenta with fetus obscuring the relationship of the margin to the cervix; *B,* Fetus moved revealing a clear-cut placenta previa.

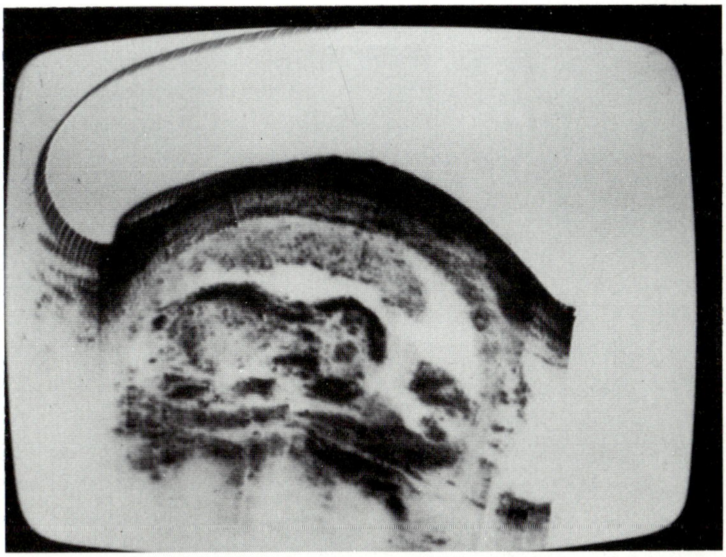

Figure 5.7. Second trimester pregnancy with apparent partial detachment of the placenta from the uterine wall.

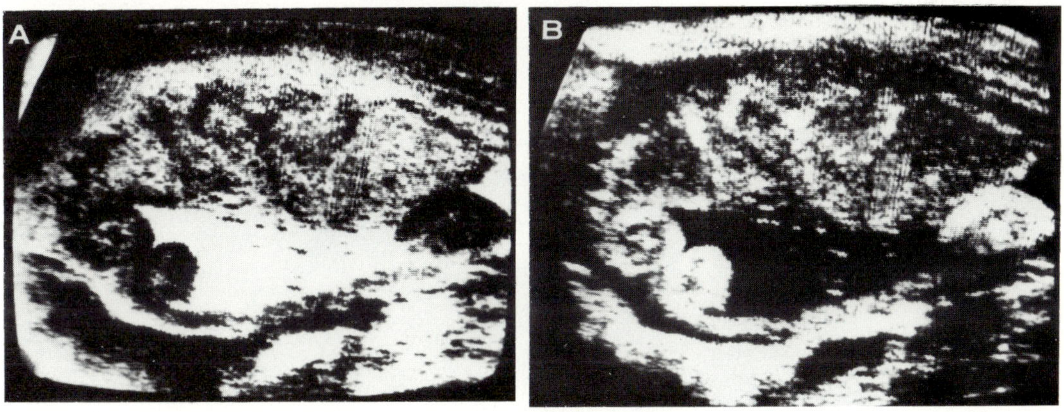

Figure 5.8. A, mature placenta (black on white); *B,* mature placenta (white on black). (Reprinted from Hobbins, J. C., Winsberg, F.: *Ultrasonography in Obstetrics and Gynecology*. Baltimore, The Williams & Wilkins Co., 1977.)

be visualized as being displaced from the uterine wall unless the separation is massive. In less dramatic situations, however, a small amount of retroplacental blood may dissect down to the lower portion of the uterus where it can be observed to accumulate under the membranes (Figure 5.11, *A* and *B*). The demonstration of blood elevating the membranes can be compatible with the normal progression of a pregnancy.

Multiple Gestation

Whenever one is evaluating a uterus which is large for dates, the possibility of a multiple gestation must be considered. This diagnosis can be somewhat difficult with ultrasound because of the restricted view offered by each scanning slice. Two circular structures can be identified as fetal heads when, in reality, they are the head and thorax of the same fetus. Conversely, one fetus can be a breech with its head very high or displaced laterally or a vertex which is deep in the pelvis, and in these situations a multiple gestation may be diagnosed as a singleton. The only way to avoid such pitfalls is to be meticulous in the scanning routine and be sure to trace

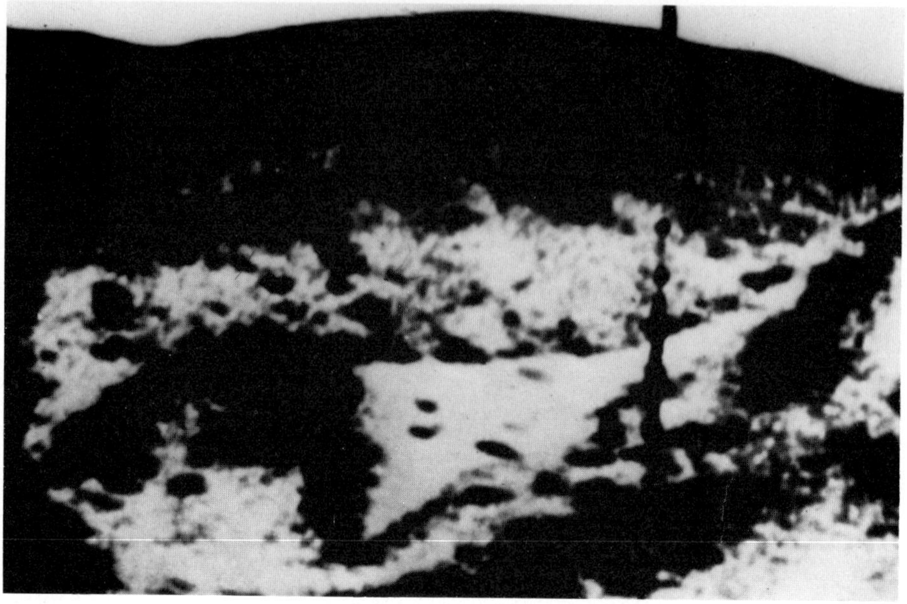

Figure 5.9. Placenta of a severe pre-eclamptic at 32 weeks. Note the premature textural maturation.

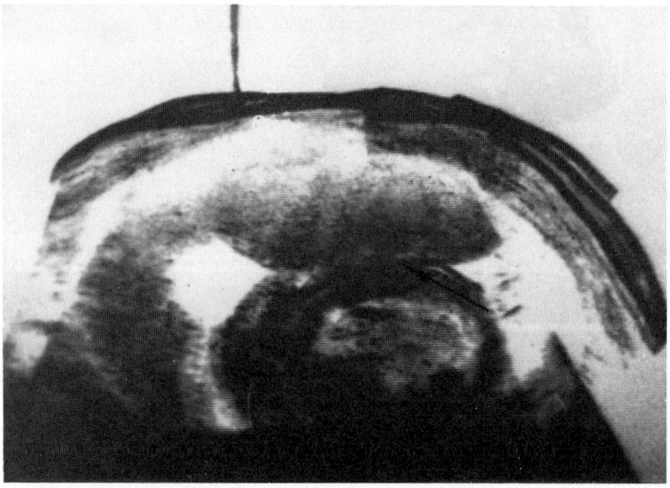

Figure 5.10. Hydropic placenta in a case of erythroblastosis fetalis. Note the double skull outline (arrow) indicative of scalp edema. (Reprinted from Hobbins, J. C., Winsberg, F.: *Ultrasonography in Obstetrics and Gynecology*. Baltimore, The Williams & Wilkins Co., 1977.)

the relationship of all visible parts to each other on multiple cuts. This is easier to do with the real-time scanner because the long arm of the transducer allows for orientation along the fetal longitudinal axis. Once the spine is traced, the relationship of two circular structures becomes obvious. When the gray scale is used, multiple slices must be made until all the various echoes become sorted out. Occasionally, two completely separated placentas will be observed (Figure 5.12). If the ultrasonographer is hasty in diagnosing or ruling out multiple gestations, he will eventually be

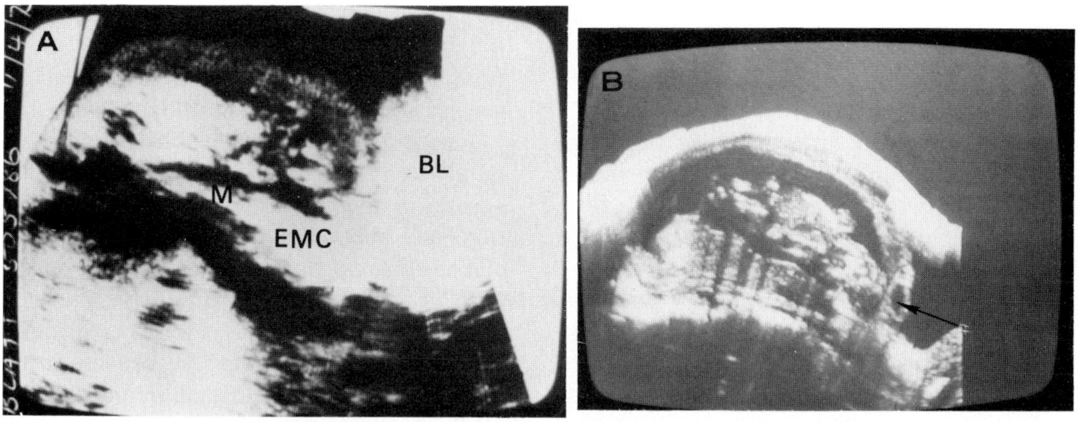

Figure 5.11. *A*, abruptio placentae with extramembranous dissection of blood and elevation of the membranes over the posterior aspect of the uterus. M, membranes; EMC, extramembranous clot; Bl, bladder. *B*, small abruptio placenta with a collection of blood beneath the anterior aspect of the lower uterine segment (arrow).

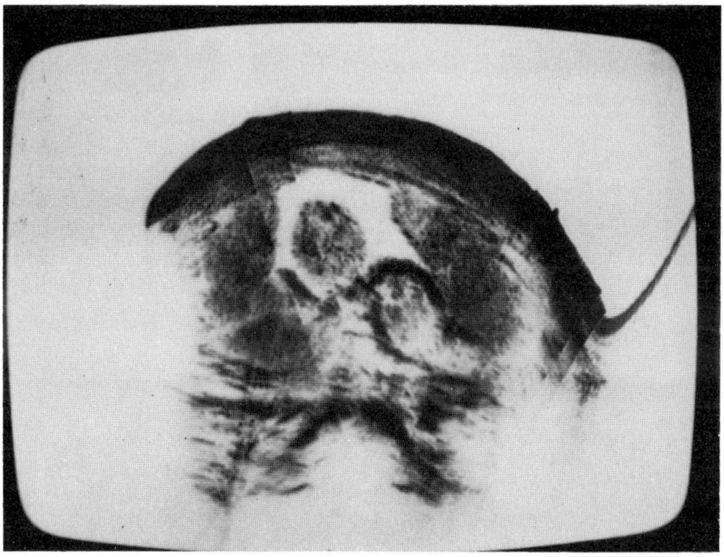

Figure 5.12. Twin gestation with two distinct placentas.

mistaken in his assessment. Few errors in obstetrics are more obvious at the time of delivery, and the referring physician can be counted on to report back to the ultrasonographer and to make reference to the case for quite some time thereafter.

Once a diagnosis of a multiple gestation has been made, the growth of the fetuses should be followed with serial scans. Monozygotic twins with a monochorial placenta can suffer from the twin-to-twin transfusion syndrome. In this situation the donor twin becomes growth retarded while the recipient twin becomes plethoric. Either twin can die in this high risk situation, and so it is important to make the diagnosis in utero as quickly as possible. The biparietal diameters should be no smaller than those of singletons up to 33 weeks of gestation, and there should be no more than a 3-mm difference in the BPD's of a normal set of twins. The diagnosis of a twin-to-twin transfusion can be suspected if the BPD's are discrepant, if there is a disparity in weight as predicted by abdominal circumferential measurements or if there are marked differences in the fetal urine production rates. Both of the latter techniques will be discussed in another section of this chapter. We have made the diagnosis of fetal death in a donor twin 4 weeks after noting a discrepancy between BPD's. After the demise of one twin, disseminated intravascular coagulation developed in the mother. Heparin was administered; when the maternal fibrinogen level had returned to an acceptable range, the patient was delivered of a healthy infant and a mascerated stillborn. The liveborn recipient in this twin-to-twin transfusion syndrome was hematologically normal because the placental vascular communication had been sealed off by thrombosis in the communicating vessels.

Amniocentesis in twins is made easier by utilizing ultrasonic localization of the intrauterine contents. Frequently, the membranes separating the two sacs can be seen with gray scale. After the first sac has been tapped, a small amount of dye such as indigo carmine is instilled to serve as a marker. If clear fluid is obtained in the next attempt, one can be sure that the second sac has been entered.

Locking is a situation which can occur when the first twin is a breech and the second is a vertex. The twins must be facing each other. During delivery, the chin of the aftercoming head is caught on the chin of the vertex. Fortunately, this only occurs about once in every 900 twin deliveries or once in every 85 breech-vertex combinations. The setup can be appreciated ultrasonically, but we would then advise a flat plate of the abdomen to better assess the relative position of the two chins.

Fetal Lie

Ultrasound can diagnose unerringly whether the fetus is in a vertex, breech, olique or transverse presentation. When the lie is transverse, one can determine whether the back is up or down. With a vertex presentation, the position of the occiput can also be ascertained (Figure 5.13).

Footling breeches can be differentiated from frank breeches, and frequently the location of loops of cord in the lower por-

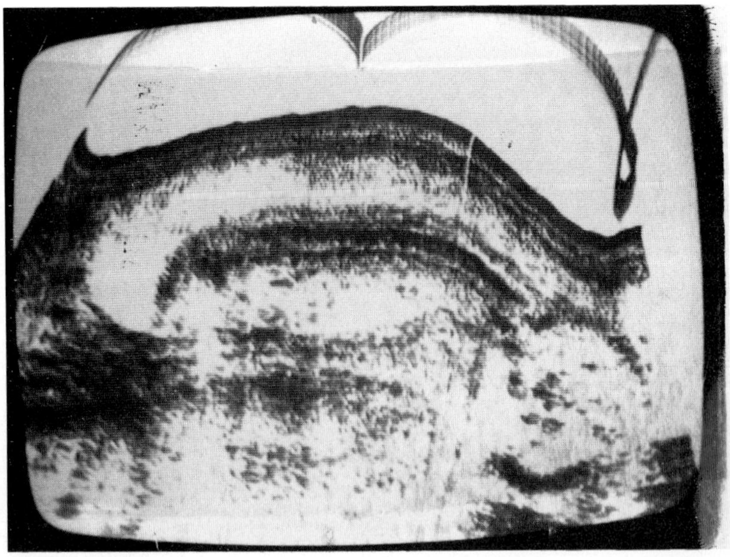

Figure 5.13. Vertex presentation. Since this scan was taken 1 cm to the left of the midline, the position is left occiput posterior.

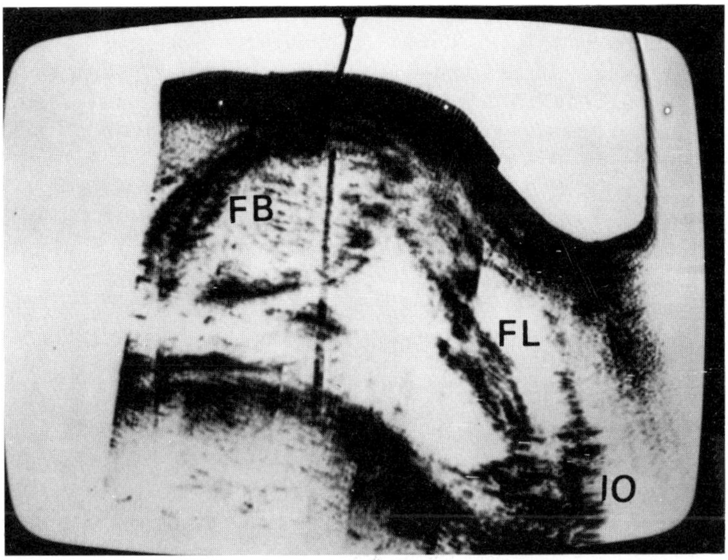

Figure 5.14. Footling breech. FB, fetal body; FL, fetal leg; IO, internal os. (Reprinted from Ablow, R. C., Taylor, K. J. W., Hobbins, J. C.: Diagnostic radiography and ultrasound in the perinatal intensive care unit. Clin Perinatol 2: 403–424, 1976.)

tion of the uterus can be demonstrated in the former instance (Figure 5.14). Extension of the head can be suspected ultrasonically, but this should be confirmed with a flat plate.

X-ray pelvimetry is necessary if any patient with a breech is to be delivered vaginally. These bony measurements cannot be made with the ultrasound equipment currently available. The size of the maternal pelvis, however, is only half of the story when one is considering the possibility of cephalopelvic disproportion. Although BPD's at term do not accurately correlate with fetal weight, we feel that a measurement of 9.6 cm or greater is associated with large enough babies that they should never by delivered vaginally as breeches, regardless of the size of the maternal pelvis. If the BPD falls between 9.3 and 9.6 cm, we would recommend vaginal delivery of a breech only if the pelvic measurements are very large.

Fetal Death

The classic findings of fetal death on x-ray examination include overriding of the fetal skull bones (Spaulding's sign), abnormal positioning of the fetal spine and gas in the fetal body. The latter sign is the earliest which can be detected radiographically and can be seen approximately 48 to 72 hr after the death has occurred. Garrett claims that he can detect "star-shaped echoes" which correspond to these collections of gas, but to our knowledge this has not been described by anyone using equipment available commercially in the United States. The Spaulding sign and abnormal fetal position are detectable ultrasonically, but these are relatively late phenomena occurring about 7 to 10 days after the demise.

The easiest and earliest way to diagnose fetal death is to demonstrate the absence of a fetal heart beat. This can be done reliably by an experienced ultrasonographer utilizing the real-time scanner.

Congenital Anomalies

The possibility of congenital anomalies should be considered whenever a patient has either increased or decreased amounts of amniotic fluid. The quantity of fluid can be determined most accurately by ultrasonically measuring the total intrauterine volume. This will be discussed further in another section. Gross deviations from the norm, however, can be picked up by a simple perusal of the ultrasound scans.

Cranial and spinal anomalies make up about 10% of all major fetal anomalies. The two most common entities in this category are anencephaly and hydrocephaly. After having a child with a neural tube defect, the chance of having another affected infant is about 5%. Hopefully, most of the women at risk for this occurrence will have second trimester amniocentesis for alpha-fetoprotein studies and will abort the affected fetuses. Unfortunately, however, about 95% of fetuses with neural tube defects are born to patients with no prior history of having affected children. This means that the clinician and ultrasonographer will continue to be confronted

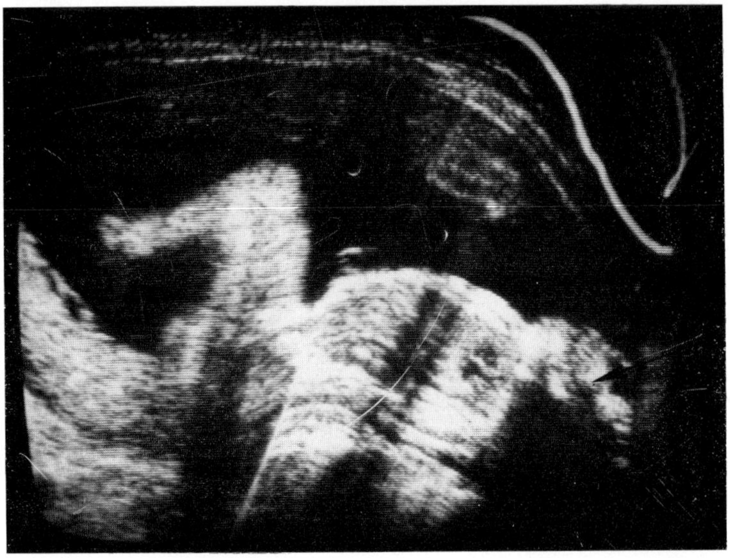

Figure 5.15. Anencephalic fetus. Arrow, primordial head. (Reprinted from Hobbins, J. C., Winsberg, F.: *Ultrasonography in Obstetrics and Gynecology*. Baltimore, The Williams & Wilkins Co., 1977.)

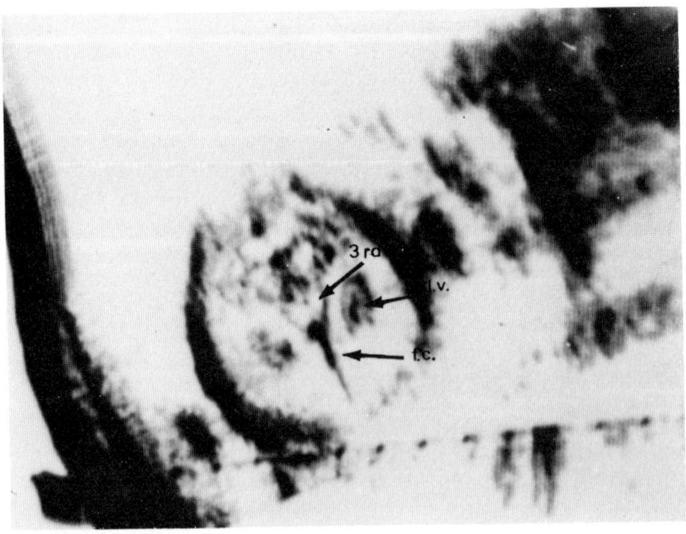

Figure 5.16. Ventricular system of the skull. 3rd v., third ventricle; l.v., lateral ventricle; f.c., falx cerebri.

by this diagnostic possibility until better screening tests are developed.

Anencephaly is frequently associated with hydramnios. This may be due to increased secretion from the exposed choroid plexus. With the real-time scanner, fetal activity and heart beat can be demonstrated, but only a primordial head will be present (Figure 5.15). The patient's bladder must be full in order to be sure that the fetal head is not being missed because it is deep in the pelvis. We believe that this diagnosis always should be confirmed with a flat plate of the abdomen before termination of the pregnancy.

The hydrocephalic fetus will have a BPD greater than dates and out of proportion to the fetal body. The cranial volume will vary depending on the severity of the condition, but a strong suspicion exists that, at least in some cases, abnormal biparietal diameters are not encountered until late in the gestation. There should be little question about the diagnosis with BPD's in excess of 10.5 cm. With gray scale, frequently it is possible to visualize the ventricular system (Figure 5.16). If this can be done in a case of hydrocephalus, one should be able to demonstrate enlargement of the third and lateral ventricles with secondary compression of cerebral tissue. One-third of hydrocephalic fetuses also have associated spinal defects. These can be very difficult to visualize ultrasonically. Up to 24 weeks of gestation, the fetal spine is relatively straight, and one can see the entire length in one scan. After this time, the fetal position is more tucked and many scanning cuts are necessary to see the spine along its whole length. It can be done, however, and Campbell has been able to diagnose at least five cases of spina bifida by taking multiple serial transverse scans.

The definition provided by the newer scan converters and real-time machines permit excellent visualization of a number of fetal structures. In addition to head, limbs, thorax and abdomen, one can see the rib cage, heart, stomach, umbilical vein, kidneys and bladder (Figures 5.17 to 5.20). Furthermore, with real-time, one can appreciate heart valve and wall motion, aortic pulsations and chest wall as well as diaphragmatic movements. The in utero diagnoses of fetal ascites, oomphalocoele, hydrops with scalp edema and polycystic kidneys all have been made ultrasonically at our institution (Figure 5.21). Others have reported diagnosing pulmonary and renal cysts as well as pericardial effusions in utero. Garrett and his group in

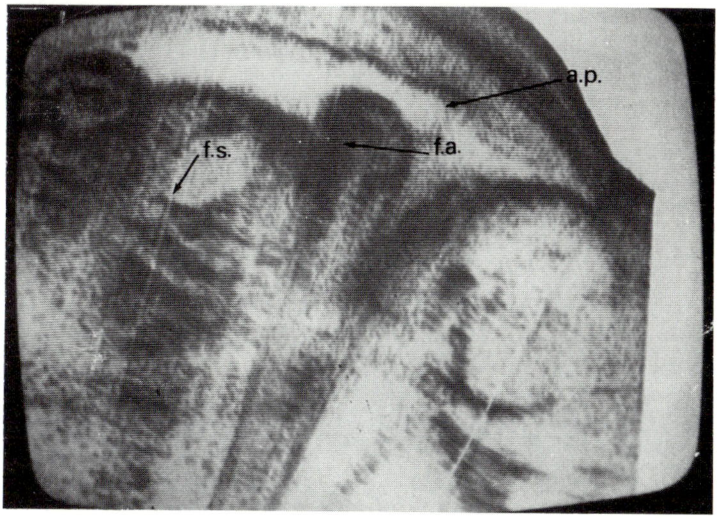

Figure 5.17. Vertex presentation with limbs and stomach visible. f.s., fetal stomach; a.p., anterior placenta; f.a., fetal arm. (Reprinted from Hobbins, J. C., Winsberg, F.: *Ultrasonography in Obstetrics and Gynecology*. Baltimore, The Williams & Wilkins Co., 1977.)

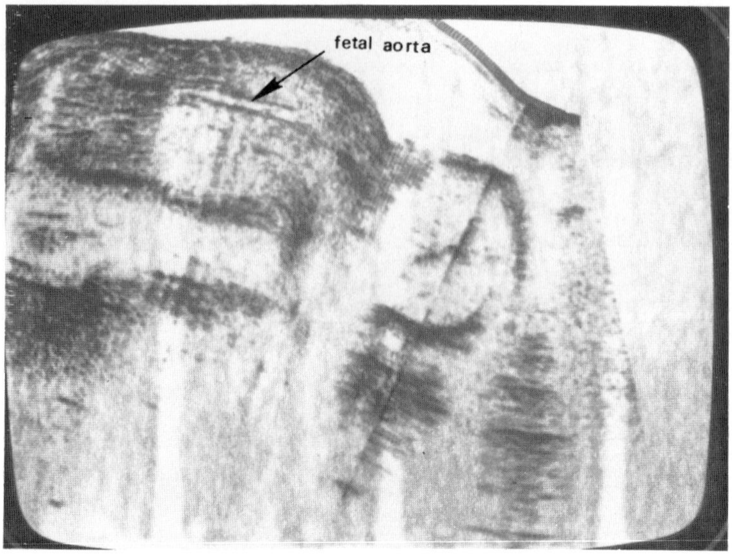

Figure 5.18. Vertex presentation with fetal ribs and aorta visible.

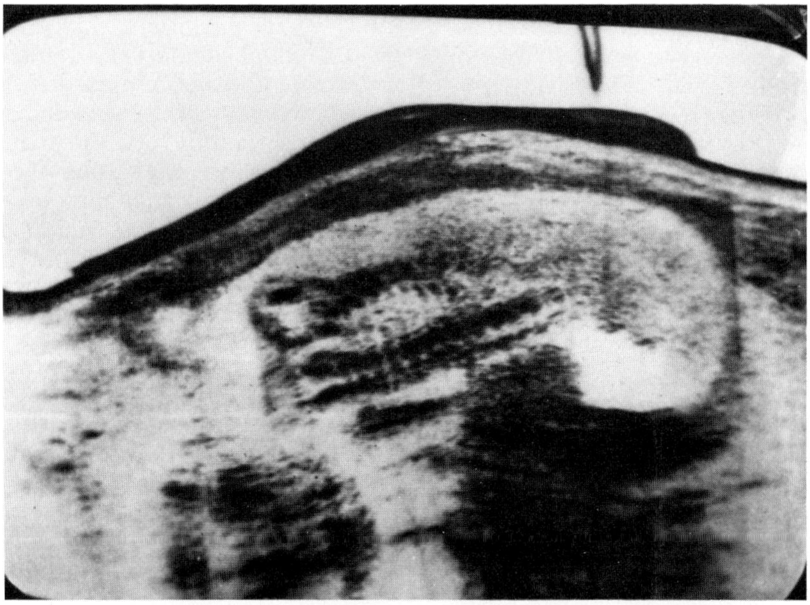

Figure 5.19. Fetal spine and ribs. (Reprinted from Hobbins, J. C., Winsberg, F.: *Ultrasonography in Obstetrics and Gynecology*. Baltimore, The Williams & Wilkins Co., 1977.)

Australia[14-16] have at their disposal sophisticated machinery which is not marketed in the United States at this time. With their equipment, they have been able to diagnose fetal hydrops with a teratoma of the lung, jejunal atresia, diaphragmatic hernia, and bilateral hydronephrosis secondary to urethral stenosis. Their equipment not only has the capacity to demonstrate such features as the fetal gallbladder, but also to mechanically and rapidly take multiple scanning cuts at short measured distances.

A word of caution should be inserted about the diagnosis of congenital anomalies. The interpretation of intrafetal structures is a relatively new development in ultrasonic scanning, and more expertise must be accumulated before confidently acting upon subtle findings. Fluid-filled loops of bowel or stomach can masquerade as hydronephrotic kidneys, and an otherwise healthy growth-retarded baby with a small bladder at the time of the scan can be confused with an infant with Potter's syndrome. The ultrasonographer must be sure of his diagnosis when he reports a congenital anomaly because a normal gestation might be terminated inappropriately if he is wrong.

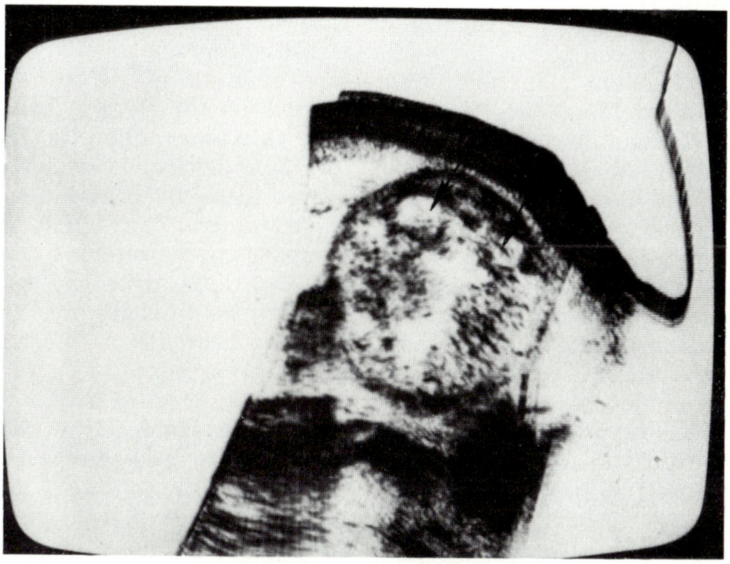

Figure 5.20. Normal kidneys (arrows).

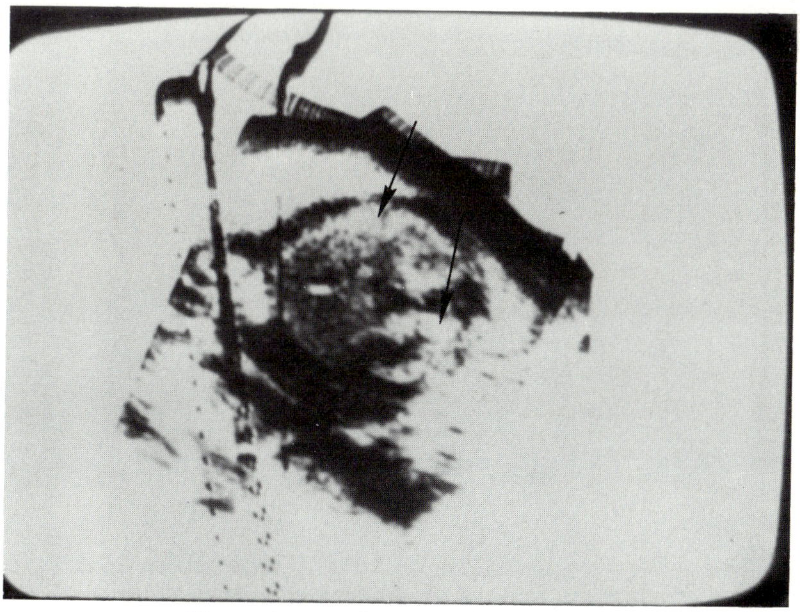

Figure 5.21. Polycystic kidneys (arrows).

Intrauterine Growth Retardation

Intrauterine growth retardation (IUGR) complicates 3 to 7% of all pregnancies in the United States. A baby is considered growth retarded when it is in or below the 10th percentile of mean weight for gestational age at birth. These babies have at least a 3-fold increase in perinatal mortality and are at significant risk for intrapartum asphyxia and neonatal hypoglycemia, acidosis, hypocalcemia and polycythemia. In addition, it is of concern that they may have developmental problems later in infancy. In order to change the course of this condition, IUGR must be diagnosed early in pregnancy, rather than at birth.

IUGR can be caused by maternal nutritional deficiency, diseases affecting placental capacity to transfer nutrients (e.g., toxemia, severe diabetes mellitus, etc.) or constitutional abnormalities of the fetus secondary to genetic aberrations, viral infections or exposure to biochemical agents. Campbell[6] has described two types of abnormal growth patterns in the human fetus. In approximately 25% of the IUGR babies he studied, both head and body were decreased symmetrically throughout the third trimester. Some of the fetuses in this group were anomalous. The remainder of the small-for-dates babies only showed decreased BPD growth late in the gestation. This phenomenon of "head sparing" resulted in asymmetric babies with disproportion between head and body.

In an ongoing study performed at the Yale-New Haven Hospital we have noted that in most cases of IUGR the fetus will initially demonstrate disproportionate slowing of body over cranial growth. The exception to this situation is the congenitally deformed fetus, which may demonstrate symmetric growth lag from the earliest examination. In all other cases, regardless of the etiology of the IUGR, it is very rare to see impaired BPD growth before 30 weeks of gestation. We have observed the following sequence of events in the development of IUGR. First there is a decrease in the amount of amniotic fluid present. This gives the fetus a crowded appearance on scanning. The next occurrence is decrease in the amount of body mass as represented by a disturbed head to body ratio (Figure 5.22). The circumference of the head at the level of the BPD normally exceeds that of the abdomen at the level of the umbilical vein until about 32 weeks. From 32 to 36 weeks these measurements are approximately the same, and for the remainder of the pregnancy the abdominal circumference is larger than that of the head. In the growth-retarded

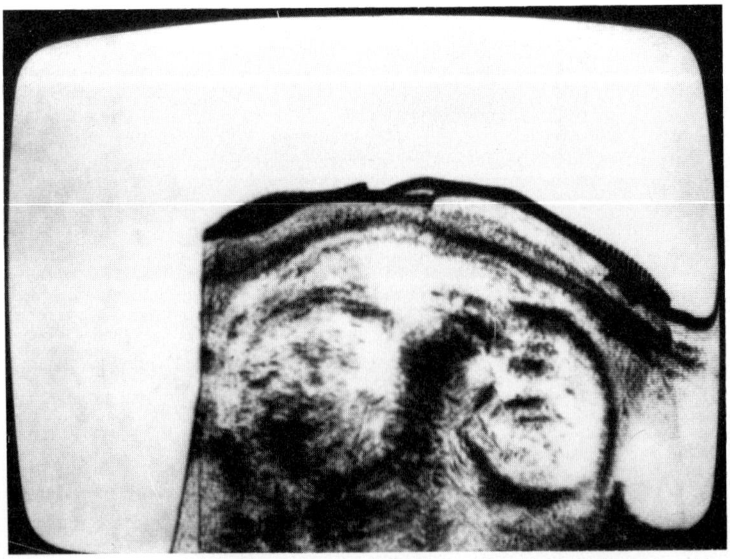

Figure 5.22. Intrauterine growth retardation with "crowding" and disproportion between head and body.

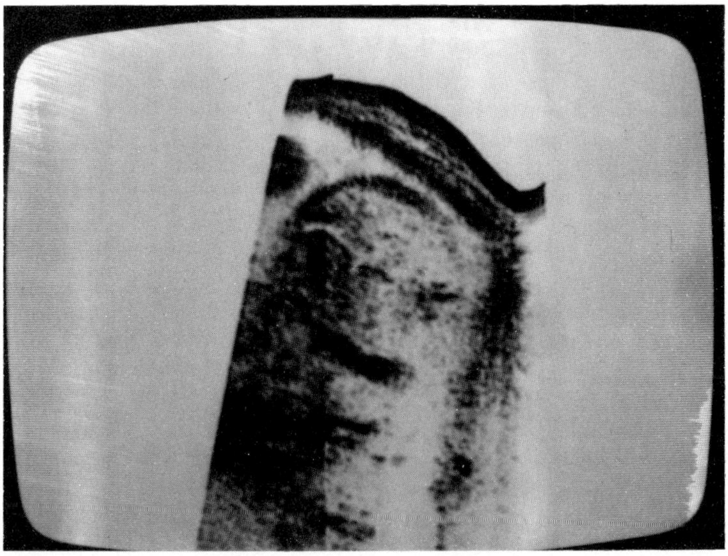

Figure 5.23. Fetal abdomen at the level of the umbilical vein. This is the site for obtaining circumferential measurements.

baby this proportionate increase in body size does not occur. Finally, if the growth-retarding process exceeds some ill defined fetal threshold, the growth of the head is decreased. This occurs in the most severely affected babies.

Fetal weight corresponds reasonably well to BPD's only up until about 30 weeks of gestation. Before this time, the biparietal diameter accurately assesses gestational age, and there is a good correlation between age and weight. For reasons mentioned earlier, the predictive accuracy of the BPD for gestational age is diminished after 30 weeks. Even more important is the fact that there are significant deviations from the mean weights of age during the last 10 weeks of pregnancy, and this is particularly true when there is asymmetric growth retardation. For these reasons, the biparietal diameter is a very crude tool with which to attempt an early diagnosis of IUGR.

By measuring the abdominal circumference at the level of the umbilical vein, fetal weight can be estimated with more accuracy than by using the BPD (Figure 5.23). Campbell[9] has constructed a nomogram for this relationship which gives a broad weight range in large babies but is considerably more accurate for infants weighing 2700 g or less. This nomogram requires extensive testing to see whether it applies to American populations and, more importantly, whether it is accurate in infants who are growth retarded. Preliminary results on normal patients at the Yale-New Haven Hospital are encouraging. It does seem that one can get a reasonable approximation of fetal weight for a given gestational age by measuring abdominal circumference.

Longitudinal, transverse and anteroposterior diameters of the fetal bladder can be measured on sagittal and transverse scans. The bladder volume can then be computed by utilizing the same formula described below for total intrauterine volume. By taking two sets of measurements 30 min apart, the hourly fetal urine production rate can be determined (Figure 5.24, *A* and *B*). Normal values for various gestational ages have been published, and patients with IUGR have been shown to have diminished rates. This is a time-consuming technique, however, and can be technically difficult to perform. At this time, it cannot be recommended as a routine part of the IUGR workup.

As mentioned above, the intrauterine contents are not affected in a parallel fashion by the growth-retarding process. Nevertheless, unless compensatory changes occur, a diminution of incremental growth of any of the component parts should be reflected by a decrease in the total intrauterine volume (TIUV). This is computed by ultrasonically measuring the greatest longitudinal (L), transverse (T) and anteroposterior (AP) diameters (Figure 5.25, *A* and *B*) and utilizing the formula for the volume of an ellipse

$$V = 4/3\,\pi\,(\frac{L}{2} \times \frac{H}{2} \times \frac{AP}{2}) = 0.5233 \times L \times H \times AP$$

Since the endpoints of the scans can be somewhat inexact, the TIUV measurement is not extremely precise. The method has been tested, however, by measuring the TIUV before and after tapping several patients with hydramnios. With volumes of fluid in excess of 1500 cc, the differential amount calculated was within 75 cc of the quantity removed.

A nomogram has been constructed at the YNHH for TIUV's plotted against weeks of gestation (Figure 5.26). To date, all of those infants whose TIUV's fell more than 1.5 SD below the mean were growth retarded at birth. All infants who were less than 1 SD below the mean were not growth retarded. The area between 1 and 1.5 SD was a "gray zone" in which some infants were growth retarded and others were not. Interestingly, those growth-retarded infants in this zone were symmetrically growth retarded and hence the most severely affected of the entire series. This is probably because the small BPD's secondary to cranial involvement in the deprivational process were not appreciated as such and, consequently, the pregnancies were dated as being earlier than they actually were. If the growth-retarded pregnancies in the gray zone were dated correctly, all of their TIUV's would have been well below 1.5 SD from the mean.

It is possible that a patient could have pure oligohydramnios with a normally developing baby. Since a large proportion of the uterine volume is comprised of amniotic fluid, this could result in a TIUV which was below 1.5 SD from the mean and a baby that was not growth retarded. We have not seen this situation yet, but it certainly could occur. We therefore recommend that BPD determinations be performed as early as possible when uterine size is not compatible with gestational age as calculated from the last menstrual period. If the BPD is 4 weeks less than the dates would suggest and the amount of fluid appears normal, then the dates are probably wrong. In any other situation the TIUV should be calculated and compared with the age as suggested by the BPD. If there is a discrepancy, abdominal circumferential measurements and head to body ratios should be determined. Serial scans should be performed thereafter to follow the progress of the pregnancy. When growth retardation is diagnosed, biophysical and biochemical parameters must be used to monitor fetal well-being, and delivery should be effected as soon as pulmonic maturity can be demonstrated. The inter-

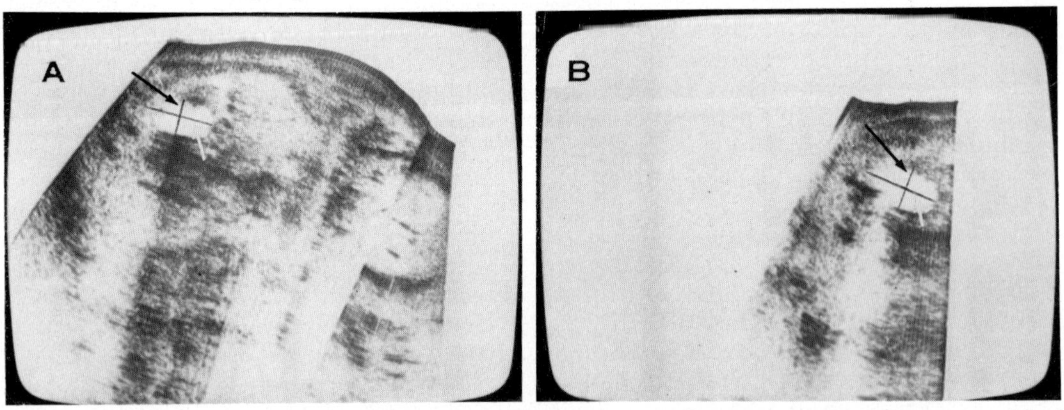

Figure 5.24. A, vertex presentation with longitudinal (white arrow) and AP diameters (black arrow) of the bladder marked (10:00 AM); *B*, same bladder at 10:20 AM.

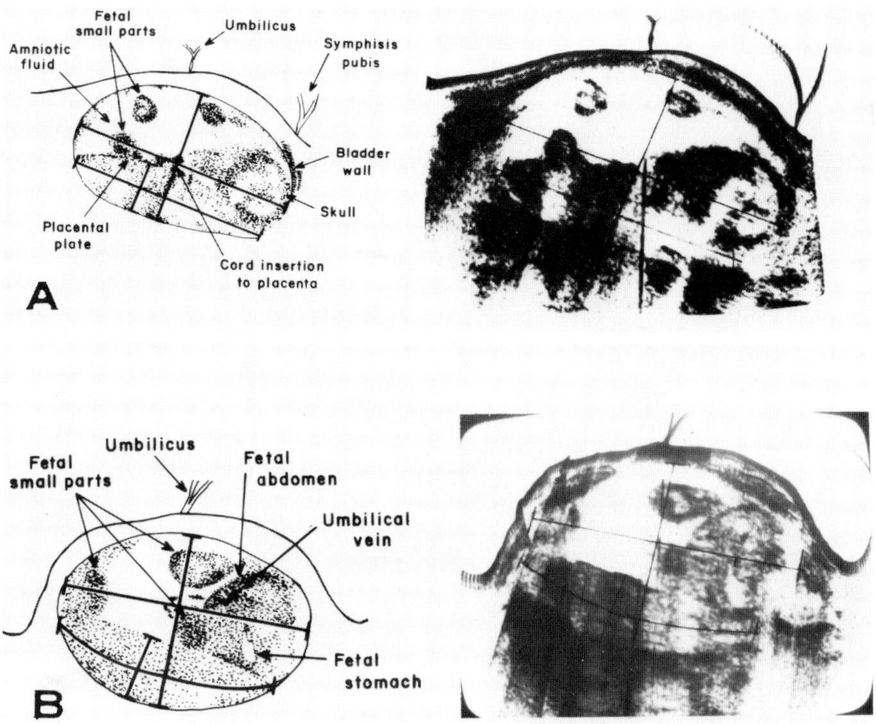

Figure 5.25. *A*, total intrauterine volume (sagittal scan); *B*, total intrauterine volume (transverse scan). (Reprinted from Gohari, P., Berkowitz, R. L., Hobbins, J. C.: Prediction of intrauterine growth retardation by determination of total intrauterine volume. Am J Obstet Gynecol 127: 255–260, 1977.)

ested reader is referred to the review article by Gohari, Berkowitz and Hobbins[17, 18] in which a more detailed description of our suggested management of the IUGR patient is presented.

Special Procedures

AMNIOCENTESIS

Amniocentesis is being performed more and more frequently these days for a variety of indications. In the second trimester, the procedure is usually done to obtain fluid for genetic studies. Cells are grown for 14 to 24 days from the fluid obtained, and then enzyme or karyotype investigations are performed. Most cell culture attempts are successful, and in those instances when they are not it is usually evident several days after the initial culture is started. For this reason, one can wait until 16 weeks of gestation to do the tap and be confident that the results will be back in time to perform an abortion, if that is appropriate. Before 16 weeks, the taps are technically more difficult to perform and offer more potential fetal morbidity. At 16 weeks, there should be approximately 175 cc of fluid in the amniotic sac.

At Yale-New Haven Hospital all second trimester genetic taps are performed in the ultrasound room. In 40% of the cases the placenta is anterior, but in half of these cases a placenta-free area can be found with ultrasound. When it is not possible to avoid the placenta, the cord insertion can be identified and a peripheral extension traversed rather than going through a central area which contains the largest fetal vessels. In addition, the fetal position is noted, and the tap is directed into an empty part of the uterus. If the fetus is lying under a placenta-free portion of the anterior uterine wall, it can be moved manually and the tap performed quickly. In our institution the incidence of bloody

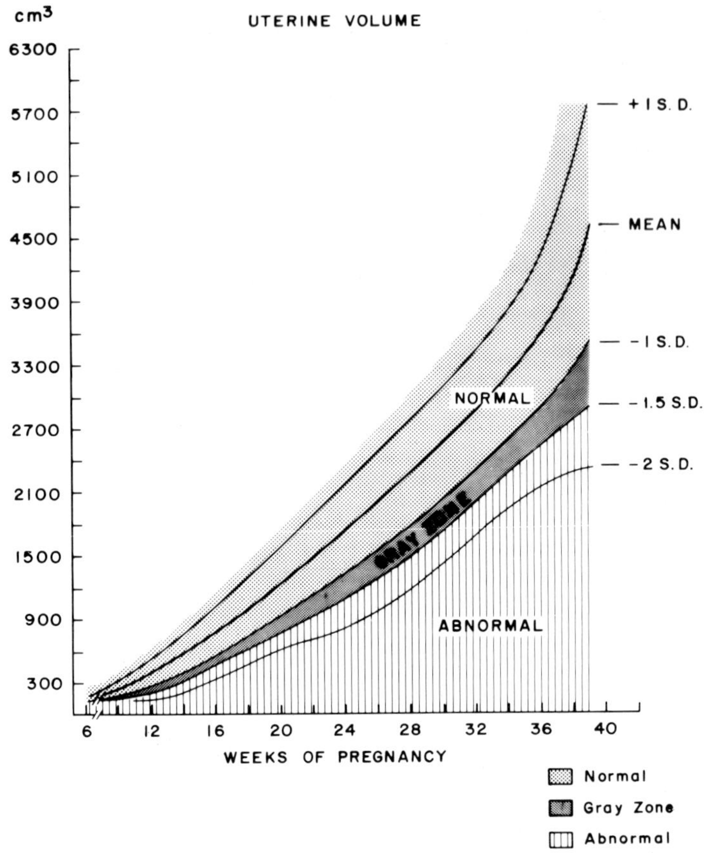

Figure 5.26. Total intrauterine volume vs. gestational age (Reprinted from Gohari, P., Berkowitz, R. L., Hobbins, J. C.: Prediction of intrauterine growth retardation by determination of total intrauterine volume. Am J Gynecol 127: 255–260, 1977.)

taps has been decreased 50% by the routine use of ultrasound.

A large multicenter collaborative study of second trimester amniocenteses has demonstrated the increased incidence of vaginal bleeding associated with increasing numbers of needle insertions into the uterus. Unfortunately, this study was unable to show a decreased number of insertions in cases where ultrasound was used as compared to patients having "blind taps." Despite this finding, we believe that ultrasound makes second trimester amniocentesis an easier and safer procedure. Subscribing to the principle that, when it comes to surgical manipulations, it is better to see what you are doing than to do it blindly, we will continue to do our midtrimester taps with the help of ultrasonic scanning.

Our technique involves the location of the amniocentesis site by longitudinal and transverse scanning. The site is marked on the patient's abdomen, and the scan is left on the viewing screen for reference (Figure 5.27). The depth to the center of the fluid pocket is measured, and after infiltrating the patient's skin with 1% lidocaine, a 9-cm long 22-gauge spinal needle with stylet is used and clear fluid usually is obtained. If the fluid is bloody, 2 or 3 cc are aspirated and discarded. This is repeated until the fluid clears, which usually happens very rapidly. Blood can interfere with cell culture growth and, if it is fetal in origin, can falsely elevate the alphafetoprotein levels. If the fluid has not cleared of blood after 8 or 9 cc are aspirated, a Kleihauer-Betke analysis for fetal cells should be made on the amniotic fluid. Fetal loss of significant quantities of blood is rare, but not impossible. It is good to remember that a given quantity of blood constitutes a greater percentage of the blood volume of a small fetus than a larger one (e.g., 1 cc represents 6% of the blood volume of a 16-week fetus and 15% of that of a 14-week fetus). This is why the potential morbidity of second trimester taps is greater in very early pregnancies than in those which are more advanced.

In the third trimester, amniocentesis is

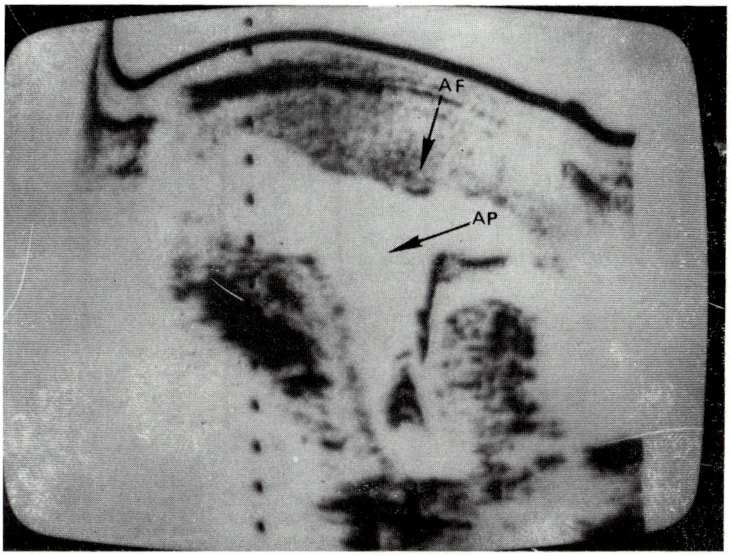

Figure 5.27. Amniocentesis site with marker perpendicular to skin surface. Dots are 1 cm apart. AF, amniotic fluid; AP, anterior placenta. (Reprinted from Hobbins, J. C., Winsberg, F.: *Ultrasonography in Obstetrics and Gynecology,* Baltimore, The Williams & Wilkins Co., 1977.)

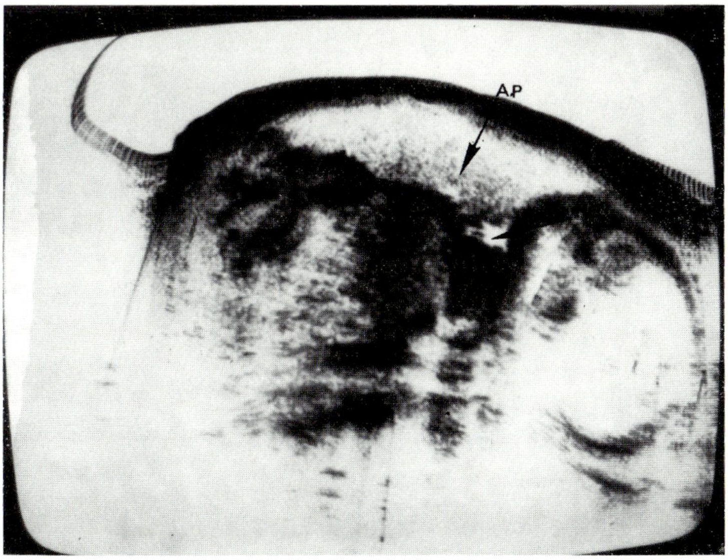

Figure 5.28. Sagittal scan. Vertex presentation with an anterior placenta (AP) and a nuchal cord (NC).

done to obtain fluid for culture, to test for indices of maturity, to follow the progress of Rh incompatible pregnancies and to look for the presence of meconium. With the aid of ultrasound, the operator can observe the position of the fetus, the location of pockets of fluid and the presence or absence of loops of cord in those pockets. Often the cord is observed next to or around the neck within a small collection of fluid (Figure 5.28). When such is the case, no attempt should be made to obtain fluid from the nuchal area. Blind tapping in this situation might well result in spearing the cord because of its inability to move away from the needle. In patients with oligohydramnios, we have been able to locate and obtain fluid from tiny pockets which simply would have been impossible to find without scanning. We have also been able to identify patients with so little fluid that amniocentesis was felt to be contraindicated. The advantages of using ultrasound to avoid hitting fetal vital parts, the cord and the placenta seem so obvious that they only need be mentioned.

INTRAUTERINE TRANSFUSION

Traditional techniques for transfusing the fetus in utero have required the use of multiple x-rays along with image-intensified fluoroscopy. Since patients often require several intrauterine transfusions during a given pregnancy, the total amount of radiation exposure can become a source of concern. By utilizing ultrasound to perform the procedure, the radiologic exposure to the mother and fetus is significantly reduced.

With careful scanning, the position of the fetal spine, bladder and umbilical vein are located. If the spine is up, the fetus can be manipulated until it is lateral or down. When this has been done, the angle of introduction of the needle is determined and the site of entrance marked on the maternal abdomen (Figure 5.29). The distance between the mark on the maternal abdominal wall and the center of the fetal abdominal cavity at a point between the umbilicus and the bladder is then calculated. The target point in the fetal cavity is electronically recorded as a mark on the A Mode oscilloscope (Figure 5.30). After infiltrating the maternal skin with 1% lidocaine, a 16-gauge Touhy needle is passed through a needle aspiration transducer which lies on the abdominal wall immediately over the site of entry. The tip of the needle emits an echo which is clearly visible on the A Mode oscilloscope. The needle

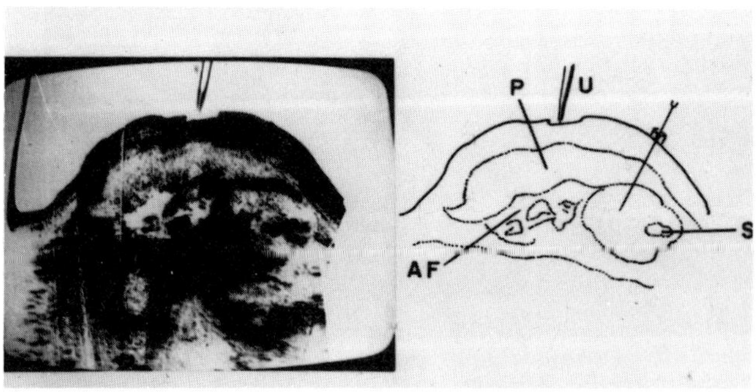

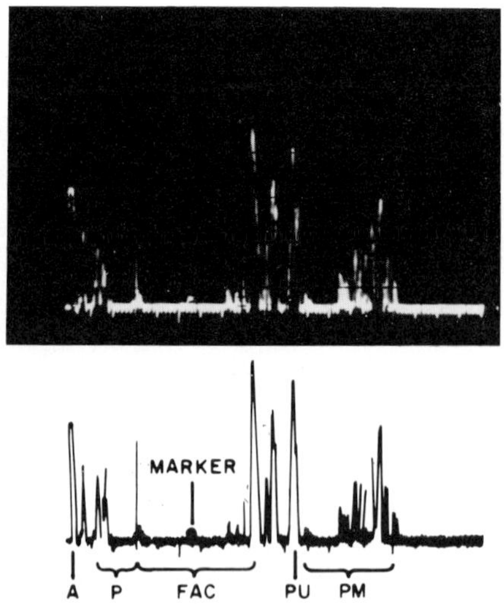

Figure 5.29 *(left)*. Transverse scan for an intrauterine transfusion.

Figure 5.30 *(right)*. A Mode scan for intrauterine transfusion. The marker is in the center of the fetal abdominal cavity. A, abdominal wall; P, placenta; FAC, fetal abdominal cavity; PU, posterior uterine wall; PM, posterior aspects of maternal tissue. (Reprinted from Hobbins, J. C., Winsberg, F.: *Ultrasonography in Obstetrics and Gynecology,* Baltimore, The Williams & Wilkins Co., 1977.)

is advanced until it is felt to enter the fetal abdomen and is pushed forward until it lies over the electronic marker on the A Mode screen. At this point 2 to 5 cc of radiopaque contrast media are injected, and with a few seconds of x-ray image intensification, the characteristic pattern of dye spilling around loops of bowel assures the operator that he is in the correct place. After this, the appropriate amount of Rh-negative blood is injected into the fetal peritoneal cavity. A more detailed description of this technique has been published by Berkowitz and Hobbins.[3]

FETOSCOPY AND FETAL BLOOD DRAWING

Studies on amniotic fluid are valuable because they are done on a substance which is one step removed from the fetus. There has been considerable interest, however, in getting even closer to the fetus itself in utero. Direct visualization would provide an opportunity to diagnose some types of congenital anomalies, and fetal biopsies could provide better material for cell culture and microanalysis. Finally, the ability to obtain fetal blood would permit the diagnosis of major hemoglobinopathies and provide white blood cells and plasma for a variety of studies.

A fiberoptic "needlescope" with a diameter of 1.7 mm has been marketed by the Dyonics Corporation, Woburn, Mass. This fits inside a cannula with a diameter of 2.2 mm, which is approximately that of a 14-gauge needle.

The area of the fetus to be observed or biopsied is located with ultrasound. The scope is introduced through a needle-aspiration transducer so that its tip can be seen on the A Mode oscilloscope. The optics of the system are such that the field of vision is very limited, and the operator must get extremely close to the object being viewed in order to see it clearly. The scope is, therefore, not good for a general overall surveillance of the fetus. It is capable, however, of visualizing the entire spine if it is introduced appropriately.

Skin biopsies are performed on the scalp. After scanning and introducing the scope through the needle aspiration transducer, an area completely covered with hair is located. Holding the cannula in place, the scope is then removed and a biopsy instrument inserted. With visualization on the A Mode, the few millimeters to the scalp are advanced, and a 1-mm biopsy is taken.

When the placenta is posterior or fundal, fetal vessels are easily visualized running over its surface. A cannula has been

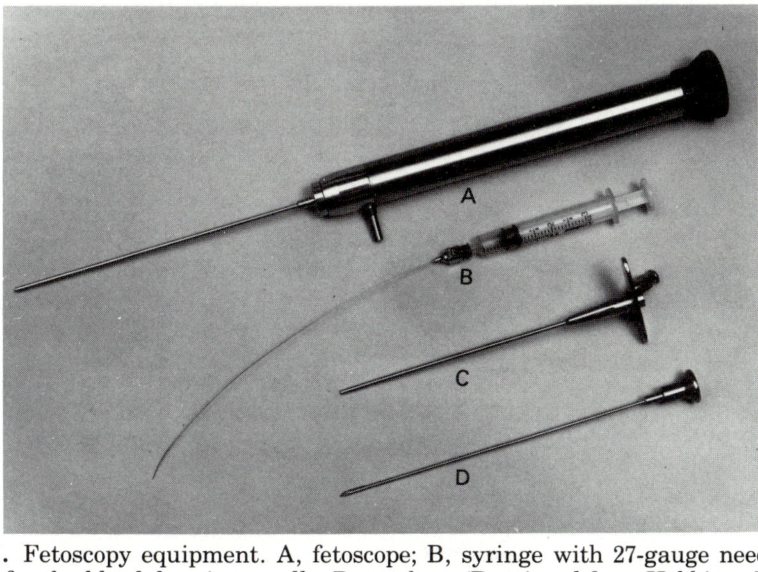

Figure 5.31. Fetoscopy equipment. A, fetoscope; B, syringe with 27-gauge needle; C, cannula with side arm for the blood drawing needle; D, trochar. (Reprinted from Hobbins, J. C., Mahoney, M. J.: Fetoscopy and fetal blood sampling: the present state of the method. Clin Obstet Gynecol 19(2), 1976.)

devised which admits the scope and has a side arm through which a 27-gauge needle can be inserted (Figure 5.31). The diameter of this cannula is 2.2 by 2.7 cm. For fetoscopic blood drawing, the operator begins by scanning the patient and identifying an area in which the fetus is not covering the placenta. The scope is then inserted and the 27-gauge needle passed through the side arm. A fetal vessel is located and under direct vision pierced by the needle (Figure 5.32). Blood is aspirated, as well as adjacent amniotic fluid, when the needle is pulled back out of the vessel.

Because the scope is not flexible, the above technique cannot be used on anterior placentas. To obtain blood in that situation, the placental aspiration technique is employed. In this method the chorionic plate is identified on the gray scale, and its distance from the abdominal wall is measured. A 20-gauge needle is then passed to and through the plate several times in a blind fashion. Blood and amniotic fluid are aspirated on multiple occasions during this procedure.

These techniques are still in their infancy and are currently being performed only in a few centers. The initial work with ongoing pregnancies, however, has been encouraging. Fetal blood has been obtained in almost all of the cases attempted, and globin chain synthesis analysis has made accurate in utero diagnoses of major hemoglobinopathies possible. To date, the morbidity has been minimal with the fetoscopy patients, but more marked with those having placental aspiration. The interested reader is referred to the articles in the reference section for a more detailed discussion of this new area of endeavor.[27–32]

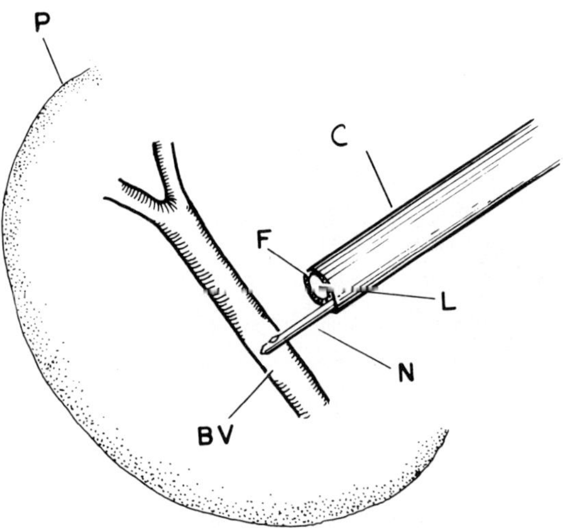

Figure 5.32. Schematic diagram for fetoscopic blood drawing. P, placenta; BV, blood vessel; C, cannula; F, fiberoptic system; L, fetoscope lens; N, blood drawing needle. (Reprinted from Hobbins, J. C., Mahoney, M. J.: In utero diagnosis of hemoglobinopathies. N Engl J Med 290: 1065–1067, 1974.)

Conclusion

This chapter has attempted to give the reader a feel for the work currently being done in obstetric ultrasound. The usefulness of this modality to the obstetrician is becoming increasingly more evident as new avenues of investigation are explored. Ultrasound is already an invaluable diagnostic tool, and its potential for the future seems to be limited only by our imaginations.

REFERENCES

1. Barker, P., Cashman, D.: Diagnosis of multiple pregnancy. Br Med J 2: 487, 1973.
2. Bartsch, P. K., Lundberg, J., Wahlstrom, J.: The technique, results and risks of amniocentesis for genetic reasons. J Obstet Gynaecol Br Commonw 81: 991, 1974.
3. Berkowitz, R. L., Hobbins, J. C.: Current concepts in the management of Rh incompatibility. Contemp Ob/Gyn 9: 3, 1977.
4. Campbell, S.: Ultrasonic fetal cephalometry during the second trimester of pregnancy. J Obstet Gynaecol Br Commonw 77: 1057, 1970.
5. Campbell, S.: Fetal urine production. J Obstet Gynaecol Br Commonw 80: 680, 1973.
6. Campbell, S.: Physical methods of assessing size at birth. *Size at Birth*. Ciba Foundation Symposium No. 27, Amsterdam, Associated Scientific Publishers, 1974.
7. Campbell, S., Dewhurst, C. J. Diagnosis of the small-for-dates fetus by serial ultrasonic cephalometry. Lancet 2: 1002, 1971.
8. Campbell, S., Johnstone, F. D., Holt, E. M., May, P.: Anencephaly: Early ultrasonic diagnosis and active management. Lancet 2: 1226, 1972.
9. Campbell, S., Wilkin, D.: Ultrasonic measurement of fetal abdomen circumference in the estimation of fetal weight. Br J Obstet Gynaecol 82: 689, 1975.
10. Campbell, S., Wladimiroff, J. W., Dewhurst, C.

J.: The antenatal measurement of fetal urine production. J Obstet Gynaecol Br Commonw 80: 680, 1973.
11. Curtis, J. D., Cohen, W. N., Richerson, H. B., White, C. A.: The importance of placental localization preceding amniocentesis. Obstet Gynecol 40: 194, 1972.
12. Davison, J. M., Lind, T., Farr, V., Whittingham, T. A.: The limitations of ultrasonic fetal cephalometry. J Obstet Gynaecol Br Commonw 30: 769, 1973.
13. Fisher, C. C., Garrett, W., Kossoff, G.: Placental aging monitored by gray scale echography. Am J Obstet Gynecol 124: 483, 1976.
14. Garrett, W. J., Grunwald, G., Robinson, D. E.: Prenatal diagnosis of fetal polycystic kidney by ultrasound. Aust NZ J Obstet Gynaecol 10: 7, 1970.
15. Garrett, W. J., Kossoff, G., Osborn, R. A.: The diagnosis of fetal hydronephrosis, megaureter and urethral obstruction by ultrasonic echography. Br J Obstet Gynaecol 82: 115, 1975.
16. Garrett, W. J., Robinson, D. E.: Assessment of fetal size and growth rate by ultrasonic echoscopy. Obstet Gynecol 38: 525, 1971.
17. Gohari, P., Berkowitz, R. L., Hobbins, J. C.: In utero prediction of intrauterine growth retardation by determination of total intrauterine volume. Am J Obstet Gynecol 127: 255, 1977.
18. Gohari, P., Berkowitz, R. L., Hobbins, J. C.: Intrauterine growth retardation—A review with suggestions for diagnosis and management. Contemp Ob/Gyn 8: 79, 1976.
19. Golbus, M. S., Kan, Y. W., Naglich-Craig, M.: Fetal blood sampling in midtrimester pregnancies. Am J Obstet Gynecol 124: 653, 1976.
20. Goldberg, B., Kotler, M., Ziskin, M., Waxham, R.: *Diagnostic Uses of Ultrasound*. New York, Grune & Stratton, Inc., 1975.
21. Goldberg, B., Pollack, A. M.: Ultrasonic aspiration-biopsy transducer. Radiology 108: 667, 1973.
22. Goldstein, P., Gershenson, D., Hobbins, J. C.: The reliability of fetal biparietal diameter as a predictor of a mature lecithin-sphingomyelin ratio. Obstet Gynecol 48: 667, 1976.
23. Gottesfeld, K. R.: The ultrasonic diagnosis of intrauterine fetal death. Am J Obstet Gynecol 108: 623, 1970.
24. Grove, C. S., Trombea, G. C., Amstey, M. S.: Fetal complications of amniocentesis. Am J Obstet Gynecol 115: 1154, 1973.
25. Hallman, M., Kulovich, M., Kirkpatrick, E., Sugarman, R. G., Gluck, L.: Phosphatidylinositol and phosphatidyl glycerol in amniotic fluid: Indices of lung maturity. Am J Obstet Gynecol 125: 613, 1976.
26. Herschlein, H. J.: Diagnosis of abruptio placentae in normally located placentae by means of ultrasonic technique. Aerztl Forsch 24: 210, 1970.
27. Hobbins, J. C.: Amniocentesis. *Dr./No. 3—Perinatal Medicine*. Medcom, Inc., 1975.
28. Hobbins, J. C., Mahoney, M. J.: In utero diagnosis of hemoglobinopathies: Technic for obtaining fetal blood. N Engl J Med 290: 1065, 1974.
29. Hobbins, J. C., Mahoney, M. J.: Experience with fetal blood drawing. Lancet 2: 107, 1975.
30. Hobbins, J. C., Mahoney, M. J.: Fetoscopy and fetal blood sampling: The present state of the method Clin Obstet Gynecol 19 (12), 1976.
31. Hobbins, J. C., Mahoney, M. J., Goldstein, L. A.: New method of intrauterine evaluation by the combined use of fetoscopy and ultrasound. Am J Obstet Gynecol 118: 1069, 1974.
32. Hobbins, J. C., Winsberg, F.: *Ultrasonography in Obstetrics and Gynecology*. Baltimore, Williams & Wilkins Co., 1977.
33. Holländer, H. J.: Ultrasound in the prenatal diagnosis of Rh erythroblastosis. Vienna, World Congress of Ultrasound in Medicine, 1969.
34. Holländer, H. J., Mast, H.: Ultrasonic measurement of the placental thickness in normal pregnancies and Rh incompatibility. Geburts Frauen 28: 662, 1968.
35. Jouppila, P.: Ultrasound in the diagnosis of early pregnancy and its complications. Acta Obstet Gynecol Scand (Suppl) 53: 3, 1971.
36. King, K. L.: Placental migration demonstrated by ultrasonography: A hypothesis of dynamic placentation. Radiology 109: 167, 1973.
37. Kobayashi, M., Hellman, L. M., Fillisti, L.: Placental localization by ultrasound. Am J Obstet Gynecol 106: 279, 1970.
38. Kohorn, E., Kaufman, M.: Sonar in the first trimester of pregnancy. Obstet Gynecol 44: 473, 1974.
39. Kossoff, G., Garrett, W. J.: Intracranial detail in fetal echograms. Invest Radiol 7: 159, 1972.
40. Kratochwil, A., Schaller. A.: Obstetric diagnostics of anencephalus using ultrasound. Geburtshilfe Frauenheilk 31: 564, 1971.
41. Levi, S.: Ultrasonic diagnosis in obstetrics: Clinical value of measuring the biparietal diameter of the fetus. Gynecol Obstet (Paris) 69: 227, 1970.
42. Lunt, R. M., Chard, T.: Reproducibility of measurement of fetal biparietal diameter by ultrasonic cephalometry. J Obstet Gynaecol Br Commonw 81: 682, 1974.
43. Mahoney, M. J., Hobbins, J. C.: Ultrasound and growth of amniotic fluid cells. Lancet 2: 454, 1973.
44. Micell, R. C., Bradley-Watson, P. J.: The detection of fetal meningocoele by ultrasound B scan. J Obstet Gynaecol Br Commonw 80: 1100, 1973.
45. NICHD National Amniocentesis Registry Study Group: The safety and accuracy of midtrimester amniocentesis for prenatal diagnosis. JAMA (In press.)
46. Robinson, H. P.: Sonar measurement of fetal crown-rump length as means of assessing maturity in first trimester of pregnancy. Br Med J 4: 28, 1973.
47. Robinson, H. P.: Gestation sac: Volumes as determined by sonar in the first trimester of pregnancy. Br J Obstet Gynaecol 82: 100, 1975.
48. Sanders, R. C.: Letter: Fetal biparietal diameters correlated with gestational age. J Clin Ultrasound 1: 344, 1973.
49. Sanders, R. C.: Localization of the cervix in ultrasonic placentography with the use of a fluid-filled pessary. Am J Obstet Gynecol 118:

566, 1974.
50. Watmough, D.: A critical assessment of ultrasonic foetal cephalometry. Br J Radiol 46: 566, 1973.
51. Wells, P. N. T.: *Physical Principles of Ultrasonic Diagnosis*. New York, Academic Press, 1969.
52. Winsberg, F.: Echographic changes with placental aging. J Clin Ultrasound 1: 52, 1973.

RONALD J. BOLOGNESE, M.D.

6

Amniotic Fluid

Introduction

In 1934 Albano[2] injected sodium phenolsulfonaphthalate into the amniotic cavity and reported its gradual disappearance. The classic isotope studies of Vosburgh et al[117] in 1948 offered further proof that amniotic fluid is not a stagnant pool, but functions as a reservoir in constant flux providing interchange between maternal and fetal circulations. The investigations of Brevis[12] in Rh-sensitized pregnancies demonstrated the first clinical application of data obtained from amniotic fluid.

This chapter will focus on identification and measurement of biochemical components and circulatory dynamics of amniotic fluid which may be used to monitor fetal growth, maturity and well-being in the management of high risk pregnancies.

Origin and Fate of the Amniotic Fluid

ORIGIN OF FLUID

The existence of fluid in the presence of blighted ova and formation of an amniotic cavity before functional activity of embryonic tissue would suggest that the embryo contributes little to amniotic fluid production. Hippocrates proposed that amniotic fluid was a product of the fetal kidneys; however, the amnion is separated from the early embryo and cannot receive waste products. The fetal kidneys begin to function by the 12th to 14th week of gestation with the formation of urine in utero. The bladder achieves coordinated contractile activity by the fifth month. Abramovich calculated that 7 to 17 cc of urine are excreted daily by midpregnancy.[1]

Numerous reports correlate the association between bilateral renal agenesis and oligohydramnios with the inference that the absence of fetal urine results in a reduction of amniotic fluid formation.[41,52,90,106,107] The increasing involvement of fetal micturition in amniotic fluid production is supported by the association of elevated urea and creatinine concentration in amniotic fluid and fetal urine as pregnancy advances. Furthermore, fetal urine is hypotonic compared to amniotic fluid and during pregnancy a progressive reduction occurs in the tonicity and total osmotic pressure of amniotic fluid.[89]

Liley[65] reported puncture of the fetal bladder during intrauterine transfusion and drainage of 60 cc of dilute urine. After injection of 3 to 4 ml of radiopaque dye into the bladder, its outline was restored rapidly, demonstrating fetal ability to produce a large quantity of urine within a short time. Seeds[107] has proposed that near term in excess of 500 cc of hypotonic fetal urine is produced each day.

The fetus may contribute to amniotic fluid formation by other mechanisms. Reynolds[97] collected large quantities of fluid with a composition similar to that of amniotic fluid from the lungs of fetal lambs. The presence of lecithin in amniotic fluid as term approaches would support contribution of fetal lung fluids to the formation of amniotic fluid.

The isotope studies of Hutchinson et al[51] and in vitro perfusion experiments suggest that the umbilical cord may contribute 40 to 50 ml of water and other ions hourly to the amniotic fluid.[87] Between 10 and 18 weeks of gestation, fetal skin contributes to amniotic fluid production by secretion from the peridermal cells; however, degeneration of these cells and keratinization in the epidermis later in pregnancy reduces the transfer of water across the skin. The early amniotic epithelium has secretory characteristics which become insignificant during the later stages of pregnancy as the membranes become avascular. Amniotic epithelial cell degeneration corresponds to the time of maximum increase in fluid volume.

Ultimately, all the constituents of amniotic fluid must be derived from the mother. However, the explanation that amniotic fluid represents an ultrafiltrate of maternal serum is contradicted by differences in composition.

FATE OF FLUID

Amniotic fluid is replaced totally during a 3-hr period and the biologic half-life of water in the fluid is estimated to be 90 min.[27,50] This represents a rapid exchange of water between mother and fetus approaching 3 to 4 liters per hr at term.[51]

In 1651 Harvey suggested that fetal swallowing accounted for removal of amniotic fluid. Normally, the fetus swallows approximately 20 cc of fluid per hr or 450 cc per day.[91,92] This represents only 5 to 10% of the actual transfer of water that occurs during the same time interval.

Clinical observations suggest that fetal swallowing is more important in the removal of amniotic fluid than is demonstrated experimentally. Radiopaque dye injected into the amniotic fluid can be detected in the fetal stomach by x-ray within 20 min.[71] Since only 10 to 15 cc of dye are necessary to outline the gastrointestinal tract, the fetus must swallow a substantial quantity of fluid to allow x-ray visualization. The association of hydramnios and congenital upper gastrointestinal abnormalities will be discussed later in the chapter.

Numerous in vitro studies have demonstrated amniotic fluid transfer to the maternal circulation via the sinusoidal vessels of the decidua.[9–11] Movement of water and sodium is by passive rather than active transport mechanisms. A pressure in the lumen of decidual vessels greater than surrounding tissue is necessary to maintain patency and creates a hydrostatic gradient in the direction of the amniotic cavity. Since amniotic fluid contains much less protein than maternal plasma, an osmotic gradient exists which is in excess of the hydrostatic gradient. Recent studies have demonstrated that the amnion is not a simple semipermeable membrane and that ionic movement may be controlled actively by the epithelium.[49]

The fetal lung, skin and umbilical cord are possible sources for removal of amniotic fluid; however, there is no evidence to substantiate such involvement.

Amniotic Fluid Volume

Measurement of amniotic fluid volume has been the subject of numerous investigations utilizing various dilutional techniques: dyes, chemical and radioactive substances.[20,21,36,83,95] Late in the first trimester the volume increases by 25 ml per week while the weekly rate of production doubles from 15 to 28 weeks of gestation.[75,98,118] At 14 weeks the average volume is 100 ml, which rises to 400 ml by midpregnancy and 670 ml at 25 to 26 weeks.[46,95]

Charles and associates[20,21] report a volume peak of approximately 1000 ml at 38 weeks in normal pregnancies. More recent studies by Queenan and coworkers,[95] however, demonstrate a mean volume peak of 984 ml by 33 to 34 weeks, a slight decrease to 836 ml at term and a continued decline to 544 ml by 41 to 42 weeks. Beischer et al[4] serially measured amniotic fluid volume in 17 prolonged pregnancies. The average volume decreased from 484 ml at 42 weeks to 162 ml by 44 weeks.

Amniotic fluid volume is not static and demonstrates a wide range of normal which increases as the gestation advances. (Figure 6.1) Fifty percent of the patients in Queenan's study[95] demonstrated a volume increase at some stage in pregnancy with values rising as late as term in several cases. A definite decrease in fluid volume occurred in one-third of the gestations as

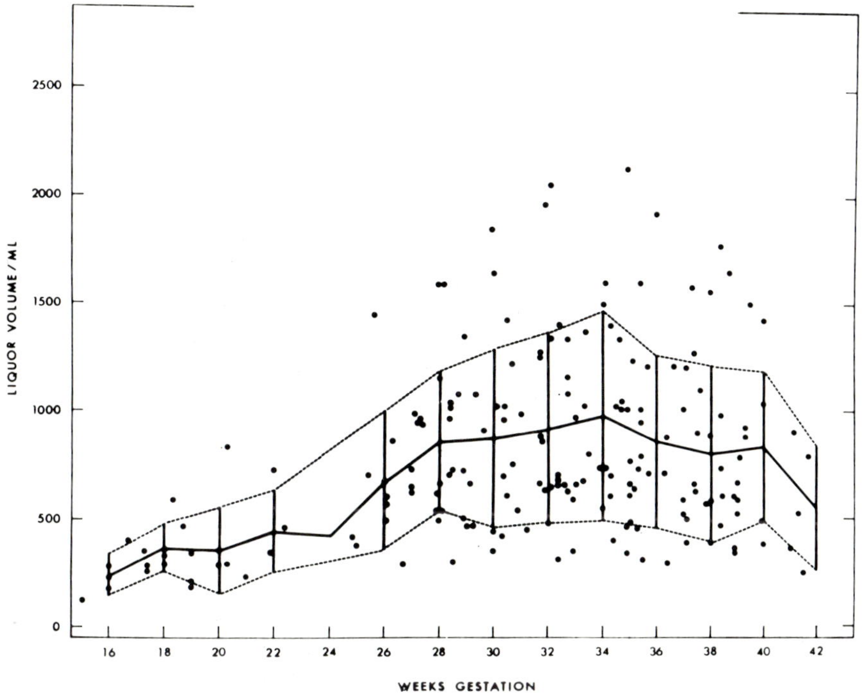

Figure 6.1. The graph shows 187 amniotic fluid volume determinations plotted against weeks of gestation. The mean values ± 1 SD were calculated for each 2-week period from 15 to 16 weeks through 41 to 42 weeks. (Reprinted from Queenan, J. T., Thompson, W., Whitfield, C. R., Shah, S. I.: Amniotic fluid volumes in normal pregnancies. Am J Obstet Gynecol 114: 34, 1972.)

early as 28 weeks. In 8 of 16 pregnancies serial determinations revealed a reversal of the initial upward or downward volume trend.

HYDRAMNIOS

Hydramnios represents an excessive amount of amniotic fluid; however, little evidence exists to define the upper limits of normal. Queenan and associates[95] recorded volumes of 2070 ml (32 weeks) and 2136 ml (35 weeks) in two gravidas who clinically appeared to be normal. Since fluid volume varies with gestational length and is subject to a wide normal range, it seems reasonable to define hydramnios as more than double the expected normal mean volume for the particular period of pregnancy.

Hydramnios may be acute or chronic. The acute form requires vigorous therapy and portends a poor prognosis. Similarly, in the chronic type, severe hydramnios is associated with an unsatisfactory fetal outcome. Depending upon the accuracy of clinical diagnosis (often overestimated), the frequency of hydramnios varies considerably. Yordan and D'Esopo,[111] in 1955, reported a 0.59% incidence. More recent data from the Collaborative Perinatal Study indicates the association of hydramnios in 1.5% of white and 1.3% of black gestations.[84]

The etiology of hydramnios remains unclear. The association of congenital upper gastrointestinal tract abnormalities or anencephaly with hydramnios implicates the absence of fetal swallowing or lack of fluid absorption as a cause of excessive volume.[18] Lloyd and Clatworthy[66] examined neonates with congenital gastrointestinal tract obstruction. Fourteen percent with esophageal atresia and 66% with atresia of the upper small bowel were associated with hydramnios. Equally important was the presence of normal fluid volume in the remaining cases. In a study by Stevenson[111] anencephaly existed in 53% of the hydramnios-associated malformations; however, a wide spectrum of congenital anomalies—hydrocephaly, spina bifida, Downs syndrome, talipes, etc.—also were observed.

Queenan and Gadow[94] reviewed 352 cases of chronic polyhydramnios of which 34% were idiopathic, 24.6% were related to diabetes, 11.5% were associated with Rh sensitization, 20% demonstrated congenital abnormalities and 8.4% involved multiple pregnancy.

Perinatal mortality parallels the severity of the hydramnios. The most significant cause of mortality is the 20 to 30% incidence of fetal malformations incompatible with life. Coexisting diabetes, erythroblastosis fetalis, twin gestations and increased risk of premature labor contribute to reduced perinatal survival.

OLIGOHYDRAMNIOS

This condition may occur at any stage of pregnancy. Fetal urinary tract anomalies are associated with oligohydramnios; the etiology is thought to be absent or reduced urine production.[41,52,90,106,107]

Oligohydramnios also is observed with amnion nodosum. In 1950 Landing[63] described small nodular masses on the fetal aspect of the amnion most numerous on the membranes covering the placenta. The nodules consist of keratinized squamous cells replacing amniotic epithelium. Five of the eight cases reported by Landing demonstrated major fetal urinary tract abnormalities. Jeffcoate and Scott[52] observed a similar association of amnion nodosum, oligohydramnios and renal agenesis.

Reduced amniotic fluid is noted with the syndrome of placental insufficiency: severe pre-eclampsia, essential hypertension and dysmaturity.[31,32,36] Elliot and Inman[31] state that the peak fluid volume in such cases occurs earlier and approaches only half that of normal pregnancy.

Amniotic Fluid Composition

Amniotic fluid is a heterogenous solution suspension. It consists of 98 to 99% water with 1 to 2% solids; about one-half of the solids are organic; of this 50% is protein. The inorganic components are similar to extracellular fluid with high concentrations of sodium (Na), chloride (Cl) and carbon dioxide (CO_2) and small amounts of potassium, calcium, magnesium and phosphate.

ELECTROLYTES

During the first half of pregnancy Na and Cl concentrations are more similar to fetal than maternal serum, suggesting that amniotic fluid may be an extension of fetal extracellular fluid. Later, the fluid becomes progressively hypotonic with decreasing Na and Cl values and a corresponding fall in total osmotic pressure. These changes, associated with a gradual rise in urea, uric acid and creatinine levels, reflect the contribution of maturing fetal renal function to amniotic fluid.

Potassium values remain constant during pregnancy. Calcium magnesium, phosphorus, zinc, iron and sulfur also are present with no significant change in concentrations as pregnancy advances.

GASES

The partial pressure of oxygen (PO_2) of amniotic fluid is quite variable.[96] Vasicka[116] investigated the effect of maternal administration of 100% oxygen for 13 to 26 min; no significant increase in amniotic fluid PO_2 was observed. A positive correlation between maternal hematocrit values and amniotic fluid PO_2 was reported by Johnson and Ojo.[53] Severely anemic gravidas had a significantly lower mean PO_2 compared to control patients.

CARBON DIOXIDE

Reported values for amniotic carbon dioxide tension (PCO_2) near term vary from 44.0 to 57.6 mm Hg.[60,99] Cohen[25] could not correlate amniotic PCO_2 with subsequent fetal distress or Apgar score. However, a significant association between amniotic fluid PCO_2 at birth and umbilical arterial and venous PCO_2 has been reported.[60,112]

HYDROGEN ION CONCENTRATION

The hydrogen ion content (pH) of amniotic fluid at term is more acid (7.04 to 7.11) than blood and is influenced by the PCO_2 and the presence of organic acids.[8] Since fetal urine contains such acids, am-

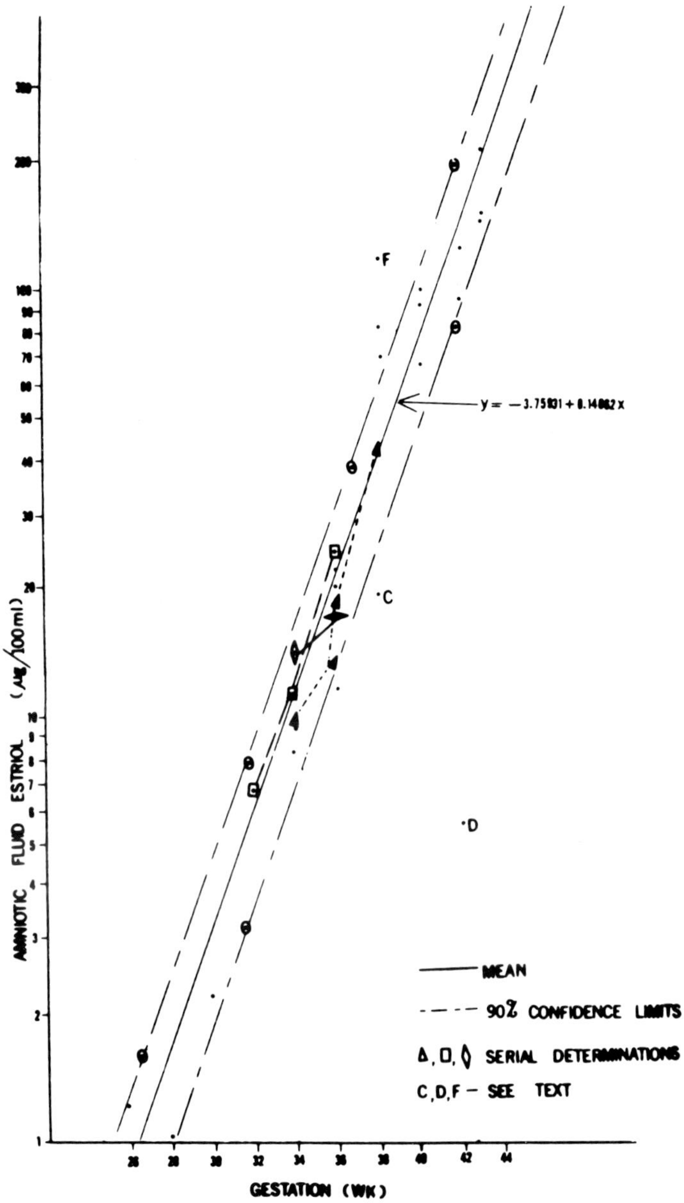

Figure 6.2. Amniotic fluid estriol concentration plotted semilogarithmically against gestational age. The semilogarithmic model, y = (−) 3.75931 + 0.14062x adequately explains ($P < 0.01$) the relationship between length of pregnancy and concentration of estriol. The plot was obtained with data from normal pregnancies. (Reprinted from Bolognese, R. J., Corson, S. L., Touchstone, J. C., Lakoff, K. M.: Correlation of amniotic fluid estriol with fetal age and well-being. Obstet Gynecol 37: 437, 1972.)

the fetus became severely affected. Imminent or actual fetal demise was associated with HPL levels approaching one-third to one-half of maternal serum values. Similar findings were noted by Crosignani and associates[28]; however, they reported a greater elevation of HCG than HPL in amniotic fluid with hydrops fetalis.

Human Prolactin

Amniotic fluid concentrations of human pituitary prolactin are 2- to 10-fold higher compared to maternal serum.[101] The source is unclear; the fetal pituitary gland, the placenta and the maternal pituitary are possible sites. Since prolactin appears to be involved in the regulation of sodium and water, it may play an important role in the regulation of amniotic fluid volume by affecting sodium transport.

Cortisol

Several studies demonstrate a rise in amniotic cortisol during the third trimester of pregnancy. Fencl and Tulchinsky[33] recorded mean concentrations of 30 ng per ml at 20 weeks and 31.8 ng per ml between 21 and 34 weeks. From 35 to 40 weeks the mean value rose to 72.4 ng per ml and continued to increase beyond term (139 ng per ml). While measuring lower mean levels (5 ng per ml at 10 to 15 weeks and 10 ng per ml from 20 to 35 weeks), Murphy and associates[78] noted an abrupt rise to 22 ng/ml during the last two weeks of pregnancy prior to the onset of labor. Cord serum values averaged twice amniotic fluid levels and a statistically significant correlation was noted between amniotic fluid and cord cortisol levels.

If amniotic fluid values reflect fetal cortisol production, these findings suggest that in the human, as in sheep, a rise in fetal cortisol may precede the spontaneous onset of labor. Recently, labor has been initiated in prolonged gestations by the intra-amniotic instillation of dexamethasone and cortisol.[70,85]

Nwosu and associates[86] measured amniotic fluid cortisol concentrations in premature, normal and post-term gestations. A rising trend in cortisol occurred from 31 to 40 weeks. No abrupt elevation was apparent before term (Figure 6.3). Most intriguing was the observation of high cortisol concentrations in 7 of 10 cases of premature labor. Since significantly increased adrenal weights have been observed in premature neonates, the authors speculated that premature fetal adrenal hyperactivity could account for early labor.

The relationship of amniotic fluid cortisol and the lecithin/sphingomyelin (L/S) ratio has been studied with conflicting results. Fencl and Tulchinsky[33] observed that cortisol levels higher than 60 ng per ml generally were associated with an L/S ratio greater than 2.0; values below 40 ng per ml were accompanied by an L/S ratio of less than 1.5. Tan and associates[113] also reported a significant correlation between amniotic fluid cortisol concentrations and L/S ratios in uncomplicated gestations of 30 weeks and greater. Although noting an increasing trend in cortisol levels, Sivakoumaran et al[108] failed to demonstrate a significant correlation.

LIPIDS

In 1969 Nelson[81] demonstrated low quantitative lecithin levels in the amniotic fluid from infants who subsequently developed respiratory distress syndrome (RDS). The major phospholipids, lecithin and

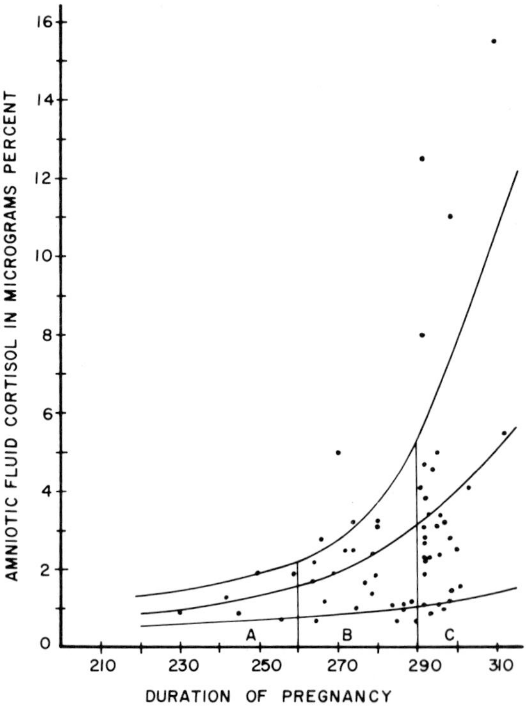

Figure 6.3. Amniotic fluid cortisol concentrations in uncomplicated pregnancy. Lines represent mean and ±1 SD above and below. A, B and C represent the preterm, term, and postterm zones. (Reprinted from Nwosu, U., Bolognese, R. J., Wallach, E. E., Bongiovanni, A. M.: Amniotic fluid cortisol concentrations in normal and premature labor: Comparison with levels in postmature pregnancy. Obstet Gynecol (In press.))

sphingomyelin, are important components of the surfactant system of the lung. These compounds line the alveoli, reducing surface tension on expiration and preventing collapse of the alveoli. Similarity of the phospholipid composition of term amniotic fluid and lung surfactant supports the contention that fetal lung effluent is transported into amniotic fluid. In 1971 Gluck and associates[37] observed changes in amniotic fluid phospholipids which reflected those of the fetal lung. Before 35 weeks, concentrations of lecithin and sphingomyelin were nearly equal; however, beyond this gestational length lecithin levels increased sharply to 4 times those of sphingomyelin. This surge of amniotic fluid lecithin heralded pulmonary maturity.

Lecithins are synthesized by two primary pathways: Pathway I, cytidine diphosphocholine + D-α,β-diglyceride $\rightarrow$ lecithin; Pathway II, phosphatidyl ethanolamine + $3CH_3 \rightarrow$ lecithin. Pathway I is the major pathway, becoming significantly active at 35 weeks; it generally is unaffected by hypoxia, acidosis and hypercapnea and marks fetal lung maturation. Pathway II predominates from 22 to 24 weeks, increases activity during pregnancy and achieves maximal function at and beyond birth; it is exquisitely sensitive to inhibition at pH 7.0 to 7.1.

Various methods of amniotic fluid lipid or phospholipid analysis have been reported including determinations of total lipids, colorimetric evaluation of phospholipids and alterations of the original technique employed by Gluck and associates.[43, 80] The significance, interpretation and potential pitfalls of these procedures for determination of the L/S ratio are reviewed by Gluck and coworkers.[39]

Although some studies are less enthusiastic, the majority of reports confirm the usefulness of the L/S ratio in predicting neonatal pulmonary maturity.[39, 43, 73, 82, 109] The L/S ratio, however, can be affected by blood or meconium contamination of the amniotic fluid specimen. Gluck and associates[38] observed that a packed red cell volume greater than 0.05 ml for 3 ml of amniotic fluid will produce L/S ratios in the range of 2. Since they reflect the acetone-precipitable material in maternal blood, these ratios are uninterpretable. By adding increasing concentrations of maternal blood, Wagstaff and associates[119] converted an immature ratio (1.0) into a mature ratio ($\geq$2.0). Buhi and Spellacy[16] determined that maternal or fetal serum has an L/S ratio of approximately 1.31 to 1.46. The addition of serum lowered high L/S ratios and raised low L/S ratios. Therefore, the effects of blood appear to be dependent on the original L/S ratio and the quantity of blood contamination. A contaminated specimen with an L/S ratio of less than or equal to 2.0 is not valid; however, an L/S ratio greater than 2.0 generally indicates fetal lung maturity.

Hallman and associates[45] correlated L/S ratios with amniotic fluid phosphatidylinositol (PI) and phosphatidylglycerol (PG), which are minor (compared to lecithin) components of surfactant phospholipids. An increase in PI closely paralleled the L/S ratio to 2.0. When the ratio exceeded 2.0, PG initially appeared as PI concomitantly decreased. Substantial levels of PG indicated fetal lung maturity. Since these acidic phospholipids are present in very small amounts in blood compared to lecithin and sphingomyelin, analysis of PI and PG in amniotic fluid may prove useful in specimens contaminated with blood.

The presence of meconium in amniotic fluid is reported to increase or decrease the L/S ratio.[16, 62] Obvious meconium contamination renders a specimen unsuitable for L/S determination. The presence of bilirubin and vernix caseosa does not affect the validity of the L/S ratio.[119]

In 1972 Clements and associates[23] described a rapid test for amniotic fluid pulmonary surfactant dependent upon the ability of the fluid to form a stable foam in the presence of ethanol. When the foam or shake test is compared to the L/S ratio, false positive and negative rates are reported; however, a good correlation exists between a positive (three tubes positive) shake test and the absence of respiratory distress syndrome.[16, 73] As an emergency or screening procedure, the foam test appears to identify with reliability fetal lung maturity. When a positive (three tubes positive) result is obtained, the L/S ratio seems unnecessary; however, if a less mature value is observed, a routine L/S ratio should follow to assess accurately pulmonary maturity. Although the presence of bilirubin and vernix caseosa do not affect the shake test, meconium contamination may contribute to a false positive result.[119]

PROSTAGLANDINS

Prostaglandins (PG) are a family of closely related unsaturated hydroxy fatty acids based on the molecule prostanoic acid (Figure 6.4). In 1966 Karim[56] extracted lipids after acidifying amniotic fluid to a pH of 3. These acidic lipids demonstrated smooth muscle-stimulating activity and further studies led to the identification of four prostaglandins: PGE_1, PGE_2, PGF_{1a} and PGF_{2a}. High concentrations of PGE_2, PGF_{1a} and PGF_{2a} were detected in amniotic fluid during labor and spontaneous abortion.[57, 58]

Salmon and Amy[100] observed relatively constant levels of PGF_{2a} between 15 and 35 weeks of gestation whereas an increase occurred after 36 weeks. A significant elevation developed during labor which paralleled cervical dilatation. Hillier and associates[47] reported similar results. A rise in amniotic fluid PGF_{2a} was recorded in all patients during labor but the extent of the increase was variable. In the early stage of oxytocin-induced labor Keirse et al[59] found PGF concentrations greater than before the onset of labor but lower than during spontaneous labor.

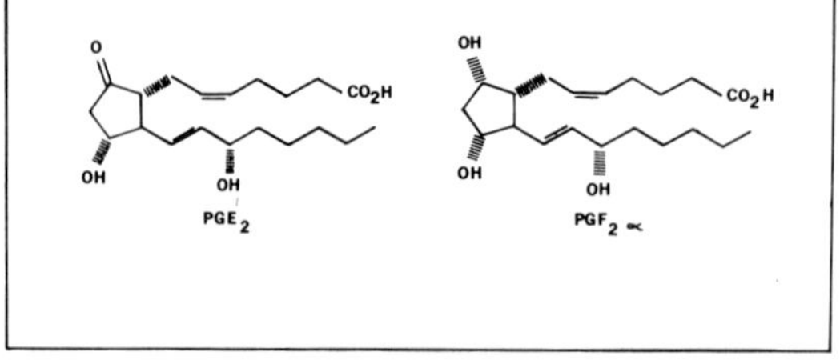

Figure 6.4. Prostanoic acid and structure of PGE_2 and PGF_{2a} (Reprinted from Bolognese, R. J., Corson, S. L.: *Interruption of Pregnancy*. Baltimore, The Williams & Wilkins Co., 1975.)

The decidua appears to be the source of amniotic fluid PG. Decidua obtained during labor demonstrates concentrations of PGE_1, PGE_2, PGF_{1a} and PGF_{2a} 10 to 30 times greater than found in amniotic fluid.[57] Unesterified or free arachidonic acid is the obligatory precursor of PGE_2 and F_{2a}. Human fetal membranes and uterine decidua are rich in esterified arachidonic acid.[103] The mean concentration of this fatty acid in fetal membranes obtained after spontaneous labor and delivery is slightly but significantly less than in membranes evaluated prior to labor or at the time of elective cesarean section. These observations support the theory that the storage form of PG precursor, arachidonic acid, is in the fetal membranes.

Schwarz and associates[104] propose that before labor an accelerated release of arachidonic acid occurs which is caused by the fetal membrane enzyme, phospholipase A_2. Recent investigations demonstrated the presence of phospholipase A_2 in the lysosomes of human fetal membranes.[104] The liberated arachidonic acid diffuses from the chorion to the uterine decidua serving as the PG precursor. PG inhibits the ATP-dependent sequestration of calcium by the sarcoplasmic reticulum of human myometrium.[17] This PG action increases intracellular free calcium which is a necessary event for the initiation of myometrial contractions and labor.

Amniocentesis

Amniocentesis generally is an innocuous and simple technique; however, indications and complications should be weighed carefully before proceeding. Ultrasound B scan is both a safe and accurate procedure for placental and fetal localization and should be employed routinely before amniocentesis (Chapter 5). Identification of an anterior placenta may require reassessment of the procedure, particularly in an Rh-negative patient, in view of the risks involved with transversing the placenta.

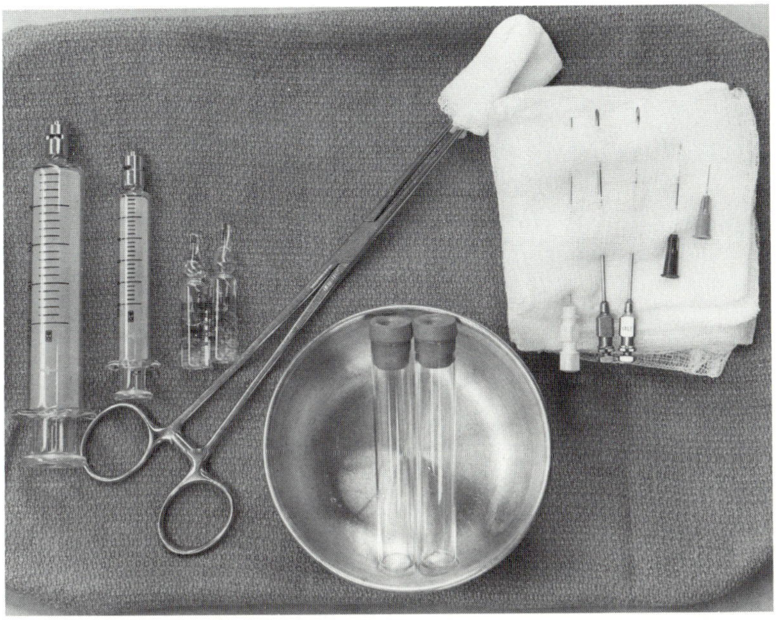

Figure 6.5. Amniocentesis tray. (Reprinted from Bolognese, R. J., Corson, S. L.: *Interruption of Pregnancy*. Baltimore, The Williams & Wilkins Co., 1975.)

Amniocentesis performed under ultrasound guidance may be important in an obese gravida. A special transducer is available through which the needle can be passed and the depth of penetration judged by A Mode evaluation.[120] Because of possible reduced amniotic fluid volume, ultrasound direction is essential in cases of suspected dysmaturity or postmaturity.

After voiding, the patient lies supine with legs extended. The fetal head and extremities are identified by abdominal examination and the heart rate is monitored with Doppler ultrasound. The lower abdomen is cleansed with an antiseptic solution and draped with sterile towels.

In advanced pregnancies the fetal extremities or neck crease are favored sites for amniocentesis; however, the best location may be dictated by ultrasound placentography. The needle site is anesthetized with any fast-acting local anesthetic agent. A 22- to 18-gauge, 3.5-inch spinal or 16- or 17-gauge Touhy needle with stylet in place is introduced through the abdominal wall (Figure 6.5). A sensation of different tissue layers is encountered as the needle is advanced firmly. A sudden reduction in needle resistance indicates entrance into the amniotic sac. The stylet is removed and a sterile plastic syringe is used to withdraw amniotic fluid. Forty to 50 ml of fluid can be obtained safely at this stage of pregnancy. If blood-tinged fluid initially is encountered, a second syringe is attached to obtain a less contaminated specimen. The needle then is quickly withdrawn and a sterile dressing is applied to the puncture site. Fetal heart sounds again are monitored.

The Rh type of all patients undergoing amniocentesis should be determined before the procedure. A bloody tap in an unsensitized Rh-negative patient raises the hazard of a fetomaternal bleed. Rh immunoglobulin should be administered to all unsensitized gravida undergoing amniocentesis. If a significant fetomaternal bleed is detected by the Kleihauer-Betke technique, 10 to 20 μg of immunoglobulin per 1 ml of red cell transfer should be given.

Summary

CLINICAL USES

The clinical uses of amniotic fluid for the management of Rh isoimmunization and the diagnosis of chromosomal abnormalities and metabolic defects are presented in Chapters 8 and 2.

FETAL MATURITY

Cytology

The presence of lipid-laden cells (fat cells) in amniotic fluid was described by Brosens in 1966.[13] Derived from the maturing fetal sebaceous gland, these anucleated polygonal cells stain metachromatically orange with Nile blue sulfate. Bishop and Corson[6] reported that all infants weighed over 2500 g and had a gestational age of 36 weeks or more when the fat cell count exceeded 20%.[4] Normal gestations as well as those complicated by Rh disease, toxemia, diabetes and sickle cell disease were studied by Morrison and associates.[77] No infant developed respiratory distress syndrome if the fat cell count was greater than 10%. In addition, the method was not affected by blood, meconium or vaginal secretions in amniotic fluid.

Creatinine

During pregnancy amniotic fluid creatinine rises progressively as a result of fetal kidney maturation and increasing fetal muscle mass. In normal pregnancies a concentration greater than 2.0 mg per 100 ml reflects a gestational age of 37 weeks or more.[88] Creatinine levels may be elevated prematurely in diabetes with associated maternal vascular disease.[19] With toxemia creatinine is higher than normal at corresponding weeks of gestation in the absence of elevated maternal serum levels.[72] Lower concentrations may be observed in gestations complicated by Rh disease and retarded fetal growth.[48, 76]

Bilirubin

In the absence of Rh sensitization, as fetal bilirubin metabolism and excretion matures, the amniotic fluid optical density (OD) at 450 mμ approaches zero. Mandelbaum and associates observed that the disappearance of the 450 mμ peak was constant at or after 36 weeks.[68] Defining maturity as a gestational age of 37 weeks and/or a birth weight of 2500 g, Myers and coworkers recorded a 56% and 69% rate of accuracy for an OD of 0.02 or less in normal and high risk pregnancies.[79] Fernandez de Castro et al[34] correctly predicted a gestational age of greater than 36 weeks in 81% of cases when the OD was less than or equal to 0.025. Only the L/S ratio offered a more accurate parameter of maturity (84%).

Phospholipids

A surge in surfactant synthesis as measured by the L/S ratio indicates fetal lung maturity. Generally, this occurs in normal pregnancies at approximately 35 weeks and is associated with an L/S ratio of 2:1 or greater.[37] Gluck and associates[39] observed acceleration of the L/S ratio in gestations complicated by maternal hypertension, sickle cell disease, narcotic addiction, intrauterine growth retardation and prolonged ruptured membranes. A delay in fetal lung maturation is seen in diabetes (class A, B, C) and the more severe cases of erythroblastosis fetalis.[39, 122]

Diagnosis of Ruptured Membranes

Leakage of amniotic fluid may be diagnosed by several techniques. Extreme alkalinity or a characteristic abortization pattern of vaginal secretions is suggestive of amniotic fluid contamination. If Nile blue sulfate mixed with vaginal fluid demonstrates orange-stained fetal cells, the diagnosis of ruptured membranes is established.[14]

Fetal Stress

The presence of meconium in amniotic fluid indicates fetal stress and is associated with increased perinatal mortality and morbidity.[69] This prenatal finding should suggest further evaluation of the fetal status by other parameters: fetal stress testing, estriol determinations, etc. During labor the combination of meconium and fetal hypoxia as evidence by late decelerations and a low scalp pH is ominous because of the increased risk of meconium aspiration. The significance of meconium-stained amniotic fluid in suspected postmature gestations is discussed in Chapter 10.

REFERENCES

1. Abramovich, D. R.: Fetal factors influencing the volume and composition of liquor amnii. J Obstet Gynaecol Br Commonw 75: 728, 1968.
2. Albano, G.: The repeated disappearance of the liquor amnii in the human ovum. Zbl Gynakol 58: 975, 1934.
3. Aleem, F. A., Pinkerton, J. H. M., Neill, D. W.: Clinical significance of the amniotic fluid estriol level. J Obstet Gynaecol Br Commonw 76: 200, 1969.
4. Beischer, N. A., Brown, J. B., Townsend, L.: Studies in prolonged pregnancy. Am J Obstet Gynecol 103: 496, 1969.
5. Berman, A. M., Kalchman, G. C., Chattoraj, S. C., et al: Relationship of amniotic fluid estriol to maternal urinary estriol. Am J Obstet Gynecol 100: 15, 1968.
6. Bishop, E. H., Corson, S. L.: Estimation of fetal maturity by cytologic examination of amniotic fluid. Am J Obstet Gynecol 102: 654, 1968.
7. Bolognese, R. J., Corson, S. L., Touchstone, J. C., Lakoff, K. M.: Correlation of amniotic fluid estriol with fetal age and well-being. Obstet Gynecol 37: 437, 1970.
8. Bonsnes, R. W.: Composition of amniotic fluid. Clin Obstet Gynecol 9: 440, 1966.
9. Brame, R. G., Harbert, G. M., McGaughey, H. S., Thorton, W. N.: Fetomaternal exchange of sodium: A possible mechanism of the formation of hydramnios. Obstet Gynecol 32: 241, 1968.
10. Brame, R. G., Overby, J. R.: Metabolism in human amnion. Obstet Gynecol 36: 425, 1970.
11. Brame, R. G.: Quantitation of transport of sodium across the amnio-chorion. Am J Obstet Gynecol 113: 1085, 1972.
12. Brevis, D. C. A.: The antinatal prediction of haemolytic disease of the newborn. Lancet 1: 395, 1952.
13. Brosens, I. A.: Cytologic study of amniotic fluid with blue nile sulfate. Acta Cytol 10: 159, 1966.
14. Brosens, I., Gordon, H.: The cytological diagnosis of ruptured membranes using Nile blue sulphate staining. J Obstet Gynaecol Br Commonw 72: 342, 1965.
15. Bruner, J. A.: Distribution of chorionic gonadotrophin in mother and fetus at various stages of pregnancy. J Clin Endocrinol 11: 360, 1951.
16. Buhi, W. C., Spellacy, W. N.: Effects of blood or meconium on the determination of the amniotic fluid lecithin/sphingomyelin ratio. Am J Obstet Gynecol 121: 321, 1975.
17. Carsten, M. E.: Prostaglandins and cellular calcium transport in the pregnant human uterus. Am J Obstet Gynecol 117: 824, 1973.
18. Cassady, G., Cailliteau, J.: The amniotic fluid in anencephaly: preliminary report. Am J Obstet Gynecol 97: 395, 1967.
19. Cassady, G., Hinkley, C., Bailey, P., Blake, M., Younger, B.: Amniotic fluid creatinine in pregnancies complicated by diabetes. Am J Obstet Gynecol 122: 13, 1975.
20. Charles, D., Jacoby, H. E., Burgess, F.: Amniotic fluid volumes in the second half of pregnancy. Am J Obstet Gynecol 93: 1042, 1965.
21. Charles, D., Jacoby, H. E.: Preliminary data on the use of sodium amniohippurate to determine amniotic fluid volumes. Am J Obstet Gynecol 95: 266, 1966.
22. Cherry, S. H., Filler, M., Harvey, H.: Lysozyme content of amniotic fluid. Am J Obstet Gynecol 116: 639, 1973.
23. Clements, J. A., Platzker, A. C. G., Tierney, D. F., et al: Assessment of the risk of the respiratory distress syndrome by a rapid test for surfactant in amniotic fluid. N Engl J Med 286: 1077, 1972.
24. Clements, J. A., Reyes, F. I., Winter, J. S. D., Faiman, C.: Studies on human sexual development. III. Fetal pituitary and serum and amniotic fluid concentrations of LH, HCG and FSH. J Clin Endocrinol Metab 38: 612, 1974.
25. Cohen, B. M.: The relationship between the fetal condition and biochemical analysis of the amniotic fluid at induction of labor. J Obstet Gynaecol Br Commonw 77: 496, 1970.
26. Corson, S. L., Bolognese, R. J.: Amniotic fluid pH as an indicator of fetal asphyxia. Obstet Gynecol 31: 397, 1968.
27. Cox, L. W., Chalmers, T. A.: The transfer of sodium to the amniotic fluid in normal and abnormal cases, determined by Na_{24} tracer methods. J Obstet Gynaecol Br Commonw 60: 222, 1953.
28. Crosignani, P. G., Nencioni, T., Brambati, B., Polvani, F.: The prognostic value of HCG and HPL in Rh-sensitized women. Abstracts of Proceedings of the Second European Congress of Perinatal Medicine, London, 1970.
29. Dicfalusy, E., Tillinger, K. G., Wiqvist, N., et al: Disposition of intraamniotically administered oestriol-16-C-oestrone-16-C sulfate by women. Clin Endocrinol (Tokyo) 23: 503, 1963.
30. Drazancic, A., Kuvacic, I.: Amniotic fluid glucose concentration. Am J Obstet Gynecol 120: 40, 1974.
31. Elliot, P. M., Inman, W. H. W.: Volume of liquor amnii in normal and abnormal pregnancy. Lancet 2: 835, 1961.
32. Elliot, P. M.: The relationships of liquor volume and placental insufficiency. Aust NZ J Obstet Gynaecol 4: 113, 1964.
33. Fencl, M. D., Tulchinsky, D.: Total cortisol in amniotic fluid and fetal lung maturation. N Engl J Med 292: 133, 1975.
34. Fernandez de Castro, A., Usategui-Gomez, M., Spellacy, W. N.: Amniotic fluid components as determinants of fetal maturity. Obstet Gynecol 46: 76, 1975.
35. Fischbacher, P. H., Quinlivan, W. L.: Qualitative and quantitative analysis of the proteins in human amniotic fluid. Am J Obstet Gynecol 108: 1051, 1970.
36. Gadd, R. L.: The volume of liquor amnii in normal and abnormal pregnancies. J Obstet Gynaecol Br Commonw 73: 11, 1966.
37. Gluck, L., Kulovich, M. V., Borer, R. C., Brenner, P. H., Anderson, G. G., Spellacy, W. N.: Diagnosis of the respiratory distress syndrome by amniocentesis. Am J Obstet Gynecol 109: 440, 1971.

38. Gluck, L., Kulovich, M. V., Borer, R. C.: Estimates of fetal lung maturity. Clin Perinatol 1: 125, 1974.
39. Gluck, L., Kulovich, M. V., Borer, R. C., Keidel, W. N.: The interpretation and significance of the lecithin/sphingomyelin ratio in amniotic fluid. Am J Obstet Gynecol 120: 142, 1974.
40. Goebelsmann, V., Wiqvist, N., Dicfalusy, E., et al: Fate of intra-amniotically administered oestriol-15-3H-3-sulfate oestriol-16-14C-16-glucosiduronate in pregnant women at mid-term. Acta Endocrinol (Kobenhavn) 52: 550, 1966.
41. Green, G. H.: Foetal renal hypoplasia and the origin of amniotic fluid. J Obstet Gynaecol Br Commonw 62: 592, 1955.
42. Guibaud, S., Bonnet, M., Thoulon, J. M., Dumont, M.: Alpha 1 antitrypsin in amniotic fluid. Obstet Gynecol 45: 34, 1975.
43. Gusdon, J. P., Waite, B. M.: A colorimetric method for amniotic fluid phospholipids and their relationship to the respiratory distress syndrome. Am J Obstet Gynecol 112: 62, 1972.
44. Hall, P. W., Roux, J. F.: Amniotic fluid beta-2 microglobulin concentration—An index of gestational age. Am J Obstet Gynecol 120: 56, 1974.
45. Hallman, M., Kulovich, M., Kirkpatrick, E., Sugarman, R. G., Gluck, L.: Phosphatidylinositol and phosphatidylglycerol in amniotic fluid. Indices of lung maturity. Am J Obstet Gynecol 125: 613, 1976.
46. Haswell, G. L., Morris, J. A.: Amniotic fluid volume studies. Obstet Gynecol 42: 725, 1973.
47. Hillier, K., Calder, A. A., Embrey, M. P.: Concentrations of prostaglandin F_{2a} in amniotic fluid and plasma in spontaneous and induced labours. J Obstet Gynaecol Br Commonw 81: 257, 1974.
48. Hinkley, C., O'Neil, L., Cassady, G.: Amniotic fluid creatinine in the Rh-sensitized pregnancy. Am J Obstet Gynecol 117: 544, 1973.
49. Hoyes, A. D.: Fine structure of human amniotic epithelium following short-term preservation in vitro. J Anat 111: 43, 1972.
59. Hutchinson, D. L., Hunter, C. B., Neslen, E. D., Plentl, A. A.: The exchange of water and electrolytes in the mechanism of amniotic fluid formation and the relationship to hydramnios. Surg Gynecol Obstet 100: 391, 1955.
51. Hutchinson, D. L., Gray, M. J., Plentl, A. A., Alvarez, H., Caldeyro-Barcia, R., et al: The role of the fetus in the water exchange of the amniotic fluid of normal and hydramniotic patients. J Clin Invest 38: 971, 1959.
52. Jeffcoate, T. N. A., Scott, J. S.: Polyhydramnios and oligohydramnios. Can Med Assoc J 80: 77, 1959.
53. Johnson, J. W. C., Ojo, O. A.: Amniotic fluid oxygen tensions in severe maternal anemia. Am J Obstet Gynecol 97: 499, 1967.
54. Josimovich, J. B., Kosor, B., Boccella, L.: Human placental lactogen (chorionic somatomammotropin). *Advances in Obstetrics and Gynecology,* Vol. II. Edited by S. L. Marcus, C. Marcus, Baltimore, The Williams & Wilkins Co., 1971.
55. Kaplan, S. L., Grumbach, M. M.: Immunoassay for human chorionic growth hormone-prolactin in serum and urine. Science 147: 751, 1965.
56. Karim, S. M. M.: Identification of prostaglandins in human amniotic fluid. J Obstet Gynaecol Br Commonw 73: 903, 1966.
57. Karim, S. M. M., Devlin, J.: Prostaglandin content of amniotic fluid during pregnancy and labor. J Obstet Gynaecol Br Commonw 74: 230, 1967.
58. Karim, S. M. M., Hillier, K.: Prostaglandins and spontaneous abortion. J Obstet Gynaecol Br Commonw 77: 837, 1970.
59. Keirse, M. J. N. C., Flint, A. P. F., Turnbull, A. C.: F prostaglandins in amniotic fluid during pregnancy and labour. J Obstet Gynaecol Br Commonw 81: 131, 1974.
60. Kittrich, M.: Changes in the acid-base balance of amniotic fluid during labour. J Obstet Gynaecol Br Commonw 75: 1138, 1968.
61. Koren, Z.: The significance of mono-amine oxidase in amniotic fluid in human foetal development. J Obstet Gynaecol Br Commonw 74: 775, 1967.
62. Kulkarni, B. D., Bieniarz, J., Burd, L., Scommegna, A.: Determination of lecithin-sphingomyelin ratio in amniotic fluid. Obstet Gynecol 40: 173, 1972.
63. Landing, B. H.: Amnion nodosum. Lesion of placenta apparently associated with deficient secretion of fetal urine. Am J Obstet Gynecol 60: 1339, 1950.
64. Larsen, B., Galask, R. P., Snyder, I. S.: Muramidase and peroxidase activity of human amniotic fluid. Obstet Gynecol 44: 219, 1974.
65. Liley, A. W.: Physiological observations in foetal transfusion. *Studies in Physiology*. Berlin, Springer-Verlag, 1965.
66. Lloyd, J. R., Clatworthy, H. W.: Hydramnios as an aid to the early diagnosis of congenital obstruction of the alimentary tract. Pediatrics 21: 903, 1958.
67. Loose, R., Paterson, W. G.: 5-hydroxyindole acetic acid in amniotic fluid and foetal 5-hydroxytryptamine metabolism. J Obstet Gynaecol Br Commonw 73: 647, 1966.
68. Mandelbaum, B., LaCroix, G. C., Robinson, A. R.: Determination of fetal maturity by spectrophotometric analysis of amniotic fluid. Obstet Gynecol 29: 471, 1967.
69. Mandelbaum, B.: Gestational meconium in the high risk pregnancy. Obstet Gynecol 42: 87, 1973.
70. Mati, J. K. G., Horrobin, D. F., Bramley, P. S.: Induction of labor in sheep and in humans by single doses of corticosteroids. Br Med 2: 149, 1973.
71. McLain, C. R., Jr.: Amniographic studies of the gastrointestinal motility of the human fetus. Am J Obstet Gynecol 86: 1079, 1963.
72. Merkatz, I. R., Aladjem, S., Little, B.: The value of biochemical estimations of amniotic fluid in management of high risk pregnancy. Clin Perinatol 1: 301, 1974.
73. Merola, J. C. L., Johnson, L. M., Bolognese, R.

J., Corson, S. L.: Determination of fetal pulmonary maturity by amniotic fluid lecithin/sphingomyelin ratio and rapid shake test. Am J Obstet Gynecol 119: 243, 1974.
74. Midgley, A. R., Jr., Jaffe, R. B.: Gel filtration radioimmunoassay to distinguish human chorionic gonadotrophin from luteinizing hormone. Nature 213: 733, 1967.
75. Monie, I. W.: The volume of the amniotic fluid in the early months of pregnancy. Am J Obstet Gynecol 66: 616, 1953.
76. Moore, W. M. O., Murphy, P. J., Davis, J. A.: Creatinine content of amniotic fluid in cases of retarded fetal growth. Am J Obstet Gynecol 110: 908, 1971.
77. Morrison, J. C., Morrison, D. L., Lovett, F. A., Whybrew, W. D., et al: Nile blue staining of cells in amniotic fluid for fetal maturity. Obstet Gynecol 44: 363, 1974.
78. Murphy, B. E. P., Patrick, J., Denton, R. L., et al: Cortisol in amniotic fluid during human/ gestation. J Clin Endocrinol Metab 40: 164, 1975.
79. Myers, J. L., Harrell, M. J. P., Hill, F. L.: Fetal maturity: Biochemical analyses of amniotic fluid. Am J Obstet Gynecol 121: 961, 1975.
80. Nakamura, J., Roux, J. F., Brown, E. G., Sweet, A. Y.: Total lipids and the lecithin-sphingolmyelin ratio of amniotic fluid: An antenatal test of lung immaturity. Am J Obstet Gynecol 113: 363, 1972.
81. Nelson, G. H.: Amniotic fluid phospholipid patterns in normal and abnormal pregnancies. Am J Obstet Gynecol 105: 1072, 1969.
82. Nelson, G. H.: Relationship between amniotic fluid lecithin concentration and respiratory distress syndrome. Am J Obstet Gynecol 112: 827, 1972.
83. Neslen, E. D., Hutchinson, D. L., Hallet, R. L., Plentl, A. A.: Dilution methods for determination of amniotic fluid volume. Obstet Gynecol 3: 598, 1954.
84. Niswander, K. R., Gordon, M.: *The Women and Their Pregnancies*. Philadelphia, W. B. Saunders, 1975.
85. Nwosu, U., Wallach, E. E., Bolognese, R. J.: Initiation of labor by intraamniotic cortisol instillation in prolonged human pregnancy. Obstet Gynecol 47: 137, 1976.
86. Nwosu, U., Bolognese, R. J., Wallach, E. D., Bongiovanni, A. M.: Amniotic fluid cortisol concentrations in normal and premature labor: Comparison with levels in postmature pregnancy. Obstet Gynecol (In press.)
87. Plentl, A. A.: Transfer of water across the perfused umbilical cord. Proc Soc Exp Biol Med 107: 622, 1961.
88. Pitkin, R. M., Zwirek, S. J.: Amniotic fluid creatinine. Am J Obstet Gynecol 98: 1135, 1967.
89. Pitkin, R. M., Reynolds, W. A., Burchell, R. C.: Fetal contribution to amniotic fluid: A preliminary report. Am J Obstet Gynecol 100: 834, 1968.
90. Potter, E. L.: Bilateral absence of ureters and kidney: A report of 50 cases. J Obstet Gynaecol Br Commonw 25: 3, 1965.
91. Pritchard, J. A.: Deglutition by normal and anencephalic fetuses. Obstet Gynecol 25: 289, 1965.
92. Pritchard, J. A.: Fetal swallowing and amniotic fluid volume. Obstet Gynecol 28: 606, 1966.
93. Queenan, J. T., Gadow, E. G., Bachner, P., Kubarych, S. F.: Amniotic fluid proteins in normal and Rh-sensitized pregnancies. Am J Obstet Gynecol 108: 406, 1970.
94. Queenan, J. T., Gadow, E. L.: Polyhydramnios. Am J Obstet Gynecol 108: 349, 1970.
95. Queenan, J. T., Thompson, W., Whitfield, Shah, S. I.: Amniotic fluid volumes in normal pregnancies. Am J Obstet Gynecol 114: 34, 1972.
96. Quilligan, E. J.: Amniotic fluid gas tension. Am J Obstet Gynecol 84: 20, 1962.
97. Reynolds, S. R. M.: Source of amniotic fluid in the lamb: Nasopharyngeal and buccal cavities. Nature 172: 307, 1953.
98. Rhodes, P.: The volume of liquor amnii in early pregnancy. J Obstet Gynaecol Br Commonw 73: 23, 1966.
99. Rooth, G., Sjostedt, S., Caligara, F.: Acid-base balance of the amniotic fluid. Am J Obstet Gynecol 81: 4, 1961.
100. Salmon, J. A., Amy, J. J.: Levels of prostaglandin F_{2a} in amniotic fluid during pregnancy and labour. Prostaglandins 4: 523, 1973.
101. Schenker, J. G., Ben-David, M., Polishuk, W. Z.: Prolactin in normal pregnancy: Relationship of maternal, fetal and amniotic fluid levels. Am J Obstet Gynecol 123: 834, 1975.
102. Schindler, A. E., Ratanosopa, V., Lee, T. Y., Herrmann, W. L.: Estriol and Rh-isoimmunization: A new approach to the management of severely affected pregnancies. Obstet Gynecol 29: 625, 1967.
103. Schwarz, B. E., Schultz, F. M., MacDonald, P. C., Johnston, J. M.: Initiation of human parturition. Obstet Gynecol 46: 564, 1975.
104. Schwarz, B. E., Schultz, F. M., MacDonald, P. C., Johnston, J. M.: Initiation of human parturition. IV. Demonstration of phospholipase A_2 in the lysosomes of human fetal membranes. Am J Obstet Gynecol 125: 1089, 1976.
105. Sciarra, J. J., Tagatz, G. E., Notation, A. D., Depp, R.: Estriol and estetrol in amniotic fluid. Am J Obstet Gynecol 118: 626, 1974.
106. Scott, J. S., Bain, A. D.: Amnion nodosum. Proc Roy Soc Med 51: 512, 1958.
107. Seeds, A. E., Jr.: Amniotic fluid and fetal water metabolism. *Intrauterine Development*. Edited by A. C. Barnes, Philadelphia, Lea & Febiger, 1968.
108. Sivakoumaran, T., Duncan, M. L., Effer, S. B., Younglai, E. V.: Relationship between cortisol and lecithin/sphingomyelin ratios in human amniotic fluid. Am J Obstet Gynecol 122: 291, 1975.
109. Spellacy, W. N., Buhi, W. C.: Amniotic fluid lecithin/sphingomyelin ratio as an index of fetal maturity. Obstet Gynecol 39: 852, 1972.
110. Spellacy, W. N., Buhi, W. C., Bradley, B.,

Holsinger, K. K.: Maternal, fetal and amniotic fluid levels of glucose, insulin and growth hormone. Obstet Gynecol 41: 323, 1973.
111. Stevenson, A. C.: Association of hydramnios with congenital malformations. Ciba Foundation Symposium on Congenital Malformations, Boston, Little, Brown, 1960.
112. Symonds, E. M., Williams, S. S., Cellier, K. M.: Maternal and fetal influences on the acid-base balance of human amniotic fluid. Obstet Gynecol 37: 742, 1971.
113. Tan, S. Y., Gewolb, I. H., Hobbins, J. C.: Unconjugated cortisol in human amniotic fluid: Relationship to lecithin/sphingomyelin ratio. J Clin Endocrinol Metab 43: 412, 1976.
114. Touchstone, J. C., Glazer, L. G., Bolognese, R. J., Corson, S. L.: Gestational age and amniotic fluid protein patterns. Am J Obstet Gynecol 114: 58, 1972.
115. Troen, P., Nilsson, B., Wiqvist, N., Diczfalusy, E.: Pattern of oestriol conjugates in human cord blood, amniotic fluid, and urine of newborns. Acta Endocrinol 38: 361, 1961.
116. Vasicka, A.: Oxygen in the amniotic fluid. Clin Obstet Gynecol 9: 461, 1966.
117. Vosburgh, G. J., Flexner, L. B., Cowie, D. G., Hellman, L. H., Proctor, N. K., Wilde, W. S.: The rate of renewal in women of the water and sodium of the amniotic fluid as determined by tracer techniques. Am J Obstet Gynecol 56: 1156, 1948.
118. Wagner, G., Fuchs, F.: The volume of amniotic fluid in the first half of human pregnancy. J Obstet Gynaecol Br Commonw 69: 131, 1962.
119. Wagstaff, I. I., Whyley, G. A., Freedman, G.: Factors influencing the measurement of the lecithin/sphingomyelin ratio in amniotic fluid. J Obstet Gynaecol Br Commonw 81: 264, 1974.
120. Weiner, S.: An ultrasound aspiration transducer for diagnostic amniocentesis. Obstet Gynecol 47: 113, 1976.
121. Weingold, A. B., Southern, A. L.: Diamine oxidase as an index of the feto-placental unit. Obstet Gynecol 32: 593, 1968.
122. Whitfield, C. R., Sproule, W. B., Brudenell, M.: The amniotic fluid lecithin: Sphingomyelin area ratio (LSAR) in pregnancies complicated by diabetes. J Obstet Gynaecol Br Commonw 80: 918, 1973.

Part II

LABOR

WAYNE R. COHEN, M.D.
BARRY S. SCHIFRIN, M.D.

7

Diagnosis and Treatment of Fetal Distress

Diagnosis of Fetal Distress

Advances in our knowledge of fetal and placental physiology have made it clear that a substantial proportion of perinatal mortality and morbidity can be ascribed to previously unrecognized traumatic, infectious or pharmacologic insults to the fetus during pregnancy, labor and the neonatal period. The most common, best understood and most readily measured are those insults associated with fetal asphyxia.

It long has been recognized that severe hypoxic insults can cause fetal death. In fact, death most frequently is ascribed in perinatal autopsies to asphyxial central nervous system damage.[99] However, it has been appreciated only recently that sublethal asphyxia may be associated with a spectrum of transient or permanent neurologic disabilities, including cerebral palsy and some kinds of mental retardation. Fetal hypoxia may well be the leading preventable cause of perinatal mortality and morbidity.

The precise toll exacted by hypoxic damage to the perinate is difficult to quantitate. This relates not only to the limitations of objective neurologic follow-up but, even more pertinently, to the relatively recent introduction of reliable clinical methods for recognizing hypoxia. Several statistics are nevertheless quite sobering; it has been estimated that the incidence of hypoxic neurologic damage in the United States is 30 per 1000 live births and that cerebral palsy alone occurs in 6 per 1000.[101] The fact that many of these children asphyxiated at birth appear to be "normal" at 4 years of age is of some comfort but it is likely that the brain lesions presumed responsible for these early abnormalities persist and may be manifested later during the individual's life.[80] Thus, the individual may compensate for damaged brain tissue by adaptation, but there is no evidence that he can bring about structural repair.[78]

The availability of methods that would enable the obstetrician to predict reliably the extent and the etiology of fetal hypoxia would be of enormous benefit. Continuous fetal heart rate monitoring and fetal capillary blood sampling for fetal surveillance during labor appear to have brought us closer to this goal.

In this report, we will explain the use of these techniques in the diagnosis and treatment of fetal distress during labor. The term "fetal distress" universally is defined in terms of the manifestations of fetal hypoxia. A number of observations, such as the appearance of meconium in amniotic fluid and auscultatory fetal bradycardia, long have been thought to reflect such compromise. These classic signs of fetal distress are notoriously inaccurate. Even modern techniques which form the basis of the ensuing discussion are not good predictors of fetal distress. The great clinical benefit of these new techniques, in sharp contrast to the old, lies in their ability to predict the normal fetal condition, i.e., the absence of hypoxia.

It is acknowledged that no data presently exist which demonstrate that the application of the methods described herein improves fetal outcome. However, because the techniques provide direct, reliable and recoverable fetal information, because they are founded in established physiologic principles and because of persuasive suggestions of improved perinatal care and outcome associated with their use, it seems appropriate to employ them.

Pathophysiology of Fetal Hypoxia

It has been appreciated for some time that fetal blood has a lower pH and oxygen tension than maternal blood. This observation was judged previously to be indicative of a pathologic condition in the fetus, and contributed to the belief that the fetus developed in a state of chronic acidosis and hypoxia. Recent evidence has shown that this is not in fact so.

Only small gradients for hydrogen ion and carbon dioxide tension exist across the placenta, and there is a close correlation between maternal and fetal acid-base balance.[2, 57] Thus, in the absence of stress, the fetus is neither acidotic nor hypercapneic but well adjusted to its environment. Although the prevailing fetal PO_2 (20 to 25 mm Hg) is much lower than that of the adult, adequate oxygenation of tissues readily is maintained by the high fetal cardiac output and systemic blood flow rates.[58] In addition, although less important, the oxygen-carrying capacity of fetal blood is higher than that of the adult. This is because fetal blood has a higher hematocrit and contains a large proportion of fetal hemoglobin, which has a greater affinity for oxygen than does adult hemoglobin A. These factors, in addition to an increased concentration of erythrocyte 2,3-diphosphoglycerate and other effects on hemoglobin-oxygen dissociation, insure adequate transfer of oxygen to the fetus under most circumstances.[59]

The fetus depends primarily upon glucose for its energy requirements, and has some capability to utilize ketones, although this is limited. Glucose is derived partly from fetal gluconeogenesis, but primarily from transfer of maternal glucose across the placenta. The oxidation of glucose to pyruvate occurs via the Embden-Myerhoff-Parnas pathway. This pathway does not require oxygen but yields only 2 moles of ATP per mole of glucose. In the presence of adequate oxygen, the pyruvate thus formed enters the Krebs citric acid cycle and the electron transport system to yield a total of 38 moles of ATP for every mole of glucose totally oxidized to carbon dioxide and water. This carbon dioxide is transferred rapidly across the placenta and excreted by the mother. Because the fetal lungs do not function in gas exchange and the fetal kidneys have a limited ability to excrete fixed acid, the placenta serves virtually all of the fetal needs in acid-base homeostasis.

When perfusion of the intervillous space is decreased as a result of impaired uterine or umbilical blood flow, the transfer of oxygen to the fetus is diminished.[22, 81, 105] The immediate consequence of this decrease in flow is an accumulation of carbon dioxide in the fetus. This yields an increase in fetal PCO_2 and a concomitant fall in pH, the analog of respiratory acidosis in the adult. Continued hypoxia deprives the fetus of sufficient oxygen to carry out the aerobic reactions of intermediary metabolism. Glucose can be oxidized only to pyruvate and lactate, a relatively inefficient mode of energy production. These free organic acids accumulate, causing an increase in hydrogen ion concentration and a further fall in pH analogous to a metabolic acidosis. Thus, transient falls in fetal or uterine perfusion generally cause a short lived respiratory acidosis, whereas more prolonged or profound falls result in a combined respiratory and metabolic acidosis which may persist for some time even after the insult has been removed. Although many factors influence the placental transfer of respiratory gases, this process is largely flow dependent, and most clinical situations in which fetal acidosis develops are associated with decreases in uterine or umbilical blood flow.

Data concerning fetal acid-base balance during human labor are obtained by sampling capillary blood from the fetal scalp.[89] There is general agreement that the fetal capillary pH in labor is lower than that observed in adults, ranging from 7.25 to 7.35 in the first stage.[56, 65, 90] Somewhat higher values have been obtained in fetuses that have not yet been subjected to labor, as well as neonates delivered by cesarean section.[7, 14, 29, 60] The gradual decline in pH observed during labor is accentuated in the second stage.[16, 56, 74] This decline is felt to be a result of both increased uterine activity and expulsive efforts of the mother which combine to reduce exchange of oxygen and carbon dioxide across the placenta. Recent evidence suggests that this terminal fall in pH is less likely to be observed when women labor and deliver in the lateral position, presumably because this maternal posture maximizes uterine blood flow.[54] There is generally good agreement between scalp blood pH, cord pH and Apgar scores.[16, 48, 71, 106] Moreover, in fetal rhesus monkey preparations, there is excellent correlation between scalp pH and the simultaneous pH of the carotid artery and jugular vein.[1] It should be emphasized that in the absence of drugs, no etiology for fetal acidemia other than that related to hypoxia or maternal acidemia has been described in the human fetus.

Clinical Diagnosis of Fetal Asphyxia

TRADITIONAL METHODS

Observation of meconium passage during labor and detection of fetal bradycardia by intermittent auscultation of the fetal heart rate long have been considered evidence of fetal jeopardy.[28] It now is apparent that relying on these two signs for evaluation of the fetus has resulted in a set of arbitrary and frequently paradoxical criteria for the clinical intrapartum diagnosis of fetal distress.[9] Moreover, obstetric management based upon these criteria has provided little improvement in fetal outcome; the criteria are of limited value for either the diagnosis of fetal hypoxia or the *absence of hypoxia*. The development of new methods for fetal surveillance during labor has enabled us to define with considerable accuracy the normal fetus and to a lesser extent determine the presence and degree of fetal asphyxia. Moreover, it is no longer appropriate to define fetal compromise on the basis of maternal condition. Although diseases such as pre-eclampsia are more commonly associated with asphyxia, each fetus must be judged individually.

FETAL BLOOD SAMPLING

Interpretation of fetal blood pH levels has not been completely uniform, but most authors consider values less than 7.20 to be suggestive of significant asphyxia and those between 7.20 and 7.24 "preacidotic," requiring further evaluation.[16, 65, 72, 88] Furthermore, since lactate and carbon dioxide readily cross the placenta when fetomaternal exchange is adequate, a low fetal pH may reflect severe maternal acidosis.[27] Thus, if the pH of the mother is low, fetal acidemia need not necessarily reflect an asphyxial insult, and considerable numbers of such babies are born without depression. Maternal acidemia scrupulously should be avoided however, for it may decrease uterine blood flow,[10] poison fetal enzyme systems, deplete buffer base reserves and lower the oxygen-carrying capacity of fetal blood, rendering the fetus vulnerable to a subsequent episode of asphyxia.

Fetuses with a primarily respiratory acidosis (high PCO_2, near normal base deficit, moderate fall in pH) usually respond very well as neonates. Those with combined respiratory and metabolic acidosis and large base deficits recover much more slowly. In explanation, the neonate achieves acid-base stability primarily by pulmonary excretion of carbon dioxide. Renal mechanisms for handling hydrogen ion are incompletely developed in the newborn.

A number of investigators have analyzed the use of blood sampling in the management of fetal distress.[7, 14, 15, 23, 26, 37, 40, 47, 48, 82, 103, 104] The ability to predict Apgar scores using fetal capillary pH alone is only about 80%. Falsely normal pH values occur with a frequency of 6 to 20% and spuriously low pH values in approximately 8 to 10%.[6, 14, 15]

Several possible explanations exist for the falsely normal values in the presence of low Apgar scores. Depression from sedatives or anesthetics could be reflected in poor respiratory effort and flaccidity at birth but normal *in utero* pH. The same could apply to prematurity, fetal infection or to any traumatic insult or meconium aspiration that occurs at delivery. Most false normal values probably result from a hypoxic episode that has occurred between the sampling period and delivery.

Spuriously low pH values may occasionally be related to maternal acidosis, to a period of hypoxemia from which the fetus recovers prior to delivery or may be a result of local scalp edema or vasoconstriction. In the latter instance, fetal capillary blood values will not accurately reflect the pH of the central circulation. We have found blood sampling to be most useful when employed in conjunction with the technique of continuous fetal heart rate monitoring.

FETAL HEART RATE MONITORING

The introduction of bioelectronic techniques for the reliable recording of the instantaneous fetal heart rate during labor has vastly expanded our knowledge of fetal cardiovascular physiology and its response to stress.[94] Several investigators have confirmed the similarity between autonomic nervous system control of the fetal and adult heart rates. In the human fetus heart rate decreases during pregnancy[55]; at term the rate is usually between 120 and 160 beats per minute (bpm). On the other hand, beat-to-beat irregularity (*variability*) increases as term approaches. These features likely reflect the increasing vagal influence which accompanies maturation of the fetal nervous system. Beat-to-beat variability appears to represent the continuous and subtle interaction of sympathetic and parasympathetic nervous systems as they determine the appropriate heart rate and cardiac output in response to continuous minor changes in venous return or perhaps metabolic demands (Figure 7.1).[31, 107] Fetal activity, as well as various central nervous system inputs, such as those related to fetal breathing movements, influence variability.[33, 102] The role of local cardiac factors, such as sinus node artery pressure, has not been investigated in the fetus.[39] Decreased variability (see below) may signify loss of fine autonomic control of the heart rate. It must be emphasized that in order to interpret variability one must employ a cardiotachometer capable of determining heart rate on a beat-by-beat basis.[52] External ultrasonic techniques or monitors which average the rate may obscure critical changes in variability.

Baseline heart rate and variability are helpful in evaluating fetal oxygenation. Good short term variability, even in the presence of other signs suggesting hypoxia, usually presages a good outcome (Figures 7.2 and 7.3).[76] Although acute hypoxia may transiently increase baseline

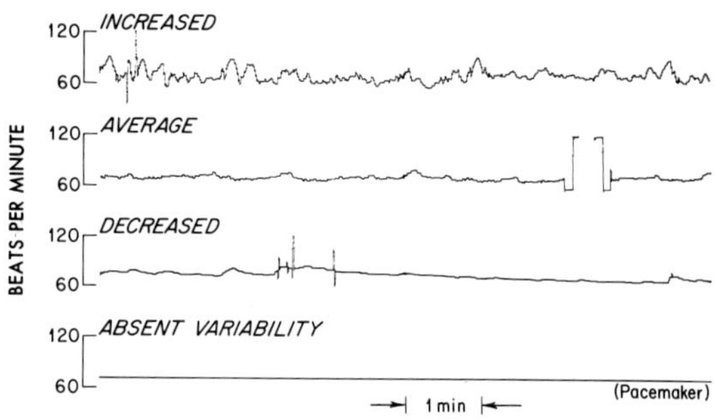

Figure 7.1. Instantaneous heart rate. Examples of variations in beat-to-beat variability. The lower tracing is taken from an adult with a cardiac pacemaker, and illustrates absolute absence of variation in R-R intervals.

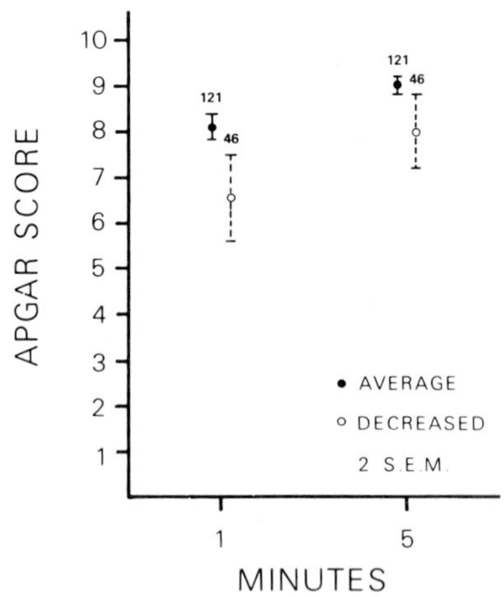

Figure 7.2. FHR variability. Heart rate patterns associated with decreased variability more frequently are associated with low Apgar scores. (Reprinted from Paul, R. H., Suidan, A. K., Yeh, S., Schifrin, B. S., Hon, E. H.: Clinical fetal monitoring. VII. The evaluation and significance of intrapartum baseline FHR variability. Am J Obstet Gynecol 123: 206, 1975.)

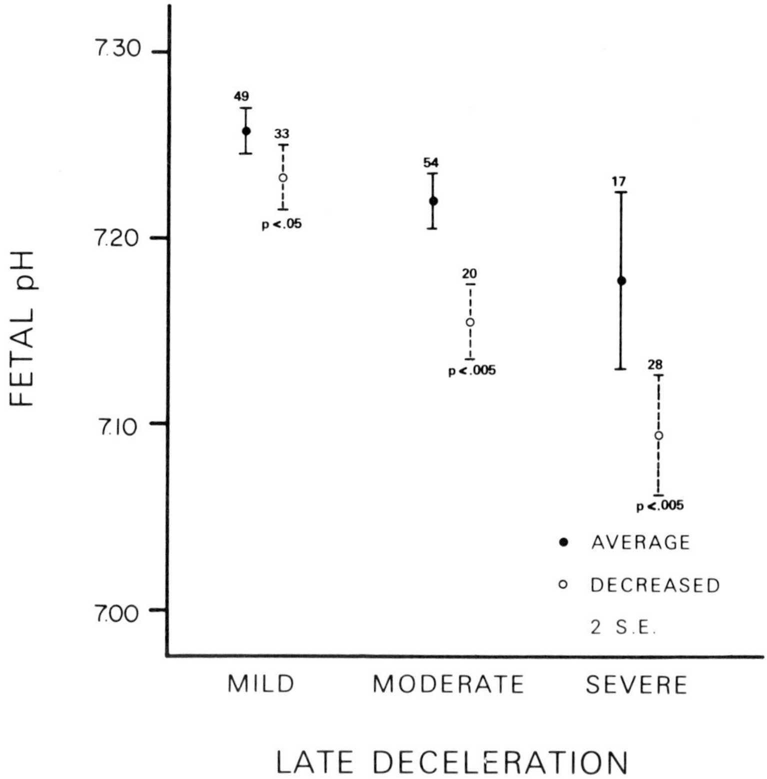

Figure 7.3. FHR variability. Late decelerations accompanied by decreased variability are associated with more severe acidosis than those with average variability. (Reprinted from Paul, R. H., Suidan, A. K., Yeh, S., Schifrin, B. S., Hon, E. H.: Clinical fetal monitoring. VII. The evaluation and significance of intrapartum baseline FHR variability. Am J Obstet Gynecol 123: 206, 1975.

variability,[17] significant chronic hypoxia is usually associated with its marked diminution.[36, 84] Decreased variability, however, frequently is seen with adequately oxygenated premature fetuses and in any fetus after the administration to the mother of certain drugs such as atropine or ataractic agents[12, 45, 107] (Figure 7.4). In addition, normal fetuses seem to undergo physiologic periods of rest or "sleep" in utero, during which time the variability is diminished.[36] Stimulation of a fetus in this condition often will cause a transient increase in variability and/or a baseline acceleration and thus assure the obstetrician of a reactive fetus whose decreased variability has occurred for nonasphyxial reasons (Table 7.1).

Heart rate responses to hypoxia are varied depending upon the frequency of contractions and the nature of the asphyxial insult. In the absence of intense uterine activity the fetus frequently compensates for *slowly* developing asphyxia with tachycardia, presumably mediated through discharge of sympathomimetic amines from the adrenal medulla.[24, 66] Tachycardia, however, especially during labor and in the absence of decelerations, is associated more often with nonasphyxial conditions, the most common being maternal fever (Table 7.2). When contractions are frequent, the earliest sign of fetal hypoxia is not tachycardia but late decelerations (see below). Whether contractions are present or not, acute, profound hypoxia causes slowing of the fetal heart rate. Hypoxia, however, is not the only cause of persistent fetal bradycardia (Table 7.3). Many normal babies have heart rates between 80 and 120 bpm. Bradycardia may be secondary to cord compression or paracervical block or secondary to drugs such as propranolol. Persistent bradycardia may be the result of severe asphyxia, under which circumstances it will be associated with a

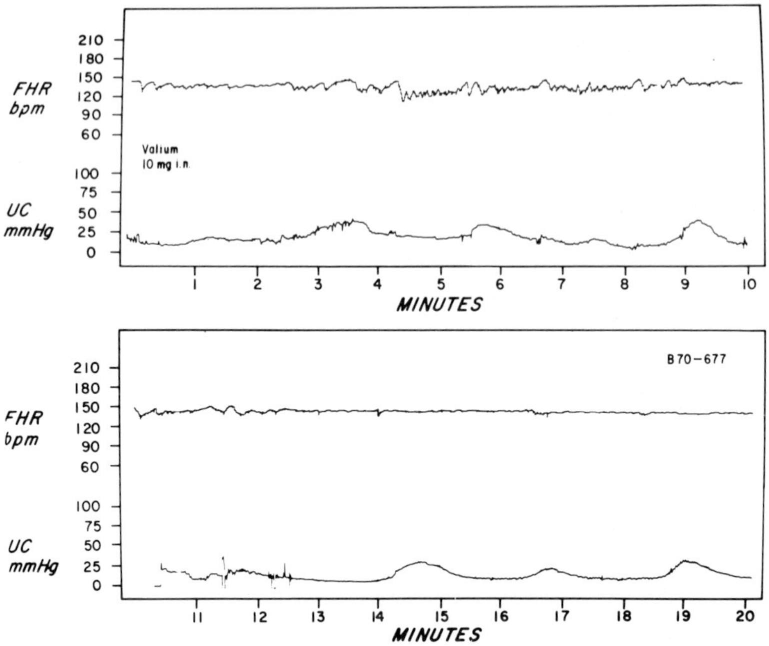

Figure 7.4. Diminution of long and short term variability after administration of diazepam to mother. UC: uterine contractions.

Table 7.1. Decreased variability

Asphyxia
Drugs
Atropine, scopolamine
Tranquilizers
Narcotics
Barbiturates
Anesthetics
Prematurity
Tachycardia
Physiologic "sleep"
Cardiac and central nervous system anomalies
Arrhythmias

Table 7.2. Fetal tachycardia

Asphyxia
Maternal fever
Fetal infection
Prematurity
Drugs, e.g., atropine, isoxuprine
Idiopathic
Fetal stimulation
Arrhythmias
Maternal anxiety
Maternal thyrotoxicosis

marked decrease in beat-to-beat variability.[50]

Sinusoidal oscillations in the baseline have been associated with fetal jeopardy

Table 7.3. Fetal bradycardia

Asphyxia (late)
Idiopathic
Drugs
Reflex
Arrhythmias
Hypothermia

during antepartum monitoring, especially in babies affected by Rh isoimmunization.[68, 86] Although this pattern has been shown to presage a poor outcome in other clinical conditions, we have observed these patterns in a number of healthy fetuses and consider their significance uncertain except in the Rh-sensitized pregnancy.[5] Before any baseline characteristic is ascribed to hypoxia, all of the other possible etiologies should be excluded and a confirmatory fetal pH obtained.

Periodic changes in the fetal heart rate (FHR) assume importance in defining the nature and intensity of asphyxial insults.[44] Hon and Quilligan[51] have defined three patterns of periodic decelerations depending on the configuration of the waveform and the timing of the deceleration in relation to the uterine contraction (Figure 7.5).

Early deceleration patterns (head compression) begin with the onset of the contraction, rarely drop below 100 bpm and return to the baseline along with the uterine pressure curve (Figure 7.6). They are most common in the second stage of labor and rarely are seen with the membranes intact. This variety of deceleration is thought to be caused by a vagal discharge related to the increase in intracranial pressure that may accompany contractions. Early decelerations are not caused by hypoxia and do not appear to be associated with poor fetal outcome.[63]

Recurrent, symmetric decelerations that begin late in the uterine contraction cycle are called *late decelerations* and usually are found in association with acute or chronic fetoplacental vascular insufficiency (Table 7.4).[19] They are felt to be precipitated by hypoxemia, which slows the rate as a result of direct myocardial depression, central nervous system asphyxia or both.[42] Fetal hypotension has been shown to accompany this pattern. Late decelerations are associated with a mixed respiratory and metabolic acidosis.[63] Late decelerations during labor are found with increased frequency in patients with pre-eclampsia, hypertension, diabe-

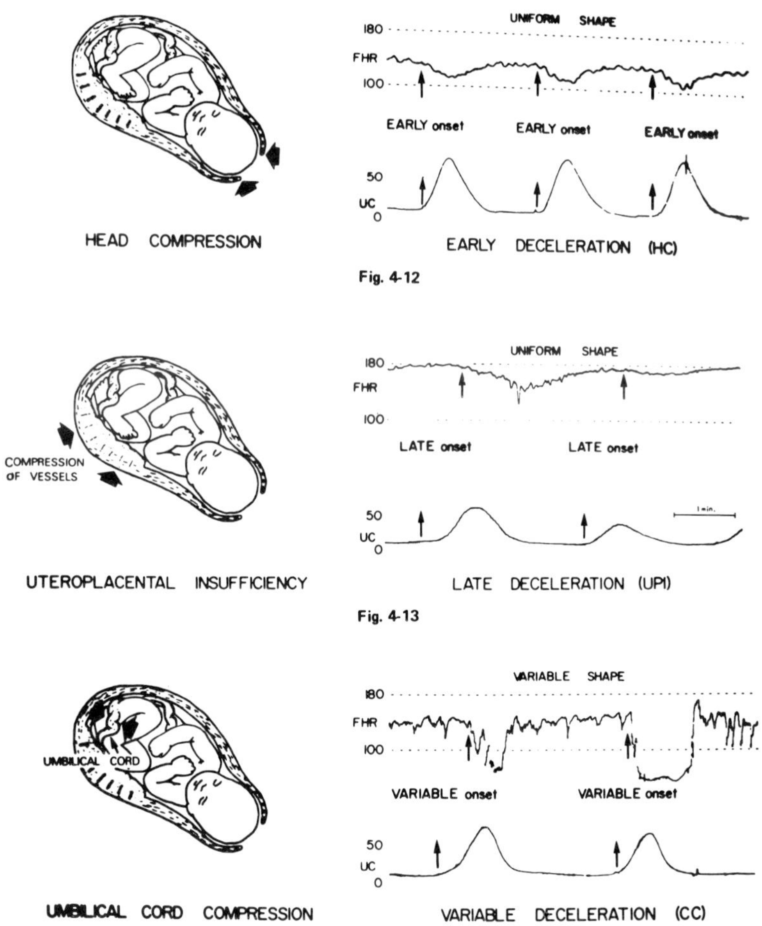

Figure 7.5. Diagrammatic representation of proposed pathogenetic mechanism of FHR deceleration patterns. In early decelerations, onset of deceleration coincides with rise in intrauterine pressure (arrows). Uniform shape of deceleration reflects shape of associated uterine pressure curve. Late deceleration is characterized by uniform shape and onset late in contraction. Variable decelerations are of variable shape and configuration. Onset is variable in relation to that of contraction. (Reprinted from Hon, E. H.: *Atlas of Fetal Heart Rate Patterns*. New Haven, Harty Press, 1968.)

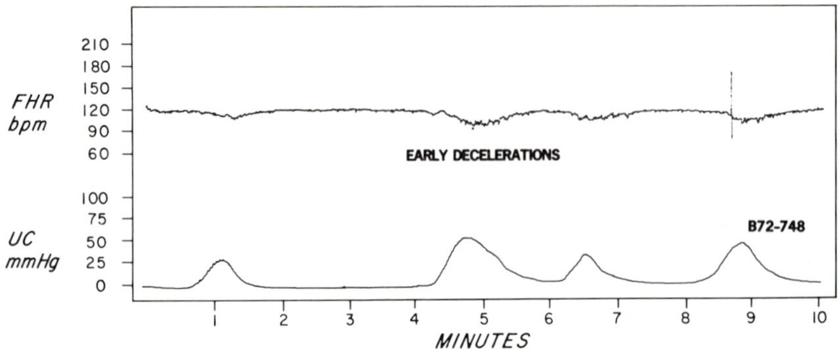

Figure 7.6. Examples of early decelerations. Note they are proportional to the amplitude of the uterine contraction (*UC*).

Table 7.4. Characteristics of late decelerations

Uniform shape
Onset late in contraction cycle
Repetitive
Duration of deceleration proportional to duration of uterine contraction
Amplitude of deceleration proportional to amplitude of uterine contraction

tes mellitus, intrauterine growth retardation or other disorders associated with chronic placental insufficiency. Presumably, the incipient decrease in placental reserve associated with these conditions may render the fetus quite vulnerable to the stress of even ordinary uterine contractions. Late decelerations also occur in situations in which there is an acute decrement in the intervillous space flow, such as abruptio placentae, maternal hypotension from conduction anesthesia or other causes or excessive uterine activity. The appearance of late decelerations under any circumstances should be of great concern because they are associated so frequently with significant asphyxia.[63, 72, 79]

Several characteristics of the late deceleration waveform have been shown by Myers et al[79] in primate experiments to correlate with the degree of hypoxia. The magnitude and initial slope of the bradycardia and the interval between the onset of the contraction and that of its late deceleration pattern bear a direct relationship with fetal oxygenation. Paul et al[84] have demonstrated that for any magnitude of late deceleration, fetal acidosis worsens as beat-to-beat variability diminishes. The development of baseline tachycardia and decreased variability between late decelerations is almost invariably an ominous sign (Figure 7.7).[6, 19] Late decelerations that are associated with good variability often are accompanied by minimal hypoxia, are frequently iatrogenic and are often remediable (Figure 7.8).

Variable decelerations (cord compression patterns) are so named because they are inconstant in configuration and bear no consistent temporal relationship to the onset of the contraction. They appear to be the result of transient compression of the umbilical cord between fetal parts or between the fetus and surrounding maternal tissues. Occlusion of the umbilical vessels removes the low resistance placental vascular bed from the circulation, increasing fetal total peripheral resistance. Presumably, this increased resistance leads to a transient rise in blood pressure, which in turn elicits a reflex deceleration by stimulation of the baroreceptors. Recent evidence, however, suggests that chemoreceptor stimulation may also play a role.[96] The initial bradycardia may be blocked or modified by atropine.[4, 43, 46] These decelerations are analogous to those observed by Barcroft[4] in cord clamping experiments in fetal goats and those produced by experimental cord compression in humans.[41] They are the most common patterns observed, particularly during the second stage of labor when descent and rotation increase the likelihood of cord entrapment. However, they may vary considerably in their impact on the fetus, depending on the duration and completeness of the cord occlusion. Mild variable decelerations cause a short lived respiratory acidosis and more prolonged patterns may be associated with profound combined acidosis.[64]

Kubli et al[63] have classified variable decelerations according to severity. Those considered to suggest fetal compromise are prolonged (longer than 1 min), and have severe bradycardias (less than 70 bpm). The mean fetal pH was found to be 7.15 in association with severe cord compression patterns defined by these criteria.[63] Poor variability and/or tachycardia between de-

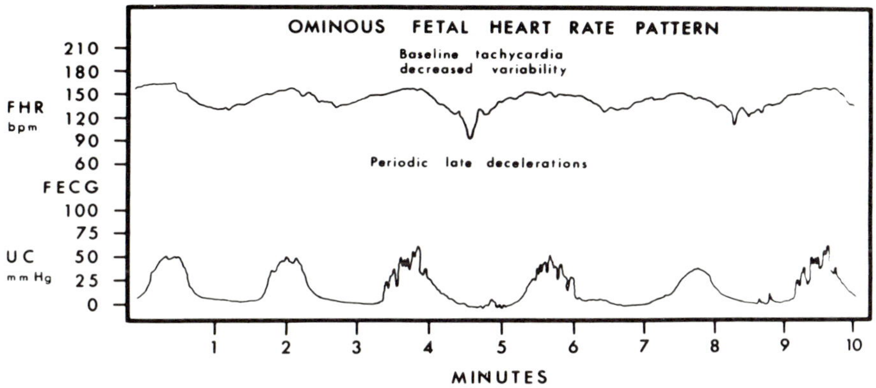

Figure 7.7. Recurrent late decelerations associated with baseline tachycardia and loss of variability usually are associated with severe hypoxia. UC: uterine contraction; FECG; fetal ECG.

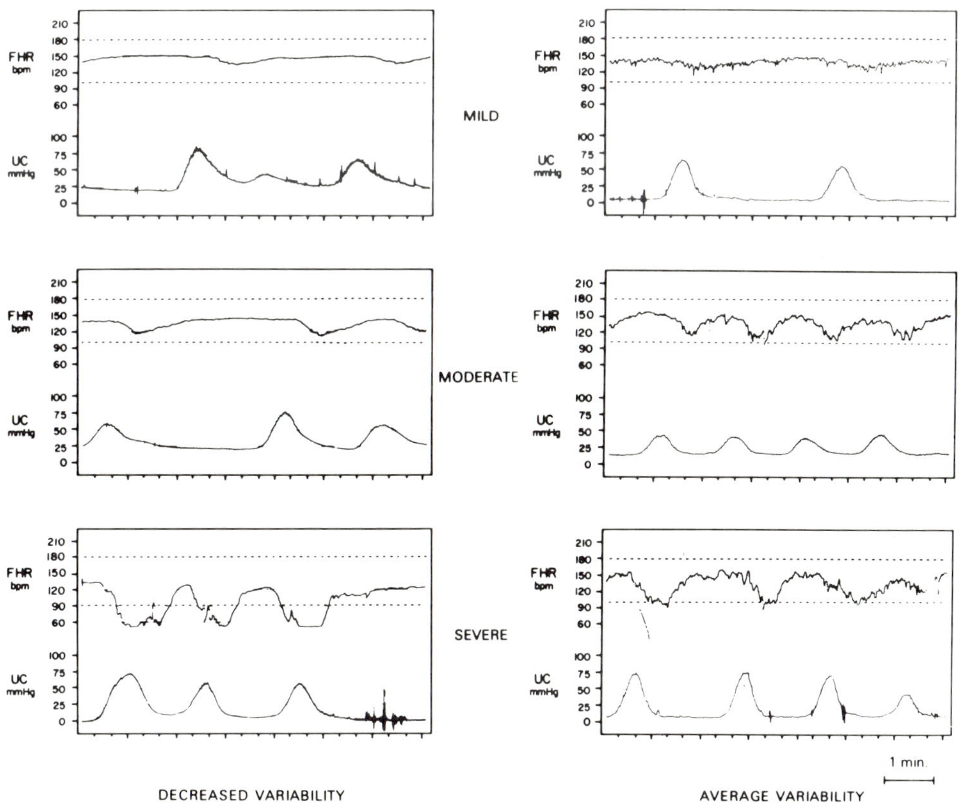

Figure 7.8. Late decelerations associated with good variability are frequently remediable and related to demonstrable insults. Those with poor variability respond less well to therapy and usually are associated with chronic placental insufficiency. UC: uterine contraction.

celerations, bradyarrhythmias (including sinus arrest) and terminal acceleration before returning to baseline are usually considered to be further indicators of severity (Figure 7.9).

Occasionally, *prolonged decelerations* of the fetal heart rate are noted. These usually consist of sudden drops of at least 30 bpm which persist for perhaps 2 min or more. This is a heterogeneous group of patterns with regard to their configuration, timing and etiology. These patterns commonly are associated with preceding variable decelerations or manipulation of the patient. In addition, uterine hypertonus, vaginal examination, scalp sampling, paracervical block anesthesia and maternal seizures may also precipitate prolonged decelerations (Figure 7.10).[11] Most of these patterns have not been associated with significant fetal hypoxia, particularly when associated with good variability.[13, 98]

Accelerations in heart rate during contractions are common. *Uniform accelerations* reflect the shape of and occur synchronously with uterine contractions (Figure 7.11). These patterns are common in early labor before membranes are ruptured and in nonvertex presentations.

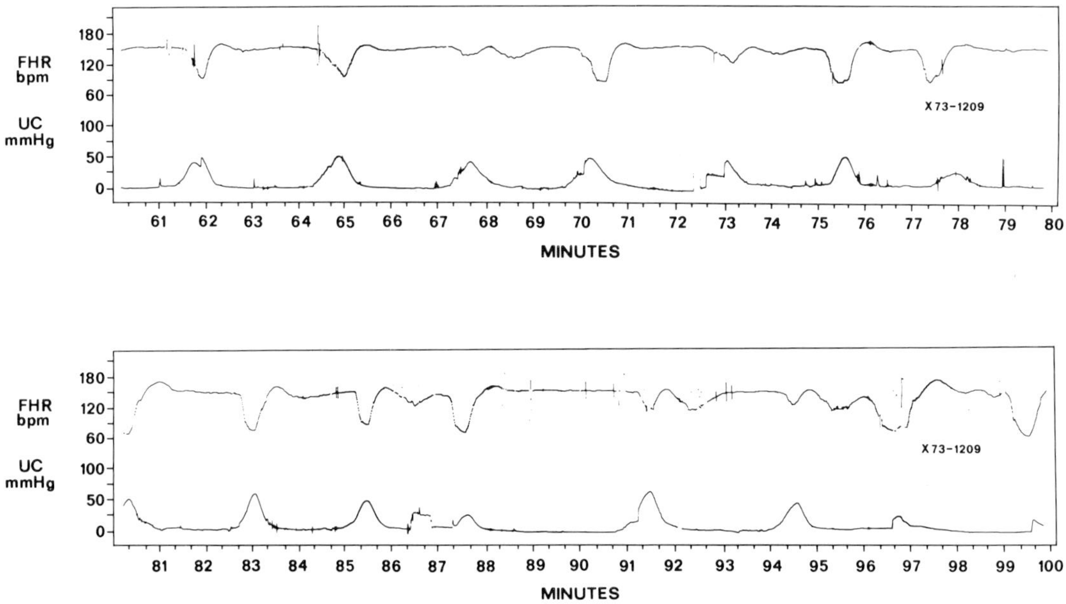

Figure 7.9. Severe recurrent variable decelerations associated with markedly diminished variability and rebound accelerations. UC: uterine contraction.

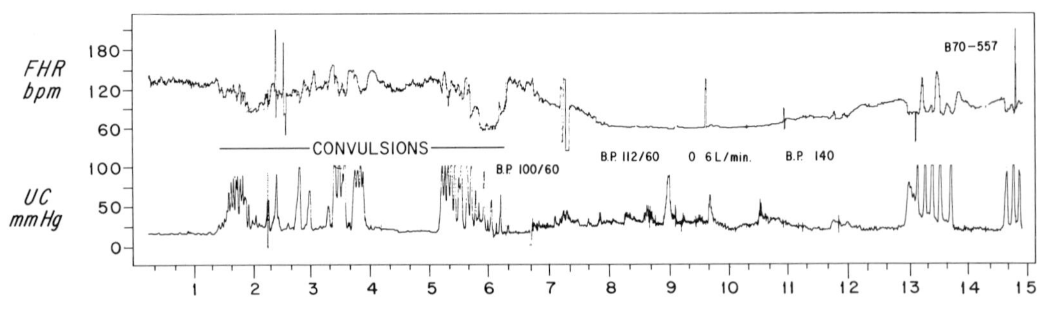

Figure 7.10. Prolonged deceleration resulting from maternal hypoxemia during seizure. If cause of such a deceleration is promptly removed, fetus will recover. UC: uterine contraction.

Such patterns usually are associated with normal baseline rate and variability and are invariably benign. They may occur in the absence of contractions and be associated with fetal movement or stimulation. *Variable accelerations* do not reflect the shape of the uterine contraction. They usually are seen immediately preceding or following variable decelerations, generally are associated with normal or increased variability and also represent an apparently benign pattern (Figure 7.12). *Rebound accelerations* ("overshoot") are accelerations which follow variable decelerations and may be of two types. Type I accelerations are the erratic accelerations associated with increased variability after a severe deceleration. Type II accelerations are recurrent accelerations associated with *absent variability* which follow a variable deceleration regardless of amplitude (Figure 7.9). Type II appears to be a most ominous pattern, probably a manifestation of impaired autonomic control, as evidenced by its appearance in immature fetuses or those given atropine.[45]

Operationally we have come to look upon baseline rate and variability as indices of *fetal reserve* and look to the deceleration waveform for insight into the *mechanism of the insult*. With this perspective we have de-emphasized consideration of the severity of decelerations, preferring instead to determine the impact of a decel-

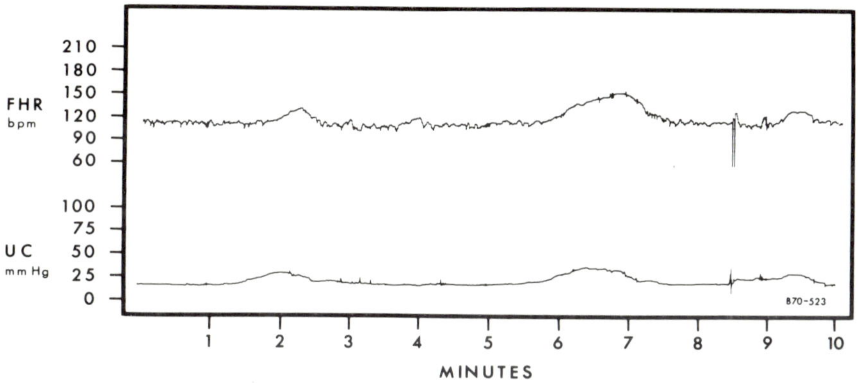

Figure 7.11. Uniform accelerations. UC: uterine contraction.

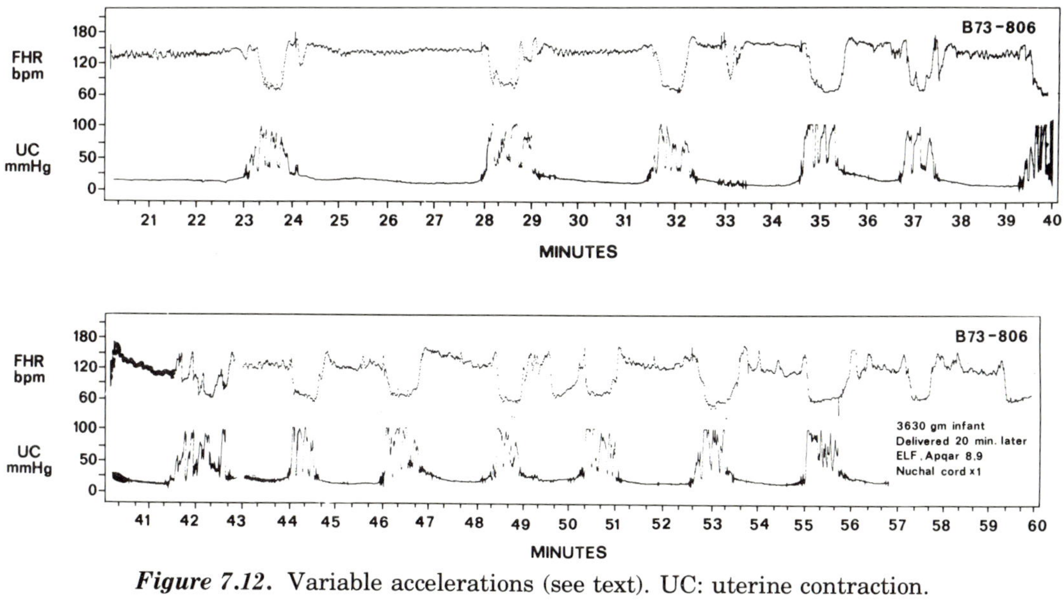

Figure 7.12. Variable accelerations (see text). UC: uterine contraction.

eration by looking at the changes it produces in rate and variability.

Several authors have shown good correlation between fetal heart rate patterns and the traditionally accepted clinical index of neonatal well-being, the Apgar score.[18, 93] Early and mild variable decelerations generally result in a normal fetal outcome. On the other hand, a significant number of babies with prolonged severe variable or late deceleration patterns are compromised at birth. Evidence suggests that such babies run a significant risk of subsequent neurologic handicap.[18] A normal FHR pattern has been shown to be an almost perfect predictor that a baby will be born in good condition.[93] Although abnormal FHR patterns are considerably less accurate in predicting low Apgar scores, virtually every depressed neonate can be anticipated.

In the foregoing discussion, we have used the term fetal distress to represent fetal hypoxia, usually resulting from a diminution in placental blood flow (giving rise to late decelerations) or umbilical blood flow (giving rise to variable decelerations). It must be borne in mind that the fetus may be compromised by a variety of nonasphyxial insults, for example, trauma, drugs or infection, which are not necessarily reflected in early changes in heart rate pattern or pH. Clinical methods of evaluating these other factors unfortunately are not widely available.

Iatrogenic Fetal Distress

Some of the lessons learned from monitoring experience and our burgeoning knowledge of obstetric physiology have made us aware of the risks inherent in many commonplace clinical practices. These have recently been reviewed by Schifrin[92] and are outlined briefly below.

MATERNAL POSITION

It has been known for some time that during late pregnancy blood flow through the abdominal aorta and inferior vena cava may be obstructed by the uterus when the mother is in the supine position. About 10% of term pregnant women experience supine hypotension and many others develop clinically undetectable falls in cardiac output and uterine blood flow.[53] The implication of this fact for the fetus, who relies on adequate uterine blood flow for nutrition and respiratory gas exchange, is self-evident. Improvement in oxygenation has been noted in babies born vaginally and by cesarean section when mothers are in the semilateral position, compared to those who are supine.[54, 100] One probably should aspire to keep all laboring and delivering women on their sides. Certainly, in any situation in which fetal distress is present or suspected, the supine position should be avoided.

OXYTOCIN STIMULATION

The use of uterotonic agents is associated with an increased incidence of late decelerations.[91] This is not surprising when excessive uterine activity has been produced. However, even when oxytocin is given in near physiologic levels under careful control, contractility may be greater than normal. The risk of hyperstimulation can be minimized with the use of both a constant infusion pump for delivery of the oxytocin and a record of uterine activity to determine the uterine response.

PERIDURAL ANESTHESIA

The sympathetic blockade which accompanies epidural anesthesia may result in diminished uterine blood flow. The incidence of late decelerations in the presence of epidural anesthesia is high, particularly when combined with the use of oxytocin (Figure 7.13).[91] Maintaining well hydrated patients in the lateral position during epidural anesthesia helps negate the potential hazards of this technique.

Intrauterine Resuscitation

Although the presence of fetal distress may occasionally demand immediate operative delivery, there is usually time to attempt intrauterine resuscitation. Based upon our understanding of the pathophysiology of abnormal heart rate patterns and fetal acidosis, methods of treating fetal distress in utero have evolved. Obstetric intervention for fetal asphyxia can be justified only when all avenues of correction have been explored and found to be of no avail.

It is convenient to divide the clinical signs of fetal distress into three categories (Table 7.5). Warning signs (tachycardia, bradycardia, decreased variability) suggest possible incipient hypoxia and should spur increased vigilance on the part of the obstetrician with employment of all available techniques to verify the presence or absence of hypoxia. He should avoid potentially compromising drugs or techniques until he is certain that another explanation for these signs probably exists. Threatening signs of fetal distress require prompt attention. They usually are related to iatrogenic insults as described above, and usually are corrected without resorting to immediate delivery. Ominous signs similarly require immediate evaluation. Although all efforts should be made to correct the ominous pattern, simultaneous preparation for cesarean section should be carried out. In the absence of immediate demonstrable benefit from conservative measures, cesarean section or immediate safe vaginal delivery is indicated.

It has been emphasized previously that late decelerations usually are related to deficits in intervillous space blood flow. Consequently, insofar as fetal hypoxia and late decelerations are related to maternal factors, they may be improved by maneuvers that maximize uterine blood flow. All patients with suspected fetal distress should be placed in the lateral position. The importance of this posture in maintaining maternal cardiac output and uterine blood flow has been emphasized previously in this chapter. Moving from the dorsal lithotomy to the lateral recumbent position can increase cardiac output by as much as 30%. The importance of adequate hydration is an equally crucial factor. It is not unusual for patients in labor to have been without oral intake for long periods of time. This can result in a total body water deficit of considerable proportions, and even though maternal pulse and blood pressure may remain relatively stable, blood may be diverted from the uterus to maintain flow in vital organs. Hence, all laboring women should have an infusion of intravenous fluids begun in early labor so

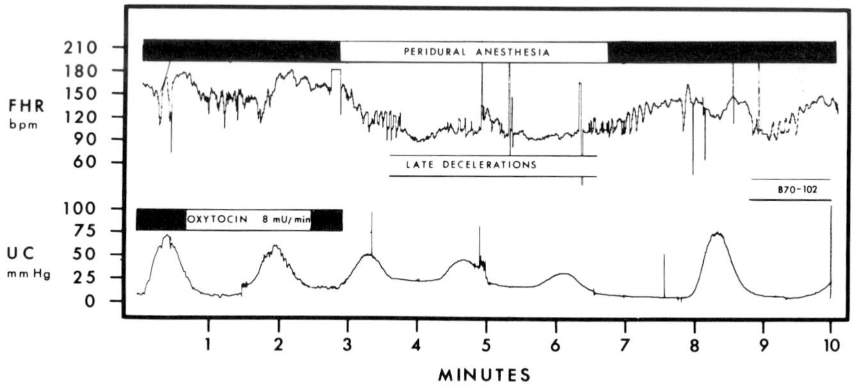

Figure 7.13. Recurrent late decelerations associated with the use of oxytocin and peridural anesthesia. UC: uterine contraction.

Table 7.5. Fetal heart rate patterns of fetal distress

	Suspicious	Threatening	Ominous
Baseline features	Decreased variability Tachycardia or bradycardia	Good variability Stable rate	Absent variability Tachycardia or bradycardia Unstable rate ("sinusoidal")
Periodic features	Decelerations absent	Late decelerations Variable decelerations	Late decelerations Variable decelerations (rebound accelerations)

that volume deficits are avoided. In the presence of late decelerations, an infusion of saline to replace depleted intravascular volume is sometimes curative. Adequate hydration is particularly vital if the use of conduction anesthesia is contemplated. The incidence of maternal hypotension and consequent fetal compromise from the peripheral vasodilatation that accompanies spinal or epidural block is reduced markedly if circulatory volume has been maintained prior to anesthetic administration.[70] In addition, maternal hypotension, hypovolemia or hypoxemia can be caused by many anesthetic agents, blood loss or underlying maternal cardiovascular, pulmonary or hematologic disease.

Increasing the concentration of inspired oxygen to the mother results in a small increment in fetal PO_2, and may be a useful measure in treating fetal distress.[3, 61, 75] However, it is of secondary importance to maneuvers that increase blood flow. Massive infusion of glucose to the mother in hopes of increasing fetal metabolic substrate has been shown to be of little value.[67] Bicarbonate does not cross the placenta readily when the fetus is acidotic. However, the use of intra-amniotic bicarbonate experimentally has been shown to have some efficacy in increasing fetal pH.[38, 95] This modality requires further investigation before it can be recommended for clinical use (Table 7.6).

Attempts to ameliorate severe variable decelerations should include all of the above measures for increasing uterine blood flow and fetal oxygenation and, in addition, maneuvers to alter the anatomic relationship of fetus, umbilical cord and uterine wall so as to relieve compression of the cord. Altering the mother's position by moving her from side to side, to Trendelenberg position or even to the knee-chest position frequently will correct or improve the patterns. When overt cord prolapse has occurred, manual elevation of the fetal head out of the maternal pelvis is an established procedure while preparations for operative delivery are carried out. It may also be efficacious in some situations in which the diagnosis of overt or occult prolapse is suspected from fetal heart rate patterns (Figure 7.14).

When recurrent severe variable decelerations do not respond to the resuscitative maneuvers described above, the patient should be readied for cesarean section, a vaginal exam performed and the presenting part gently elevated.[20] If an overt prolapse is discovered, one may proceed with abdominal delivery while maintaining elevation of the presenting part. If no cord is felt, and the heart rate pattern does not show evidence of recovery, immediate delivery becomes mandatory. However, if improvement is seen, one may allow the fetus to recover completely and then permit it to descend once again. If severe decelerations recur, elevation should be reinstituted and a cesarean section performed after the fetus recovers. If the heart rate remains stable, labor may be allowed to progress in the usual manner. Quite commonly in these situations, one is dealing with an occult prolapse of the cord which may correct itself. Our custom of placing the mother in Trendelenberg position before the vertex is elevated minimizes the potential for precipitating a cord prolapse where one was not previously present.

Table 7.6. Fetal distress: Methods of treatment

Improve uterine blood flow
Avoid supine position
Reduce uterine contractions
Decrease oxytocin
(Uterine relaxants)
Ensure adequate hydration
Correct maternal hypotension
Improve umbilical blood flow
Alter maternal position
Elevate vertex
Enhance maternal substrate
Oxygen
(Bicarbonate)

PRACTICAL CONSIDERATIONS

When warning signs of fetal distress are present, the obstetrician or nurse should examine the patient to be sure that she is in the proper posture, is well hydrated, and that any correctable factors which might contribute to fetal hypoxia are dealt with at once. All potentially compromising techniques, such as oxytocin stimulation or regional or paracervical anesthesia, should be withheld from patients with possible impending fetal distress.

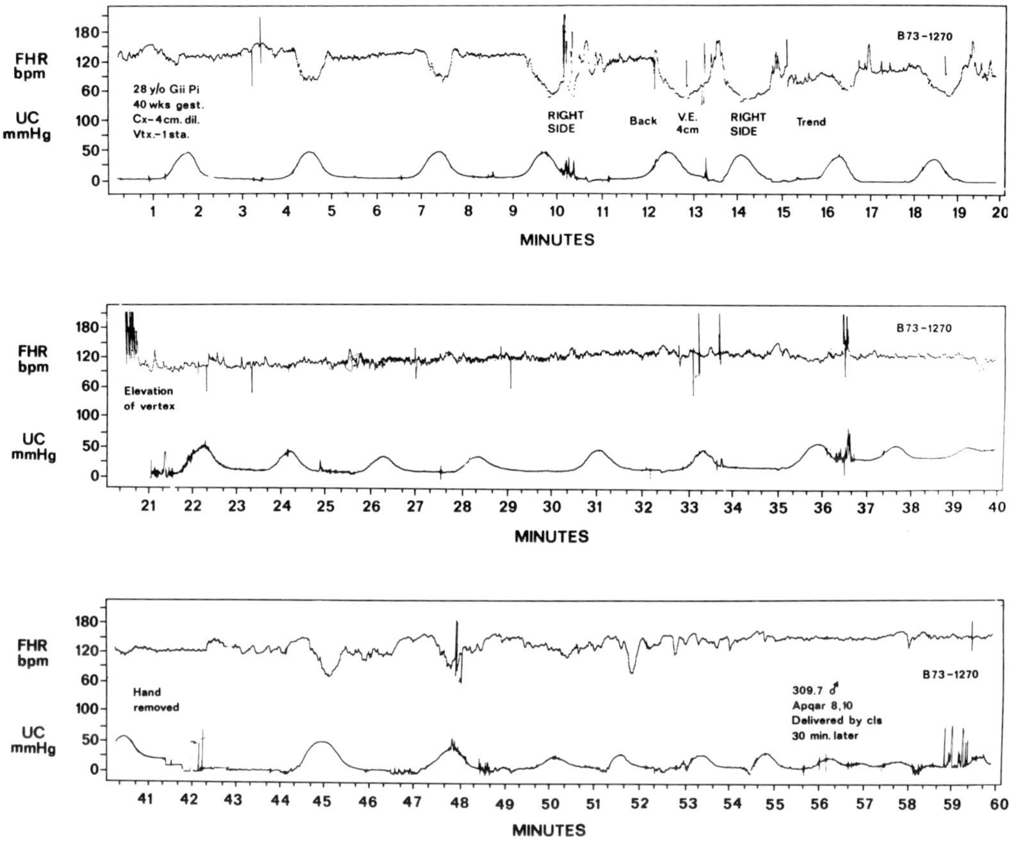

Figure 7.14. Elevation of the vertex improved recurrent severe variable decelerations. When vertex was allowed to descend again, only mild variable decelerations supervened. UC: uterine contraction.

Mild to moderate variable decelerations are generally of no serious consequence, but attempts should be made to relieve them nonetheless. Intervention need not be carried out if the baseline heart rate is stable and variability is average. Intervention should be considered if variable decelerations are accompanied by a rising baseline, loss of variability or falling pH.

During labor, tachycardia or bradycardia or decreased variability as isolated signs are usually not indications of fetal hypoxia. They assume more ominous significance if they are present with minimal uterine activity. In the latter event, a fetal blood sample should be obtained or the uterus stimulated with oxytocin in an effort to better define the fetal condition. Occasionally, a terminally asphyxiated fetus may present with absent variability as its only heart rate abnormality.

Prolonged decelerations should be treated according to the recommendations made for variable decelerations. Intervention for prolonged decelerations should be considered in the face of progressive acidosis as determined by serial sampling and/or absent short term variability without evidence of recovery in the rate.

As noted, the nature of the asphyxial insult often can be determined from the waveform of the fetal heart rate decelerations. Once the diagnosis of severe cord compression or decreased uteroplacental blood flow has been made, appropriate treatment for each should be instituted, as described above. Scrupulous attention should be paid to the condition of the baseline tracing between contractions as a measure of fetal reserve. Prompt recovery from a deceleration without tachycardia and with good variability suggests that the fetus has tolerated the insult of the contraction well. A rising baseline rate and decreasing variability are more ominous. When blood sampling is employed care should be taken that the sample is obtained between decelerations with the patient on her side so that the sample will serve as a measure of the fetus' ability to recover from stress; if taken at the nadir of a deceleration, acidosis commonly will be present.

Meconium staining of the amniotic fluid is suggestive, but never diagnostic, of hypoxia.[73] Its presence should be used as an indication for the use of fetal heart rate monitoring and/or scalp sampling to determine the presence of asphyxia. In addition, because of the risks of aspiration when meconium is present, the obstetrician should be certain that adequately trained personnel and all of the requisite equipment for neonatal resuscitation are present in the delivery room.

Uterine activity should be assessed. The use of uterotonic agents should be proscribed in the presence of fetal distress, even when uterine activity does not appear to be excessive. The use of myometrial relaxants is still experimental, but may become an important part of our armamentarium for managing in utero distress.

While maneuvers of intrauterine resuscitation are being carried out, the patient should be prepared for operative delivery. It should be stressed firmly that the indication for intervention in a case of fetal asphyxia is not simply the presence of distress, but rather the presence of *nonremediable* distress. If the inciting stimulus can be removed, the fetus will recover more quickly in utero than if it were delivered in a hypoxic condition. The success of intrauterine resuscitation can be assessed in an ongoing fashion by improvements in FHR patterns or pH. Even if intrauterine treatment of distress is only temporarily effective, it often will allow the careful delivery of a well oxygenated fetus rather than the hasty delivery of a hypoxic one. It is inappropriate to establish any arbitrary limits for the time allowable between detection of fetal distress and intervention. Rather, it is the likelihood of recovery that should determine the timing of intervention. Late decelerations accompanied by absent variability usually signify a chronically distressed baby in whom recovery is unlikely. On the other hand, a fetus with good variability who develops late decelerations with a demonstrable etiology, such as maternal hypotension, can be expected to recover. The presence of baseline variability as an indication of the fetal margin of reserve is the cornerstone of heart rate pattern interpretation.

Delivery of an asphyxiated fetus often requires a choice between cesarean section and midforceps delivery. Although each case must be judged individually, we favor cesarean section in most instances. A growing body of evidence attests to the considerable dangers of midforceps operations.[30] We prefer not to employ a potentially traumatic procedure on a fetus that is already compromised by hypoxia.

LIMITATIONS OF TECHNIQUES

Each of the available methods for diagnosing fetal asphyxia possesses limitations and strengths. Ideally, capillary blood sampling and heart rate monitoring should be employed in a complementary fashion. Numerous studies attest to the generally good correlation between pH and heart rate patterns.[6,49,62,64,85,97,105,106]

The virtues of heart rate monitoring have been explained above. The continuous nature of the information, its reliability, ease of application and ability to be employed on virtually all patients make it a clinically useful method of surveillance. We feel that all fetuses should be subjected to heart rate monitoring because many purportedly healthy babies will show evidence of fetal distress. When monitoring capabilities are limited, a high risk population, as defined by obstetric history, hormonal assays or other modes of antepartum evaluation, should receive priority. It should be emphasized that the effective employment of this technique requires reliable electronic equipment, including cardiotachometers capable of defining the instantaneous beat-to-beat rate, the use of direct fetal electrodes and personnel skilled in the interpretation of fetal heart rate patterns.

A number of potential pitfalls may preclude adequate interpretation of the fetal monitoring data. Under appropriate conditions, each technique of monitoring, either direct or indirect, may exaggerate or give spurious data about both heart rate and variability. Under certain circumstances the maternal heart rate may be counted. Ultrasound, the most widely used technique for obtaining heart rate externally, notoriously increases the amount of apparent variability. Proper monitoring requires understanding of the technical limitations of the equipment being used.

We have found fetal blood sampling especially useful in situations in which the heart rate pattern is confusing or equivocal, or when, in the presence of an abnormal heart rate pattern, one desires to follow serial pH values to determine trends in the fetal acid-base milieu. It should be remembered that the scalp pH represents the biochemical status of the fetus at one moment in time, and a single determination imparts no information about the nature of the asphyxial insult or the fetus' ability to recover from it. When employed alone, frequent serial pH values are necessary to obtain useful information. In addition, methodologic errors can occur with faulty calibration of the machine, improper temperature regulation, exposure of the sample to air or contamination with amniotic fluid.

In human fetuses, one cannot be certain that capillary pH of the presenting part invariably represents that of the central circulation. During hypoxic conditions there is peripheral vasoconstriction and diversion of blood to vital organs.[8, 21] Thus, although the scalp blood may be acidotic, the blood perfusing the heart and brain may be normally oxygenated. The local effects of scalp edema and vasocongestion are impossible to quantitate. Even excess pressure from the amnioscope could conceivably cause local obstruction to flow and hypoxia. The usual custom of placing patients in lithotomy position for fetal blood sampling may also contribute to fetal compromise and yield misleading results. Blood samples are not obtainable if cervical dilatation and fetal descent are insufficient, and are somewhat uncomfortable for the patient.

GOALS

The question of how much hypoxia can be tolerated by the human fetus before irreversible central nervous system damage occurs cannot be answered at this time. It seems reasonable that until this information is available, our present goal should be to minimize hypoxic insults to the fetus insofar as possible without jeopardizing the health of the fetus or mother. The prevention of iatrogenic distress by conservative and intelligent use of analgesia, anesthesia and uterotonic agents will bring us a long way toward this goal. Careful and continuous monitoring of every fetus beginning early in labor must become a routine aspect of obstetric care. The aggressive use of techniques of intrauterine resuscitation and the employment of nontraumatic methods when emergency delivery is indicated will help to minimize fetal damage.

Important questions concerning the efficacy of heart rate monitoring and blood sampling remain to be answered. There is no available large scale, prospective double-blind study of fetal heart rate monitoring which tests the hypothesis that outcome is improved. Paul et al[83] have reported a retrospective study in which the perinatal mortality in a large group of high risk monitored patients was lower than that of a group of unmonitored normal patients, suggesting the beneficial effect of monitoring. Others have shown a decreased incidence of stillbirths in monitored labors. Future research must proceed in several directions. It has become clear that perinatal mortality rates and Apgar scores do not permit adequate assessment of hypoxic damage. New neurologic and psychologic testing must be developed to adequately measure the effects of sublethal asphyxia and these must be applied to large populations with prolonged follow-up. Carefully controlled studies to measure the impact of our present monitoring techniques on fetal outcome are needed. There is evidence to suggest that other biophysical parameters such as fetal movements,[87] systolic time intervals,[34, 76] fetal respirations[25, 69] and electroencephalograms[66] are affected by hypoxia.[35] Techniques for accurately measuring these functions must be developed and critically evaluated. Abnormal labor may itself adversely affect fetal outcome and its effects must also be further investigated.[30] Computer analysis of data may help to clarify the interaction of the various functions evaluated.

The obstetrician must become cognizant of his enormous burden of responsibility in assuring the welfare of every fetus and neonate. Through the widespread employment of our current methods of preventing, detecting and treating fetal jeopardy, and through unrelenting research to develop new diagnostic and therapeutic techniques, we hope to improve the quality of human existence so that each individual can commence his extrauterine life without handicap and with the capability of achieving his full biologic potential.

REFERENCES

1. Adamsons, K., Beard, R. W., Myers, R. E.: Comparison of the composition of arterial, venous and capillary blood of the fetal monkey during labor. Am J Obstet Gynecol 107: 435, 1970.
2. Adamsons, K., James, L. S., Towell, M., Lucey, J.: Physiologic observations during induced anemia in utero in the rhesus monkey. Am Pediatr Soc Abst 1965.
3. Althabe, O., Jr., Schwarcz, R. L., Pose S. V., Escarcena, L., Caldeyro-Barcia, R.: Effects on fetal heart rate and fetal pO_2 of oxygen administration to the mother. Am J Obstet Gynecol 98: 858, 1967.
4. Barcroft, J.: *Researches on Prenatal Life.* Springfield, Ill. Charles C Thomas, Publisher, 1947.
5. Baskett, T. F., Koh, K. S.: Sinusoidal fetal heart rate pattern: A sign of fetal hypoxia. Obstet Gynecol 44: 379, 1974.
6. Beard, R. W., Filshie, G. M., Knight, C. A., Roberts, G. M.: The significance of the changes in the continuous fetal heart rate in the first stage of labor. J Obstet Gynaecol Br Commonw 78: 865, 1971.
7. Beard, R. W., Morris, E. D., Clayton, S. G.: pH of foetal capillary blood as an indicator of the condition of the fetus. J Obstet Gynaecol Br Commonw 74: 812, 1967.
8. Behrman, R. E., Lees, M. H., Peterson, E. N., De Lannov, C. W., Seeds, E. A.: Distribution of the circulation in the normal and asphyxiated fetal primate. Am J Obstet Gynecol 108: 956, 1970.
9. Benson, R. C., Shubeck, F., Deutschberger, J., Weiss, W., Berendes, H.: Fetal heart rate as a predictor of fetal distress. Obstet Gynecol 32: 259, 1968.
10. Blechner, J. N., Stenger, V. G., Prystowsky, H.: Blood flow to the human uterus during maternal metabolic acidosis. Am J Obstet Gynecol 121: 789, 1975.
11. Boehm, F., Growdon, J.: The effect of eclamptic convulsions on the fetal heart rate. Am J Obstet Gynecol 120: 851, 1974.
12. Boehm, F., Growdon, J.: The effect of scopolamine on fetal heart rate baseline variability. Am J Obstet Gynecol 120: 1099, 1974.
13. Boehm, F. H.: Prolonged end stage fetal heart rate deceleration. Obstet Gynecol 45: 579, 1975.
14. Bowe, E. T.: Fetal blood sampling in labor. Bull Sloane Hosp Women 15: 103, 1969.
15. Bowe, E. T., Beard, R. W., Finster, M., Poppers, P. J., Adamsons, K., James, L. S.: Reliability of fetal blood sampling. Am J Obstet Gynecol 107: 279, 1970.
16. Bretscher, J., Saling, E.: pH values in the human fetus during labor. Am J Obstet Gynecol 97: 906, 1967.
17. Bronatek, V., Scheffs, J.: The pathogenesis and significance of saltatory patterns in the fetal heart rate. Int J Gynaecol Obstet 11: 223, 1973.
18. Caldeyro-Barcia, R., Mendez-Bauer, C., Poseiro, J. J., Escarcena, L. A., Pose, S. V., Arnt, I. C., Gulin, L., Althabe, O., Bieniarz, J.: Control of human fetal heart rate during labor. *The Heart and Circulation in the Newborn Infant.* Edited by D. E. Cassels, New York, Grune & Stratton, 1966.
19. Cibils, L.: Clinical significance of fetal heart rate patterns during labor. II. Late decelerations. Am J Obstet Gynecol 123: 473, 1975.
20. Cohen, W. R., Schifrin, B. S., Doctor, G.: Elevation of the fetal presenting part, a method of intrauterine resuscitation. Am J Obstet Gynecol 123: 646, 1975.
21. Cohn, H. E., Sacks, E. J., Heymann, M. A., Rudolph, A. M.: Cardiovascular responses to hypoxemia and acidemia in fetal lambs. Am J Obstet Gynecol 120: 817, 1974.
22. Comline, R. S., Silver, M.: Placental transfer of blood gases. Br Med Bull 31: 25, 1975.
23. Coltart, T. M., Trickey, N. R. A., Beard, R. W.: Fetal blood sampling: Practical approach to management of fetal distress. Br Med J 1: 342, 1969.
24. Dawes, G.: Foetal and Neonatal Physiology. Chicago, Year Book Medical Publishers, Inc., 1968.
25. Dawes, G.: Breathing before birth in animals and man. N Engl J Med 290: 557, 1974.
26. Dela Rama, F. E., Jr., Merkatz, I. R.: Evaluation of fetal scalp pH with a proposed new clinical assessment of the neonate. Am J Obstet Gynecol 107: 93, 1970.
27. Derom, R.: Anaerobic metabolism in the human fetus. I. The normal delivery. Am J Obstet Gynecol 89: 241, 1964.
28. Fenton, A. N., Steer, C. M.: Fetal distress. Am J Obstet Gynecol 83: 354, 1962.
29. Freda, V. J., Adamsons, K.: Exchange transfusion in utero. Am J Obstet Gynecol 89: 817, 1964.

30. Friedman, E. A.: Patterns of labor as indicators of risk. Clin Obstet Gynecol 16: 172, 1973.
31. Glick, G., Braunwald, E.: Relative roles of the sympathetic and parasympathetic nervous systems in the reflex control of heart rate. Circ Res 16: 363, 1965.
32. Goodlin, R. C.: Intrapartum fetal heart rate responses and plethysmographic pulse. Am J Obstet Gynecol 110: 210, 1971.
33. Goodlin, R. C.: Fetal cardiovascular responses to stress. Washoe Seminar on Fetal Monitoring, February 1975.
34. Goodlin, R. C., Haesslein, H. C., Crocker, K., Carlson, R. G.: Fetal cardiac interval recorder. Obstet Gynecol 46: 69, 1975.
35. Goodlin, R. C., Lowe, E. W.: Multiphasic fetal monitoring: A preliminary evaluation. Am J Obstet Gynecol 119: 341, 1974.
36. Goodlin, R. C., Schmidt, W.: Human fetal arousal levels as indicated by heart rate recordings. Am J Obstet Gynecol 114: 613, 1972.
37. Grimwade, J. C.: The management of fetal distress with the use of fetal blood pH. Am J Obstet Gynecol 106: 266, 1970.
38. Hamilton, L. A., Behrman, R. E.: Intra-amniotic infusion of bicarbonate in the treatment of human fetal acidosis. Am J Obstet Gynecol 112: 834, 1972.
39. Hashimoto, L., Tanaka, S., Hirata, M., Chiba, S.: Responses of the sino-atrial node to change in pressure of the sinus node artery. Circ Res 21: 297, 1967.
40. Hobel, C. J.: Intrapartum clinical assessment of fetal distress. Am J Obstet Gynecol 110: 336, 1971.
41. Hon, E.: The electronic evaluation of the fetal heart rate. Am J Obstet Gynecol 75: 1215, 1958.
42. Hon, E.: Electronic evaluation of the fetal heart rate. VI. Fetal distress—a working hypothesis. Am J Obstet Gynecol 83: 333, 1962.
43. Hon, E.: Additional observations on "pathologic" bradycardia. Am J Obstet Gynecol 118: 428, 1974.
44. Hon, E. H.: Detection of fetal distress. Fifth World Congress of Gynaecology and Obstetrics, Sydney, Australia, 1967. London, Butterworth, 1967.
45. Hon, E. H.: *Atlas of Fetal Heart Rate Patterns*. New Haven, Harty Press, 1968.
46. Hon, E. H., Bradfield, A. N., Hess, O. W.: The electronic evaluation of the fetal heart rate. V. The vagal factor in fetal bradycardia. Am J Obstet Gynecol 82: 291, 1961.
47. Hon, E. H., Khazin, A. F.: Biochemical studies of the fetus. I. The fetal pH measuring system. Am J Obstet Gynecol 33: 219, 1969.
48. Hon, E. H., Khazin, A. F., Paul, R. H.: Biochemical studies of the fetus. II. Fetal pH and Apgar scores. Am J Obstet Gynecol 33: 237, 1969.
49. Hon, E. H., Khazin, A. F.: Observations on fetal heart rate and fetal biochemistry. I. Base deficit. Am J Obstet Gynecol 105: 721, 1969.
50. Hon, E. H., Lee, S. T.: Electronic evaluation of the fetal heart rate. VIII. Patterns preceding fetal death: further observations. Am J Obstet Gynecol 87: 814, 1963.
51. Hon, E. H., Quilligan, E. J.: The classification of fetal heart rate. II. A revised working classification. Conn Med 31: 779, 1967.
52. Hon, E. H., Yeh, S.: Electronic evaluation of the fetal heart rate. X. The fetal arrhythmia index. Med Res Eng 8: 14, 1969.
53. Howard, B. K., Goodson, J. H., Mengert, N.: Supine hypotensive syndrome in late pregnancy. Obstet Gynecol 1: 371, 1953.
54. Humphrey, M. D., Chang, A., Wood, E. C., Morgan, S., Hounslow, D.: A decrease in fetal pH during the second stage of labor when conducted in the dorsal position. J Obstet Gynaecol Br Commonw 81: 600, 1974.
55. Ibarra-Polo, A. A., Guiloff, F. E., Gomez-Rogers, C.: Fetal heart rate throughout pregnancy. Am J Obstet Gynecol 113: 814, 1972.
56. Jacobson, L., Rooth, G.: Interpretative aspects on the acid base composition and its variation in fetal scalp blood and maternal blood during labor. J Obstet Gynaecol Br Commonw 78: 971, 1971.
57. James, L. S.: Physiologic adjustments at birth: Effect of labor, delivery and anesthesia on the newborn. Anesthesiology 26: 501, 1965.
58. James, L. S., Adamsons, K.: Respiratory physiology of the fetus and newborn infant. N Engl J Med 271: 1352, 1403, 1964.
59. Jepson, J.: Factors influencing oxygenation in mother and fetus. Obstet Gynecol 44: 906, 1974.
60. Jouvenat, N. C., and Newman, R. L.: Fetal blood gas homeostasis at cesarean section. Contemp Ob/Gyn 3: 87, 1973.
61. Khazin, A. F., Hon, E. H., Hehre, F. W.: Effects of maternal hyperoxia on the fetus. Am J Obstet Gynecol 109: 628, 1971.
62. Khazin, A. F., Hon, E. H., Yeh, S.: Observations on fetal heart rate and fetal biochemistry. III. Base deficit of umbilical cord blood. J Pediatr 79: 406, 1971.
63. Kubli, F. W., Hon, E. H., Khazin, A. F., Takemura, H.: Observations on heart rate and pH in the human fetus during labor. Am J Obstet Gynecol 104: 1190, 1969.
64. Low, J. A., Boston, R. W., Pancham, S. R.: The role of fetal heart rate patterns in the recognition of fetal asphyxia with metabolic acidosis. Am J Obstet Gynecol 109: 922, 1971.
65. Lumley, J., McKinnon, L., Wood, C.: Lack of agreement on normal values for fetal scalp blood. J Obstet Gynaecol Br Commonw 78: 13, 1971.
66. Mann, L. I., Prichard, J. W., Symmes, D.: EEG, ECG, and acid-base observations during acute fetal hypoxia. Am J Obstet Gynecol 106: 39, 1970.
67. Mann, L. I., Prichard, J. W., Symmes, D.: The effect of glucose loading on the fetal response to hypoxia. Am J Obstet Gynecol 107: 610, 1970.
68. Manseau, P., Vaquier, J., Chavinine, J., Sureau, C.: Le rythme cardiaque foetal "sinusoidal." J Gynecol Obstet Biol Repr 1: 343, 1972.
69. Martin, C., Murata, Y., Petrie, R., Parer, J.: Respiratory movements in fetal rhesus monkeys. Am J Obstet Gynecol 119: 939, 1974.

70. McCrann, D., Schifrin, B. S.: Double-blind comparison of etidocaine and lidocaine for epidural anesthesia during labor. Am J Obstet Gynecol (In press.)
71. McDonald, J. S.: Evaluation of fetal blood pH as a reflection of fetal well-being. Am J Obstet Gynecol 97: 912, 1967.
72. Mendez-Bauer, C., Arnt, I. C., Gulin, L., Escarcena, L., Caldeyro-Barcia, R.: Relationship between blood pH and heart rate in the human fetus during labor. Am J Obstet Gynecol 97: 530, 1967.
73. Miller, F. C., Sacks, D. A., Yeh, S., Paul, R. H., Schifrin, B. S., Martin, C. B., Jr., Hon, E. H.: Significance of meconium during labor. Am J Obstet Gynecol 122: 573, 1975.
74. Mondanlou, H., Yeh, S., Hon, E. H., Forsythe, A.: Fetal and neonatal biochemistry and Apgar scores. Am J Obstet Gynecol 117: 942, 1973.
75. Morishima, H., Daniel, S., Richards, R., James, L. S.: The effect of increased maternal PaO_2 upon the fetus during labor. Am J Obstet Gynecol 123: 257, 1975.
76. Murata, Y., Martin C. B., Jr.: Systolic time intervals and the fetal cardiac cycle. Obstet Gynecol 44: 224, 1974.
77. Myers, R. E.: The clinical and pathological effects of asphyxia in the fetal rhesus monkey. *Diagnosis and Treatment of Fetal Disorders*. Edited by K. Adamsons, New York, Springer-Verlag, 1968.
78. Myers, R. E.: Two patterns of perinatal brain damage and their conditions of occurrence. Am J Obstet Gynecol 112: 246, 1972.
79. Myers, R. E., Mueller-Heubach, E., Adamsons, K.: Predictability of the state of fetal oxygenation from a quantitative analysis of the components of late deceleration. Am J Obstet Gynecol 115: 1083, 1973.
80. Niswander, K. R., Gordon M., Drage, J.: The effect of intrauterine hypoxia on the child surviving to 4 years. Am J Obstet Gynecol 121: 892, 1975.
81. Parer, J. T., Behrman, R. E.: The influence of uterine blood flow on the acid-base status of the rhesus monkey. Am J Obstet Gynecol 107: 1241, 1970.
82. Paul, W., Gare, D., Whetham, J.: Assessment of fetal scalp sampling in labor. Am J Obstet Gynecol 99: 745, 1967.
83. Paul, R. H., Hon, E. H.: Clinical fetal monitoring. V. Effect on perinatal outcome. Am J Obstet Gynecol 118: 529, 1974.
84. Paul, R. H., Suidan, A. K., Yeh, S., Schifrin, B. S., Hon, E. H.: Clinical fetal monitoring. VII. The evaluation and significance of intrapartum baseline FHR variability. Am J Obstet Gynecol 123: 206, 1975.
85. Quilligan, E. J., Katigbak, E., Hofschild, J.: Correlation of fetal heart rate patterns and blood gas values. II. Bradycardia. Am J Obstet Gynecol 91: 1123, 1965.
86. Rochard, F.: Le rhythme cardiaque foetal au cours de la grossesse Université de Paris. V. Rene Descartes Faculte de Medecine Cochin Port Royal, 1973. Doctoral Thesis.
87. Sadovsky, E., Yaffe, H., Wolfe, Z.: Fetal movement in normal and pathologic pregnancy. Int J Gynaecol Obstet 12: 75, 1974.
88. Saling, E.: *Foetal and Neonatal Hypoxia in Relation to Clinical Obstetric Practice*. Baltimore, The Williams & Wilkins Co., 1968.
89. Saling, E.: Amnioscopy and fetal blood sampling: Observations on fetal acidosis. *Diagnosis and Treatment of Fetal Disorders*. Edited by K. Adamsons, New York, Springer-Verlag, 1968.
90. Saling, E., Schneider, D.: Biochemical supervision of the fetus during labor. J Obstet Gynaecol Br Commonw 74: 799, 1967.
91. Schifrin, B. S.: Fetal heart rate patterns following epidural anesthesia and oxytocin infusion during labour. J Obstet Gynaecol Br Commonw 79: 332, 1972.
92. Schifrin, B. S.: Iatrogenic fetal distress. Int. Anesthesiol Clin 11: 119, 1973.
93. Schifrin, B. S., Dame, L.: Fetal heart rate patterns: Prediction of Apgar score. JAMA 219: 1322, 1972.
94. Schifrin, B. S., Suzuki, K.: Fetal surveillance during labor. Int Anesthesiol Clin 11: 17, 1973.
95. Seeds, A. E., Bissonnette, J., Lin, H., Behrman, R. L.: Changes in rhesus monkey fetal and maternal acid-base measurements following amniotic fluid bicarbonate or Tris infusions. Am J Obstet Gynecol 107: 232, 1970.
96. Siassi, B., Blanco, C., Martin, C. B.: Presented to the Society for Gynecologic Investigation, Atlanta, March 28–30, 1973, p 32 (Abstract.)
97. Tejani, N., Mann, L., Bhakthavathsalan, A., Weiss, R.: Correlation of fetal heart rate—Uterine contraction patterns with fetal scalp blood pH. Obstet Gynecol 46: 392, 1975.
98. Tejani, N., Mann, L., Bhakthavathsalan, A., Weiss, R.: Prolonged fetal bradycardia with recovery: Its significance and outcome. Am J Obstet Gynecol 122: 975, 1975.
99. Towbin, A.: Cerebral hypoxic damage in fetus and newborn. Arch Neurol 20: 35, 1969.
100. Waldron, K. W., Wood, C.: Cesarean section in the lateral position. Obstet Gynecol 37: 706, 1971.
101. Windle, W. F.: Brain damage at birth. JAMA 206: 1967, 1964.
102. Wolf, S.: Central autonomic influences on cardiac rate and rhythm. Mod Concep Cardiovasc Dis 38: 29, 1969.
103. Wood, C.: Scalp blood pH in assessing fetal well-being. Contemp Ob/Gyn 5: 87, 1975.
104. Wood, C., Ferguson, R., Leeton, J., Newman, W., Walker, A.: Fetal heart rate and acid-base status in the assessment of fetal hypoxia. Am J Obstet Gynecol 98: 62, 1967.
105. Wood, C., Lumley, J., Renou, P.: A clinical assessment of fetal diagnostic methods. J Obstet Gynaecol Br Commonw 74: 823, 1967.
106. Wood, C., Newman, W. Lumley, J., Hammond, J.: Classification of fetal heart rate in relation to fetal scalp blood measurements and Apgar score. Am J Obstet Gynecol 105: 942, 1969.
107. Yeh, S., Forsythe, A., Hon, E.: Quantification of beat-to-beat interval differences. Obstet Gynecol 41: 355, 1973.

Part III

MANAGEMENT OF SPECIFIC DISORDERS

STEPHEN L. CORSON, M.D.

8

Management of Rh Sensitization

The saga of Rh erythroblastosis has unfolded over a relatively brief span of years. The pathophysiology was documented in the 1930's and the basic immunologic factors were recognized in the next decade. One of the first exchange transfusions was performed by Wallerstein[59] in 1946 and by the 1950's effective treatment consisting of early delivery and exchange was commonplace. Diagnostic amniocentesis to assess fetal involvement was described in 1956 by Bevis.[6] Intrauterine transfusion was accomplished by Liley[30] in 1963 as a technique to avoid stillborn delivery in cases too severe to manage by early delivery and exchange transfusion. Later, Freda's group[16] demonstrated a method of passive immunization which could prevent maternal sensitization. Still, cases of first pregnancy clinical sensitization, Rh-incompatible transfusions and anti-Rh_0 failure continue to cause tragic outcomes.

The first description of erythroblastosis fetalis may have emanated from Hippocrates in 400 B.C.; the term itself was coined by Rautmann[46] in 1912. Although used synonymously with Rh sensitization, the process of erythroblastosis fetalis may been seen as a result of other antigen-antibody systems (such as Kell) activated during pregnancy.

In 1932, Diamond et al[13] proposed that hydrops fetalis, icterus gravus neonatorum and anicteric anemia were all graded manifestations of one pathologic process, erythroblastosis fetalis. ABO incompatibility was rejected by them as an etiology.

Darrow[11] reviewed the subject in a classic paper published in 1938. The pathologic findings in stillborn and early neonatal deaths were appreciated and special note was made of kernicterus, massive hypertrophy of the liver and spleen and intensive secondary hematopoietic effort. Landsteiner and Wiener's paper[25] describing the Rh antigen was still 2 years off, but Darrow's concluding sentence reads " . . . an antigen antibody reaction seems to explain best all aspects of these related disorders." In 1939 Levine and Stetson[27] postulated that maternal immunization to the fetus resulted from inheritance of a paternal antigen not found in the mother. While working with interspecies immunity to red cells, Landsteiner and Wiener evolved a system of producing antisera in rabbits injected with rhesus monkey blood. This antiserum also agglutinated human cells bearing M antigen.[25] Still another antigenic group was found on the human cell after M had been absorbed and this was labeled "Rh," although it was noted subsequently not to be identical with the monkey antigen. In the same year (1940) Wiener and Peters[67] linked the Rh antigen to clinical findings of transfusion reaction in a group O patient receiving homologous blood subsequent to initial successful transfusion. Using a modified cross-matching technique under cold conditions, clumping not observed in the standard tests at room temperature was noted. The antibody isolated in this manner was shown to parallel that produced in the rabbit to the Rh antigen. The authors described a patient (A^-) who received first A^+ and then A^- transfusions without clinical evidence of sensitization. Another A^+ transfusion triggered a hemolytic response, the mechanism of which they correctly elucidated. Further, they stated, "...why such reactions are not encountered more frequently, as many patients, of whom about one-seventh would be Rh negative, are given repeated transfusions. The probable answer is that not all Rh^- individuals are capable of producing Rh antibodies. . . . In addition, the interval between transfusions must be long enough to permit an adequate rise in titer of the antibody."

Diamond[12] presented data to the Royal Society of Medicine during 1947 which showed a lowering of newborn mortality in Rh-sensitized cases by effecting early delivery and by utilizing Rh^- transfusions in the baby. In 1950 Allen, Diamond and Vaughan[2] demonstrated the relationship between bilirubinemia and kernicterus. They lowered the frequency of kernicterus by exchange transfusion and proved statistically that this was an effective method of treatment of the affected newborn. In 1954 Allen, Diamond and Jones[1] proved the value of early delivery in reducing the stillborn rate of affected cases.

Pathology

The associated pathologic findings are detailed in Queenan's excellent text on Rh disease.[42] The gross autopsy descriptions of hideous distortion as a consequence of massive edema are encountered rarely today, and usually in undiagnosed cases allowed to go to term.

Microscopic evidence of extramedullary hematopoiesis is apparent in the liver, spleen, kidneys, adrenals and in lymphoid tissue. The liver size reflects alteration of function as well as congestion secondary to high output heart failure on an anemic basis. The heart itself shows hypertrophy and dilatation.

Stillborn fetuses demonstrate no kernicterus (bilirubin deposits in the basal nuclei) unless there is severe concomitant maternal liver impairment. However, kernicterus is marked in newborns who succumb without successful exchange transfusion.

The placenta usually undergoes marked hypertrophy and becomes edematous. Instead of the usual ratio of one-seventh fetal weight, it may weigh one-half as much as the fetus. The enlarged, pale cotyledons reflect the anemic process. The umbilical cord may be deeply stained while nucleated red cells are noted in the placental villi. Severe cases of Rh sensitization may result in cord hemoglobin values of 5 g/100 ml compared with normal levels of 16.6 ± 1.5 g/100 ml.

Serology and Immunology

The classic explanation of initial sensitization follows the line of reasoning presented earlier. A paternally inherited factor (usually Rh_0 (D)) in the fetus which is not native to the mother crosses the placenta in small amounts during early pregnancy, and in larger quantities during the second and third trimesters with major transfer occurring at delivery. We have observed passage as early as 6 weeks of gestation[7] using the standard Kleihauer-Betke technique.[24] Usually the amounts passed during the pregnancy are too small to evoke clinical or laboratory evidence of active immunization. In subsequent pregnancies specific maternal antibodies, if formed as an anamnestic response, cross the placenta and enter the fetal circulation, causing agglutination and subsequent hemolysis.

The practice, common before 1940, of injecting intramuscularly several milliliters of blood into children subject to infections no doubt promoted sensitization, since as little as 0.1 ml can initiate the process.[72]

Part of the antigenic determinant depends on the dose as well as the strength of the antigen. A and B antigens are very sensitizing and since antibodies are naturally present, ABO incompatibility actually provides a partial protective effect against development of subsequent Rh sensitization.[26, 45] Rh_0 (D) is the next strongest antigen and accidental transfusion of 1 unit of Rh^+ blood will sensitize 75% of Rh^- recipients. However, only 11%

of Rh$^-$ susceptible women will be sensitized by pregnancy judged by hemolysis in a subsequent gestation. Until recently, it was not fully appreciated that as many as 30% of Rh$^-$ subjects are nonresponders. This is better documented by tagged red blood cell (RBC) survival studies after the original challenge or sensitizing dose than by antibody detection methods. This state is not dose dependent and may be an inherited trait. Although the Kell factor is less sensitizing by a factor of approximately 15-fold, the severity of the hemolytic disease can be as great.

Of interest also is the maternal to fetal transfer during pregnancy. Taylor[52] studied 236 families in which the grandmother of the proband Rh$^+$ newborn could be typed. ABO incompatible matches were eliminated. A statistically significant excess of Rh$^+$ grandmothers was found in cases of erythroblastosis. Thus, rather than conferring immunologic tolerance, exposure to Rh$^+$ cells while in utero served to sensitize the female fetus to her own first Rh$^+$ fetus. Scott and Beer[51] quantitated the incidence of first pregnancy sensitization as 0.4 to 2.0%. They studied eight patients and noted that all affected babies were ABO compatible males. They questioned a Y-linked factor and also suggested administration of anti-D immunoglobulin to newborn Rh$^-$ females born of Rh$^+$ mothers. Supposed "first pregnancy" sensitization may also occur from immunization at the time of undisclosed previous abortion (either spontaneous or induced). It is imperative that a reproductive history be taken, and that routine antibody titers be performed during each trimester of all Rh$^-$ pregnancies except with a documented Rh$^-$ sire. The problems related to immunization with mismatched blood will be discussed later in this chapter.

The Wiener versus Fisher-Race nomenclature debate has raged for over 30 years. The original Wiener system is cumbersome, whereas the Fisher-Race system is much easier to utilize. However, there exists a deeper divergence of philosophy. Wiener[65,66] holds that multiple alleles act on a single locus to control the formed antigens, whereas Fisher and Race postulate three pairs of alleles (Cc, Dd and Ee).[44] Fisher and Race postulate genetic redistribution from crossing over whereas Wiener[66] denies this as a reasonable explanation.

Table 8.1 shows the homologs between both systems and the incidence as found in the usual North American Caucasian population. Note that the first three entries account for 93% of the phenotypes found. R^o has a 40% incidence in the black population. Utilizing test sera against the red blood cells (note: there is no "d" antiserum), a genotype frequency table based on allelic frequency can be constructed in order to predict homo- or heterozygosity, but does not supersede results of family typing studies. Table 8.2 provides information used to evaluate husbands of Rh$^-$ women referred for counseling before or early in the course of a potentially affected pregnancy. We have used this table along with the obstetric history to advise Rh$^-$ donor

Table 8.1. Prevalence of Rh chromosomal type

Chromosome	Antigens	Caucasian frequency (%)
R^1(DCe)	Rh_0(D), rh′(C), hr″(e)	40
R^2(DcE)	Rh_0(D), hr′(c), rh″(E)	15
r(cde)	hr′(c), hr″(e)	38
r′(dCe)	rh′(C), hr″(e)	2.7
r″(dcE)	hr′(c), rh″(E)	1.3
R^o(Dce)	Rh_0(D), hr′(c), hr″(e)	2.5
R^z(DCE)	Rh_0(D), rh′(C), rh″(E)	0.24
r^y(dCE)	rh′(c), rh″(E)	Low

Table 8.2. Genotype table

Reaction in test sera					Type	Not excluded	%	Homo/hetero
D	C	E	c	e				
+	+	−	+	+	R^1r		32	h
						R^1R^o	2	H
						R^or′	0.1	h
+	+	−	−	+	R^1R^1		17	H
						R^1r′	0.8	h
+	+	+	+	+	R^1R^2		12	H
						R^1r′	1	h
						R^2r′	0.3	h
+	−	+	+	+	R^2r		11	h
						R^2R^o	1	H
						R^or″	0.1	h
+	−	+	+	−	R^2R^2		2	H
						R^2r″	0.3	h
+	−	−	+	+	R^or		2	h
						R^oR^o	0.1	H

insemination in cases of immunization too severe to manage with intrauterine transfusion (IUT) when data indicates probable Rh homozygosity in the husband. Although many patients show antibodies to both "D" and "c," clinical disease as a result of "c" sensitization alone occurs less commonly (Figure 8.1).

In 1944 both Wiener[64] and Race[43] published papers dealing with the problem of a "blocking" or "incomplete" antibody. This antibody would not cause agglutination in the usual laboratory setting; however, it could be identified by inhibition of the agglutinating ability of Rh_0 antibody or by its effect on Rh^+ cells, causing them not to be agglutinated by anti-D after incubation, centrifugation, washing and resuspension in saline. The paper by Coombs et al[10] which appeared the next year was of extreme clinical import, for it described a method of detecting any antibody present, whether or not the cells were coated. The basis of this procedure is anti-human globulin produced in the rabbit. Thus, cells coated with globulin at the D receptor site react under these conditions even if the original screen against anti-D sera is negative. Cord bloods may type as Rh^- because maternal antibody coats the fetal cells interfering with added antisera. The Coombs' test allows for identification of a blocking antibody under these conditions and an eluate permits definite identification of anti-D. Maternal antibodies may be IgG, M, D or A, but only IgG has significant placental transfer. Measurement of this so called "albumin-reacting" antibody provides the most consistent clinical correlation.

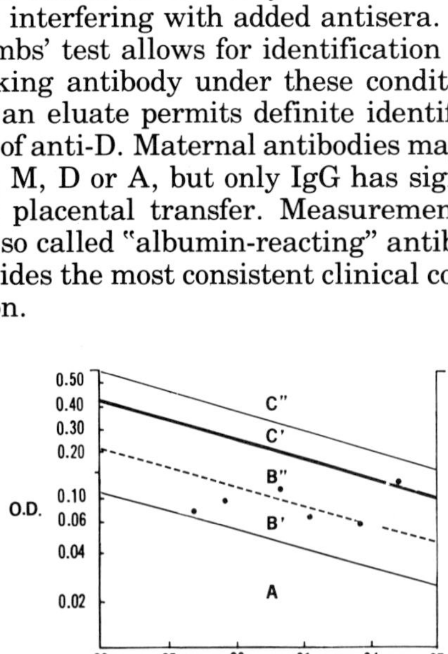

Figure 8.1. "c" sensitization requiring early delivery and four exchange transfusions.

Widespread use of serial amniocenteses has supplanted serial titer determinations as the procedure of choice to follow known sensitized pregnancies. The question remains: at what titer level should amniocentesis be considered? There are patients in whom the placental implantation site discourages or even precludes amniocentesis except in severe cases. Traumatic taps may actually make the process more severe by increasing fetomaternal bleed. Therefore, serial titer results, although frequently unreliable, may have to be employed until uterine growth allows a site for a "clean" amniocentesis. Because of variation between laboratories, it is of little value to formulate policy predicated on specific values. Our routine is outlined below as a guide.

All first pregnancies of Rh^- women are monitored by antibody detection tests at the time of the initial visit, at 20 to 22 weeks and at 32 weeks if results remain negative. Husbands are typed to determine probable zygosity. The expected incidence of primary sensitization with the initial pregnancy is low (0.4 to 2.0%). Although usually mild, if present, we have seen undiagnosed sensitization severe enough to cause stillborns. The sudden appearance of hydramnios in an Rh^- patient may signify sensitization and calls for immediate titer determination. An abrupt decrease in fetal motion may be a sign of severe fetal anemia. Should antibodies develop by 20 to 22 weeks, more intensive scrutiny is employed. Initial appearance at 32 weeks allows time for amniocentesis and possible transfusion or early delivery based on optical density (O.D.) readings and the lecithin to sphingomyelin (L/S) ratio.

At Pennsylvania Hospital titers are expressed in saline, albumin and in Coombs' serum. Saline antibodies do not pass the placenta but frequently are noted to rise just before albumin titer elevations, signifying a possible acute sensitization, particularly after traumatic amniocentesis. Albumin antibodies are most reliable and a two-tube dilutional change, e.g., 1:8 versus 1:32, is significant. Coombs' antibodies are noted to remain elevated after delivery when the albumin titers have decreased, and therefore represent a more chronic condition. Optical density of amniotic fluid is obtained if albumin titers reach 1:8 *in the first sensitized pregnancy*. Any titer elevation deserves re-evaluation at 2-week intervals.

Patients with a prior sensitization are evaluated in a more aggressive manner. An accurate medical history is essential and obstetric-nursery records relating to previous deliveries must be obtained. Any patient with a history of an affected liveborn infant has biweekly titers performed after 20 weeks. An albumin titer of ≥1:8 becomes an indication for amniocentesis. Many patients have initial titers in excess of this level. Since amniocentesis under B scan or gray scan ultrasonic guidance has proven to be a safe technique, we feel that the risk of missing a severely sensitized case by not obtaining amniotic fluid O.D. readings outweighs the risk of the procedure.

Any patient who has delivered a stillbirth or a baby requiring exchange transfusion has an amniocentesis regardless of titers. We recently cared for a patient who required IUT at 30 weeks; her albumin titers never rose beyond 1:4. Serial amniocenteses which demonstrated impending fetal death were instigated because of a prior infant needing but one exchange transfusion.

Although many authors state that they have never seen an intrauterine demise at titers <1:32 or<1:16, this does not argue against liberal use of amniocentesis to determine more accurately the fetal status. Planned early delivery, depending on L/S and O.D. values, will result in decreased neonatal mortality and morbidity. On the other hand, we do not advocate a cavalier approach to amniocentesis. Since transfusion below 25 weeks results in so few liveborn babies, there is little reason to obtain an O.D. before 22 weeks, regardless of the previous history or current titers. With the placenta occupying a greater percentage of the uterine surface early in pregnancy, amniocentesis is more likely to cause increased sensitization.

Amniocentesis and Analyses of Amniotic Fluid

Analysis of amniotic fluid as an indicator in Rh sensitization of fetal involvement and status brings us closer to the actual patient compared with maternal titers which measure the virulence of the offending party. Ideally, a technique to measure fetal hemoglobin levels directly would be preferable to currently employed methods which measure metabolic breakdown products of hemoglobin. We estimate what has been lost, but not what remains, since there is great variation in the ability of a fetus to compensate for hemolytic anemia.

Bevis originally measured amniotic fluid iron as an indicator of fetal hemoglobin degradation.[4] He added urobilinogen to the analysis in 1952[5] and produced his classic paper in 1956[6] on the correlation between amniotic fluid blood pigments and severity of erythroblastosis fetalis.

Many variations of technique have been proposed since Liley's original description.[29] We have found no reason to alter

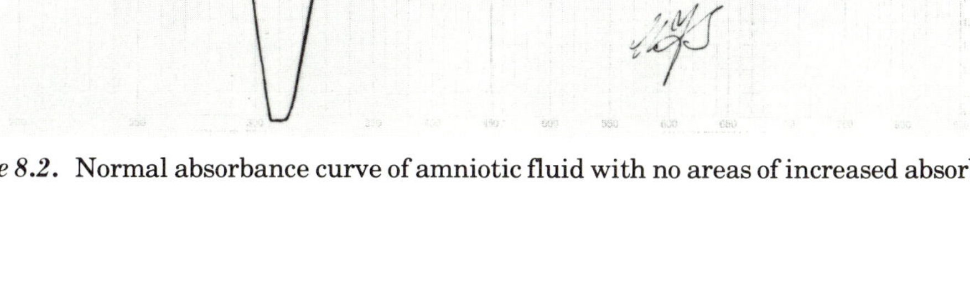

***Figure** 8.2*. Normal absorbance curve of amniotic fluid with no areas of increased absorbance.

our method which closely parallels that of Liley's. A continuous recording spectrophotometer measures absorbance over the 350- to 750-nm range plotted against an ordinate with a logarithmic scale. Normal absorbance decreases with fetal age. Bilirubin and related pigments absorb preferentially around 450 nm, producing deviation from the normal smooth absorption pattern (Figure 8.2). Smaller peaks may be caused by oxyhemoglobin at 412 nm (soret peak, Figure 8.3) and by hemoglobin at 540 nm and 575 nm (Figure 8.4). Meconium absorbs preferentially at 410 nm.

Light, especially sunlight, greatly accelerates the breakdown of bilirubin compounds. As a result, accurate analysis depends on shielding the specimen soon after collection with an opaque covering such as commercial aluminum wrap. Hydramnios dilutes the specimen and may decrease the magnitude of the 450 peak. Except in rare cases, accurate determination of amniotic volume with dye such as Evan's blue is unnecessary to calculate concentrations of heme pigments. Centrifugation of the specimen helps remove interfering blood and vernix but is less successful in dealing with meconium. Because of a marked pH effect on absorbance, adjustment of the specimen with buffer to pH 7.4 is required.

The specifics of amniocentesis will not be discussed save to emphasize that special care should be taken to avoid the placenta. Localization with ultrasonic techniques is helpful. Often, the entire placental site cannot be outlined definitely, but a pocket or pool of fluid can be observed. Placement

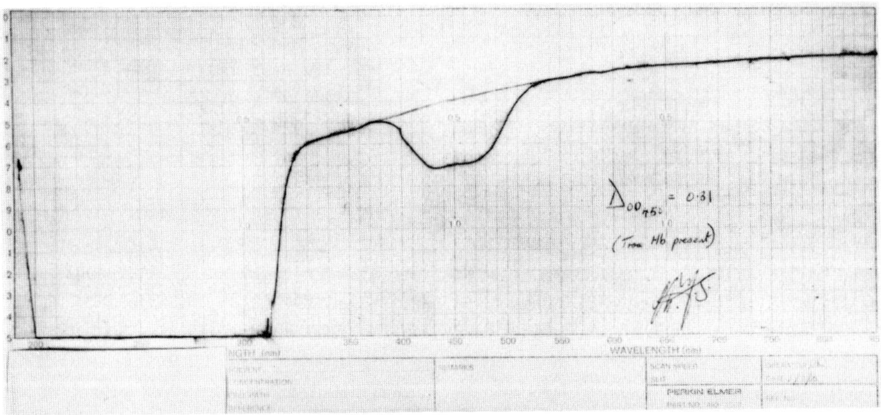

Figure 8.3. Absorbance difference at 450 nm of 0.31 with early oxyhemoglobin shoulder around 412 nm.

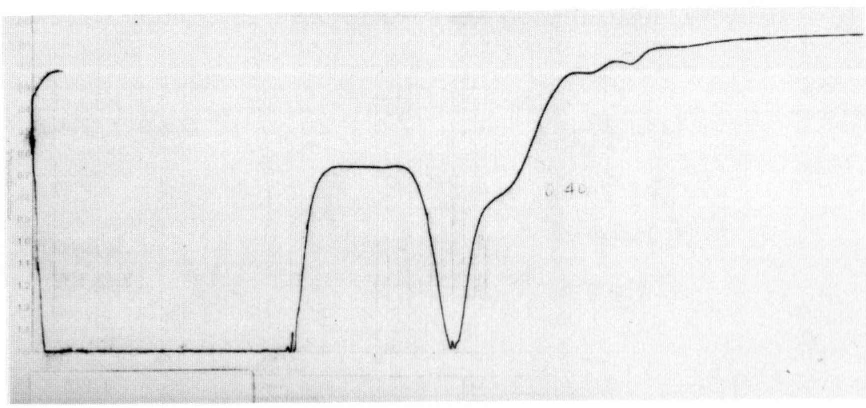

Figure 8.4. Absorbance difference at 450 nm of 0.40 with small secondary peaks at 540 and 575 nm caused by hemoglobin contamination in the specimen.

of the needle through a hollow transducer allows for a clean tap.[62] Therefore, placental as well as fetal location determines the site of amniocentesis. The scan is of great aid in multiple pregnancy with fetuses demonstrating differing degrees of involvement.

Figure 8.5 shows a simplified Liley-like optical density plot which we use to follow sensitized patients. Zone "A" values usually reflect unaffected or mildly affected fetuses. Zone "B" readings indicate minimal to marked sensitization, depending on whether values fall in the lower or upper range. Values in the "C" area imply severe fetal jeopardy requiring immediate IUT or delivery.

Unless an initial "C" value is recorded, we usually obtain readings 10 to 21 days apart in order to determine a vector to assess fetal involvement. The frequency depends on prior history as well as the initial O.D. recorded. Serial measurements may show worsening or improvement depending on the amount of maternal antibody reaching the fetus. Values do not reflect *accurately* the ability of the fetus to increase red cell production. That this indirect measurement roughly reflects the hemoglobin status of the fetus was demonstrated by Liley.[31] The proper course of action for "A" zone and lower "B" zone readings is continued observation. "C" zone fetuses need delivery as soon as possible with IUT utilized as a delaying technique. The decision as to the most propitious time for delivery is predicated on previous stillborn history, data from the current pregnancy, the skill of the transfusion operator but, most of all, on the ability of the neonatologist to deal with a severely ill premature newborn. Thus, management of a pregnancy at 32 to 33 weeks with high "B" readings must be a team decision. To deliver or transfuse must be decided for each case on all the available data. Urinary or plasma estriol levels have been of little aid. Serial ultrasonic biparietal measurements can be used to plot fetal growth but the L/S ratio and the O.D. values are of prime importance. Ward et al[60] employed plasma placental lactogen as a prognostic aid; we have had no experience with this approach or with amniotic fluid diamine oxidase levels in the management of immunized pregnancies.[61]

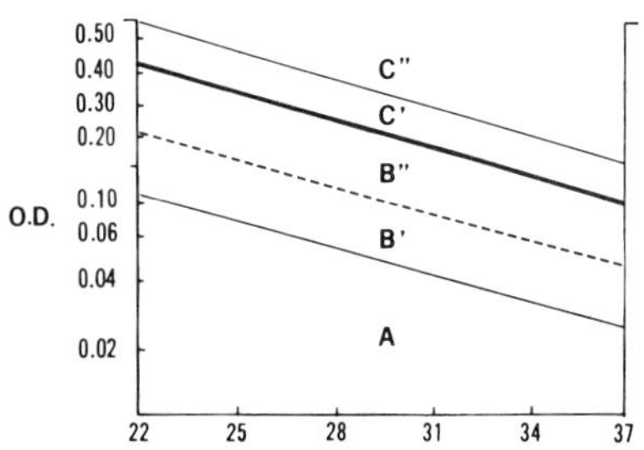

Figure 8.5. Semilogarthmic O.D. difference plot versus weeks after Liley.

Injection of Hypaque 50 at the time of amniocentesis is recommended if the fluid grossly is pigmented, suggesting the need for IUT. Films taken 24 hr later show concentration of the dye in the fetal intestine, providing a target for placement of the transfusion needle. Lack of dye ingestion suggests a moribund fetus or associated congenital gastrointestinal defects (high atresias). Care must be taken not to inject over 15 ml since the intense hygroscopic action of the dye may increase the amniotic volume, causing premature rupture of the membranes.

Even if transfusion is not contemplated, an amniogram can give valuable information. Loss of the typical fetal folded position with extension of the limbs and straightening of the spine is a poor prognostic sign and suggests ascites. This may be confirmed by the finding of the ribs in a flared or horizontal position. Fetal scalp edema can be seen with the dye contrast. On occasion the fetal abdomen may be outlined (ultrasound is a better technique). Radiographic signs of fetal demise are no longer needed because of the availability of Doppler units and fetal EKG machines. Reinjection of dye prior to each IUT is not necessary since there is enough present from the original administration and the preceding IUT to outline the fetal intestinal tract.

After the initial paper by Gluck and associates in 1971,[18] many investigators have reported salutary results in the timing of delivery based on this test of fetal pulmonary maturation. Not only does the L/S ratio usually increase sharply at 34 to 36 weeks, but the generation of lecithin changes from the α-palmitic/β-myristic acid methylation pathway to favor the production of α-palmitic/β-palmitic acid by the CDP-choline pathway. This latter phospholipid is more stable, especially in hypothermic conditions.[8] Hypoxia and low pH, commonly found in premature neonates, may inhibit methylation, explaining the vulnerability of the smaller newborn to respiratory distress syndrome (RDS).[19]

Because cesarean section may predispose to development of RDS,[56] it is particularly important to assess fetal lung maturity in Rh problems since severe cases usually are delivered by the abdominal route. Using Gluck's technique, we rarely encounter significant RDS with an L/S ratio in excess of 2.5:1.

After the work of Liggins and Howie,[28] we began to use betamethasone intramuscularly to induce fetal lung maturity in cases of premature labor and other high risk situations. That the fetal lung is a target organ for glucocorticoids has been demonstrated by tbe identification of numerous specific binding sites in fetal lung.[17, 53] We have been impressed with results in gestations of less than 33 weeks. There are cases with no apparent response, but overall, our experience has mirrored that of Liggins and Howie[28] and Avery[3] in that gains seem to outweigh both theoretic and actual risks. Treatment of the fetus via the mother with potent steroids, however, greatly affects the fetal adrenal-placental axis, causing dramatic drops in estriol production, which usually recovers 72 hr after the last injection.[36, 63]

We *routinely* give intramuscular betamethasone, 6 mg, daily for 3 days during the 31st week of gestation when IUT is employed. A large proportion of the patients will spontaneously initiate labor secondary to transfusion; others may rupture membranes without labor. Prophylactic administration before either of these two events provides sufficient time to elapse for potential stimulation of lung maturity. This plan also allows for elective delivery in some cases at 33 to 34 weeks as an alternative to another IUT.

Intrauterine Transfusion

With publication of Liley's account of IUT,[30] a new modality of treatment for severe Rh isoimmunization became a reality. This first reported case (two transfusions 10 days apart) culminated in a successful outcome. The physiology was founded on work performed a century previously by von Recklinghausen,[57] who documented transperitoneal absorbance of defibrinated blood in the rabbit. Rochlin, Zill and Blakemore[49] used ^{51}Cr-tagged red cells to demonstrate that dogs could absorb 70% of intraperitoneally injected blood. Their data showed no reduction in survival time of cells compared with intravenous infusion, and proved that resorption took place entirely via lymphatics. Pritchard and Adams[41] documented absorption of two-thirds of ^{51}Cr-tagged intraperitoneal blood (with acid-citrose-dextose solution) deposited at laparotomy. Niesert,[35] in a series of 800 infants less than 1 year of age, demonstrated good absorption of whole fresh blood given as an intraperitoneal transfusion. Kleihauer staining and ^{51}Cr studies in intrauterine transfusions have led to the conclusion that 60 to 90% of packed red cells are absorbed (in the absence of ascites) with completion of the process by 6 days, although most of the erythrocytes enter the fetal circulation in the first 48 hr. Ascites modifies both absorption and the amount of cells that can be safely deposited in an already distended cavity, but is not a contraindication to IUT.

Indications for IUT are predicated on prior obstetric history and the optical density readings during the 25th to 35th week of gestation. With the exception of acute emergency referrals, we hesitate to perform IUT based on one reading since values occasionally decrease markedly, offering observation with early delivery or transfusion at a later date. Figure 8.6 demonstrates the zones of the Liley plot which serve as a guide to transfusion. A history of a previous stillborn or hydropic newborn argues for earlier transfusion in borderline cases. In the later stages, the L/S ratio is the most important factor in deciding whether to transfuse (initially or again) or deliver. Also to be considered are

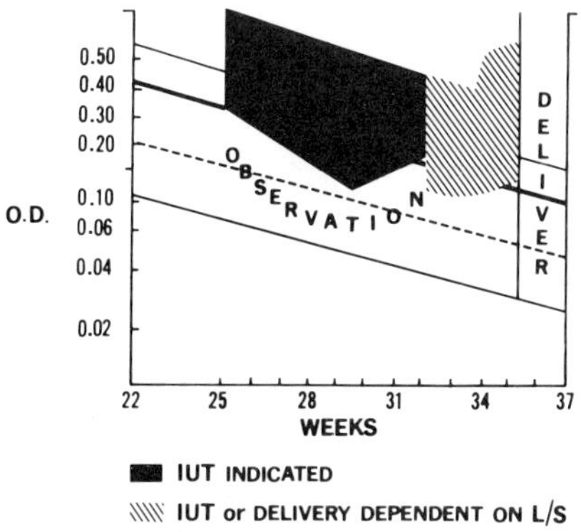

Figure 8.6. Guide to IUT dependent on O.D. and gestational length.

the skill of the operator and the capabilities of the neonatologist and intensive care nursery to handle not only the hematologic and pulmonary complications of these premature infants, but central nervous system apnea and necrotizing enterocolitis as well.

The questions of how much packed cells to give and how often are intertwined. The volume is further dependent on fetal blood volume and peritoneal capacity at a given stage during gestation. Figure 8.7 demonstrates the curve we use to determine (according to gestational age) the volume of packed cells transfused. It closely resembles figures employed by the group at Queen Charlotte's Maternity Hospital in London, whose results are discussed later in this chapter.[21] Deposition of an excessive volume of packed cells will cause rigid peritoneal distension and result in acute cardiac embarrassment with fetal death. Too little has a transient effect and does not justify the fetal risk. Although cells are absorbed rapidly, fetal growth rate between 26 to 34 weeks is such that transfusion is usually scheduled at 12- to 16-day intervals.

Blood (O, Rh negative) is obtained from a donor who will satisfactorily cross-match with the mother. Serologic testing of the specimen for syphilis and hepatitis antigens is performed routinely. We prefer to use erythrocytes which are as fresh as possible, not only for increased survival, but to reduce fetal potassium load caused by erythrocyte breakdown. Cells are centrifuged and packed to achieve a hematocrit near 90%. The buffy coat containing most of the white cells is removed. The fear of "runting" caused by foreign white cells (lymphocytes) acting in a graft versus host fashion is theoretic and can be produced in laboratory animals whose fetal immunologic competence is low; this has not been demonstrated in the human under these circumstances.

On the day prior to the first transfusion 12 to 15 ml of 50% Hypaque is injected transabdominally into the amniotic cavity so that the fetus may swallow and concentrate dye in the colon. Too much Hypaque rapidly increases amniotic volume by its hygroscopic action, causing rupture of the membranes. The patient is admitted a few hours prior to the procedure for preliminary fetal monitoring to evaluate baseline heart rate and spontaneous beat-to-beat variability. One hour before transfusion intramuscular sedation such as meperidine and diazepam or morphine sulfate is administered to decrease spontaneous fetal activity. A sufficient quantity of donor cells are packed to allow for the transfusion, the volume of the tubing and container and the inadvertent loss during the process of attaching a syringe.

The patient is positioned supine on the radiology table in a room with a fluoroscopic vision intensifier unit and a televi-

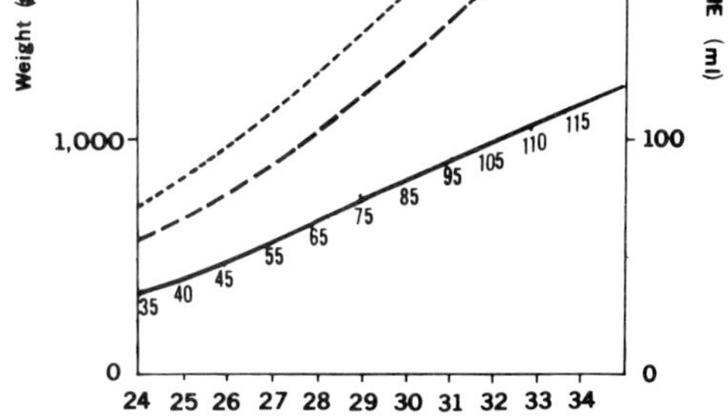

Figure 8.7. Guide to volume of packed cells necessary for IUT according to gestational length.

sion monitor. Numbered markers are placed on the abdomen with one over the umbilicus. Preliminary full sized films (Figures 8.8 and 8.9) are taken in anterior-posterior and lateral planes. Concentration of dye in the fetal gut is noted as well as the presence or absence of scalp edema. Fetal ascites is suggested by an increased volume of the fetal abdominal shadow and horizontal flaring of the ribs. The lie and attitude of the fetus then is determined in order to choose the appropriate site of entry and trajectory of the needle.

An IUT tray is shown in Figure 8.10. The abdomen is prepared with povidone-iodine and aseptically draped with sterile towels. A small skin wheal is raised with local anesthesia and carried down to the fascia with a 25-gauge needle. An elongated 16-gauge Tuohy needle is inserted through the skin wheal in a direction agreed upon by the operator and radiologist after inspection of the films. It is important to start the procedure as soon as possible after the scout films to avoid major positional changes of the fetus.

Upon entry into the amniotic sac, the stylet is removed and fluid can be withdrawn for O.D. or L/S studies. Although Mennuti et al[32] have suggested that O.D. readings remain a valid indicator of the hemolytic process after IUT, our experience does not confirm their contention. Significant amounts of blood may leak from the fetal needle tract ino the amniotic fluid causing a spurious high O.D. reading. L/S ratios, however, seem to remain valid after IUT if specimens are prepared properly.

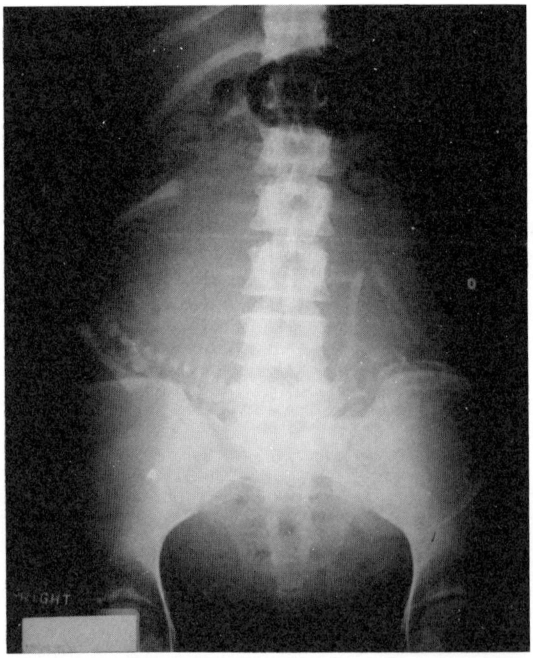

Figure 8.8. Anterior-posterior radiograph of fetal position.

The stylet is replaced and the needle advanced until the fetus is touched. Fluoroscopic guidance then is employed to determine the relationship of the needle to the fetus. If a correction is necessary, the needle must be totally withdrawn from the uterus (but not necessarily the maternal abdomen) to effectively change the direction. When satisfactory alignment of the needle and fetal dye shadows have been achieved, the fetus is touched with the needle and usually will float away only to return in a ballotment-type maneuver. On the recoil the operator must sharply impale the fetus on the needle. Characteristically, one can feel the needle pass through the fetal abdomen into a free space. The stylet is withdrawn and gentle aspiration is attempted with a syringe. If blood is noted, the needle is removed immediately. Since one cannot grossly differentiate between amniotic fluid and fetal ascitic fluid, the next step in the process is performed.

One or 2 ml of 50% Hypaque is injected under fluoroscopic guidance through a rubber tubing and triple stopcock attached to the needle. The tubing removes the operator's hands from the fluoroscopic field. A characteristic spreading pattern of dye over the loops of bowel is seen if the needle is free in the peritoneal cavity (Figure 8.11). If the needle is in soft tissue or a solid organ, such as the liver, a solid dense spot of dye which does not diffuse is evident (Figure 8.12). Entry into fetal gut shows a tubular pattern of dye spread (Figure 8.13). If the needle is in the amniotic sac, the dye rapidly diffuses in an obviously large space. Placental placement shows maternal runoff through the uterine veins. Figure 8.14 demonstrates placement of dye in the fetal bladder; Figure 8.15 shows a fetal myelogram.

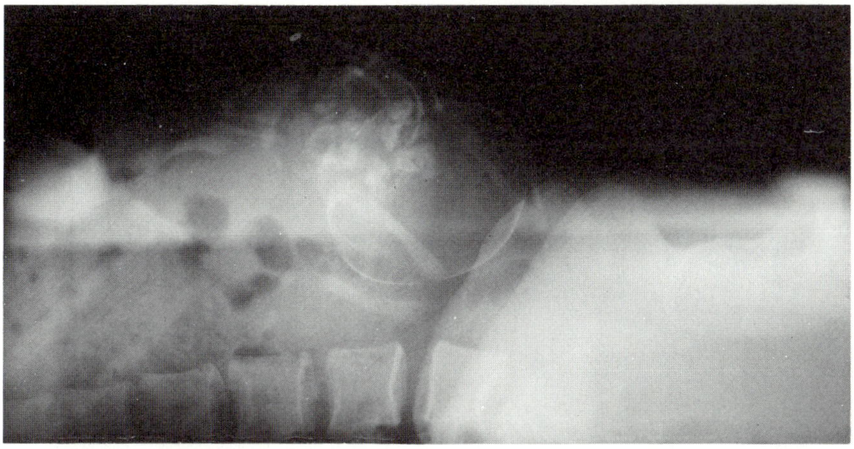

Figure 8.9. Lateral radiograph of fetal position.

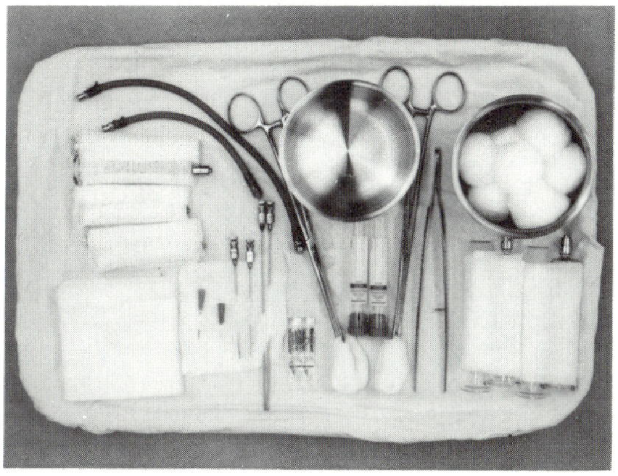

Figure 8.10. Tray used for IUT.

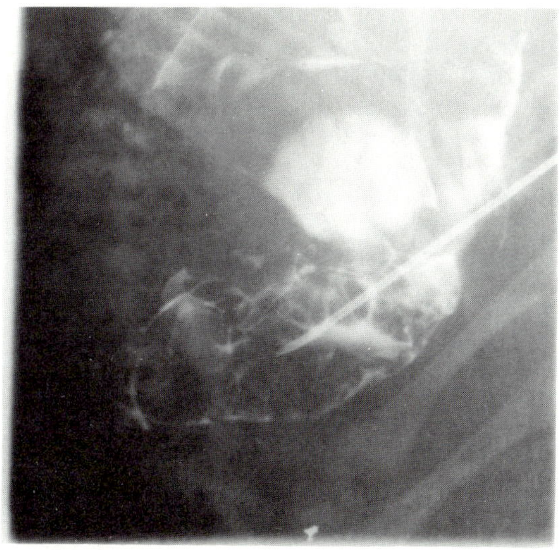

Figure 8.11. Needle and radiopaque dye in fetal peritoneal cavity just before IUT.

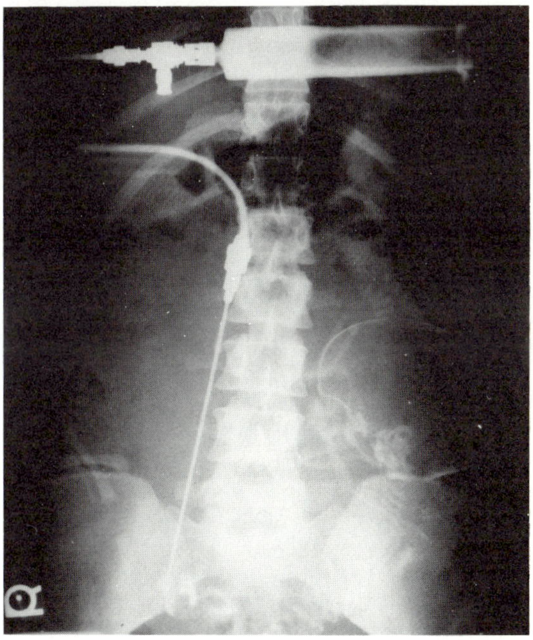

Figure 8.12. Injection of dye into solid abdominal organ of fetus.

With satisfactory localization the blood administration set and tubing is attached to the other side of the triple stopcock and the packed cells are given over a 5-min period via a 30-ml plastic syringe. We do not use a catheter threaded through the needle since this technique prolongs transfusion time and the operator loses his feel for end-pressure via the syringe. If fetal ascites is encountered, the fluid is allowed to run out of the needle (without suction)

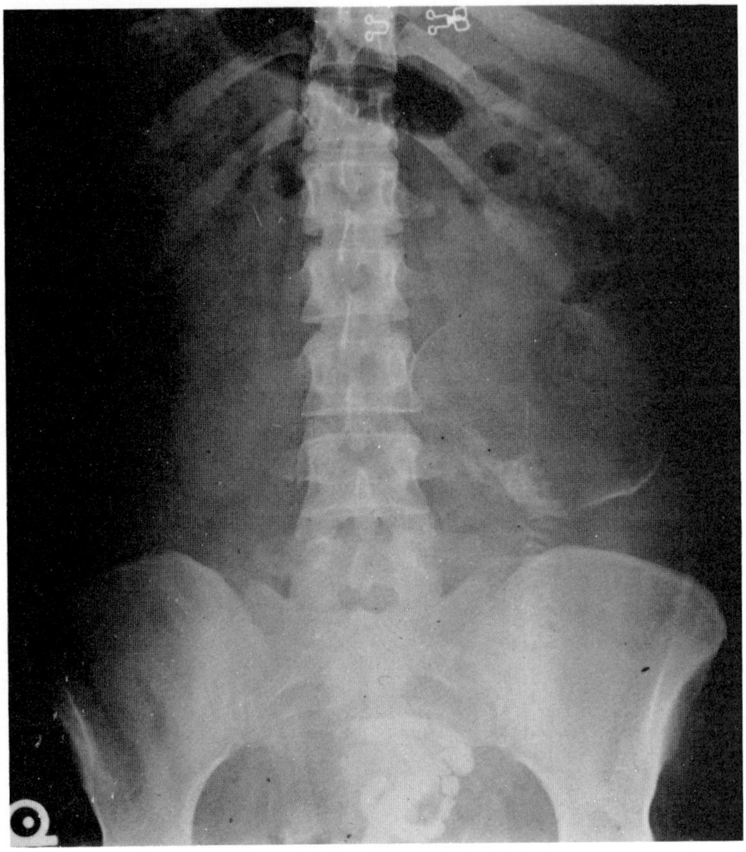

Figure 8.13. Fetal intraintestinal placement of dye.

before infusion of the packed cells in order to decrease fetal peritoneal distension and to increase absorption of the cells. Attempts at aspiration usually result in bowel blocking the needle. Because powder from sterile gloves can jam glass barrels, we now use plastic syringes. As soon as a sensation of increased pressure is noted, the procedure is halted even if short of the intended volume. If, during the transfusion, gross fetal movement occurs, 1 or 2 ml of Hypaque is reinjected to verify needle position. Hobbins et al[20] have described transfusion using a combination of ultrasonic and radiographic approaches. This markedly reduces fetal x-ray exposure but final placement is still a radiographic diagnosis.

After transfusion, the patient is monitored by ultrasonic and external tocographic instruments. Commonly, post-transfusion fetal tachycardia is noted. Sporadic uterine contractions frequently occur and are treated with aspirin or oral alcohol if persistent. Progressive labor is an indication for intravenous alcohol or other tocolytic agents such as isoxuprine. Patients usually are discharged 4 hours after transfusion with activity restricted for 24 hr. Continued slow leaking of fluid from high needle tracts is common and innocuous, whereas a gush of fluid suggests low rupture of the sac. No prophylactic antibiotics are employed.

The risks of IUT to the mother are low, but include abruptio placenta with Couvelaire uterus, hepatitis and sepsis. Fetal morbidity and mortality result from direct needle trauma causing laceration of the liver, aorta, spleen, umbilical cord or bleeding from a major fetal vessel in the placenta. Injection of dye into joint spaces has caused contracture deformities. Data presented at the Ross conference in 1966 suggested a minimum risk factor of 6.5% mortality per procedure based on 238 fetuses receiving 399 transfusions.[50] Turner et al,[55] in 1975, reported an upper risk of

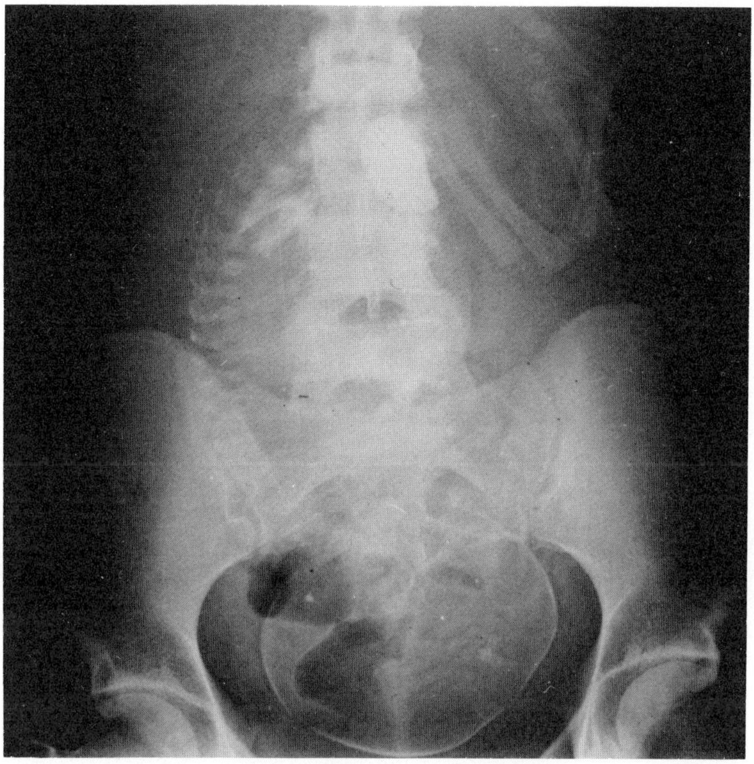

Figure 8.14. Fetal urinary cystogram.

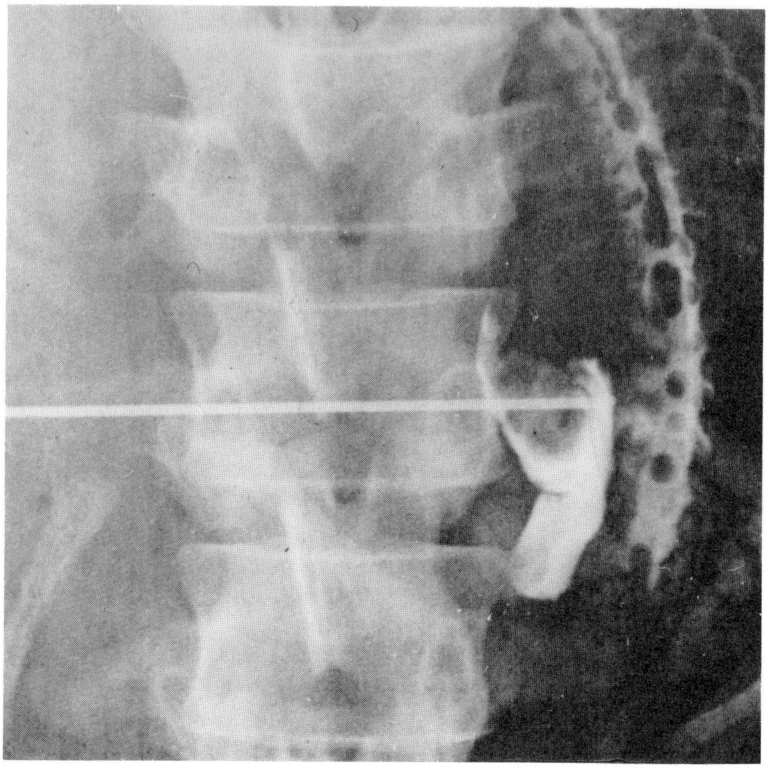

Figure 8.15. Fetal myelogram.

7.2% mortality per procedure based on 147 cases receiving transfusions. Therefore, the risk factor has not changed appreciably in 10 years and probably will not unless the ultrasonic approach proves to be of added benefit in reducing inappropriate needle placement.

The Ross conference reported an overall survival rate of 30.7%; 13.6% with hydrops and 45.3% for nonhydropic fetuses. Since this information was generated by 11 cooperating institutions, indications and techniques necessarily varied. Turner et al[55] found similar results: 14% survival with hydrops and 47% success with IUT in nonhydropic cases. The British group at Queen Charlotte's Maternity Hospital[21] reported a transfusion failure rate of 8.1% and a fetal mortality rate from the procedure of 15.4% which fell to 5% after the second transfusion. The overall survival rate was 46.3%; however, 31.5% of hydropic fetuses were salvaged. They also concluded that transfusion before 24 weeks was not indicated because of the risk to benefit ratio.

Because final statistics reflect a team approach to the problem, we evaluated our data over the last 2 years when certain changes were made in the management of respiratory complications in the intensive care nursery and at the same time we began to use betamethasone routinely at 30 to 31 weeks. During this interval 18 fetuses had one or more IUT (43 total) for erythroblastosis fetalis as detailed in Table 8.3. Thirteen cases resulted in live infants who survived. Of the failures, one died of RDS in the nursery, three were stillborns with hydrops and "C" zone O.D. readings and one may represent a procedure death. Our overall salvage rate of 72%, with only one respiratory death as the sole liveborn that succumbed, attests to the interplay which must exist between the obstetrician and the neonatologist in the formulation of a therapeutic program. In only 4 cases of 13 liveborn infants did rupture of membranes or spontaneous labor ensue prior to 33 weeks. Still, this rate of roughly one-third not completing the projected program argues, we believe, for the prophylactic use of betamethasone.

Although follow-up of these infants has usually shown good physical and mental development,[48] Turner's group reports a 50% abnormality rate in physical, intellectual and/or social maturation. One patient developed lymphocytic leukemia at 4.5 years of age associated with persistent donor white blood cells. Unfortunately, at this time there is no good alternative treatment for the severely sensitized fetus.

Prophylaxis

As is frequently the case, two independent groups, starting with slightly different premises, came to a major discovery at the same point in time. Freda and Gorman,[15] using anti-D globulin prepared by Pollack at Ortho, administered this preparation prior to a test challenge of D-positive cells in male Rh-negative volunteers. Since their idea was to use this preparation *during* pregnancy to prevent sensitization, they were interested primarily in the 19S component which would not cross the placenta. The 7S portion was felt to be useful at delivery when most of the fetomaternal bleed occurs. Finn's English group began from the opposite direction, injecting the D-positive cells first.[14] Finn used the Kleihauer technique for estimating the amount of fetal cells leaking into the maternal circulation.

Freda and associates[16] went on to produce a 7S anti-D gammaglobulin, and challenged males monthly for 5 months with 2 ml of Rh-positive whole blood following antibody administration. Four of the 5 who acted as control subjects were sensitized, but none of the 4 receiving antibody showed isoimmunization. Woodrow et al[70] used ^{51}Cr-tagged cells to demonstrate that Rh-positive cells exposed to 7S antibody were sequestrated in the spleen, compared with ABO-incompatible cells, which were concentrated in the liver. Presumably, coating of Rh-incompatible cells by macrophages in the spleen prevented sensitization. Because the liver contains fewer immunologically active cells, they theorized that this might explain ABO-incompatible protection of Rh-negative females. In the same paper they statistically correlated Kleihauer counts around delivery with subsequent antibody production.

Results of a combined English-American study from 4 centers were pub-

Table 8.3. Evaluation of 18 cases of erythroblastosis fetalis with IUT over 2-year period

Patient No.	Previous Rh history	No. of IUT	Week at 1st IUT	Liley zone	Outcome
1	Exchange transfusion with first pregnancy	1	32	C′	RDS at L/S 2.1; possible amnionitis; Atony at CS refractive to treatment led to hysterectomy. Baby and mother well, exchange transfusions (3)
2	Initial sensitization last delivery CS for placenta previa	1	28	C′	Stillborn hydropic, possible Down's syndrome
3	Exchange transfusion	1	32	B″	Planned delivery at 34 weeks, CS, phototherapy
4	Initial sensitization, class A diabetes	1	34	B″	Transfused because of low L/S at 34 weeks and vaginal del at 35 weeks; exchange transfusions (7)
5	Initial sensitization	1	32	C″	Blood bank or physician error resulted in no Rh_0-Gam 1971, stillborn hydropic, spontaneous labor
6	Initial sensitization	1	30	B″	32 weeks; CS; ascitic at IUT. Exchange transfusion (1)
7	Initial sensitization in 4th pregnancy	2	30	C′	CS at 35 weeks, L/S 2.3, mild RDS; exchange transfusions (3)
8	Prior stillborn	2	25	C″	Stillborn hydropic at 28 weeks
9	Prior stillborn	2	26	C′	Rupture of membranes at 30 weeks; labor and CS delivery at 31 weeks; exchange transfusions (5)
10	Exchange transfusion	2	29	C′	Rupture of membranes and labor at 32 weeks; CS for monitor changes; exchange transfusions (4)
11	Exchange transfusion	2	27	B″	Stillborn at 30 weeks; possibly trauma of IUT
12	Prior stillborn	3	29	C′	CS at 35 weeks; exchange transfusions (2)
13	Prior stillborn (Rh_0Gam failure)	3	28	B″	CS at 34 weeks; exchange transfusions (4)
14	Prior stillborn with IUT	3	27	C′	CS hydropic at 33 weeks. RDS; death
15	Exchange transfusion	4	26	C″	CS at 34 weeks after course of betamethasone; meconium staining of fluid; exchange transfusions (4)
16	Prior stillborn	4	27	B″	CS at 35 weeks. L/S 2.3:1; moderate RDS; exchange transfusions (4)
17	Prior neonatal demise	5	25	C″	CS at 34 weeks; exchange transfusions (2)
18	Prior neonatal hydropic demise	5	26	B″	CS at 36 weeks after 2 courses of betamethasone; L/S 1.8:1; severe RDS; exchange transfusions (2)

lished in 1966.[39] The women included were all judged to be at high risk as determined by Kleihauer tests. Serologic testing 6 months after pregnancy demonstrated that 22% of the control subjects became sensitized versus none of the group treated with 5 ml of high titer anti-D given within 36 hr of delivery. Pollack et al[38] used two dose levels (300 and 1000 μg) in a large study and showed one sensitization with the 300-μg dose in 781 gravidas. Moreover, 145 patients were followed into a second pregnancy; 1 of 82 treated became sentitized versus 7 of 63 control subjects. Pollack et al[37] also quantitated in male volunteers the amount of blood that can be neutralized by a standard dose of anti-D globulin. This proved to be 35 ml of blood per 267 μg.

Mollison et al[34] demonstrated the sensitivity of ^{51}Cr-tagging compared with antibody detection methods by showing altered RBC survival curves in 6 of 13 patients challenged with Rh-positive cells who did not demonstrate antibody after a "priming" dose of Rh-positive cells. However, anti-D (75 μg) was effective in preventing this response in those treated.

Woodrow et al[71] in 1971 reported a "low risk" group of 844 gravidas with minimal fetomaternal bleed (<0.2 ml) as suggested by Kleihauer counts. After 200 μg of anti-D, 1.8% developed titers after the next Rh-positive pregnancy, compared with 10.2% of the control subjects. Thus, a protection rate of about 82% was achieved at this dose. Sensitization initiated during the second pregnancy incorrectly would be included in this figure since antibody detection between pregnancies is not sufficiently sensitive to document priming. On the other hand, statistics generated by antibody studies at 6 months may be faulted because passive antibody may still be measured at that time. Table 8.4 gives data presented by Woodrow[68] in 1973. A protection rate of 93% has been achieved in high risk studies with 1000 μg.[40]

If failure is caused by persistent transfer of cells during pregnancy, only routine prepartum administration of anti-D might help. Such an approach was taken by Bowman and associates, who employed anti-D at 28 weeks of gestation in women at risk in addition to the usual postpartum dose.[22] The investigators calculated that 6.7% of sensitizations occurred before 29 weeks rather than at delivery. Review of 3532 Rh-negative women who delivered Rh-positive infants showed that 1.7% had no antibody at the beginning of the pregnancy but were found to be sensitized late in pregnancy or after delivery. Indirect Coombs screening would have missed 41 of these 60 cases (68%). Since the program was begun in 1968, no treated patient has shown sensitization.

Even if failure with passive antibody should occur, the initial sensitized pregnancy may be less severely affected. This was the finding of Tovey and Robinson[54] in a study of 2459 women. Failure to protect occurred in 1.6%. Follow-up of 53 of these subsequent Rh-positive affected pregnancies showed reduced morbidity (only one loss) compared with a similar series not given immunoglobulin. The exact mechanism is unclear but may have to do with the total amount of antigen and the time of exposure to the host's immune systems. Woodrow et al[69] administered D-positive, K-positive cells to D-negative, Kell-negative volunteers. Half then were given IgG anti-K. Anti-D developed in 11 of 31 control subjects and in only 1 of 31 treated subjects. The suppression of D immunization was associated with rapid clearance of the foreign red cells in the spleen. Therefore, the process is not antigen specific but, rather, involves the entire red cell, probably via splenic macrophages.

A shortage of anti-D globulin some years ago in the United Kingdom made the question of "how much is enough" of more than passing academic interest. Background control figures were 8% of women sensitized by 6 months and an additional 9% by the end of the next Rh-positive pregnancy. Doses of 200 μg, 100 μg, 50 μg and 20 μg were evaluated.[47] Failure rates at 6 months judged by indirect antiglobulin detection were 0.22%, 0.23%, 0.44% and 1.35%, respectively, and the correlation with dose was significant at $P = 0.02$. Failure rates generated by antibody detection in the next potentially affected pregnancy were 1.5%, 1.1%, 1.5% and 2.9%. These results indicated a surprisingly high level of effectiveness of the 20-μg dose, but one which is probably too low for general use. The authors advocated 100 μg for routine cases. The problem of passive versus active antibody detection at 6 months was discussed. After a dose of 1000 μg, Wallace[58] measured passive anti-

Table 8.4. Controlled clinical trials: Efficacy of anti-D administration after delivery and in subsequent pregnancy

Center	Antibodies (%) months later		Antibodies (%) next pregnancy	
	Control	Treated	Control	Treated
England				
1000 μg*	21.6	0.58	30.7	2.4
200 μg†	3.6	0.0	10.2	2.3
United States	6.9	0.18	13.4	1.1
West Germany	3.9	0.49	7.8	0.0

* High risk group.
† Low risk group.

body with an AutoAnalyzer in three of eight subjects at 9 months. Using [^{125}I]IgG, he calculated a $t_{0.5}$ of 26 days over a 5-month period. Levels following a 200-μg dose would be expected to be just measurable at 6 months by automatic methods but not with enzymatically treated cells and manual methods.

A summary of the 1974 Brighton workshop[33] which was chaired by Clarke, appears in his excellent book, *Rhesus Hemolytic Disease*.[9] Hungarian data demonstrated that 3.8% of women at risk who had pregnancy termination at 3 months without passive antibody administration developed titers. Sampson reported on delayed administration of anti-D up to 2 weeks after injection of D-positive red cells; immunization was suppressed in half. Actually, the 72-hour limit commonly employed was based on the week-end hiatus during the original volunteer studies.

Keith et al[23] report a survey of 2286 transfusion facilities over a 1-year span. Of 203 patients receiving Rh-incompatible transfusions, 44 were women 49 years of age or younger. Fifty percent received volumes in excess of 250 ml. Immunoglobulin was given to only 22 patients. Ratios of globulin (micrograms) to cells (milliliters) ranged from 9.0 to 36.0. None of the three patients receiving globulin at a 20 μg per ml or more ratio developed anti-D titers. Four patients received <20 μg per ml and one developed antibodies; five of seven women who received no treatment were immunized.

Recommendations for routine administration of anti-D immunoglobulin in nonsensitized women at risk are as follows.

1. A standard dose of 200 to 300 μg should be given intramuscularly after abortion beginning at 8 weeks or delivery of intrauterine or extrauterine pregnancy. This should be given within 72 hr but will be of benefit if given later. Trophoblastic tumors have not been shown to be capable of initiating isoimmunization.
2. After inadvertent administration of Rh-incompatible blood, anti-D should be given intramuscularly or intravenously in a ratio of 20 μg per ml of *cells* absorbed. Follow-up screening is essential.
3. Larger doses should be given in cases where increased fetomaternal transfer is documented by Kleihauer quantitation. Suspicion of an increased bleed as in cases of multiple gestation, placenta previa, abruptio or difficult extraction of the placenta should be given a double dose in the absence of quantitation.
4. Provided that no titers already exist, we recommend routine use of 100 μg of anti-D at the time of amniocentesis whether performed early or late in the gestation. Suspicion of placental trauma should be documented with serial maternal peripheral smears and anti-D dosage should be determined appropriately.

REFERENCES

1. Allen, F. H., Jr., Diamond, L. K., Jones, A. R.: Erythroblastosis fetalis. IX. Problems of stillbirth. N Engl J Med 251: 453, 1954.
2. Allen, F. H., Jr., Diamond, L. K., Vaughan, V. C., III: Erythroblastosis fetalis. VI. Prevention of kernicterus. Am J Dis Child 80: 779, 1950.
3. Avery, M. E.: Prenatal diagnosis and prevention of hyaline membrane disease. N Engl J Med 292: 151, 1975.
4. Bevis, D. C. A.: Composition of liquor amnii in haemolytic disease of the newborn. Lancet 2: 443, 1950.
5. Bevis, D. C. A.: The antenatal prediction of haemolytic disease of the newborn. Lancet 1: 395, 1952.
6. Bevis, D. C. A.: Blood pigments in haemolytic disease of the newborn. J Obstet Gynaecol Br Emp 63: 68, 1956.
7. Bolognese, R. J., Corson, S. L., Lakoff, K. M., Klein, J.: Transplacental passage of fetal cells at the time of suction D&E. J Repr Med 6: 260, 1971.
8. Brown, B. J., Gabert, H. A., Stenchever, M. A.: Respiratory distress syndrome, surfactant biochemistry, and acceleration of fetal lung maturity: A review. Obstet Gynecol Surv 30: 71, 1975.
9. Clarke, C. A.: Rhesus Hemolytic Disease. Baltimore, University Park Press, 1975, p 313.
10. Coombs, R. R. A., Mourant, A. E., Race, R. R.: Detection of weak and "incomplete" Rh agglutinins: A new test. Lancet 2: 15, 1945.
11. Darrow, R. R.: Icterus gravis (erythroblastosis) neonatorum: Examination of etiologic considerations. Arch Pathol 25: 378, 1938.
12. Diamond, L. K.: Erythroblastosis foetalis or haemolytic disease of the newborn. Proc Roy Soc Med 40: 546, 1947.
13. Diamond, L. K., Blackfan, K. D., Baty, J. M.: Erythroblastosis fetalis and its association with universal edema of fetus, icterus gravis neonatorum, and anemia of the newborn. J Pediatr 1: 269, 1932.
14. Finn, R., Clarke, C. A., Donohoe, W. T. A., McConnell, R. B., Sheppard, P. M., Lehane, D., Kulke, W. Experimental studies on the prevention of Rh haemolytic disease. Br Med J 1: 1486, 1961.
15. Freda, V. J., Gorman, J. G. Current concepts:

Antepartum management of Rh hemolytic disease. Bull Sloane Hosp Women 8: 147, 1962.
16. Freda, V. J., Gorman J. G., Pollack, W.: Successful prevention of experimental Rh sensitization in man with an anti-Rh gamma$_2$-globulin antibody preparation. Transfusion 4: 26, 1964.
17. Giannopoulos, G., Malay, S., Solomon, S.: Glucocorticoid receptors in lung. J Biol Chem 248: 5016, 1973.
18. Gluck, L., Kulovich, M. V., Borer, R. C., Brenner, P. H., Anderson, G. G., Spellacy, W. N.: The diagnosis of respiratory distress syndrome (RDS) by amniocentesis. Am J Obstet Gynecol 109: 440, 1971.
19. Gluck, L., Sribney, M., Kulovich, M. V.: The biochemical development of surface activity in mammalian lung. II. The biosynthesis of phospholipids in the lung of the developing rabbit fetus and newborn. Pediatr Res 1: 247, 1967.
20. Hobbins, J. C., Davis, C. D., Webster, J.: A new technique utilizing ultrasound to aid in intrauterine transfusion. J Clin Ultrasound 4: 135, 1975.
21. Holt, E. M., Boyd, I. E., Dewhurst, C. J., Murray, J., Naylor, C. H., Smitham, J. H. Intrauterine transfusion: 101 consecutive cases treated at Queen Charlotte's Maternity Hospital. Br Med J 3: 39, 1973.
22. IgG at 28 weeks for Rh protection. Med World News p 23, February 23, 1976.
23. Keith, L., Berger, G. S., Pollack, W.: The transfusion of Rh-positive blood into Rh-negative women. Am J Obstet Gynecol 125: 502, 1976.
24. Kleihauer, E., Braun, H., Betke, K. Demonstration von getalem hemoglobin in den erythrocytes eines blutausstrichs. Klin Wochenshr 35: 637, 1957.
25. Landsteiner, K., Wiener, A. S.: An agglutinable factor in human blood recognised by immune sera for Rhesus blood. Soc Exp Biol New York 43: 223, 1940.
26. Levine, P.: Serological factors as possible causes in spontaneous abortions. J Hered 34: 71, 1943.
27. Levine, P., Stetson, R. E.: Unusual cases of intragroup agglutination. JAMA 113: 126, 1939.
28. Liggins, G. C., Howie, R. N.: A controlled trial of antepartum glucocorticoid treatment for prevention of the respiratory distress syndrome in premature infants. Pediatrics 50: 515, 1972.
29. Liley, A. W.: Liquor amnii analysis in management of pregnancy complicated by rhesus sensitization. Am J Obstet Gynecol 82: 1359, 1961.
30. Liley, A. W.: Intrauterine transfusion of foetus in haemolytic disease. Br Med J 2: 1107, 1963.
31. Liley, A. W.: Errors in assessment of hemolytic disease from amniotic fluid. Am J Obstet Gynecol 86: 485, 1963.
32. Mennuti, M. T., Branca, P., Schwarz, R. H. Amniotic fluid evaluation after intrauterine transfusion. Obstet Gynecol 42: 823, 1973.
33. Mollison, P. L.: Rh and iso-immunisation. Summary of a workshop held at the 2nd International Congress of immunology at Brighton, England, in July 1974. Vox Sang (In press.)
34. Mollison, P. I., Hughes-Jones, N. C., Lindsay, M., Wessely, J.: Suppression of primary Rh immunisation by passively-administered antibody: Experiments in volunteers. Vox Sang 16: 421, 1969.
35. Niesert, F. J.: Die intraperitoneale Bluttransfusion im Säuglingsalter. Dtsch Med Wochenshr 75: 619, 1950.
36. Ohrlander, S. A. V., Gennser, G. M., Gennert, L.: Impact of betamethasone load given to pregnant women on endocrine balance of fetoplacental unit. Am J Obstet Gynecol 123: 228, 1975.
37. Pollack, W., Ascari, W. Q., Kochesky, R. J., O'Connor, R. R., Ho, T. Y., Tripodi, D.: Studies on Rh prophylaxis. 1. Relationship between doses of anti-Rh and size of antigenic stimulus. Transfusion 11: 33, 1971.
38. Pollack, W., Gorman, J. G., Freda, V. J., Ascari, W. Q., Allen, A. E., and Baker, W. J.: Results of clinical trials of RhoGAM in women. Transfusion 8: 151, 1968.
39. Prevention of Rh-haemolytic disease: Results of the clinical trial. A combined study from centres in England and Baltimore. Br Med J 2: 907, 1966.
40. Prevention of Rh-haemolytic disease: Final results of the "high risk" clinical trial. A combined study from centres in England and Baltimore. Br Med J 2: 607, 1971.
41. Pritchard, J. A., Adams, R. H.: The fate of blood in the peritoneal cavity. Surg Gynecol Obstet 105: 621, 1957.
42. Queenan, J. T.: *Modern Management of the Rh Problem*. New York, Harper & Row, 1967, p 303.
43. Race, R. R.: An "incomplete" antibody in human serum. Nature (London) 153: 771, 1944.
44. Race, R. R.: Some notes on Fisher's contributions to human blood groups. Biometrics 20: 361, 1964.
45. Race, R. R., Sanger, R.: Blood Groups in Man, First edition. Oxford, Blackwell Scientific Publications, 1950, pp 234–236.
46. Rautmann, H.: Über Blutbildung bei fötaler allgemeiner Wassersucht. Beitr Pathol Anat 54: 332, 1912.
47. Report of MRC Anti-D Working Party. Controlled trial of various anti-D dosages in suppression of sensitisation following pregnancy. Br. Med J 2: 75, 1974.
48. Richings, J.: Later progress of infants who received transfusions *in utero* for severe rhesus haemolytic disease. Lancet 1: 1220, 1973.
49. Rochlin, D. B., Zill, H., Blakemore, W. S.: Studies of the resorption of chromium-51 tagged erythrocytes from the peritoneal cavity; the absorption of fluids and particulate matter from the peritoneal cavity. *Surgery, Gynecology and Obstetrics International Abstracts of Surgery*, Vol. 107. Chicago, Franklin H. Martin Memorial Foundation, 1958, p 1.
50. Ross Conference on Pediatric Research. *Intrauterine Transfusion and Erythroblastosis Fetalis*. Aspen, Colorado, March 1966.
51. Scott, J. R., Beer, A. E.: Immunological factors in first-pregnancy Rh isoimmunisation. Lancet 1: 717, 1973.
52. Taylor, J. F.: Sensitization of Rh-negative daughters by their Rh-positive mothers. N Engl J Med 276: 547, 1967.
53. Toft, D., Chytil, F.: Receptors for glucocorticoids

in lung tissue. Arch Biochem Biophys 157: 464, 1973.
54. Tovey, L. A. D., Robinson, A. E.: Reduced severity of Rh-haemolytic disease after anti-D immunoglobulin. Br Med J 4: 320, 1975.
55. Turner, J. H., Hutchinson, D. L., Hayashi, T. T., Petricciani, J. C., Germanowski, J.: Fetal and maternal risks associated with intrauterine transfusion procedures. Am J Obstet Gynecol 123: 251, 1975.
56. Usher, R. H., Allen, A. C., McLean, F. H.: Risk of respiratory distress syndrome related to gestational age, route of delivery and maternal diabetes. Am J Obstet Gynecol 111: 826, 1971.
57. von Recklinhausen, F. V.: Zur fettresorption. Virchow's Arch Pathol Anat 26: 172, 1863.
58. Wallace, J.: Personal communication, 1971. Cited in Report of MRC Anti-D Working Party. Controlled trial of various anti-D dosages in suppression of sensitisation following pregnancy. Br Med J 2: 75, 1974.
59. Wallerstein, H.: Treatment of severe erythroblastosis by simultaneous removal and replacement of blood of newborn infant. Science 103: 583, 1946.
60. Ward, R. H. T., Letchworth, A. T., Niven, P. A. R., Chard, T.: Placental lactogen levels in rhesus isoimmunization. Br Med J 1: 347, 1974.
61. Ward, H. Whyley, G. A., Millar, M. D.: The value of amniotic fluid diamine oxidase estimations in the management of severe rhesus isoimmunization. Acta Obstet Gynecol Scand 55: 63, 1976.
62. Weiner, S.: An ultrasound aspiration transducer for diagnostic amniocenteses. Obstet Gynecol 47: 113, 1976.
63. Whitt, G. G., Buster, J. E., Killam, A. P., Scragg, W. H.: A comparison of two glucocorticoid regimens for acceleration of fetal lung maturation in premature labor. Am J Obstet Gynecol 124: 479, 1976.
64. Wiener, A. S.: A new test (blocking test) for Rh sensitization. Proc Soc Exp Biol Med 56: 173, 1944.
65. Wiener, A. S.: Heredity of the Rh blood types. VIII. Proceedings of The Eighth International Congress on Genetics, Stockholm, July 1948. 1949.
66. Wiener, A. S.: Elements of blood group nomenclature with special reference to the Rh-Hr blood types. JAMA 199: 131, 1967.
67. Wiener, A. S., Peters, H. R.: Hemolytic reactions following transfusions of blood of the homologous group, with three cases in which the same agglutinogen was responsible. Ann Intern Med 13: 2306, 1940.
68. Woodrow, J. C.: Effectiveness of Rh prophylaxis. Paper given at Bonn Working Party, 1973. Haematologia 8: 281, 1973.
69. Woodrow, J. C., Clarke, C. A., Donohoe, W. T. A., Finn, R., McConnell, R. B., Sheppard, P. M., Lehane, D., Roberts, F. M., Gimlette, T. M. D.: Mechanism of Rh prophylaxis: An experimental study on specificity of immunosuppression. Br Med J 2: 57, 1975.
70. Woodrow, J. C., Clarke, C. A., Donohoe, W. T. A., Finn, R., McConnell, R. B., Sheppard, P. M., Lehane, D., Russell, S. H., Kulke, W., Durkin, C. M.: Prevention of Rh-haemolytic disease: A third report. Br Med J 1: 279, 1965.
71. Woodrow, J. C., Clarke, C. A., McConnell, R. B., Towers, S. H., Donohoe, W. T. A.: Prevention of Rh-haemolytic disease: results of the Liverpool "low-risk" clinical trial. Br Med J 2: 610, 1971.
72. Zipursky, A.: Personal communication to Queenan, J. T., 1966. Cited in Queenan, J. T. *Modern Management of the Rh Problem*. New York, Harper & Row, 1967, p 21.

RICHARD H. AUBRY, M.D.
SAMIR BEYDOUN, M.D.
M. THERESA CABALUM, M.D.
MARGARET L. WILLIAMS, M.D.

9

Fetal Growth Retardation

Introduction

As perinatal medicine addresses itself to the challenge of further reducing perinatal mortality and morbidity, it seems clear that the major focus must be on low birth weight ("prematurity"), since it is the major finding in over half of perinatal mortality and is associated with a striking increase in immediate as well as long term perinatal morbidity. However, as the discipline has focused more sharply on the problem, it has become increasingly clear that at least one-third of low birth weight infants are actually small for gestational age (SGA) and are the result of intrauterine fetal growth retardation (IUGR). This component of low birth weight infants is especially challenging because the definitions are not sufficiently clear, the etiologies are many and interrelated, the prenatal diagnosis and management are difficult and the long term prognosis is a matter of some conjecture.

It will be the purpose of this chapter to make a concise and practical presentation of the definition, etiology, prenatal diagnosis, management and outcome of fetal growth retardation.

Normal Fetal Growth

STANDARD FETAL GROWTH CURVES

The definition of fetal growth retardation must start from acceptable standards describing the "normal" relationship between birth weight and gestational age. The newborn whose weight deviates significantly from the "normal standard" can then be diagnosed and evaluated. An increasing number of such normal fetal growth curves have been published in North America[7, 42, 48, 79, 94, 111, 114] and other parts of the world.[24, 66] Although these curves are in agreement as far as showing that the changes in fetal weight during gestation follow a similar sigmoid pattern, the mean fetal weight at a particular week of gestation differs from study to study. The disparity is exemplified in Figure 9.1, which compares the established norms of intrauterine growth as derived from obstetric populations in Baltimore, Denver, Melbourne and Vancouver. This observation causes one to look more closely into the validity of the growth curves themselves as well as to examine the factors which affect the construction of these individual curves.

Intrinsic Validity of Growth Curve

The weight of the same fetus can not be measured sequentially in utero and, therefore, the intrauterine growth standards are constructed from birth weights of infants born at various stages of gestation. This introduces the probably erroneous assumption that the weight of a premature newborn is the same as that of a fetus in utero at the same gestational age. That assumption overlooks the fact that premature delivery itself is probably part of an

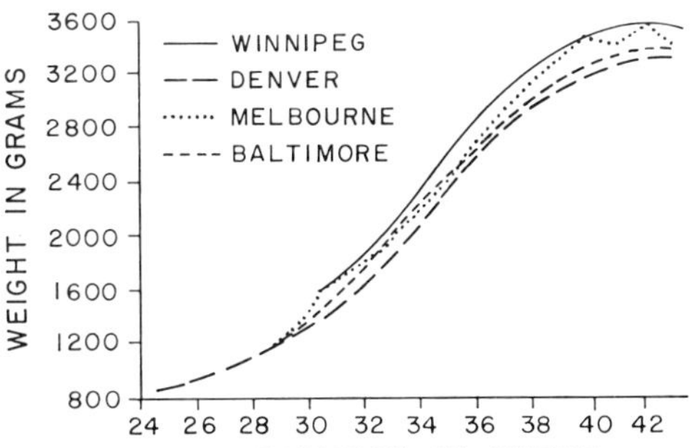

Figure 9.1. Comparison of the fiftieth percentile birth weight curves for males and females combined from Denver, Baltimore, Winnipeg and Melbourne.[48, 66, 79, 94] (Reprinted from Pusey, V. A., Haworth, J. C.: The relation between birth weight and gestational age for a Winnipeg hospital population. Can Med Assoc J 100: 842, 1969.)

"unphysiologic" state involving both the mother and/or her conceptus for variable durations.[79]

The plotting of the fetal growth data is totally dependent on the validity of the last normal menstrual period (LNMP). Unfortunately, wide individual variations in the length of the menstrual cycle, the 20% incidence of postconception bleeding, the delay in ovulation that often occurs immediately after the cessation of oral contraceptive therapy and, finally, inaccurate recollection of the LNMP, combine to make the foundation of these standard curves somewhat insecure.

Heterogeneity of Sample Populations Studied

This encompasses two major problems: the geographic location and the socioeconomic state of the population from which each curve was constructed, and the variable criteria used in the selection of data to be included in the development of a particular growth curve. Discussion of Figure 9.1 will shed some light on these potential problems. The figures of Lubchenco et al,[79] for example, are derived from a predominantly indigent population of Caucasian and Spanish-Americans living in Denver, Colorado at 5,000 feet above sea level. Indeed, 30.8% of the population studied were referred from a community living at 10,000 feet. These figures, furthermore, included neonates who were admitted to their medical center selectively because of low birth weight; and excluded those neonates whose weight was above the 90th percentile, as being "not compatible" with their gestational ages as determined by LNMP. All these factors would tend to depress the resultant fetal growth curve, especially in that portion of the curve reflecting earlier fetal growth.

Although the majority of Gruenwald's population[48] used in the construction of his intrauterine growth curves was also from a low socioeconomic group, the subjects differed from those of Lubchenco[79] in that they were born in Baltimore, at sea level, and were comprised of a higher proportion of Negroes. He also included perinatal deaths in his calculations (where theoretically the majority, if not all, fetal deaths cannot be considered as normal) and used 250-g weight increments in contrast to the 100-g increments used by Lubchenco. All of these variables contribute to the differing mean birth weight at each gestational age by the two investigators.

The subjects used by Kitchen[66] in development of the Melbourne fetal growth curve were selected from a hospital that attends to a predominantly low socioeconomic status population of Anglo-Saxon, Italian and Greek ethnic backgrounds. The housing, nutritional and medical care status of the parents of the infants were felt by the author to be of a better quality than that of those patients studied in the Denver and Baltimore reports. Kitchen, furthermore, included neonatal deaths and congenital anomalies that do not distort body proportions, as well as twins and infants delivered of certain complicated pregnancies, asserting that these factors "made no practical difference to the weight charts."

Finally, the material used in constructing the Winnipeg growth standards[94] came from a combined indigent and private population with no racial or ethnic predilection mentioned. Pregnancies prior to 30 weeks of gestation based on the LNMP were excluded because of insufficient numbers. Furthermore, an in contrast to Lubchenco[79] and Gruenwald,[48] the authors did not exclude infants who were deemed too heavy for their gestational ages, hence contributing to the higher mean birth weight obtained at each stage of gestation.

From the discrepancies in the fetal growth curves discussed above, one is therefore entitled to conclude that some newborns, considered of "normal" weight by Denver standards, may "become" growth retarded if the Vancouver or Melbourne curves are applied. It is clear that in order to obtain a meaningful understanding of the prior growth pattern of a particular fetus or newborn, great care must be taken in comparing the birth weight to a properly developed and comparable standard fetal growth curve.

Table 9.1 provides recommendations regarding the ideal criteria, as modified by Freeman et al,[42] to be used in the construction of future growth standard curves.

MAJOR PHYSIOLOGIC FACTORS INFLUENCING FETAL GROWTH

Ideally, the rate of fetal growth should be determined by its genetically established growth potential, but in fact that intrinsic potential for growth is modified by the more variable support the fetus receives via its mother and placenta. The sigmoid shape noted in standard fetal growth curves probably reflects uninhibited fetal growth at its maximum genetic potential from the 20th to 32nd week, followed by increasing impairment by limited maternal or placental resources. This is especially noticeable beyond 36 weeks of gestation.

Many factors have been known to influence intrauterine growth.[3, 63, 65] The following group may be considered "physiologic."

Fetal Sex

Influence of fetal sex on subsequent birth weight begins to become apparent after the 24th week of gestation and, by term, results in male fetuses weighing 150 to 200 g more than females. This sexual difference in growth rate is poorly understood, but may be due either to the influence of the sex hormones or the genetically determined Y-chromosome, making the male fetus more antigenically dissimilar from the mother than its female counterpart.

Table 9.1. Criteria for accurate standard fetal growth curves

The study population should be defined and should be homogeneous as to Geographic location (altitude, mean environmental temperature, etc.) Socioeconomic status Nutritional status (food habits)
All newborn infants included should be born in that particular population. Newborn transfers should be excluded.
Newborns should be included *only* if their stage of gestation is established by two or more independent criteria such as LNMP, sonogram, uterine size early in pregnancy, Dubowitz, etc.
Once stage of gestation is established, all newborns should be included regardless of birth weight at each stage of gestation. Only stillbirths should be excluded.
Each week of gestation should be analyzed separately based on established criteria, i.e., nearest week, week completed, etc.; no grouping of weeks should occur.
Individual birth weights should be analyzed separately rather than grouping the weights in increments of 100, 250 and 500 g.
Separate curves should be devised for each race, ethnic group, newborn sex and for twin gestations within the population studied.
Other natural factors that might influence birth weight in members of each defined population should be considered, i.e., parental height, maternal weight and weight gain in pregnancy, etc.
A universal agreement should prevail whether to use percentiles or standard deviations when the growth standard curves are finally constructed.

Maternal Age and Parity

Maternal age has little influence on birth weight apart from its association with parity, whereas it is generally agreed that firstborn infants are the lightest, followed by a gradual increase in birth weight until the third pregnancy, after which the effect disappears.[11, 16, 64, 114]

Race and Ethnic Background

Racial and ethnic background differences in mean term birth weight may be greater than 1000 g. For instance, the highest mean birth weight so far recorded in the literature is that of the Cheyenne American Indian tribe in the United States (3830 g) and the lowest mean birth weight occurs in mothers from the Wapi ethnic group of Lumi in the South Pacific (2400 g).[58] Although various factors, such as altitude, ambient temperature, nutritional status, etc, may play a role in these differences, real genetically based racial differences probably do occur. For example, Fujikura and Froehlich[43] observed that Negro fetuses are consistently heavier than Caucasians until the 35th week of pregnancy, after which the trend is reversed, resulting in a lower term mean birth weight among Negroes. It is impossible to be certain but the preponderance of evidence suggests that deceleration near term is predominantly environmental rather than genetic.

Parental Size

Cross-breeding and fertilized ova transplant experiments in animals document clearly that a positive correlation exists between maternal size and birth weight.[109, 118] In the human, the rate of intrauterine fetal growth is directly proportional to the weight of the mother, and her inter- and intrapregnancy weight gain.[12, 36, 114] Although a positive correlation also exists between maternal weight and birth weight, this correlation may in fact be simply the result of the greater weight of the taller mother.[73]

Finally, it is worth mentioning that there is growing evidence that paternal height may have a positive influence on fetal weight, although to a much less degree than the weight of the mother.[68]

Immunology

Although there is consistent evidence that the trophoblast, as a consequence of the unique surface properties of its cells, is an ineffective elicitor of the cellular component of transplantation immunity,[70] animal studies have shown that fetomaternal histoincompatability can influence fetal weight.[13, 52] In man, no such data are yet available. Preliminary results of our prospective study evaluating the influence of fetomaternal incompatability to the human leukocyte antigen (HLA) on fetal weight determine that only 1 out of the 39 pregnant women studied possessed antibodies against a major HLA locus of her fetus, and that infant showed no apparent birth weight difference from the mean of the total group.[10]

Intrauterine Fetal Growth Retardation

DEFINITION AND INCIDENCE

Recognizing the fact that we must base our judgments on some clinically ascertainable yardstick, we use the Standard Fetal Growth Curve of Lubchenco (Figure 9.2). An intrauterine growth-retarded fetus is, therefore, currently defined retrospectively and arbitrarily as that fetus whose newborn weight falls below the normal range of birth weight appropriate for its gestational age. Weight below the 10th percentile is considered clinically signifi-

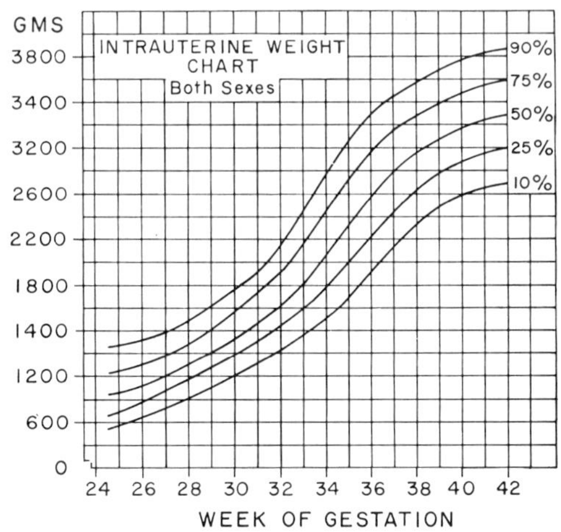

Figure 9.2. The weights of liveborn Caucasian infants at gestational ages from 24 to 42 weeks are graphed as percentiles. (Reprinted from Lubchenco, L. O., Hansman, C., Dresser, M., Boyd, E.: Intrauterine growth as estimated from liveborn birth weight data at 24–42 weeks of gestation. Pediatrics 32: 793, 1963.)

cant fetal growth retardation, weights below the 3rd percentile or more than 2 SD below the mean is considered severe fetal growth retardation. The incidence of intrauterine growth retardation, therefore, can be stated to be 8% moderate, and 2% severe.

Because of the arbitrary nature of these definitions, and since growth retardation may develop at different stages of gestation, based on the etiology and timing of the insult, a new and more specific classification of fetal growth retardation which relates to the age of onset and the possible etiology may be much more meaningful and useful.[1]

PATHOPHYSIOLOGY OF INTRAUTERINE GROWTH RETARDATION

Cellular Growth

At the outset, it is pertinent to define the different phases of cellular growth in order to have a better understanding of the nature of the effects of certain forces that can affect fetal growth. Winick[123, 124] described three phases of cellular growth in fetal organs: (*a*) the phase of hyperplasia, wherein there is a proportional increase in weight, protein and DNA content; (*b*) the phase of concomitant hyperplasia and hypertrophy, where there is an increase in DNA, but it is a slower increase than in protein and weight; (*c*) the phase of hypertrophy, wherein there is not a further increase in DNA content, but the net protein and weight continue to increase at the same rate.

It is therefore possible that factors which affect growth may result in different effects depending upon whether they exert their influence on the rate of cell division or whether they affect the subsequent increase in cell size. The embryonic and early fetal growth is predominantly hyperplasia, whereas late fetal growth includes some hypertrophy.[61] However, all fetal organs are to some extent perpetually involved with the hyperplasia phase of growth. Therefore, it is understandable that they are not only highly susceptible to the effects of certain environmental factors, but that the resultant effects will be long lasting since they will result in an absolute reduction of total cell number.

The detailed effects of certain specific stresses on fetal growth are clearly documentable in animal studies; however, in human studies this is difficult since the placenta is the only organ readily accessible for detailed study after birth. Nevertheless, observations in the placenta have shown that it has the same pattern of growth as fetal organs, so that examination of the placenta can give us inferential information as to the effects of stresses on human fetal growth. It must be recalled, however, that in the human placenta, cell division continues until the 34th or 36th week of gestation; hence, stress before the 36th week of gestation can lead to a permanent reduction in placental cell number, whereas stimuli that are active only after cell division has ceased can affect cell size but not cell number.[123]

Causes of Fetal Growth Retardation

Most fetal growth retardation occurs after the 28th week of pregnancy, with increasing frequency toward term. However, impairment of fetal growth may occur at any time in gestation. During the first half of pregnancy, growth retardation is most likely due to a genetic defect or embryonic injury, such as viral invasion of the embryo or early fetus.[5] During the second half of pregnancy, growth impairment is usually associated with a reduction in the flow of nutrients and/or oxygen to the fetus. This latter phenomenon may be brought about by factors which cause a decrease in the transport across the placenta to the fetus, by a deficiency in the ability of the mother to supply these substances to the fetus or by inadequacy of the mother's external environment. Figure 9.3 illustrates an overview of these mechanisms.

Specific stress factors that are associated with intrauterine growth impairment are detailed here.

Chromosomal Abnormalities. Some chromosomal aberrations are known to be associated with impairment of fetal growth rate. Whether this represents retardation of embryologic development has not been documented.[97] Growth failure caused by this stress factor appears to be

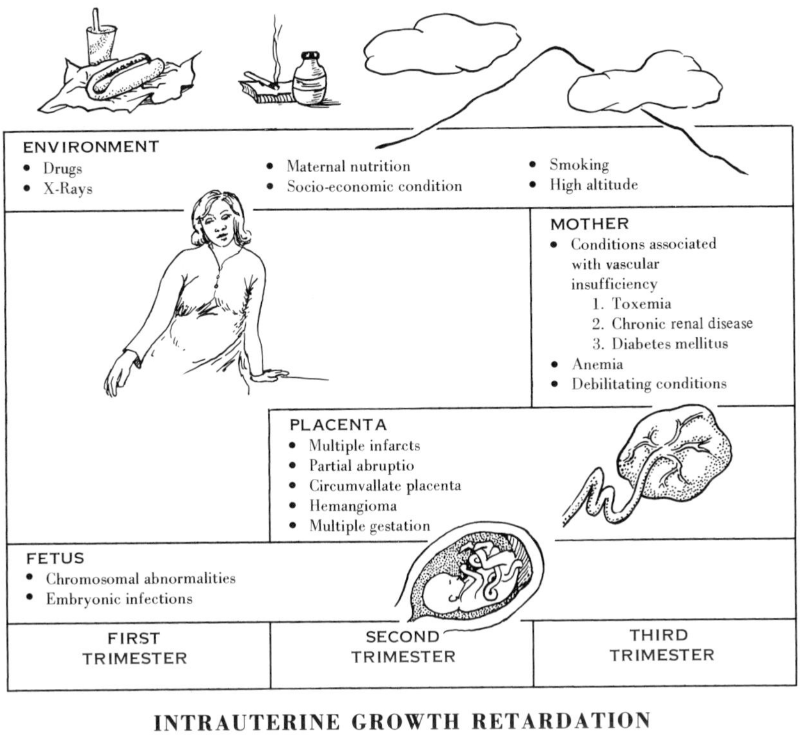

Figure 9.3. Overview of the mechanisms causing intrauterine growth retardation.

intrinsic to the fetus itself as observations of the placentas of these fetuses show them to have normal weights and morphology. It appears that the chromosomal abnormality as well as the genetic imbalance disturbs the development of the fetus by causing a generalized embryologic chaos. Examples include the following.

Down's syndrome. Most studies have indicated that the birth weights of children with Down's syndrome show a 10 to 15% decrease from the normal average weight. Birth weight of these infants is about 400 g lower than the normal average weight.

Trisomy 18. The relationship of infants with trisomy 18 and low birth weight has been documented. Average birth weights of 2100 to 2300 g have been found despite an average gestational age of 40 weeks.

Trisomy 13, Chromosomal Deletion Syndromes and Sex Chromosomal Aberrations. Seventy percent of infants with *cri de chat* syndrome show deletion of part of the short arms of chromosome 5 and have a birth weight below the 10th percentile. Infant's with Turner's (45,XO) are small for gestational age and one-third of these infants are under 2500 g at birth.

Embryonic Infections.[56] Low birth weights have been associated with several infections acquired in utero by the fetus including rubella, CMV, herpes simplex, toxoplasma, malaria and congenital syphilis as well as rare bacterial infections.

During the rubella epidemic of 1964, 60% of affected newborns had a birth weight less than the 10th percentile. Despite attaining a full 40 weeks of gestation, the birth weight averaged 2100 to 2200 g.

The mechanism by which rubella, as well as other viral agents, cause IUGR is complex. It appears, however, that during the phase of maternal viremia, the virus reaches the placenta, causing a villous placentitis and subsequent damage to the vascular endothelium. This leads to obliterative angiopathy of small placental blood vessels, resulting in subsequent poor placental function. Fetal viremia also occurs and has direct effect on fetal cells. It has been shown in cultures of human embryonic tissue that rubella virus will arrest mitotic activity, so that fetal growth retardation and specific anomalies may result from direct inhibition of cell division by the virus. An arrest in cellular proliferation occurs, such that certain organs may remain at the embryonic stage of development. Generally, it appears that the earlier in gestation a viral infection occurs, the greater the risk of damage to the fetus. With earlier infections, the types of defects are numerous; and with later infections, the variety and seriousness of fetal abnormalities are more limited.

Placental Pathology. This may include multiple infarcts, chronic partial separation of the placenta, circumvallate placenta, hemangiomas and multiple gestation. All of these conditions involve reduction in the surface area necessary for placental transport of nutrients and oxygen.

Maternal Pathology. Vascular insufficiency, maternal conditions associated with toxemia, chronic renal disease, and diabetes mellitus with vascular involvement may result in fetal growth retardation. Serious maternal heart disease, especially the cyanotic variety, is often associated with growth retardation. Maternal anemia, especially that due to folate deficiency or hemoglobinopathy, may interfere with oxygen supply to the conceptus.[50] Growth retardation due to other types of anemia is harder to document. Nutritional anemias are frequently associated with chronic debilitating conditions or chronic infection in the mother. Whether the effect on fetal growth is due to the anemia or to conditions associated with chronic maternal infection or debilitation remains to be resolved.

Faulty Maternal Environment. *Maternal Nutrition*. Perhaps this is the most common cause of mild to moderate intrauterine growth retardation and this factor can exert its influence on the fetus at any stage in pregnancy. It has been shown both in animal and human studies that fetal malnutrition, particularly protein deficiency, leads to retardation of fetal growth and brain development. The role of nutrition in the pathogenesis of intrauterine growth retardation has been studied by several investigators, but the exact mechanism by which it works is still poorly understood.

It has been shown in recent studies in Guatamala that adequate caloric and/or protein supplementation to mothers with subclinical protein/calorie malnutrition causes an increase in the birth weight of their babies amounting to 400 g.[103] Likewise, other studies in developing countries wherein malnutrition is a prevalent problem have shown the same association between intrauterine growth retardation and malnutrition.

A striking correlation has been noted between maternal plasma amino acid concentration, birth weight, length and cranial volume.[1] These studies suggested that fetal growth and development in stunted when insufficient amino acids are available to the fetus.

Smoking. Growth retardation has been directly related to the number of cigarettes smoked and is generally observed when 10 or more cigarettes are consumed per day. The effect of smoking on fetal growth may be due to excessive carbon monoxide in the blood, which decreases the ability of the blood to transport oxygen since it competes with oxygen for available hemoglobin.[4] It is likewise postulated that this high carbon monoxide concentration may interfere with normal placental enzyme activity. Excessive smoking also causes a reduction in maternal food intake and the effect of malnutrition on fetal growth has been previously discussed. In addition, nicotine is observed to affect uteroplacental circulation, leading to a decrease in placental blood flow.

High Altitude. As already discussed, several studies have shown that birth weight is inversely proportional to the degree of elevation. The relationship of ischemia or chronic hypoxia to progressive fetal stunting has been demonstrated experimentally in rats by compromising the uteroplacental circulation.[4] Usually, this causes an asymmetric growth retardation which may be due to preferential distribution of the better oxygenated blood to the fetal brain, leading to the brain-sparing effect of this growth failure.

Poor Socioeconomic Conditions. Innumerable studies show that poverty predisposes to a higher rate of mild to moderate fetal growth retardation. The precise mechanisms remain obscure, but seem to be wrapped in the Gordian knot of repeated pregnancies, disadvantageous age, nutrition, general poor health and recurrent infection.

PRENATAL DIAGNOSIS AND CLINICAL MANAGEMENT OF FETAL GROWTH RETARDATION

Diagnosis

High Index of Suspicion. The diagnosis of fetal growth retardation must begin with the clinician's having a high index of suspicion. The high perinatal mortality and morbidity associated with this disorder and the potential benefits of judicious intervention warrant diligent surveillance of the total obstetric population. Specifically, the discovery of certain factors known to be associated with a higher rate of growth retardation—poor obstetric history, especially a history of prior fetal growth retardation, multiple gestation, toxemia, malnutrition and other factors reviewed earlier—should be followed by an especially careful search for the disorder. A number of prenatal risk assessment systems are widely utilized which successfully identify the high risk obstetric population which will contribute the majority of perinatal mortality and morbidity.[45, 55, 86, 96] These same scoring systems also identify the patients who have a high risk for fetal growth retardation. Approximately 50 to 60% of patients with a growth-retarded fetus demonstrate one or more factors, diagnosable prenatally, which are known to be associated with a greater risk of growth retardation.[8, 75, 82]

Estimated Date of Confinement (EDC). The proper care of all obstetric patients requires the careful documentation of the correct EDC. This is especially important in those at risk for growth retardation. The subsequent interpretation of clinical and laboratory findings is greatly affected by accurately established dates. Many practical steps can be taken.

LNMP: Fully 15 to 20% of pregnancies are associated with bleeding or spotting at the time of the first missed period. Therefore, careful history of the nature of the LNMP is important. Patients who conceive in the first cycle off of birth control pills frequently are incorrectly suspected of having a poorly growing fetus when in reality the ovulation and conception occurred 2 to 3 weeks later than in a normal spontaneous cycle.[98] Documentation of the date of the first positive pregnancy test or review of the BBT chart among infertility patients will sometimes help.

Early Uterine Size. A careful assessment of uterine size (with an empty bladder) between 6 and 12 weeks, perhaps on two occasions, will often refine the gestational age assessment to ±2 weeks without difficulty.

Fetal Heartbeat (FH), Quickening and Uterine Size. It is helpful to remember that the appearance of the FH (by using a standard clinical fetoscope), quickening and the arrival of the uterine fundus at the umbilicus occurs at 20 weeks ± 2 weeks. Of course, FH by ultrasound is present much earlier and quickening occurs earlier in multipara than in primigravida, but when these features of a 20-week gestation coincide with the LNMP and early uterine size, a great deal of security regarding the EDC is established.

Sonography. In the first 2 to 4 months, sonographic measurement of the size of the gestational sac[31, 100] or, even more accurately, the fetal crown rump diameter[34, 99] is quite reliable in establishing the correct EDC. However, determination of the biparietal diameter (BPD) at 20 to 28 weeks is probably the best prediction of the correct EDC because of the relatively small range of BPD at each week of gestation at this point in pregnancy.[19, 104] The BPD is considerably less valuable in this respect after 32 weeks because of the increasingly wide range of BPD as term approaches. Our policy is to do a sonogram at 20 to 24 weeks in all of our high risk cases. If the sonogram result fits with the LNMP, early uterine size, FH and quickening, we consider the EDC confirmed. If it does not fit, we repeat the sonogram at 24 to 28 weeks and use the two sonogram results exclusively to establish the EDC.

Clinical Signs

Once the risk group is identified, careful and frequent observations will help to identify the poorly growing fetus.[67, 72] Poor maternal weight gain is a common correlate of fetal growth retardation. This is especially true after 32 weeks. A persistent gain of less than one-half pound per week is reason for concern. Poor fundal growth is probably the most frequent clinical finding in fetal growth retardation. Serial and frequent measurements from 20 weeks and using the same measuring techniques is important. We use the centimeter tape measure which has the advantage that generally the number of centimeters equals the gestational weeks, especially between 24 and 36 weeks. Unfortunately, severe obesity introduces a serious interpretive problem.[9] The use of "fingers above the umbilicus" is to be condemned. The suspicion of oligohydramnios in the last 4 to 6 weeks of pregnancy is an ominous sign and is a frequent concomitant of fetal growth retardation.

It is known that good placentation and optimal placental function are critically important for proper fetal growth. These same processes also result in many of the alterations of maternal physiology which occur in normal pregnancy: the fall in blood pressure, hematocrit, blood urea-nitrogen, and the rise in glomerular filtration rate, insulin resistance, etc. There is often a *lack* of these changes in the face of poor placentation, therefore, the absence can be a subtle indication of faulty fetal growth. One example of this is Page's observation[91] that the higher the diastolic blood pressure is at midpregnancy, the greater the incidence of fetal growth retardation.

Laboratory Signs

Many laboratory signs of fetal growth retardation have been reported. None of them alone are highly reliable in every instance; however, when used in combination, they may be very reliable.

Ultrasound. The serial measurement of BPD is probably the most often used and reported.[17, 18, 101, 121, 127] Indeed, values plotted on standard graphs of BPD growth[20, 40, 44] are very useful and can pick out perhaps 40 to 70% of growth-retarded fetuses.[17, 95, 121] Unfortunately, a sizable proportion of growth retardation is late in onset (>34 weeks) and/or vascular in origin. These types of growth retardation tend to be associated with relative sparing of the fetal head such that the body suffers earlier and to a greater degree than is reflected in even serial BPD's. Increasingly better techniques are being reported for quantitation of body growth as reflected in thoracic or abdominal measurements.[21, 44, 53] These measurements, especially when compared to head size, can give more precise estimations of fetal weight or growth.[69, 80] Fetal urine production rates can be determined by ultrasound and significant decreases have been found in the presence of fetal growth retardation.[125] Even further uses of ultrasound in the detection and quantitation of fetal growth retardation are being explored.[54] Hopefully, the costs of ultranic procedures will decrease so as to make their utilization a practical clinical approach.

Estrogens. Estrogen measurements are frequently followed in high risk obstetric populations and many studies have found low urinary estrogen excretion in 50 to 70% of the cases of fetal growth retardation.[84, 93, 101, 126] Edwards[37] has found decreased plasma estrogens in 58% of such cases. One would suppose that since estrogen levels are a function of combined fetal-placental endocrine activity, such levels would be quite reliable and be universally low in the face of growth retardation. Unfortunately, errors in both directions are not uncommon. Many other factors (drugs, wrong dates, posture, maternal-renal impairment, improper urine collections, etc.) can produce low estrogen excretion in the face of normal fetal growth. In addition, about one-third of the cases of intrauterine growth retardation are found to have normal estrogen excretion. Clearly, the reflection of fetal growth in urinary estrogens must be highly affected by the etiology, timing and severity of growth retardation. Nevertheless, with these observations in mind, it is worthwhile to measure urinary estrogens in patients at risk for fetal growth retardation. Such tests should be done at least weekly from the 25th week on. Quite aside from their utility in the diagnosis of intrauterine growth retardation, Wallace and Michie[117] as well as Yogman et al[129] found a high incidence of neurologic impairment in infants born to mothers who exhibited low estrogen excretions. Greene[46] did not find such a relationship, but had few babies of less than 2500 g in his study.

Human Placental Lactogen. Since HPL is a function of placental integrity, it would not be expected to correlate closely with fetal growth retardation. However, since many of the etiologies also affect placental growth, it does indirectly relate to fetal growth. Studies have shown that one-third to one-half of cases of fetal growth retardation have low levels of plasma HPL.[37, 60, 71] Our experience indicates that HPL is even more commonly decreased if the growth retardation is due to a chronic vascular etiology such as toxemia. Therefore, the presence of low HPL levels in a chronic hypertensive is highly associated with fetal growth retardation.

Oxytocinase (CAP). This enzyme is also a function of placental integrity and yields information similar to HPL. Except for Curzen and Varma[29] investigators have found that CAP has been particularly useful in identifying fetal growth retardation occurring in relation to placental insufficiency.[22, 23, 29, 51, 57, 89, 101] More studies are needed to clarify its true value in clinical practice.

Radiology. Delayed appearance of ossification centers or hyperflexion of the fetal spine have been reported in the fetus with growth retardation.[26, 27] These are probably late findings and are not helpful in our experience.

Progesterone. Studies on urinary pregnanediol and serum progesterone in patients with fetal growth retardation indicate that these tests are of little value diagnostically.[30, 126]

Management

Using various combinations of the above tests and procedures, it is possible to detect one-half to two-thirds of all fetal growth retardation in the prenatal period.[14, 18, 37, 82, 93, 101, 126, 127] It is well established that perinatal mortality and morbidity are increased 2- to 6-fold in the face of fetal growth retardation.[49, 57, 75, 87, 92, 128] Mann et al[82] have shown that the perinatal mortality and morbidity can be reduced drastically in diagnosed and treated patients. This opens the opportunity for intervention. Since this diagnosis has been possible only recently, the specific interventions and their impact have not been studied sufficiently to warrant strong recommendations. However, the following appear to be indicated based on current knowledge.

Detailed Evaluation. Once fetal growth retardation has been identified, a great effort at dissection of the clinical problem is justified. Hospitalization is often necessary. A search for each of the known etiologies requires a repeat and detailed history and physical, careful cardiovascular renal evaluation, dietary assessment and many laboratory studies. Not only must the etiology be clarified, but also the extent of the problem and a careful subsequent pregnancy management plan must be established.

Bed Rest. Probably the most dramatic help is bed rest, although only a few studies have documented its value.[59, 62] This does not have to be in the hospital or necessarily even in bed. Lying on the side much of the day, and the avoidance of work, trips or quiet standing is strongly recommended.

Nutrition. Not only dietary evaluation but also dietary therapy often is helpful. Nutritional supplementation, especially high protein, high carbohydrate diets are useful. Some have claimed to show increasing fetal growth and a rise in urinary estrogens as a result of bed rest and an improved diet.[59] Introduction of nutrients directly into the amniotic sac has been suggested but the techniques are not sufficiently practical at the present time.

Antihypertensive Medication. If toxemia is the problem, careful administration of antihypertensives appears to be helpful. Aldomet is especially to be recommended and is most valuable if begun early in pregnancy. Care must be taken not to produce too marked a lowering of mean arterial blood pressure.

Constant Surveillance of Fetal Growth Oxygenation and Welfare. Since fetal growth retardation is associated with such a risk of fetal death or perinatal asphyxia, the fetus must be observed carefully for signs of hypoxia and acidosis. The use of serial sonography, urinary estrogens, oxytocin challenge tests and periodic amniocentesis or amnioscopy for meconium detection is essential. With abnormality in two of these measurements, at any time after 32 weeks the fetus is better delivered regardless of the lecithen to sphingomyelin (L/S) ratio.

Periodic Assessment of Fetal Maturity. Fortunately, many of the causes of fetal growth retardation are associated with acceleration of fetal maturity (lungs, kidneys, etc.). Since infants with IUGR are at such high and unpredictable risk in late fetal life, we choose to deliver our patients with this problem as soon as pulmonary maturation is assured by an L/S ratio >2.

Delivery. Often the uterus is hyperirritable in the face of fetal growth retardation and therefore, induction of labor is relatively easy. Careful monitoring in labor is mandatory.[74] Any sign of fetal distress such as repeated type II dips or loss of baseline variability, especially if either is combined with the appearance of stained amniotic fluid, is reason to go to cesarian section. We think prophylactic high flow maternal oxygen is helpful but have no hard evidence to support this. The patient should labor on her side and have a relatively high intravenous fluid intake throughout her labor. Naturally, all drugs are to be avoided, anesthesia should be local, the episiotomy wide and the neonatal team available and ready to care for the newborn.

NEONATAL ASPECTS OF FETAL GROWTH RETARDATION

Postnatal Assessment of Fetal Growth

The infant who is inappropriately small for gestational age (SGA) may be either symmetrically undergrown or disproportionately so, and thus there is no one typical appearance. The former group whose inadequate growth dates from early in pregnancy shows decreased weight, length and head circumference which leads to approximately normal body proportions. The second or disproportionate group of infants has grown normally during the early months of intrauterine life but suffers acute malnutrition or other insults in the last few weeks before delivery. The head circumferences generally correlate well with gestational age, but length is somewhat reduced and the weight is markedly reduced. There is actual wasting of subcutaneous tissue; the face appears "pinched"; the skin fits loosely; the color is a muddy gray; and the infants often appear hypertonic. A third group of infants who do not fit either of the above categories is comprised of those whose head size is relatively smaller than would be expected for length or weight as a result of intrauterine infection.

Examination of organ weights in infants who have suffered fetal malnutrition shows the brain weight to be closer to appropriate value for gestational age than weight of other organs. Heart, lung and kidney are also heavier in SGA infants than in prematures of similar birth weight, whereas the liver, spleen, adrenals and thyroids of the SGA fetus are smaller than those of the appropriate for gestational age (AGA) counterpart.[47, 77, 85]

Assessment of degree of abnormality is made by comparison of weight, length and head circumference to statistical tables for normal growth. The best known of these is the Denver Intrauterine Growth Chart with the original definition of the SGA infant being one with weight below the 10th percentile for gestational age.[78] The accuracy of estimated gestational age is of course critical in the assessment and this has led to the development of clinical criteria of maturity, e.g., the Dubowitz scale.[35] to be used in conjunction with the EDC.

After identification of a newborn as SGA, an intensive effort should be made to discover the etiology by review of maternal data and complete screening tests of the newborn. This is critical since not only will knowledge of the etiology affect the prognosis, but, more importantly, also will greatly help the neonatal management.

Clinical Course

The infant who has suffered intrauterine deprivation is deserving of most careful observation during the birth process and for several hours thereafter. At any gestation, the risk of death in the newborn period is 5 to 10 times higher than that of the appropriately grown newborn. The maternal placental or fetal pathology originally responsible for the growth retardation may compromise oxygenation at the time of delivery and severe metabolic acidosis is common. The malnourished infant with poor cardiac glycogen reserves is in a particularly poor position to withstand this insult.[107] The incidence of severe hypoxic damage is high in this group of children with manifestations in the kidney, heart and brain.[102, 115] Renal shutdown may occur, as may cerebral edema. The most severely asphyxiated infants may show marked generalized edema related to a failing heart. Others may have pulmonary or cerebral hemorrhage occurring in conjunction with coagulation abnormality and thrombocytopenia.

Even those infants who escape intrapartum asphyxia may present other problems in the newborn period. Hypoglycemia is one of the most common and may be present as early as 2 hr of life. This has been attributed to deficiency of stored glycogen in the liver[108] but reduced gluconeogenesis in these infants, as demonstrated by Mestyan[83] and others,[122] may play a role of equal importance. The relatively large size of the brain and possible hyperinsulism may also be factors. Blood glucose should be examined by Dextrostix routinely at 4-hr intervals or more frequently if symptoms of hypoglycemia occur. Low values should be checked by laboratory determination. Asymptomatic infants with blood sugar levels less than 30 mg per dl should receive an intravenous infusion of 10% dextrose. Symptomatic infants can be given 4 ml per kg of 25% dextrose by direct intravenous injection, followed by a 10% glucose infusion. All SGA infants should receive early feedings if their condition allows.

Other problems encountered in these newborns include frequent congenital anomalies, poor temperature control related to the paucity of subcutaneous tissue and polycythemia, possibly attributable to intrauterine hypoxia.[106, 110] The latter situation, if exaggerated, may lead to cerebral or other organ damage and the reduction of circulating red cell concentration by partial plasma exchange transfusion is to be recommended in infants with hematocrit levels greater than 70%.[88]

Investigation of the cause of intrauterine growth retardation entails a careful search for evidence of genetic abnormality, intrauterine infection, maternal illness or external environmental problems. Management of the infant's course should include strict attention to the provision of adequate calories, optimally at intakes providing calories in the range of 150 cal per kg per day or greater in order to facilitate any possible catch-up growth.

Long Term Prognosis

The infant who has grown poorly in utero needs careful long term scrutiny and plans for careful follow-up that should be formulated in the newborn period.

With the recognition that a significant percentage of low birth weight infants, either born at term or premature, are small for gestational age, clearer view of postnatal growth patterns has evolved.

A number of studies support the fact that the SGA infant has a reduced potential for long term postnatal somatic growth.[28, 39, 90] However, immediate postnatal growth in these infants may be rapid, generally exceeding the preceding intrauterine rate which has been restricted by physical environment. The postnatal spurt is not maintained and the weight of SGA infants slips behind that of their AGA counterparts by the second month and length by the second half of the first year.[116] Head circumference of SGA infants at 1 year of age is also significantly smaller than that of full term, normally grown infants in contrast to the catch-up head growth which is seen in prematures when size is plotted as a function of postconceptional age.[6]

The overall pattern of first year growth of the SGA infant is similar to that of the premature and normally grown term infant in that all groups show the most rapid growth in the first 13 weeks.[28] However, velocity growth for the full first year is less in SGA infants than that of AGA premature infants of 28 weeks to 36 weeks of gestation and, therefore, distance (total) growth is less ($P < 0.01$). In the second and third years the SGA infants continue to grow at a slower rate than the prematures, but this difference is not significant.

A survey Fitzhardinge and Taylor[39] of 96 infants followed for 4 years showed mean height and weight between the 10th and 25th percentile with 35% of the children below the 3rd percentile and only 8% above the 50th. The short stature in these individuals is associated with a persistent retardation of bone age as compared with height, age and retarded physical development, indicating a defect in skeletal maturation.

As with the study of growth, early reports on developmental outcome of low birth weight infants are handicapped by failure to separate AGA and SGA infants. Even follow-up studies of better defined populations are limited by the fact that they may be viewed only in relation to the time period in which the individuals were born. The radical changes in neonatal care practices over the past 5 to 10 years limit applicability of earlier data.

A further confounding factor was pointed out by Drillien[32] in the lumping of SGA babies with severe organic disease (infections, anomalies, etc.) with those who are merely undergrown. In her study of infants of birth weight less than 2000 g, mental and neurologic defects were found in much higher incidence in those children who had anomalies than those without. Drillien also described an important role for environment in the potential development of the SGA infant whereby the SGA infant showed slower development than his AGA counterpart in similarly "poor" homes, but not in "superior" homes.

A few studies[15, 25, 41, 105, 119] have reported an increased risk of handicap in SGA infants. However, the detailed prospective study by Fitzhardinge[38] of 96 full term SGA infants showed a low incidence of major deficits, including only 1 child with cerebral palsy and 6 with convulsions, all of which had a history of severe neonatal asphyxia. In addition, they reported a 25% incidence of minimal cerebral dysfunction, irritability and poor coordination in these infants, with 50% of boys and 36% of girls showing poor school performance. EEG abnormalities were also seen in a higher percentage of the SGA children than in the general population.

Thus, there appears to be a residual of intrauterine deprivation which affects a significant number of individuals. Although early recognition may minimize handicap, possible intervention at the fetal level offers the most effective help.

Conclusion

Fetal growth, both normal and retarded, is just beginning to be understood. More attention must be paid to developing more appropriate normal fetal growth curves against which retarded fetal growth may be judged and thereby, defined. Nevertheless, it is possible to identify 10% of newborns as having experienced some degree of fetal growth retardation. Careful studies in this group have indicated a wide range of possible etiologic factors residing in the fetus, placenta, mother or her environment. Prevention is the obvious ideal. Failing that, early detection and treatment in utero are possible and should result in improved survival and quality of the fetus and newborn. Early identification in the newborn period and aggressive neonatal intensive care are needed for the complex needs of these fragile neonates. Long term studies indicate that significant sequelae of fetal growth retardation do occur but not so often as to dampen an aggressive approach to care at any point the problem is identified.

Indeed, it is only by meticulous attention to detail that the diagnosis can be made. Once diagnosed, the full implementation of the perinatal team approach should reduce the toll of perinatal mortality. morbidity and long term effects of perinatal injury among this high risk group of patients.

REFERENCES

1. Abdul-Karim, R. W.: The clinical significance of deviations in fetal growth. Int J Gynecol Obstet 1976 (In press.)
2. Abdul-Karim, R. W., Beydoun, S. N.: Amniotic fluid: The value of prenatal analysis. Part I. Postgr Med, 52: 147 1972.
3. Abdul-Karim, R. W., Beydoun, S. N.: Growth of the Human Fetus. Clin Obstet Cynecol 17: 37, 1974.
4. Assali, N., Editor, *Pathophysiology of Gestation Fetal Placental Disorders,* Vol. II. New York, Academic Press, 1972.
5. Babson, G., et al: Management of High Risk Pregnancy Intensive Care of the Neonate. Sec-

ond edition, St. Louis, C. V. Mosby Co., 1971.
6. Babson, S. G.: Growth of Low birth weight infants. J Pediatr 77: 11, 1970.
7. Babson, S. G., Behrman, R. E., Lessel, R.: Fetal growth liveborn birth weights for gestational age of white middle class infants. Pediatrics 45: 937, 1970.
8. Bard, H.: Intrauterine growth retardation. Clin Obstet Gynecol 13: 511, 1970.
9. Beazley, J. M., Underhill, R. A.: Fallacy of the fundal height. Br Med J IV: 404, 1970.
10. Beydoun, S. N.: Unpublished data.
11. Biggs, J. S. G.: Pregnancy at 40 years and over. Med J Austr 1: 542, 1973.
12. Billewicz, W. Z., Thomson, A. M.: Birthweight in consecutive pregnancies. J Obstet Gynaecol Br Commonw 80: 491, 1973.
13. Billington, W. D.: Influence of immunological dissimilarity of mother and fetus size of placenta in mice. Nature (London) 202: 317, 1964.
14. Bowes, W. A., Draegemueller, W.: Identification and management of intrauterine growth retardation, *Controversy in Obstetrics and Gynecology* Vol. II. Edited by D. E. Reed, C. D. Christian, Philadelphia, W. B. Saunders Co., 1974, p 10.
15. Butler, N. R., Bonham, D. G.: *Perinatal Mortality*, Edinburgh, E. and S. Livingston, 1963.
16. Camilleri, A. P., Cremona, V.: The effect of parity on birth weight. J Obstet Gynaecol Br Commonw 77: 145, 1970.
17. Campbell, S., Dewhurst, C. J.: Diagnosis of the small-for-dates fetus by serial ultrasonic cephalometry. Lancet 2: 1002, 1971.
18. Campbell, S., Kurjak, A.: Comparison between urinary oestrogen asseys and serial ultrasonic cephalometry in assessment of fetal growth retardation. Br Med J 4: 337, 1972.
19. Campbell S., Newman, G. B.: Growth of the fetal biparietal diameter during normal pregnancy. J Obstet Gynaecol Br Commonw 78: 513, 1971.
20. Campbell, S., Newman, G.: Growth of the fetal biparietal diameter during normal pregnancy. J Obstet Gynaecol Br Commonw, 79: 304, 1972.
21. Campbell, S., Wilkin, D.: Ultrasonic measurement of fetal abdomen circumference in the estimation of fetal weight. Br J Obstet Gynaecol 82: 689, 1975.
22. Carter, E. R., Goodman, L. V., DeHaan, R., et al: Serum oxytocinase: A laboratory and clinical appraisal. Am J Obstet Gynecol 119: 76, 1974.
23. Chapman, L., Burrows-Peakin, R., Silk, E.: Serum cystine aminopeptidase and the small-for-dates baby in hypertensive pregnancy. Br J Obstet Gynaecol 83: 238, 1976.
24. Cheng, M. C. E., Chew, P. C. T., Ratnam, S. S.: Birth weight distribution of singapore, Chinese, Malay, and Indian infants from 34 weeks to 42 weeks gestation. J Obstet Gynaecol Br Commonw 79: 149, 1972.
25. Churchill, J. A.: The relationship between intelligence and birth weight in twins. Neurology 15: 341, 1965.
26. Croall, J., Grech, P.: Radiological maturity of the small-for-dates fetus. J Obstet Gynaecol Br Commonw 77: 802, 1970.
27. Croall, J., Grech, P.: Hyperflexion of the small-for-dates fetus. J Obstet Gynaecol Br Commonw 77: 808, 1970.
28. Cruise, M. O.: A longitudinal study of the growth of low-birth weight infants. I. Velocity and distance growth, birth to three years. Pediatrics 51: 620, 1973.
29. Curzen, P., Varma, R.: A comparison of serum cystine aminopeptidase and urinary estrogen as placental function tests. Am J Obstet Gynecol 115: 929, 1973.
30. Dawood, M. Y.: Circulating maternal serum progesterone in high risk pregnancies. Am J Obstet Gynecol 125: 832, 1976.
31. Donald, I.: Sonar as a method of studying prenatal development. J Pediatr 75: 326, 1969.
32. Drillien, C. M.: The small-for-dates infant: Etiology and prognosis. Pediatr Clin North Am 17: 9. 1970.
33. Drillien, C. M.: Abnormal neurologic signs in the first year of life in low brith weight infants; possible prognostic significance. Dev Med Child Neurol 14: 575, 1972.
34. Drumm, J. E., Clinch, J., Mackenzie, G.: The ultrasonic measurement of fetal crown-rump length as a method of assessing gestational age. Br J Obstet Bynaecol 83: 417, 1976.
35. Dubowicz. L Dubowicz, V., Goldberg. C.: Clinical assessment of gestational age in the newborn infant. J Pediatr 77: 1, 1970.
36. Eastman, N. J., Jackson, E.: Weight relationships in pregnancy; the hearing of maternal weight gain and pre-pregnancy weight on birth weight in full term pregnancies. Obstet Gynecol Surv 23: 1003, 1968.
37. Edwards, R. P., Diver, M. J., Davis, J. C., Hipkin, L. J.: Plasma oestriol and human placental lactogen measurements in patients with high risk pregnancies. Br J Obstet Gynaecol 83: 229, 1976.
38. Fitzhardinge, P. M., Steven, E. M.: The small-for-dates infant. II. Neurological and intellectual sequelae. Pediatrics 50: 50, 1972.
39. Fitzhardinge, P. M., Taylor, E. M.: The small-for-dates infant. I. Later growth patterns. Pediatrics 49: 671, 1972.
40. Flamme, P.: Ultrasonic fetal cephalometry: Percentiles curve. Br Med J 3: 384, 1972.
41. Francis-Williams, J., Davies, P. A.: Very low birth weight and later intelligence. Dev Med Child Neurol 16: 709, 1974.
42. Freeman, M. G., Graves, W. L., Thompson, R.: Indigent Negro and Caucasian birth weight gestation tables. Pediatrics 46: 9, 1970.
43. Fujikura, T., Froehlich, L. A.: Birth weight: Gestational age and renal glomerular development as indices of fetal maturity. Am J Obstet Gynecol 113: 627, 1972.
44. Garrett, W., Robinson, D.: Assessment of fetal size and growth rate by ultrasonic echoscopy. Obstet Gynecol 38: 525, 1971.
45. Goodwin, J. W., Dunne, J. T., Thomas, B. W.: Antepartum identification of the fetus at risk. Can Med Assoc J 101: 458, 1969.
46. Greene, J. W., Jr., Beargie, R. A., Clark. B. K Smith, K.: Correlation of estriol excretion pat-

terns of pregnant women with subsequent development of their children. Am J Obstet Gynecol 105: 730, 1969.
47. Gruenwald, P.: Chronic fetal distress and placental insufficiency. Biol Neonat 5: 215, 1963.
48. Gruenwald, P.: Growth of the human fetus. I. Normal growth and its variation. Am J Obstet Gynecol 94: 1112, 1966.
49. Gruenwald, P.: The second report of the 1958 British Perinatal Mortality Survey. *Perinatal Problems*. Edinburgh, E. and S. Livingston, 1969.
50. Harrison, K. A.: Ibeziako "Maternal anemia and fetal birth weight." J Obstet Gynaecol Br Commonw 80: 798, 1973.
51. Hensleigh, P. A., Krantz, K. E.: Oxytocinase and placental function. Am J Obstet Gynecol 107: 1233, 1970.
52. Hetherington, C. M.: The decidual cell reaction, placental weight, fetal weight and placental morphology in the mouse. J Repr Fertil 25: 417, 1971.
53. Higginbottom, J., Slatter, J., Porter, G., Whitefield, C. R.: Estimation of fetal weight from ultrasonic measurement of trunk circumference. Br J Obstet Gynaecol 82: 698, 1975.
54. Hobbins, J. C., Gohan, P.: In utero prediction of intrauterine growth retardation by determination of total intrauterine volume. Gynecol Invest (Sci Abstr) 7: 22, 1976.
55. Hobel, C. J., Hyrarinen, M. A., Okada, D. M., et al: Prenatal and intrapartal high-risk screening. I. Prediction of the high-risk neonate. Am J Obstet Gynecol 117: 1, 1973.
56. Hughes, W.: Infections and IUGR. Pediatr Clin North Am 17 (1): 119, 1970.
57. Hurry, D. J., Tovey, J. E., Robinson, D. A., et al: Cystine aminopeptidase in normal and complicated pregnancies. J Obstet Gynaecol Br Commonw 79: 788, 1972.
58. Hytten, F. E., and Leitch, I.: Mean birth weight by geographic area (Appendix D) *The Physiology of Human Pregnancy,* Second edition. Edited by F. H. Hytten, I. Leitch, Oxford, Blackwell, 1971, pp 481–513.
59. Iyenser, L.: Effects of dietary supplements late in pregnancy on the expectant mother and her newborn. Ind J Med Res 55: 85, 1967.
60. Jasimovich, J. B., Kosor, B., Bocella, L., et al: Placental lactogen in maternal serum as an index of fetal health. Obstet Gynecol 36: 244, 1970.
61. Jasper, H.: Cellular changes during fetal growth. Contemp Ob/Gyn 2 (6): 60.
62. Jeffery, R. L., Bowes, W. A., Delaney, J. J.: Role of bed rest in twin gestation. Obstet Gynecol 43: 822, 1974.
63. Karim, R. A., Beydoun, S.: Growth of human fetus. Clin Obstet Gynecol 17 (3): 1974.
64. Karn, M. N., Penrose, L. S.: Birth weight and gestation time in relation to maternal age, parity, and infant survival. Ann Eugen 16: 147, 1951–1952.
65. Kelly, J. A.: Diagnostic techniques in prepartal fetal evaluation. Clin Obstet Gynecol 17: 53, 1974.
66. Kitchen, W. H.: Austr Pediat J 4: 29, 1968.
67. Kloosterman, G. J.: On intrauterine growth: The significance of prenatal care. Int J Gynecol Obstet 8: 895, 1970.
68. Kloosterman, G. J.: As quoted by Abdul-Karim, R. W., Beydoun, S. N.
69. Kurjak, A., Breyer, B.: Estimation of fetal weight by ultrasonic abdominometry. Am J Obstet Gynecol 125: 962, 1976.
70. Lanman, J. T.: Immunological functions of the placenta and its maternal supply line. *Effect of Insufficiency on the Fetus*. Edited by P. Gruenwald, Baltimore, University Park Press, 1975.
71. Lindberg, B. S., Nilsson, B. A.: Human placental lactogen (HPL) levels in abnormal pregnancies. J Obstet Gynaecol Br Commonw 80: 1046, 1973.
72. Loeffler, F. E.: Clinical foetal weight prediction. J Obstet Gynaecol Br Commonw 74: 675, 1967.
73. Love, E. J., Kinch, R. A. H.: Factors influencing the birth weight in normal pregnancy. Am J Obstet Gynecol 91: 342, 1965.
74. Low, J. A., Boston, R. W., Pancham, S. R.: Fetal asphyxia during the intrapartum period in intrauterine growth retarded infants. Am J Obstet Gynecol 113: 351, 1972.
75. Low, J. A., Galbraith, R. S.: Pregnancy characteristics of intrauterine growth retardation. Obstet Gynecol 44: 122, 1974.
76. Lubchenco, L. O., Bard, H., Goldman, A. L., Coyer, W. B., McIntyre, C., Smith, D. M.: Newborn intensive care and long-term prognosis. Dev Med Child Neurol 16: 421, 1974.
77. Lubchenco, L. O., Delivoria-Papadopoulos, M., and Searls, D.: Long-term follow-up of prematurely born infants. II. Influence of birth weight and gestational age on sequelae. J Pediatr 80: 509, 1972.
78. Lubchenco, L. O., Hansman, C., Boyd, E.: Intrauterine growth in length and head circumference as estimated from live births at gestational ages from 26–42 weeks. Pediatrics 37: 403, 1966.
79. Lubchenco, L. O., Hansman, C., Dresser, M., Boyd, E.: Intrauterine growth as estimated from live born birth weight data at 24–42 weeks of gestation. Pediatrics 32: 793, 1963.
80. Lunt, R., Chard, T.: A new method for estimation of fetal weight in late pregnancy by ultrasonic scanning. Br J Obstet Gynaecol 83: 1, 1976.
81. Maghissi, K., (Editor, *Birth Defects and Fetal Development—Endocrine and Metabolic Factors*. Springfield, Ill., Charles C Thomas, Publisher, 1974.
82. Mann, L. I., Tejani, N. A., Weiss, R. R.: Antenatal diagnosis and management of the small-for-gestational age fetus. Am J Obstet Gynecol 120: 995, 1974.
83. Mestyan, J., Schulz, K., Horvath, M.: Comparative glycemic response to alanine in normal term and S.G.A. infants. J. Pediatr 85: 276, 1974.
84. Michie, E.: Urinary oestriol excretion in pregnancies complicated by suspected intra-uterine

growth, toxemia, or essential hypertension. J Obstet Gynaecol Br Commonw 74: 896, 1967.
85. Naeye, R. L., Kelly, J. A.: Judgment of fetal age. III. The pathologist's evaluation. Pediatr Clin North Am 13: 849, 1966.
86. Nesbitt, R. E. L., Aubry, R. H.: High risk obstetrics. II. Value of semiobjective grading system in identifying the vulnerable group. Am J Obstet Gynecol 103: 972, 1969.
87. Odenall, H.: Fetal heart rate patterns in patients with intrauterine growth retardation. Obstet Gynecol 48: 187, 1976.
88. Oski, F. A., Naiman, J. L.: Hematologic problems in the newborn. Philadelphia, W. B. Saunders, 1972, p 81.
89. Ounsted, M., Ounsted, C.: *On the Fetal Growth Rate*. London, Heinemann, 1973, pp 72–82.
90. Ounsted, M., Taylor, M. E.: The postnatal growth of children who were small-for-dates or large-for-dates at birth. Devel Med Child Neurol 13: 421, 1971.
91. Page, E., Christianson, R.: The impact of mean arterial pressure in the middle trimester upon the outcome of pregnancy. Am J Obstet Gynecol 125: 740, 1976.
92. Perry, C. P., Harris, R. E., DeLemos, R. A., Null, D. M.: Intrauterine growth retarded infants. Obstet Gynecol 48: 182, 1976.
93. Petrucco, O. M., Cellier, K., Fishtall, A.: Diagnosis of intrauterine fetal growth retardation by serial serum oxytocinase, urinary oestrogen, and serum heat-stable alkaline phoshatose estimations in uncomplicated and hypertensive pregnancies. J Obstet Gynaecol Br Commonw 80: 499, 1973.
94. Pusey, V. A., Haworth, J. C.: The relation between birth weight and gestational age for a Winnipeg hospital population. J Can Med Assoc 100: 842, 1969.
95. Queenan, J. T., Kubarych, S. F., Cook, L. N., Anderson, G. D., Griffin, L. P.: Am J Obstet Gynecol 124: 865, 1976.
96. Rantakallio, P.: Groups at risk in low birth weight infants and perinatal mortality. Acta Pediatr Scand (Suppl.) 218: 1971.
97. Reisman, L.: Chromosomal abnormalities and intrauterine growth retardation. Pediatr Clin North Am 17 (1): 101, 1970.
98. Rice-wray, E., Corren, S., Gorodousky, J., Esquinel, J., Goldzicher, J. W.: Return of ovulation after discontinuance of oral contraceptives. Fertil. Steril. 18: 212, 1967.
99. Robinson, H. P.: Sonar measurement of fetal crown-rump length as a means of assessing maturity in the first trimester of pregnancy. Br Med J IV: 28, 1973.
100. Robinson, H. P.: "Gestation sac" volumes as determined by sonar in the first trimester of pregnancy. Br J Obstet Gynaecol 82: 100, 1975.
101. Robinson, H. P., Chatfield, W. R., Logan, R. W., et al: A scoring system for the assessment of multiple methods of monitoring fetal growth. J Obstet Gynaecol Br Commonw 80: 230, 1973.
102. Robinson, R.: The small-for-dates baby. II. Br Med J 4: 480, 1971.
103. Rosso, L., Winick, M.: Intrauterine growth retardation. J Perinatal Med 2: 1974.
104. Sabbagha, R. E., Turner, H., Rockette, H., Mazer, H., Orgill, J.: Sonar BPD and fetal age: Definition of the relationship. Obstet Gynecol 43: 7, 1974.
105. Sabel, K. G., Ologard, R., Victorin, L: Remaining sequelae with modern perinatal care. Pediatrics 57: 652, 1976.
106. Scott, K. E., Usher, R., MacLean, R.: Postnatal study of fetal malnutrition syndrome. J Pediatr 63: 734, 1963.
107. Shelley, H. J.: Carbohydrate reserves in the newborn infant. Br Med J 1: 273, 1964.
108. Shelley, H. J., Neligan, G. A.: Neonatal hypoglycemia. Br Med Bull 22: 34, 1966.
109. Smidt, D., Steinbach, J., Scheven, B.: Die beeinflussung per Pra-und postnatalen entwicklung durch grosse and korpergewicht der mutter, largstellt an ergebnissen reziproker eitransplantonen zwischen Zwergschweinen und grossen hausschweinen. Monatsschr Kinderheilkd 115: 533, 1967.
110. Sinclair, J. C: Heat production and thermoregulation in the small-for-dates infant. Pediatr Clin North Am 17: 147, 1970.
111. Sterky, G.: Swedish standard curves for intrauterine growth. Pediatrics 46: 7, 1970.
112. Stevenson, R.: *The Fetus and Newly Born Infant*. St. Louis, C. V. Mosby Co., 1973.
113. Stimler, L.: Infants who are small for gestational age. Proc Roy Soc Med 63: 500, 1970.
114. Thomson, A. M., Billewicz, W. Z., Hytten F. E.: The assessment of fetal growth. J Obstet Gynaecol Br Commonw 75: 903, 1968.
115. Usher, R. H.: Clinical and therapeutic aspects of fetal malnutrition. Pediatr Clin North Am 17: 169, 1970.
116. Van den Berg, B. J., Yerushalmy, J.: The relationship of rate of intrauterine growth of infants of low birth weight to mortality, morbidity, and congenital anomalies. J Pediatr 69: 531, 1966.
117. Wallace, S. J., Michie, E. C.: A follow-up study of infants born to mothers with low estriol excretion during pregnancy. Lancet 2: 560, 1966.
118. Walton, A., Hammond, J.: The maternal effects of growth and conformation in Shir horse-Shetland pony crosses. Proc Roy Soc Lond 125: 311, 1938.
119. Weiner, G.: The relationship of birth weight and length of gestation to intellectual development at ages 8 to 10 years. J Pediatr 76: 694, 1970.
120. Weingold, A. B.: Intrauterine growth retardation: obstetrical aspects. J Repr Med 14 (6): 244, 1975.
121. Whetham, J. C. G., Muggah, H., Davidson, S.: Assessment of intrauterine growth retardation by diagnostic ultrasound. Am J Obstet Gynecol 125: 577, 1976.
122. Williams, P. R., Fiser, R. H., Jr., Sperling, M. A., Oh, W.: Effects of oral alanine in small-for-gestational age infants. N Engl J Med 292: 612, 1975.
123. Winick, M.: Cellular growth in intrauterine

malnutrition. Pediatr Clin North Am 17: 69, 1970.
124. Winick, M., Brasel, J. A., et al: Effects of prenatal nutrition upon pregnancy risk. Clin Obstet Gynecol 16 (1): 1973.
125. Wladimiroff, J. W., Campbell, S.: Fetal urine production rates in normal and complicated pregnancy. Lancet 1: 151, 1974.
126. Wolfrum, R., Bordasch, C., Holweg, J.: An endocrine model for the diagnosis of intrauterine growth retardation as demonstrated by the determination of total estrogen and pregnondial 24-hour urinary excretion in 222 at risk pregnancies. J Perinatal Med 3: 248, 1975.
127. Yarma, T. R.: A comparison between serial cephalometry and maternal urinary oestrogen excretion in assessing fetal pregnancies. Austr NZ J Obstet Gynaecol 13: 191, 1973.
128. Yerushalmy, J. Relation of birth weight, gestational age, and the rate of intrauterine growth to perinatal mortality. Clin Obstet Gynecol 13: 107, 1970.
129. Yogman, M., Speroff, L., Huttenlocher, P., Kase, N.: Child development after pregnancies complicated by low urinary estriol excretion and preeclampsia. Am J Obstet Gynecol 114: 1069, 1972.

UCHENNA C. NWOSU, M.D.

10

Post-term Pregnancy

Scope of Problem

About 10% of all pregnancies continue for 14 or more days beyond term.[1, 2] Of these prolonged pregnancies 20–40% will result in the delivery of postmature neonates,[1] with some or all of the following features: apparent loss of subcutaneous tissue, dry skin with deep creases and desquamation, elongated nails and alert facies.[1] Meconium staining of the skin and integument occur in the worst cases. The perinatal mortality of postmature neonates is 3 times that of term newborns. Average mortality collated from five reports shows that about 35% of the deaths occur before the onset of labor, 47% during labor and 18% in the neonatal period.[3] Autopsy generally fails to reveal any cause of death except in a few cases where the alveoli are stained with meconium and the terminal bronchioles impacted with meconium plugs.

Etiology

It is widely accepted that the syndrome of postmaturity is caused by placental insufficiency. First proposed by Ballantyne in 1902,[4] this viewpoint reached its zenith in the 1950's following Clifford's classic papers on the subject.[5, 6] According to this theory the placenta has a finite lifespan beyond which it begins to degenerate to the point where the transport mechanism is impaired. Evidence of degenerative changes such as excessive fibrosis and calcification has been found in some, but by no means in all postmature placentas. Furthermore, similar changes have been observed with equal frequency in placentas from normal term newborns.[7–10]

Although the concept of placental insufficiency could be invoked to explain the physical signs of fetal inanition observed in this syndrome, it does not account for the cause of prolongation beyond term. In the long run the etiology of postmaturity will have to be related to the causation of spontaneous labor.

Initiation of Labor

The mechanism of onset of spontaneous labor continues to be elusive and we are probably no nearer the truth than when Hippocates (460 B.C.) suggested that the fetus plays a large part in determining its own destiny. Many theories have been proposed from time to time, but only the leading ones will be reviewed.

"PROGESTERONE BLOCK" THEORY

Based upon extensive work with the rabbit, Csapo[11] has proposed that the pregnant uterus is capable of spontaneous activity at any point in gestation, but remains inhibited by progesterone. As pregnancy advances the increasing volume of the uterus stretches the uterine muscle fibers. As with muscles elsewhere, changes in the length of myometrial cell control spontaneous membrane activity, the contractile threshold and the force developed. Therefore, the effect of the stretch tends to counteract the progesterone block until a critical volume to progesterone ratio is reached, at which point the progesterone block is overridden and spontaneous uterine activity initiated. This theory has been more recently modified to a see-saw concept in which the blocking effect of progesterone is balanced by the stimulating effect of stretch-dependent prostaglandin $F_2\alpha$ which is endogenously produced in the myometrium.[12] Csapo[13] and Turbull et al[14] have found evidence of progesterone withdrawal in the peripheral plasma during the last weeks of human pregnancy. However, this has not been a consistent observation prior to onset of labor.

OXYTOCIN THEORY

Many obstetricians assume that oxytocin release from maternal neurohypophysis plays a role in the initiation of labor. The origin of this concept dates back to the discovery in the 1920's of uterine-stimulating effects of extracts from the posterior pituitary. By the following decade numerous authors were investigating a possible relationship between neurohypophysis and onset of labor in animals. During the 1940's Canadian obstetricians brought attention to the fact that ethyl alcohol could inhibit spontaneous uterine activity. Subsequently, Fuchs demonstrated that intravenous alcohol could abolish uterine contractions in the rabbit[15] and human.[16] Based on these experimental observations, it has been proposed that labor is initiated by an unknown signal emanating from the fetal compartment and stimulating the maternal hypothalamus to synthesize oxytocin and vasopressin. These octapeptides are known to travel via the neuronal axons to the posterior pituitary. Upon release the oxytocin is blood-bourne to the uterus where it stimulates contractile activity.

Although this theory may be tenable under certain conditions, it should be stated that the onset or maintenance of labor is not abnormal in cases of diabetes insipidus.[17] Furthermore, oxytocin may or may not be demonstrable in maternal plasma during early labor.[18] On the other hand, oxytocin can be found consistently at relatively high levels in the cord blood, the level being higher in the arterial than the venous plasma. This suggests that oxytocin may be released by the fetus during labor. Whether the release of fetal oxytocin initiates labor remains to be determined. However, it should be noted that normal delivery may occur with an anencephalic fetus who lacks a posterior pituitary.

FETAL ADRENOCORTICAL THEORY

That the genotype of the fetus is a factor influencing the duration of intrauterine life is demonstrated in the reciprocal cross between the horse and the donkey (Table 10.1). Recent studies suggest that this determination may occur through a hormonal platform in which the fetal adrenal cortex plays a key role. Table 10.2 summarizes the various conditions which have been associated with either prolongation or shortening of pregnancy.

A sudden rise in fetal plasma corticosteroids has been observed a few days before the onset of labor in the sheep, a rise which is unrelated to the levels of maternal corticoids. This phenomenon was demonstrated in 1969 by Bassett and Thorburn[24] through in utero blood sampling of the fetal lamb. The recent investigations of Murphy[25] offer some support that a rise in fetal cortisol levels may precede labor in the human. She noted a rise in cortisol levels of mixed umbilical cord blood between the 20th week of pregnancy and term. Infants delivered after spontaneous labor demonstrated mean cord plasma cortisol levels higher than those of infants delivered by elective cesarean section or elective induction of labor. Measurement of arterial and venous cord plasma cortisol levels has shown the source of cortisol to be fetal rather than maternal.[26]

Several years ago we measured the cord and neonatal plasma cortisol levels in postmature neonates and compared values

Table 10.1. Approximate duration of gestation in horse-donkey crosses

Stallion × Mare	340 days
Stallion × Jennett	350 days
Jack × Mare	355 days
Jack × Jennet	365 days

Table 10.2. Factors associated with alteration of pregnancy duration in various species

Condition	Result	Species
Fetal pituitary ablation	Prolonged pregnancy	Sheep,[19] monkey[20]
Fetal adrenalectomy	Prolonged pregnancy	Sheep[21]
Anencephaly	Prolonged pregnancy	Human[22]
Fetal cortisol infusion	Premature delivery	Sheep[23]
Fetal ACTH infusion	Premature delivery	Sheep[23]

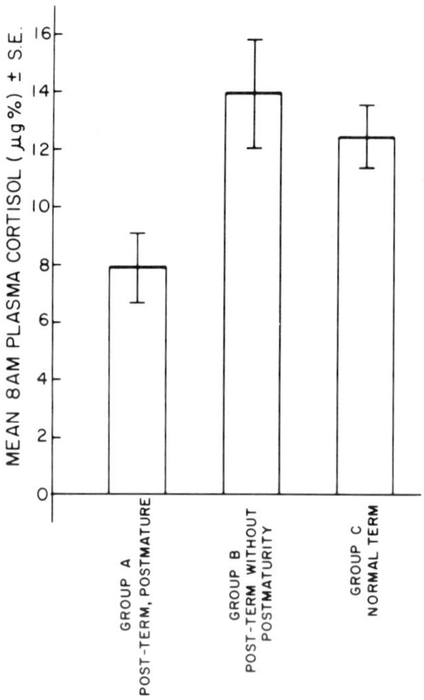

Figure 10.1. Plasma cortisol levels of postmature, post-term and normal neonates.

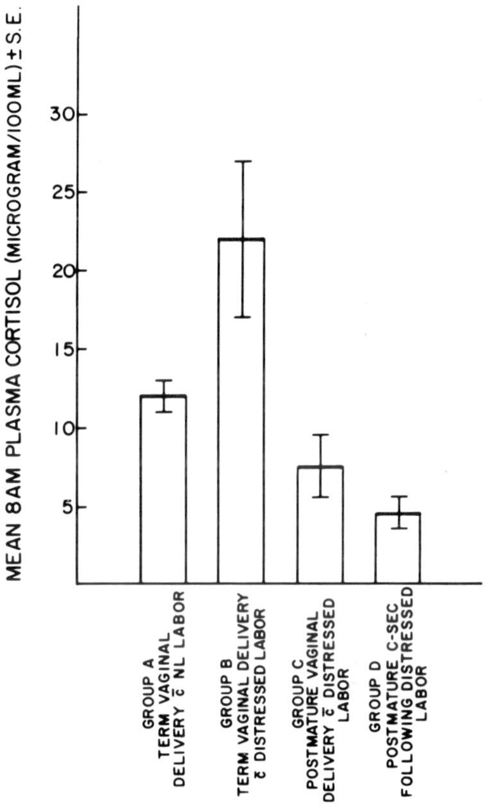

Figure 10.2. Plasma cortisol levels of postmature neonates who had undergone fetal distress during labor compared with those of normal term neonates with and without fetal distress.

with those of normal term newborns, as well as post-term newborns who showed no physical signs of postmaturity.[27] Although no difference was observed among the cord blood samples, the neonatal cortisol levels were significantly lower in the postmature newborns when compared with the normal term newborns or the merely post-term newborns (Figure 10.1). We then measured the cortisol levels in postmature neonates who had undergone fetal distress during labor and compared values with those of normal term neonates with and without fetal distress during labor.[28] Again, no differences were found in the cord levels. The differences observed in the neonatal levels are summarized in Figure 10.2. The mean neonatal cortisol level of the distressed term group was found to be almost twice that of the control group ($P < 0.01$). In contrast, the mean value found in post-term, postmature neonates with mild to moderate fetal distress was significantly lower than that of the control group ($P < 0.05$). When the mean level in post-term, postmature group with severe fetal distress was compared with that of the control group, the former value was found to be significantly lower ($P < 0.005$).

Since the enzyme Δ^5-3_B-hydroxysteroid dehydrogenase has been shown to be relatively deficient in human fetal adrenal glands, and since this enzyme is required for cortisol synthesis from Δ^5 precursors, the hypothesis of a bell curve distribution of this enzyme activity was advanced, such that the post-term, postmature neonates may fall at the extreme end of the curve, where the enzyme activity is severely limited (Figure 10.3). Consequently, such a fetus might be unable to trigger labor by an abrupt cortisol production.

This speculation prompted a third study in which an attempt was made to initiate labor in prolonged human pregnancy by iatrogenic elevation of fetal cortisol level.[29] Patients without prenatal complication other than prolongation of pregnancy were assigned to two groups on an alternating basis. Our criterion for prolonged gestation was a well established due date as calculated by Naegle's rule. Bishop's scoring system[30] was used to assess the degree of pelvic readiness for labor. Those patients with a Bishop's induction score of 9 or more, as judged by two independent examiners, were excluded.

Five hundred milligrams of cortisol, dissolved in the accompanying diluent of bacteriostatic water to form 4 ml of solution, was injected into the amniotic sac in group A patients, whereas group B patients received 4 ml of bacteriostatic water intra-amniotically to serve as controls. The age, gravidity, pregnancy duration and Bishop's score were comparable in both groups at the initiation of the study.

Of the 10 patients who received cortisol, 8 began spontaneous labor within 120 hr compared with 2 out of 9 in the control group. This represented a significant difference by chi square test ($P < 0.01$). The mean instillation-labor interval in those patients receiving intra-amniotic cortisol was 86 hr as compared with 228 hr in the control group ($P < 0.001$). These results were in harmony with the data reported by Mati et al,[31] who used betamethasone instead of cortisol and had a mean instillation labor interval of 78.9 hr for the experimental group and 323 hr for control patients. Although these findings are encouraging, the data reported are nonetheless too small to be anything but preliminary. It is hoped that further work will be done in the area.

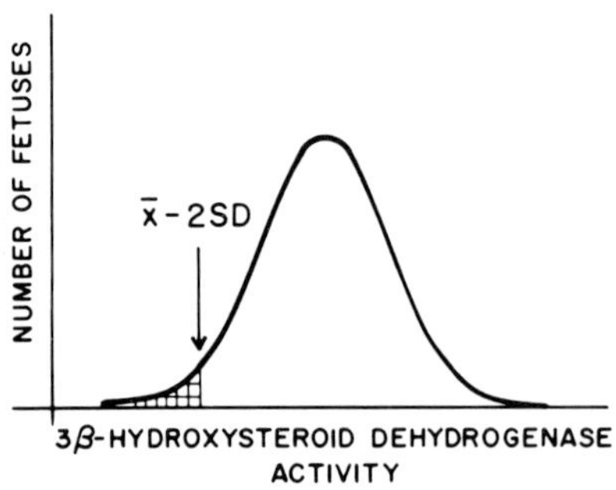

Figure 10.3. Theoretical curve of distribution of 3β-hydroxysteroid dehydrogenase in infinite number of fetal adrenal glands.

Teleologically, we can assume that labor initiation is so important in the preservation of the species that it has no single mechanism. There may well be a primary mechanism for each species as well as multiple back-up mechanisms.

Clinical Diagnosis

Postmaturity is a neonatal diagnosis. The term should not be used interchangeably with "postdatism" or post-term pregnancy." The latter terms refer to a pregnancy which has been prolonged beyond its due date as calculated by Naegle's rule. A post-term pregnancy may or may not eventuate in the delivery of a postmature neonate. The obstetrician's present challenge is to make postmaturity a prenatal rather than postnatal diagnosis.

Published data on postmaturity are difficult to analyze because of confusion in terms, with postmaturity often referring to postdatism. However, it appears that both nulliparous and multiparous gravidas are at risk, although the elderly gravida is at increased risk. In the same gravida the risk varies from one pregnancy to another.

Since postdatism is the first sign of possible postmaturity, it is essential to ascertain the last menstrual period (LMP) as accurately as possible upon registration of the patient. Because of postpill amenorrhea and delayed ovulation, the last withdrawal bleeding following discontinuation of oral contraceptives should be suspect when pregnancy occurs without an intervening spontaneous menses. Nonspecific LMP is not infrequently encountered, especially in lower socioeconomic groups. Wenner and Young[32] have shown this phenomenon to be associated with poor reproductive outcome in general.

For confirmation of LMP gravidas should be instructed upon registration to note the day of quickening (19th week in primigravidas and 17th week in multigravidas). The growth of the uterine fundus should be carefully followed, with progression to the umbilical level being regarded as 20 weeks' gestation. When a patient is examined by multiple examiners, fundal height is best recorded in centimeters above the superior border of the pubic bone. Early determination (24 to 28 weeks) of fetal biparietal diameter, using the B-scan ultrasound, will accurately date a pregnancy. This technique becomes less reliable as term is approached, and cannot be used for differentiating a term from a post-term pregnancy. Cervical softening and effacement occur in most gravidas as term approaches, occurring earlier in primigravidas. However, absence of cervical ripeness does not exclude postdatism.

Diagnostic Tests

At present there is no single prenatal test that would accurately diagnose a postmature fetus. However, a combination of tests has been found useful. Optimum management of post-term pregnancy can be achieved by the combined use of urinary estriol, amniocentesis and oxytocin challenge test. Novel applications of B scan may also prove useful in the management of this entity.

B-SCAN ULTRASOUND

Fetal Biparietal Diameter

At present, the principal application of B-scan ultrasound in the management of post-term pregnancy is to arrive at an accurate dating before term. Since dating is most accurate between the 20th and 30th weeks of pregnancy, the B scan should be used prospectively whenever the expected date of confinement (EDC) by history is uncertain. If a pregnancy has not been dated by B-scan biparietal diameter before term, it is worthless attempting to do so post-term.

Amniotic Fluid Volume

A noticeable decrease in the abdominal girth may occur post-term as a result of a gradual decrease in the amniotic fluid volume. The average amniotic fluid volume at 42, 43 and 44 weeks of gestation have been estimated at 484 ml, 332 ml and 162 ml, respectively.[33] Since there is a significant correlation between oligohydramnios (<200 ml) and postmaturity,[33] serial measurement of total intrauterine volume by using B-scan ultrasound, as recently reported by Hobbins and Gohari,[34] may well prove a novel and useful method for prenatal diagnosis of postmaturity.

ESTRIOL

Estriol is produced by the placental action on fetal steroid precursors. The availability of these precursors is dependent upon fetal size and well-being. Several reports have shown that urinary estriol levels might be of value in the prenatal diagnosis of postmaturity. Persistent low or falling sequential values may be indicative of the syndrome,[35–39] although normal levels do not exclude it.[28] In our laboratory a 24-hr urinary post-term estriol level below 12 mg is considered low whereas a 40% decrease between sequential values is considered significant. The estriol to creatinine ratio is the basis for comparison of sequential values.

OXYTOCIN CHALLENGE TEST (OCT)

Although the relationship between postmaturity and placental insufficiency is controversial and poorly established, the OCT has been found moderately helpful in the management of post-term pregnancy. In a recent study at Pennsylvania Hospital,[40] 46 post-term gravidas were monitored with both OCT and sequential urinary estriols. Eleven of the 46 delivered newborns that were considered postmature by the usual criteria. Three (27%) of the 11 had a positive OCT whereas 8 (73%) had a negative OCT. Two other post-term gravidas with a positive OCT were delivered of normal appearing newborns. Ten of the 11 gravidas had sequential estriol determinations. Five (50%) were diagnosable by low or falling estriols. Two other post-term gravidas with low estriol excretion did not have postmature neonates. Only 1 of the 11 postmature newborns showed both poor estriols and a positive OCT. On the other hand, two gravidas with both a positive OCT and falling estriols were delivered of newborns showing no evidence of clinical postmaturity.

AMNIOCENTESIS

The primary purpose of amniocentesis in post-term pregnancy is to exclude the presence of meconium. Presence of meconium in post-term pregnancy is often indicative of fetal distress and postmaturity. This is reflected in Clifford's[5] classification of the syndrome into three stages as follows:

> *Stage I,* loss of subcutaneous tissue plus desquamation, long nails, abundant hair and alert facies. Amniotic fluid is clear but shows loss of vernix.
> *Stage II,* Stage I plus green meconium-stained amniotic fluid with meconium staining of membranes, placenta and cord.
> *Stage III,* Stage II changes plus yellow meconium staining, indicative of long exposure.

Amnioscopy may be substituted for amniocentesis, although the former requires a certain degree of cervical dilatation, and may be falsely negative. Presence of scanty vernix in clear amniotic fluid may be indicative of either prematurity or postmaturity. In the former, the vernix has not been fully formed, whereas in the latter it is precipitated out onto the choroidal plate to form vernix caeseosa. Therefore, such fluid should be subjected to lecithin/sphingomyelin (L/S) ratio determination. Scanty fluid or dry tap should raise the suspicion of postmaturity, especially if such a tap was done using the B-scan ultrasound.

Management

When a pregnancy extends 7 days beyond term, the prenatal chart should be reviewed for confirmation of EDC. The uterine fundus at the umbilical level accurately reflects 20 weeks of gestation in most cases, and may be used to project the EDC. Subsequent fundal progression and B scan (if obtained before 30 weeks) are used to confirm that the true EDC has been exceeded.

If the chart review confirms that the EDC has been exceeded, a pelvic examination is performed to evaluate pelvic readiness for induction. Bishop's pelvic score[30] may be helpful in judging pelvic readiness. Elective induction with intravenous oxytocin is performed if the cervix is inducible (Bishop score 9), otherwise twice weekly urinary estriol determinations are initiated. Sequential urinary estriol levels would show a rising trend, falling trend or a pleateau. If a rising trend is noted, a false EDC should be suspected and estriol determinations continued weekly instead of twice weekly. If a plateau is noted over two determinations or if a decline of 40% is noted between any two estriol/creatinine values, amniocentesis is performed.

With an unfavorable cervix, the presence of meconium-stained fluid in the face of falling estriols, or the absence of fluid is an indication for primary cesarean section. The approach of subjecting a post-term fetus in such an unfavorable intrauterine environment to a protracted course of induction, or a 2-day induction with overnight rest is to be decried. Meconium aspiration or sudden fetal demise is apt to occur during such a prolonged period of hypoxic stress.

On the other hand, if amniocentesis reveals clear fluid, an oxytocin challenge test is carried out immediately. *A primary cesarean section is performed for type II decelerations in the presence of an unfavorable cervix.* With a negative OCT, however, a pelvic examination is repeated for reassessment of cervical inducibility, and the management cycle repeated as charted in Figure 10.4.

When a patient is encountered at 42 or more weeks without previous estriol values, the management protocol is modified as shown in Figure 10.5. The prenatal records again must be reviewed to ascertain the accuracy of the EDC. Should pelvic examination reveal an uninducible cervix,

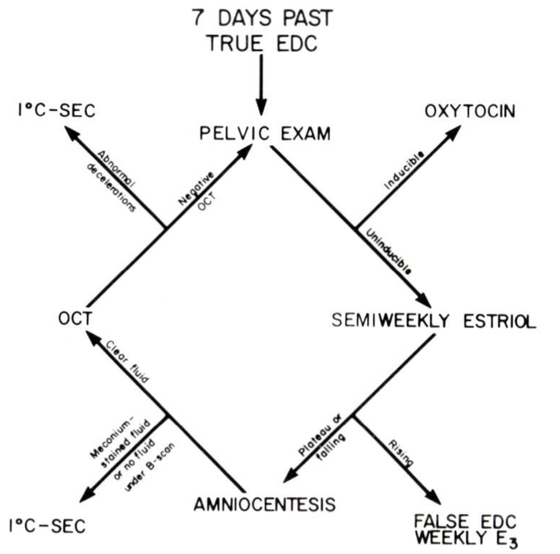

Figure 10.4. Flowsheet for pregnancy management at 41 weeks.

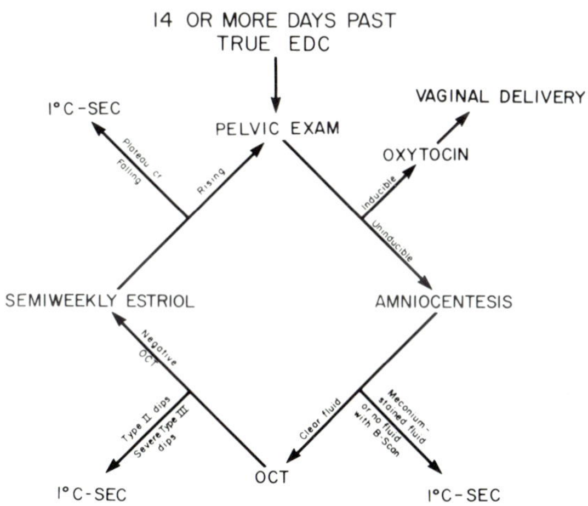

Figure 10.5. Flowsheet for management of prolonged pregnancy encountered at 42 or more weeks without previous evaluation.

one should proceed to amniocentesis prior to an OCT. *The presence of meconium in a confirmed post-term pregnancy with an unfavorable cervix constitutes an indication for cesarean section.* If, however, the amniotic fluid is clear, an OCT will give additional reassurance before the patient is discharged, to start 24-hr sequential urine collections for estriol determination. (Figure 10.5).

The sequence of fetal testing is especially important in the management of a post-term pregnancy without previous urinary estriols. The fetus could be in such a precarious state of well-being that oxytocin stimulation, even at 4 drops (2.4 mμ per min), could precipitate rapid fetal demise by some unknown mechanism. Whenever this has occurred in our experience, the amniotic fluid has been found to be thick with meconium.

Summary

1. Although placental insufficience may contribute to the stigmata of postmaturity, it is incorrect to assume that it causes the syndrome.
2. The etiology of postmaturity may be related to a dysfunction in the mechanism of labor initiation.
3. No single theory of labor initiation successfully has accounted for all the experimental observations in various species.
4. Potential management of prolonged pregnancy must be initiated *prior to* term by accurate dating of every pregnancy.
5. Falling sequential estriol levels, meconium-stained amniotic fluid or a positive OCT justify obstetric intervention in post-term pregnancy.

REFERENCES

1. Strand, A.: Prolonged pregnancy. Acta Obstet, Gynecol Scand 35: 76, 1956.
2. Lindell, A.: Prolonged pregnancy. Acta Obstet Gynecol Scand 35: 136, 1956.
3. Vorherr, H.: Placental insufficiency in relation to postterm pregnancy and fetal postmaturity. Am J Obstet Gynecol 123: 67, 1975.
4. Ballantyne, J. W.: The problem of the postmature infant. J Obstet Gynecol Br Emp II: 521, 1902.
5. Clifford, S. H.: Postmaturity—with placental dysfunction: clinical syndrome and pathologic findings. J Pediatr 44: 1, 1954.
6. Clifford, S. H.: Pediatric aspects of placental dysfunction syndrome in postmaturity. JAMA 165: 1663, 1957.
7. Reynolds, F. N.: The problem of postmaturity. Proc Roy Soc Med 31: 781, 1938.
8. Masters, M., Clayton, S. G.: Calcification of the human placenta. J Obstet Gynecol Br Emp 47: 437, 1940.
9. Flemming, A. M.: The clinical significance of the degree of calcification of the placenta as demonstrated by X-ray photography. J Obstet Gynecol 50: 135, 1943.
10. Malpas, P.: Criticism of the hypothesis of placental insufficiency. J Obstet Gynecol Br Emp 63: 199, 1956.

11. Csapo, A.: Ciba symposium. Progesterone and the defense mechanism of pregnancy, London, Churchill, Ltd., 1961, p 3.
12. Csapo, A.: The prospect of PGs in postconceptional therapy. Prostaglandins 3: 245, 1973.
13. Csapo, A. I., Knobil, E., van der Molen, H. J., Wiest, W. G.: Peripheral plasma progesterone levels during human pregnancy and labor. Am J Obstet Gynecol 110: 630, 1971.
14. Turnbull, A. C., Patten, P. T., Flint, A. P. F., Keirse, M. J. N. C., Jeremy, J. Y., Anderson, A. B. M.: Significant fall in progesterone and rise in estradiol levels in human peripheral plasma before onset of labor. Lancet 1: 101, 1974.
15. Fuchs, A. R.: The inhibitory effect of ethanol on the release of oxytocin during parturition in the rabbit. J Endocrinol 35: 125, 1966.
16. Fuchs, R., Fuchs, A. R., Poblete, V. F., Rizk, A.: Effect of alcohol on threatened premature labor. Am J Obstet Gynecol 99: 627, 1967.
17. Hendricks, C. H.: The neurohypophysis in pregnancy. Obstet Gynecol Surv 9: 323, 1954.
18. Chard, T., Boyd, N. R. H., Forsling, M. L., McNeilly, A. S., Landon, J.: The development of radioimmunoassay for oxytocin: The extraction of oxytocin from plasma and its measurement during parturition in human and goat blood. J Endocrinol 48: 223, 1970.
19. Liggins, G. C., Kennedy, P. C., Holm, L. W.: Failure of initiation of parturition after electrocoagulation of the pituitary of the fetal lamb. Am J Obstet Gynecol 98: 1080, 1967.
20. Chez, R. A., Hutchinson, D. L., Salazer, H., Mintz, D. H.: Some effects of fetal and maternal hypophysectomy in pregnancy. Am J Obstet Gynecol 108: 643, 1970.
21. Drost, M., Holm, L. W.: Prolonged gestation in lives after fetal adrenalectomy. J Endocrinol 40: 293, 1968.
22. Anderson, A. B., Lawrence, K. M., Turnbull, A. C.: The relationship in anencephaly between the size of the adrenal cortex and the length of gestation. J Obstet Gynecol Br Commonw 76: 196, 1969.
23. Liggins, G. C.: Premature parturition after infusion of corticotrophin or cortisol. J Endocrinol 42: 323, 1968.
24. Bassett, J. M., Thorburn, G. D.: Fetal plasma corticosteroids and initiation of parturition in sheep. J Endocrinol 44: 285, 1969.
25. Murphy, B. E. P.: Does the human fetal adrenal play a role in parturition? Am J Obstet Gynecol 115: 521, 1973.
26. Leong, M. K. H., Murphy, B. E. P.: Cortisol levels in maternal venous and umbilical cord arterial and venous serum at vaginal delivery. Am J Obstet Gynecol 124: 471, 1976.
27. Nwosu, U., Wallach, E. E., Boggs, T. R., Nemiroff, R. L., Bongiovanni, A. M.: Possible role of the fetal adrenal glands in the etiology of postmaturity. Am J Obstet Gynecol 121: 366, 1975.
28. Nwosu, U., Wallach, E. E., Boggs, T. R., Bongiovanni, A. M.: Possible adrenocortical insufficiency in postmature neonates. Am J Obstet Gynecol 122: 969, 1975.
29. Nwosu, U. C., Wallach, E. E., Bolognese, R. J.: Initiation of labor by intraamniotic cortisol instillation in prolonged human pregnancy. Obstet Gynecol 47: 137, 1976.
30. Bishop, E. J.: Pelvic scoring for elective induction. Obstet Gynecol 24: 266, 1964.
31. Mati, J. K. G., Horrobin, D. F., Bramley, P. S.: Induction of labor in sheep and in humans by single doses of corticosteroids. Br Med J 2: 149, 1973.
32. Wenner, W. H., Young, E. B.: Nonspecific date of last menstrual period: An indication of poor reproductive outcome. Am J Obstet Gynecol 120: 1071, 1974.
33. Beischer, N. A., Brown, J. B., Townsend, L.: Studies in prolonged pregnancy. III. Amniocentesis in prolonged pregnancy. Am J Obstet Gynecol 103: 496, 1969.
34. Hobbins, J. C., Gohari, P.: In utero prediction of intrauterine growth retardation by determination of total intrauterine volume. Gynec Invest (Sci Abstr) 7: 22, 1976.
35. Smith, K., Greene, J. W., Touchstone, J. C.: Urinary estriol determination in the management of prolonged pregnancy. Am J Obstet Gynecol 96: 901, 1966.
36. Lundwall, F., Stakeman, G.: The urinary excretion of estriol in postmaturity. Acta Obstet Gynecol Scand 45: 301, 1966.
37. Beischer, N. A., Brown, J. B., Smith, M. A., Townsend, L.: Studies in prolonged pregnancy. II. Clinical results and urinary estriol excretion in prolonged pregnancy. Am J Obstet Gynecol 103: 483, 1969.
38. Jenkins, D. M., Farquhar, J. B., Oakey, R. E.: Urinary estrogen excretion in prolonged pregnancies. Obstet Gynecol 37: 442, 1971.
39. Aubry, R. H., Pennington, J. C.: Identification and evaluation of high-risk pregnancy: The perinatal concept. Clin Obstet Gynecol 16: 3, 1973.
40. Cooper, J. M., Soffronoff, E. C., Bolognese, R. J.: Oxytocin challenge test in monitoring high-risk pregnancies. Obstet Gynecol 45: 27, 1975.

TOM P. BARDEN, M.D.

11

Prematurity

There is abundant evidence that neonatal survival is influenced independently by birth weight and gestational age. From most studies, it is evident that low birth weight is a higher mortality risk factor than short gestational age. The prognosis for the neonate is worse when low birth weight results from preterm interruption of normal pregnancy than when it relates to intrauterine maldevelopment. The term "premature" has generally been applied to infants with birth weight less than 2,500 g, and yet approximately 15% of these infants have achieved maturation consistent with term, or gestation of 37 weeks or more. Evaluation of the neonate by physical or neurologic developmental factors, contrasted with birth weight, frequently reveals considerable disparity. Thus, it is meaningful to describe the fetus or newborn on a basis of growth patterns and gestational age or maturation, in addition to weight.

Preterm, low birth weight delivery has remained the foremost obstetric problem in the United States despite significant reduction of the pregnancy rate, improved standards of living and medical advances. The 8% of infants with birth weight of less than 2,500 g at birth rarely survive without some neurologic residual or compromise of intellectual ability. There is growing evidence that the use of neonatal intensive care concepts will reduce this morbidity. The availability of these techniques of newborn management will be extended by the use of regional intensive care nursery facilities. However, despite these advances, the greatest potential for improved outcome lies in prevention of low birth weight delivery. Traditional obstetrical management of premature labor has been supportive at best. Management precepts have included bed rest, avoidance of drugs with potential depressant effects and atraumatic birth. Generally, the employment of drugs to inhibit premature labor was based on anecdotal evidence. There were no convincing studies to support the efficacy of various neuromuscular relaxants, hormonal substances or psycholeptics in common use. The identification of uterine-relaxing properties of intravenous ethanol and various sympathomimetic amines provided clinicians with more specific pharmacologic approaches to the treatment of premature labor. However, with more effective treatment methods came the frequent clinical dilemma of which labors to stop. Unless improvement of intrauterine environment is concomitant to uterine relaxation, the fetus of a compromised pregnancy may, by treatment of premature labor, be doomed to death in utero. The search for effective and safe uterine relaxants is inexorably related to an understanding of the mechanism of labor and its relation to the condition of the fetus.

Labor is characterized by increasing uterine activity and progressive changes of the cervix which may lead to vaginal delivery of the fetus. The onset of labor is more a culmination of pre-existing changes than an abrupt event. Thus, the components of the mechanism of labor may be present in some degree throughout pregnancy. Until recently, the most prevalent hypothesis of the mechanism of labor onset held that it primarily involved release of oxytocin from the maternal pituitary gland through some type of reflex mechanism. Ferguson[45] observed that the uterine contractility which occurred after stimulation of the cervix in rabbits failed to occur after either transection of the spinal cord or destruction of the pituitary. Thus, he suggested that cervical stimulation produced a cord-mediated reflex which triggered release of oxytocin from the pituitary. Yet, in humans, it is well known that labor onset is not consistently affected by spinal cord lesions or by a nonfunctioning pituitary. From studies in rabbits, Fuchs[46] reported evidence that intravenous infusion of ethanol blocked the pituitary release of oxytocin. Subsequently, further studies revealed that intravenous ethanol was capable of inhibiting uterine activity in humans.[47, 130] The implication of these observations was that a surge of oxytocin occurred at the onset of labor, but at that time there was no practical method to measure blood levels of oxytocin. The more recent development of the radioimmunoassay technique provided the necessary methodology to learn that there is no measurable rise in the level of oxytocin in maternal peripheral blood at the onset of labor in humans. However, at the time of delivery, Chard and coworkers[32] found significantly higher levels of oxytocin in fetal blood from the umbilical cord than in maternal blood. Kumaresan and associates,[74] using a more sensitive antiserum, found comparable levels of oxytocin in maternal venous and umbilical artery blood. In both studies, oxytocin levels were higher in umbilical artery versus umbilical vein blood, implying that the fetus is an active producer of oxytocin.[32, 74] Seppala and associates[113] reported that meconium-stained amniotic fluid contained more oxytocin than clear fluid. Also, Seppala and Aho[112] reported that the presence of meconium-stained amniotic fluid was associated with shorter labor, in contrast to the length of labor in patients with clear amniotic fluid. By passing meconium in response to intrauterine asphyxia, the fetus may be triggering labor to effect an escape from a hostile environment. Ethanol may inhibit labor by its influence on fetal pituitary release of oxytocin, for it readily crosses the placenta to the fetus. The concept of fetal oxytocin production in labor onset is supported by the common association of fetal anencephaly and delayed onset of labor. Without a pituitary gland, the anencephalic fetus is unable to signal labor onset at term.

In addition to stimulation of labor by oxytocin, the relaxing influence of progesterone on the uterus has long been considered a plausible component of the control mechanism. The administration of progesterone during pregnancy will delay the onset of labor in several animal species. Csapo[34, 35] introduced the concept that placental production of progesterone produces a local block of myometrial activity. This block subsequently is released as placental production of progesterone decreases prior to the onset of labor. Bengtsson[13] reported that the injection of medroxyprogesterone into the anterior wall of the uterus successfully inhibited labor in 9 of 10 patients in clinical premature labor. Csapo's hypothesis was further supported when Kumar and associates[71] found a consistently higher concentration of progesterone in myometrium from the placental site than elsewhere in the uterus. Csapo and associates[40] found decreasing plasma progesterone levels after intra-amniotic hypertonic saline injection for induction of abortion. Turnbull and coworkers[122] detected falling peripheral plasma levels of progesterone, when measured serially, in a series of patients in late pregnancy. The role of progesterone block in maintenance of pregnancy was further supported by a report of Scommegna and associates[111] in which spontaneous labor was temporarily inhibited during intravenous infusion of pregnenolone, the immediate precursor of progesterone. In contrast, Lanman and associates[78] reported that in rhesus monkeys there was no decrease of progesterone in peripheral plasma, but a sharp fall in uterine vein levels prior to the onset of labor.

Such evidence of the potential pregnancy maintenance role of progesterone has stimulated several therapeutic trials, as well as rather common usage of progesterone in clinical management of patients predisposed to premature labor. Brenner and Hendricks[21] found no evidence that medroxyprogesterone, taken orally in late human pregnancy, had any effect on the timing of labor onset. In contrast, Johnson and associates[62] reported on a double blind prospective study of 17α-hydroxyprogesterone caproate to prevent premature labor. In 36 patients at risk for premature labor, the 14 who received the progestational drug all delivered after 36 weeks, whereas 9 of 22 patients in the placebo group delivered before 36 weeks. If further studies support the efficacy and safety of this preventive approach, we may anticipate reducing the incidence of premature labor by identification and treatment of those at risk, or perhaps by prophylactic treatment of all patients.

The studies of Caldeyro-Barcia and associates[27] suggested that the increased levels of estrogen during pregnancy were responsible for increasing sensitivity of myometrium to oxytocin. Pinto and coworkers[101, 102] reported an oxytocic effect of intravenous or intra-amniotic 17β-estradiol administered in late human pregnancy. More recently, Raja and associates,[104] using the radioimmunoassay technique, reported increased levels of plasma estradiol in patients subsequently developing spontaneous premature labor. In agreement with the initial report of Siiteri and MacDonald,[115] it is now well established that estrogen in pregnancy is produced by the placenta from fetal adrenal precursors. The role of estrogen in labor onset is further suggested by the frequent prolongation of human pregnancy with anencephaly, where adrenal hypoplasia is associated with markedly depressed estrogen levels. From studies in sheep, Liggins and associates[84] reported prolongation of pregnancy after destruction of the fetal pituitary, whereas Drost and Holm[43] found the same result after fetal adrenalectomy. Liggins[81] subsequently reported that injection of fetal lambs with ACTH, cortisol or dexamethasone was followed by premature labor. Further studies in sheep[6, 82] revealed an elevation of fetal cortisol starting about 10 days prior to labor, followed by a sudden rise in estrogen and fall in progesterone during the 24 hr prior to labor. Nwosu and associates[99] reported successful induction of labor in most of a small series of postterm patients by intra-amniotic injection of 500 mg of hydrocortisone. In contrast, similar patients receiving only intra-amniotic sterile water generally failed to develop labor. Urinary estriol excretion progressively declined after injection of hydrocortisone, but not after water. Similarly, Mati and associates[90] reported successful induction of labor in six patients after intra-amniotic injection of betamethasone, whereas in one patient with an anencephalic fetus, the same treatment failed to induce labor. Gennser and associates[51] reported that large doses of betamethasone in late human pregnancy did not reduce the gestational period, but did reduce fetal blood cortisol levels. This reduction of fetal cortisol levels, however, was not associated with prolonged pregnancy. In contrast to the results in sheep, Mueller-Heubach and associates[93] reported that fetal adrenalectomy in a series of rhesus monkeys had no significant influence on the timing of labor onset. From observations in human pregnancy, Nwosu and associates[97, 98] reported that newborn plasma cortisol levels were depressed in postmature infants.

The role of fetal adrenal function in the mechanism of labor onset is further supported by numerous studies of maternal and fetal cortisol levels related to the characteristics of labor and delivery. Several studies have reported elevated levels of cortisol in cord blood after spontaneous labor, as contrasted with labor induced by oxytocin.[31, 52, 94] However, other investigators have found similar levels of cortisol in cord blood in the same two categories of patients.[120, 121] Although maternal blood ACTH is higher with induced versus spontaneous labor,[121] maternal cortisol levels are similar between the two groups.[52, 121] Another report states that maternal cortisol levels are lower in spontaneous labor than in oxytocin-induced labor.[100] Fetal blood cortisol levels are higher after vaginal delivery than cesarean section, with or without labor,[31, 52, 119] and levels are even further elevated when there is fetal asphyxia during labor.[119] Thus, there are many factors which influence maternal and fetal cortisol levels. Although there is no evidence that maternal ACTH is transferred from mother to fetus, changes of maternal cortisol levels may influence fetal blood ACTH levels. In a study reported by Simmer and associates,[114] administration of cortisol to the mother resulted in a 57% decrease of ACTH in umbilical artery blood.

The onset of labor is almost certainly influenced by the complex relationships of maternal and fetal adrenal function and placental steroid production. Although extrapolation of animal data to humans may be misleading, available evidence rather strongly suggests that fetal cortisol production plays an important role in parturition. The relationships between glucocorticoids and placental functions are not yet fully understood. However, recent reports indicate that cortisol induces a steroid 17α-hydroxylase in the sheep placenta, which may serve to reduce progesterone and elevate estrogen.[5, 117]

The role of prostaglandins in parturition is suggested by their oxytocic activity and their appearance in amniotic fluid and blood at the onset of labor.[65–67] In studies of sheep, Liggins and associates[82] found a rise in prostaglandin $F_2\alpha$ in uterine venous blood shortly before the onset of labor. They observed a similar rise after the administration of estrogen. The production of prostaglandins may also occur in response to myometrial stretch with increasing uterine volume in late pregnancy. Kloeck and Jung[69] reported that stretch of in vitro myometrial strips influenced their release of prostaglandins. During spontaneous activity, the muscle strips released small quantities of prostaglandins E and F, but after stretching, there was an increase of prostaglandin E and a decrease of prostaglandin F. The effect of uterine volume on myometrial activity was studied by Csapo and associates,[39] who observed increased uterine activity after addition of 150 ml of isotonic solution to the amniotic fluid of patients at term.

Unesterified arachidonic acid is the obligatory precursor for the synthesis of prostaglandin $F_2\alpha$. MacDonald and associates,[86] utilizing a series of patients requesting abortion, demonstrated that intra-amniotic injection of arachidonate consistently triggered labor. From several recent studies, there is evidence that arachidonic acid is stored in fetal membranes and decidua in its esterified inactive form as glycerophospholipids.[4, 55, 68, 86, 109, 110] Progesterone serves to stabilize lysosomal phospholipase A_2, located in fetal membranes and/or decidua. With progesterone withdrawal, phospholipase A_2 is released and in turn catalyzes the hydrolysis of phospholipids, releasing unesterified arachidonate. Liberated arachidonic acid serves as the precursor of prostaglandin formation in the decidua. Vane[123] described the ability of certain nonsteroidal anti-inflammatory drugs, including aspirin and indomethacin, to block the biosynthesis of prostaglandins by their inhibitory effect on the prostaglandin synthetase enzyme system. In subsequent studies, several of these aspirin-like drugs were shown to be capable of delaying the onset of labor.[2, 38, 96, 131] The oxytocic effects of prostaglandins are probably mediated through alterations of myometrial cell calcium flux. Carsten[28, 29] reported that prostaglandins inhibit the ATP-dependent sequestration of calcium by sarcoplasmic reticulum, leading to an increase of intracellular free calcium.

Although its pathogenesis is often obscure, there are a number of specific and general clinical factors related to preterm onset of labor. Of these, socioeconomic deprivation is by far the most common. In this circumstance, it is likely that the complex mechanism of labor onset is prematurely triggered through the influence of inadequate nutrition, infection of the genitourinary tract, life-stress factors or the effects of reproductive excess. Some of these factors may act by influencing the delicate enzymatic mechanism related to pregnancy maintenance. The clinical conditions most often identified with preterm labor include urinary tract infection, hypertensive disease, multiple pregnancy and situations which distort the shape of the uterine cavity, such as placenta previa, uterine anomalies and uterine fibroids. The resultant crowding of intrauterine contents may trigger a fetal response to stress or produce excessive myometrial stretch. Goodlin and associates[53] reported a higher incidence of preterm labor in patients who achieve sexual orgasm during pregnancy. Perhaps it is significant that prostaglandin has been implicated in the mechanism of orgasm. Premature labor is also more common in sexually active patients, where it may be triggered in part by the oxytocic activity of prostaglandins in male seminal fluid. Despite our awareness of these clinical relationships, there is very little evidence that the current concept of optimal prenatal care, if extended to all patients, would significantly reduce the incidence of preterm labor. A more promising outcome could be expected from a general upgrading of socioeconomic standards.

The initial management of preterm labor should involve a judgment based on the clinical circumstances for either supportive care or active intervention. From our current understanding of the mechanisms of labor onset, it becomes obvious that fetal factors may serve to trigger labor. If labor is inhibited without correcting these factors, the fetus may be doomed to intrauterine death. For example, at present it is inappropriate to attempt inhibition of preterm labor associated with intrauterine infection, abruptio placenta or chronic fetal distress. However, a patient developing premature labor with evidence of a urinary tract infection may benefit from inhibition of labor to permit specific therapy of the infection. The clinical experience of many has indicated that inhibition of labor is generally ineffective when cervical effacement is advanced, or dilatation is beyond 4 cm. Evidence is mixed regarding the advisability of inhibiting premature labor associated with premature rupture of membranes. Delay presents the growing danger of intrauterine infection but the opportunity for advancement of fetal lung maturation, whereas failure to postpone labor may result in neonatal death due to pulmonary immaturity. Liggins and Howie[83] found evidence of improved neonatal pulmonary maturation after maternal administration of corticosteroids. In their studies, treatment with betamethasone was facilitated by delaying labor by the intravenous infusion of ethanol or salbutamol. In the group of infants under 32 weeks of gestation, the incidence of respiratory distress syndrome was 11.8% when treated for at least 24 hr prior to delivery, contrasted with 69.6% in those who did not receive betamethasone. Despite the promising results of this study and subsequent clinical experience, there is not yet adequate evidence to prove the long term benefit and safety of corticosteroids administered during labor.

The diagnosis of preterm labor is frequently impaired by the inherent difficulty in recognizing progressive labor versus other labor-like uterine activity. Many patients initially considered in labor will eventually be diagnosed as having false labor. A number of studies have established that bed rest, especially in the lateral position, serves to improve uterine blood flow and relax the uterus.[16, 26, 57] Thus, in a patient admitted for management of preterm labor, contractions may subside because she is placed in bed for observation. Also, the diagnosis of preterm labor is often confused by uncertainty over the question of pregnancy, or by inaccurate estimation of fetal weight. Zlatnik[129] reviewed the experience during a study of the efficacy of ethanol to inhibit preterm labor. Only 31 of 191 patients who delivered infants weighing less than 2,500 g were entered into the study. Of the 160 excluded from study 31% was due to error in judgment of fetal weight, 28% due to ruptured membranes, and 18% due to imminent delivery at the time of admission.

Until recently, the management of preterm labor consisted of bed rest, supportive care and a variety of nonspecific measures of questionable efficacy, generally based on anecdotal evidence. Of these approaches, the most common probably was the use of sedatives or, more recently, of tranquilizers. Although the influence of psychic factors on mechanisms of labor are poorly understood, there is no evidence that these agents inhibit established labor, and there is growing evidence that they have potentially adverse effects on the neonate. Neuromuscular agents such as magnesium sulfate,[56, 72] amyl nitrite[73] and succinylcholine[61] will in some circumstances relax myometrium, but none has proven effective for inhibition of preterm labor. As discussed earlier, the traditional concepts of hormonal control of uterine activity, derived from observations in various animals, prompted many investigators to examine the effect of progesterone on human labor. In most studies[36, 103, 127, 132] administration of progesterone failed to inhibit labor; however, Bengtsson[13] reported temporary inhibition of labor when progesterone was injected directly into the myometrium. Scommegna and associates[111] observed that the intravenous infusion of pregnenolone, the immediate precursor of placental progesterone, partially inhibited human labor. From the same group of investigators, Bieniarz and associates[14] reported that the relaxing effect of intravenous pregnenolone was enhanced by simultaneous infusion of ethanol and additional intravenous fluids. Until its recent withdrawal from clinical availability in the United States, lututrin, an aqueous extract of sow corpus luteum, was another hormonal substance widely used in treatment of threatened premature labor. The only reported studies of this substance failed to employ adequate controls to establish its efficacy.[87, 105, 106]

The use of catecholamine-like agents to influence uterine activity was suggested as early as 1928 when Bourne and Burn[20] reported that intravenous injection of epinephrine during labor inhibited uterine activity. In contrast, Brown and Wilder[24] reported that intravenous epinephrine stimulated uterine activity. This apparent disparity in results of similar experiments was resolved when in 1948, Ahlquist[1] reported on evidence that the action of sympathomimetic amines on smooth muscle is mediated through two sets of receptors, the "alpha" and the "beta." Uterine relaxation is mediated via beta receptor stimulation, whereas alpha receptor stimulation results in increased uterine activity. Subsequent studies revealed that the uterine response to epinephrine was dose dependent, with lower doses producing relaxation and higher doses stimulating activity.[63, 125, 134] It was also noted that a rebound excitatory response often occurred after stopping the intravenous infusion of epinephrine.[50, 134] Subsequently, Sutherland and associates[118] clarified the nature of the beta-adrenergic receptor. First, messenger hormones, such as epinephrine, interact with the target cell membrane to release adenyl cyclase within the cell.[107] Adenyl cyclase catalyzes the intracellular formation of adenosine 3′,5′-monophosphate, which serves as a second messenger to trigger the cellular action, which in this case is myometrial cell relaxation. Although epinephrine will inhibit labor, it lacks specificity for uterine beta receptors, so its cardiovascular side effects limit clinical applicability.

With further understanding of the nature of the mechanism of myometrial cell response to sympathomimetic amines, a search developed for a compound capable of inhibiting labor without producing unacceptable side effects. In 1960, Lish and associates[85] reported on the uterine-relaxing effects of isoxsuprine hydrochloride in experimental animals. Evidence suggested that isoxsuprine had a favorable balance of myometrial versus cardiovascular activity. In 1961, Bishop and Woutersz[17] reported their experience with isoxsuprine in human labor. Of 120 patients in preterm labor, 87% were delayed for more than 24 hr by administration of isoxsuprine by initial intravenous infusion, followed by intramuscular or oral doses for 1 week. However, in 10 term labor patients, they found virtually no effect of isoxsuprine on uterine activity, but observed hypotension when the dose was increased to more than 0.5 mg per min. Hendricks and associates[58] reported that isoxsuprine inhibited both spontaneous and oxytocin-induced uterine activity. Das,[41] in India, reported on treatment of 50 patients in preterm labor in a controlled study of isoxsuprine versus bed rest and sedatives. Labor was successfully delayed in 72% of the isoxsuprine group, and in only 25% of the controls. Castren and associates[30] reported on a comparative study of 194 patients in premature labor treated with isoxsuprine, ethanol, nylidrin or placebo. Nylidrin is a beta-sympathomimetic agent with a structural formula similar to isoxsuprine and ritodrine. It is not currently available for study in the United

States. When success of treatment was defined as birth weight over 2500 g, it was achieved in 86, 75, 70 and 71% of the nylidrin, isoxsuprine, ethanol and placebo groups, respectively. However, when considering patients who were delayed for at least 7 days, success was achieved in 73, 77, 62 and 56%, respectively. The investigators concluded that ethanol was no more successful than placebo.

From the experience to date, the optimal dosage of isoxsuprine hydrochloride in treatment of preterm labor is 0.25 to 0.5 mg per min, intravenously, adjusted downward or stopped on a basis of side effects. The infusion is stopped and considered a treatment failure if labor-like activity persists beyond 1 hr. The most common side effects are restlessness and palpitations. From earlier reports, it became evident that up to 10% of patients became hypotensive during the infusion.[58, 64, 116] With hypotension, there frequently was evidence of fetal distress. It is now evident that this effect is infrequent if the patient is maintained in the lateral rather than the supine position. If successful, the infusion is maintained for 8 to 12 hr, and then followed with intramuscular or oral administration of 5 to 20 mg of isoxsuprine hydrochloride every 3 to 6 hr, with the dosage schedule directed by uterine sensitivity and side effects. The intravenous infusion is repeated if labor recurs during the intramuscular or oral drug treatment. There is no concensus on the optimal length of oral drug therapy, but it should be continued at least until the patient has resumed moderate physical activity. There is no evidence that treatment with isoxsuprine, or other beta-sympathomimetic agents, is associated with subsequent prolonged pregnancy, abnormal labor, postpartum uterine atony or neonatal abnormalities.

Despite the apparent efficacy of isoxsuprine in treatment of preterm labor, others have found little evidence that its prophylactic administration during pregnancy will decrease the incidence of preterm labor. Briscoe[23] reported no significant difference in the incidence of low birth infants of 1165 patients who took either isoxsuprine, 10 mg orally four times a day, or a similar appearing placebo, throughout much of their pregnancies. Mathews and associates[89] found no significant differences in outcome of 103 patients with current multiple pregnancy or a previous preterm labor when treated with either isoxsuprine, 30 mg orally four times a day, or a similar appearing placebo.

Ritodrine hydrochloride is another sympathomimetic amine, which was specifically synthesized for its uterine-relaxing effects. From studies in animals and humans, it became evident that ritodrine was a potent uterine relaxant with fewer cardiovascular effects than most related agents.[49, 77] In 1971, Wesselius-de Casparis and coauthors[126] reported the results of a double blind, placebo-controlled study of ritodrine in human preterm labor. In a series of 81 patients, preterm labor was delayed for at least 7 days in 80% of the patients receiving ritodrine, and in 48% of the placebo group. Maternal side effects were few and mild, and there were no apparent fetal side effects. From these and other studies has emerged a favorable commentary on the safety and efficacy of ritodrine for inhibition of preterm labor.[11, 15, 95] It is likely that it will soon become clinically available in the United States.

Another of these agents is orciprenaline, which has been widely used in Europe and South America, but currently is not available in the United States. Baillie and associates[10] reported successful delay of labor to beyond 36 weeks of gestation in two-thirds of a series of preterm labor patients receiving an infusion of orciprenaline. Side effects were similar to those of isoxsuprine from other reports. Zilianti and Aller[128] studied orciprenaline in 13 patients in term labor. Contractions were effectively inhibited, but maternal cardiovascular effects, which included marked tachycardia and sinus arrhythmia, required discontinuance of the drug in four cases. Belizan and associates[12] studied orciprenaline in a series of 15 patients in labor at term. They concluded that an intravenous infusion of 10 to 20 mg per min effectively inhibited uterine contractions, with few cardiovascular effects.

Salbutamol, another beta-adrenergic

agent, has been studied predominantly in Great Britain, New Zealand and Australia. Korda and associates[70] studied salbutamol in the treatment of preterm labor in 53 patients. Despite ruptured membranes in 16, labor was delayed for more than 24 hr in 95%, and for more than 7 days in 51%. Several reports from Sweden suggested that terbutaline, another of these agents, has a favorable balance of uterine to cardiovascular effects.[3, 7, 8] It is capable of producing uterine relaxation with little effect on maternal heart rate. There have been no reports of its use in treatment of preterm labor. Berotec is closely related to orciprenaline, but is more potent and may have greater specificity for uterine smooth muscle. Lauersen and associates[79] reported that it effectively reduced uterine activity in pregnant baboons, but it also had considerable cardiovascular effects. During the search for the best of these agents, it has become apparent that there are at least two populations of beta-adrenergic receptors. The $beta_1$ receptors of cardiac muscle are distinct from the $beta_2$ receptors of uterine and bronchial smooth muscle. At present, the pharmacologic search continues for a specific $beta_2$ receptor acting agent.

The first clinical studies of intravenous ethanol treatment of preterm labor were reported by Fuchs and associates[48] in 1967. Encouraging results prompted the controlled study subsequently reported by Zlatnik and Fuchs.[130] A series of 42 patients in preterm labor, with intact membranes and no active uterine bleeding, were given either intravenous ethanol or 5% glucose solution. Labor was considered successfully delayed when delivery did not occur within 72 hr. Success was achieved in 81% of the ethanol-treated group and 38% of the glucose solution-treated group. The dosage schedule subsequently recommended consists of 7.5 ml of a 9.5% ethanol solution per kg of body weight per hr, intravenously, for 2 hr as a loading dose, and then 1.5 ml per kg body weight per hr for 10 hr or more.[133] In contrast, Graft[54] continued the maintainence dose for only 1 hr after contractions ceased, and all but 1 of 20 patients delivered within 3 days.

The most common maternal side effects of intravenous ethanol are nausea, vomiting, headache and restlessness. Animal studies have revealed decreased uterine blood flow and fetal asphyxia during intravenous ethanol administration.[42, 59, 88] However, from experience in humans, there is no evidence of adverse effects on the fetus or neonate of ethanol infusion during labor. Wagner and associates[124] reported that intravenous infusion of ethanol to six low birth weight infants produced no change in acid-base status, vital signs or psychomotor state. Generally, the treatment of preterm labor with intravenous ethanol has proven clinical efficacy and is free of serious side effects.

In 1971, Vane[123] reported that aspirin and other nonsteroidal, anti-inflammatory agents block prostaglandin production in rabbit lung preparations by interfering with their synthesis from arachidonic acid. From in vitro studies, Csapo and Csapo[37] reported that these agents inhibit myometrial activity, which may then be restored by addition of prostaglandin, but not by oxytocin. Thus, evidence suggests the obligatory presence of prostaglandin for the development of myometrial activity. From animal studies, other investigators reported that the spontaneous onset of labor could be delayed by pretreatment with aspirin, indomethacin or naproxen.[2, 38, 96] Dunn and associates[44] reported a similar delay in onset of labor in rats produced by intraperitoneal administration of prostaglandin $F_{2\alpha}$ antibody. Lewis and Schulman[80] reported that human labor was delayed and somewhat longer in a series of patients who had taken large doses of aspirin during pregnancy. Zuckerman and associates[131] reported successful inhibition of preterm labor in 40 of 50 patients given large doses of indomethacin. Despite these promising results, other evidence suggest the potential danger of these agents. In 1969, Archilla and associates[9] reported on evidence of closure of the ductus arteriosus before birth of an infant exposed to salicylates in late pregnancy. More recently, Rudolph[108] reported on growing evidence from animals and humans that aspirin and related compounds promote closure of the fetal ductus arteriosus, and that this effect is reversed by prostaglandins. Many additional studies will be necessary to establish the potential efficacy and safety of these agents in the management of preterm labor.

Diazoxide, an antihypertensive benzothiadiazine, was introduced as an antihypertensive compound, but was also found to possess smooth muscle relaxing properties.[18] Landesman and associates reported that diazoxide relaxed human myometrium in vitro,[76] and inhibited contractions of human labor at term.[75] It is also known to suppress insulin and elevate blood glucose.[18] There have been no reported studies of diazoxide treatment of preterm labor.

Aminophyllin, a methylxanthine derivative, is capable of relaxing myometrium by inhibition of the metabolic degradation of intracellular adenosine 3′,5′-monophosphate. Countinho and Vieira-Lopes[33] reported that aminophylline relaxed uterine motility in nonpregnant subjects. It has not been evaluated in the management of preterm labor.

The search for the optimal agent for treatment of preterm labor has lead to several other potential clinical applications of some of these drugs. Caldeyro-Barcia and associates[25] reported on successful use of orciprenaline to inhibit labors associated with fetal distress. After inhibition of contractions, fetal distress resolved to permit subsequent delivery by cesarean section of infants in good condition. In contrast, Zilianti and Aller[128] reported a similar case of fetal distress in which the situation further deteriorated after administration of orciprenaline. Humphrey and associates[60] reported that an infusion of ritodrine obviated the usual development of fetal respiratory acidosis in late labor. Brettes and associates,[22] using a thermistor probe implanted in the cervix to estimate uterine blood flow, found that it increased during the intravenous infusion of ritodrine in pregnancies complicated by intrauterine growth retardation and/or maternal hypertension, but found no significant changes in normal pregnancies. Miller and coworkers[92] studied the maternal and fetal responses to the infusion of ritodrine in 25 patients in labor with evidence of toxemia. After the infusion, maternal and fetal pH decreased, base deficit increased, PO_2 and PCO_2 remained stable and blood glucose rose. The disparity of results in some of these studies may be due to the variety of mechanisms producing fetal distress which are not necessarily reversed by uterine relaxation or the cardiovascular effects of these agents. The use of sympathomimetic amines as an approach to treatment of fetal distress clearly deserves further evaluation.

The administration of sympathomimetic amines in late pregnancy may serve to mimic the adrenal response to stress which may be beneficial for the fetus. There is considerable evidence that fetal lung maturation is advanced when pregnancy is chronically stressed by conditions such as maternal hypertension, drug addiction, malnutrition or premature rupture of membranes. Boog and associates[19] reported significantly less respiratory distress syndrome in a group of infants exposed to ritodrine hydrochloride in late pregnancy than in infants of similar weight who did not receive the drug. By improving uteroplacental blood flow, these agents may also prove useful in management of pregnancies at risk of fetal growth retardation, such as multiple pregnancies or pregnancies complicated by maternal hypertensive disorders. Further studies may also establish the role of tocolytic agents in preventing preterm labor after cervical cerclage procedures, to facilitate intrauterine operative procedures during pregnancy or to relax excessive uterine activity rapidly during labor.

The successful management of preterm labor with uterine relaxing agents must be premised on appropriate selection of patients who will benefit from the treatment. It is now apparent that events related to fetal compromise serve as one of several mechanisms triggering labor onset. Thus, unless the drug therapy improves the intrauterine environment, as well as inhibiting contractions, it may only serve to block the natural escape mechanism for the fetus. The role of infection, nutrition, drugs and even physical stimuli in the initiation of preterm labor remains poorly understood. Further studies are needed to elucidate the intrauterine environment before it serves to precipitate untimely clinical labor.

At present, the most widely employed agents for control of preterm labor in the

United States are ethanol and isoxsuprine hydrochloride. Neither of these agents has received approval of the Federal Drug Administration for inhibition of preterm labor; however, widespread clinical experience has indicated that each is relatively effective and reasonably safe. Indomethacin is also unapproved for treatment of preterm labor. Its recent popularity in prophylaxis or treatment of preterm labor is of considerable concern, for its safety has not been established by appropriate studies. Several of the newer sympathomimetic amines, which are not yet clinically available, may have greater efficacy and safety than isoxsuprine. Of these, only ritodrine is currently undergoing investigative trials in the United States. Merkatz and associates[91] recently reported the results of a comparative study of ethanol and ritodrine in treatment of 135 preterm labor patients. Labor was delayed for at least 72 hr in 73% of those receiving ethanol versus 90% of the ritodrine group. Furthermore, 54% and 72% of the ethanol and ritodrine groups, respectively, were delayed to term. In the future, a further understanding of the mechanism of labor will certainly lead to more effective and safer methods of preventing and/or treating preterm labor.

REFERENCES

1. Ahlquist, R. P.: A study of the adrenotropic receptors. Am J Physiol 153: 586, 1948.
2. Aiken, J. W.: Aspirin and indomethacin prolong parturition in rats: Evidence that prostaglandins contribute to expulsion of foetus. Nature 240: 21, 1972.
3. Akerlund, M., Andersson, K. E.: Effects of terbutaline on human myometrial activity and endometrial blood flow. Obstet Gynecol 47: 529, 1976.
4. Akesson, G., Gustavii, B.: Occurrence of phospholipase A_1 and A_2 in human decidua. Prostaglandins 9: 667, 1975.
5. Anderson, A. B., Flint, A. P., Turnbull, A. C.: Mechanism of action of glucocorticoids in induction of ovine parturition: Effect on placental steroid metabolism. J Endocrinol, 66: 61, 1975.
6. Anderson, A. B., Pierrepoint, C. G., Griffiths, K., Turnbull, A. C.: Steroid metabolism in the adrenals of fetal sheep in relation to natural and corticotrophin-induced parturition. J Repr Fertil (Suppl) 16: 25, 1972.
7. Andersson, K. E., Bengtsson, L. P., Gustafson, I., Ingemarsson, I.: The relaxing effect of terbutaline on the human uterus during term labor. Am J Obstet Gynecol 121: 602, 1975.
8. Andersson, K. E., Ingemarsson, I., Persson, C. G. A.: Effects of terbutaline on human uterine motility at term. Acta Obstet Gynecol Scand 54: 165, 1975.
9. Arcilla, R. A., Thilenius, O. G., Ranniger, K.: Congestive heart failure from suspected ductal closure in utero. J Pediatr 75: 74, 1969.
10. Baillie, P., Meehan, F. P., Tyack, A. J.: Treatment of premature labour with orciprenaline. Br Med J 4: 154, 1970.
11. Barden, T. P.: Effect of ritodrine on human uterine motility and cardiovascular responses in term labor and the early postpartum state. Am J Obstet Gynecol 112: 645, 1972.
12. Belizan, J. M., Diaz, A. G., Abuslene, C., Poseiro, J. J., Caldeyro-Barcia, R.: Effects of orciprenaline on uterine contractility and maternal heart rate. Obstet Gynecol 46: 385, 1975.
13. Bengtsson, L. P.: Experiments on the suppressive effect of a synthetic gestogen on the activity of the pregnant human uterus. Acta Obstet Gynecol Scand 41: 124, 1962.
14. Bieniarz, J., Burd, L., Motew, M., Scommegna, A., Lin, S., Wineman, C., Seals, C.: Inhibition of uterine contractility in labor. Am J Obstet Gynecol 111: 874, 1971.
15. Bieniarz, J., Motew, M., Scommegna, A.: Uterine and cardiovascular effects of ritodrine in premature labor. Obstet Gynecol 40: 65, 1972.
16. Bieniarz, J., Crottogini, J. J., Curuchet, E., Romero-Salinas, G., Yoshida, T., Poseiro, J. J., Caldeyro-Barcis, R.: Aortocaval compression by the uterus in late human pregnancy. II. An arteriographic study. Am J Obstet Gynecol 100: 203, 1968.
17. Bishop, E. H., Woutersz, T. B: Isoxsuprine, a myometrial relaxant, a preliminary report. Obstet Gynecol 17: 442, 1961.
18. Blackard, W. G., Aprill, C. N.: Mechanism of action of diazoxide. J Lab Clin Med 69: 960, 1967.
19. Boog, G., Ben Brahim, M., Gaudar, R.: Betamimetic drugs and possible prevention of respiratory distress syndrome. Br J Obstet Gynecol 82: 285, 1975.
20. Bourne, A., Burn, J. H.: The dosage and action of pituitary extract and of the ergot alkaloids on the uterus in labor, with a note on the action of adrenalin. J Obstet Gynaecol Br Emp 34: 249, 1927.
21. Brenner, W. E., Hendricks, C. H.: Effect of medroxyprogesterone acetate upon the duration and characteristics of human gestation and labor. Am J Obstet Gynecol 82: 1094, 1962.
22. Brettes, J. P., Renaud, R., Gaudar, R.: A double-blind investigation into the effects of ritodrine on uterine blood flow during the third trimester of pregnancy. Am J Obstet Gynecol 124: 164, 1976.
23. Briscoe, C. C.: Failure of oral isoxsuprine to prevent prematurity. Am J Obstet Gynecol 94: 885, 1966.
24. Brown, W. E., Wilder, V. M.: The response of the human uterus to epinephrine. Am J Obstet Gynecol 54: 659, 1943.

25. Caldeyro-Barcia, R., Magana, J. M., Castillo, J. B., Poseiro, J. J., Mendez-Bauer, C., Pose, S. V., Escarcena, L., Casacuberta, C., Bustos, J. R., Giussi, G.: A new approach to the treatment of acute intrapartum fetal distress. *Perinatal Factors Affecting Human Dvelopment.* Washington, D.C., Pan American Health Organization, 1969, p 248.
26. Caldeyro-Barcia, R., Noriega-Guerra, L., Cibils, L. A., Alvarez, H., Poseiro, J. J., Pose, S. V., Sica-Blanco, Y., Mendez-Bauer, C., Fielitz, C., Gonzalez-Panizza, V. H.: Effect of position changes on the intensity and frequency of uterine contractions during labor. Am J Obstet Gynecol 80: 284, 1960.
27. Caldeyro-Barcia, R., Sereno, J. A.: The response of the human uterus to oxytocin throughout pregnancy. *Oxytocin.* Edited by R. Caldeyro-Barcia, H. Heller, New York, Pergamon Press, 1971, pp 177–202.
28. Carsten, M. E.: Prostaglandins and cellular calcium transport in the pregnant human uterus. Am J Obstet Gynecol 117: 824, 1973.
29. Carsten, M. E.: Prostaglandins and oxytocin: Their effects on uterine smooth muscle. Prostaglandins 5: 33, 1974.
30. Castren, O., Gummervs, M., Saarikoski, S.: Treatment of imminent premature labor. Acta Obstet Gynecol Scand 54: 95, 1975.
31. Cawson, M. J., Anderson, A. B. M., Turnbull, A. C., Lampe, L.: Cortisol, cortisone, and 11-deoxycortisol levels in human umbilical and maternal plasma in relation to the onset of labour. J Obstet Gynaecol Br Commonw 81: 737, 1974.
32. Chard, T., Hudson, C. N., Edwards, C. R. W., Boyd, N. R. H.: Release of oxytocin and vasopressin by the human foetus during labour. Nature 234: 352, 1971.
33. Coutinho, E. M., Vieira-Lopes, A. C.: Inhibition of uterine motility by aminophylline. Am J Obstet Gynecol 110: 726, 1971.
34. Csapo, A.: Defence mechanism of pregnancy. Ciba Foundation Study Groups: Progesterone and the Defence Mechanism of Pregnancy. Boston, Little, Brown, and Company, 1961.
35. Csapo, A.: Progesterone "block." Am J Anat 98: 273, 1956.
36. Csapo, A., de Sousa, F., de Sousa, J. C., de Sousa, O.: Effect of massive progestational hormone treatment on the parturient human uterus. Fertil Steril 17: 621, 1966.
37. Csapo, A. I., Csapo, E. E.: The "prostaglandin step," a bottleneck in the activation of the uterus. Life Sci 14: 719, 1974.
38. Csapo, A. I., Csapo, E. E., Fay, E., Henzl, M. R., Salau, G.: The delay of spontaneous labor by naproxen in the rat model. Prostaglandins 3: 827, 1973.
39. Csapo, A. I., Jaffin, H., Kerenyi, T., Lipman, J. I., Wood, C.: Volume and activity of the pregnant human uterus. Am J Obstet Gynecol 85: 819, 1963.
40. Csapo, A. I., Kuobil, E., Pulkkinen, M., van der Molen, H. J., Sommerville, I. F., Wiest, W. G.: Progesterone withdrawal during hypertonic saline-induced abortions. Am J Obstet Gynecol 105: 1132, 1969.
41. Das, R. K.: Isoxsuprine in premature labor. J Obstet Gynaecol India 19: 566, 1969.
42. Dilts, P. V.: Effect of ethanol on uterine and umbilical hemodynamics and oxygen transfer. Am J Obstet Gynecol 108: 221, 1970.
43. Drost, M., Holm, L. W.: Prolonged gestation in ewes after foetal adrenalectomy. J Endocrinol 40: 293, 1968.
44. Dunn, M. V., Humphries, N. G., Judkins, G. R., Kendall, J. Z., Knight, G. W.: The effect of prostaglandin $F_2\alpha$ antibody on gestation length in the rat. Prostaglandins 3: 509, 1973.
45. Ferguson, J. K. W.: A study of the motility of the intact uterus at term. Surg Gynecol Obstet 73: 359, 1941.
46. Fuchs, A. R.: The inhibitory effect of ethanol on the release of oxytocin during parturition in the rabbit. J Endocrinol 35: 125, 1966.
47. Fuchs, A., Coutinho, E. M., Xavier, R., Bates, P. E., Fuchs, F.: Effect of ethanol on the activity of the nonpregnant human uterus and its reactivity to neurohypophyseal hormones. Am J Obstet Gynecol 101: 997, 1968.
48. Fuchs, F., Fuchs, A. R., Poblete, V. F., Jr., Risk, A.: Effect of alcohol on threatened premature labor. Am J Obstet Gynecol 99: 627, 1967.
49. Gamissans, O., Esteban-Altirriba, J., Maiques, V.: Inhibition of human myometrial activity by a new β-adrenergic drug (DU21220). J Obstet Gynaecol Br Commonw 76: 656, 1969.
50. Garrett, W. J.: The effects of adrenaline and noradrenaline on the intact human uterus in late pregnancy and labour. J Obstet Gynaecol Br Emp 61: 586, 1954.
51. Gennser, G., Ohrlander, S., Enerath, P.: Cortisol in amniotic fluid and cord blood in relation to prenatal betamethasone load and delivery. Am J Obstet Gynecol 124: 43, 1976.
52. Goldkraud, J. W., Schulte, R. L., Messer, R. H.: Maternal and fetal plasma cortisol levels at parturition. Obstet Gynecol 47: 41, 1976.
53. Goodlin, R. C., Keller, D. W., Raffin, M.: Orgasm during late pregnancy. Obstet Gynecol 38: 916, 1971.
54. Graff, G.: Failure to prevent premature labor with ethanol. Am J Obstet Gynecol 110: 878, 1971.
55. Gustavvi, B.: Release of lysosomal acid phosphatase into the cytoplasm of decidual cells before the onset of labor in humans. Br J Obstet Gynaecol 82: 177, 1975.
56. Harbert, G. M., Cornell, G. W., Thornton, W. N., Jr.: Effect of toxemia therapy on uterine dynamics. Am J Obstet Gynecol 105: 94, 1969.
57. Hendricks, C. H.: The hemodynamics of a uterine contraction. Am J Obstet Gynecol 76: 969, 1958.
58. Hendricks, C. H., Cibils, L. A., Pose, S. V., Eskes, T. K. A. B.: The pharmacologic control of excessive uterine activity with isozsuprine. Am J Obstet Gynecol 82: 1064, 1961.
59. Horiguchi, T., Suzuki, K., Comas-Urrutia, A. C., Mueller-Heubach, E., Boyer-Milic, A. M., Baratz, R. A., Morishima, H. O., James, L. S., Adamsons, K.: Effect of ethanol upon uterine

activity and fetal acid-base state of the rhesus monkey. Am J Obstet Gynecol 109: 910, 1971.
60. Humphrey, M., Cahng, A., Gilbert, M., Wood, C.: The effect of intravenous ritodrine on the acid-base status of the fetus during the second stage of labour. Br J Obstet Gynaecol 82: 234, 1975.
61. Iuppa, J. B., Smith, G. A., Colella, J. J., Gibson, J. L.: Succinylcholine effect on human myometrial activity. Obstet Gynecol 37: 591, 1971.
62. Johnson, J. W. C., Austin, K. L., Jones, G. S., Davis, G. H., King, T. M.: Efficacy of 17α-hydroxyprogesterone caproate in the prevention of premature labor. N Engl J Med 293: 675, 1975.
63. Kaiser, I. H.: The effect of epinephrine and norepinephrine on the contraction of the human uterus in labor. Surg Gynecol Obstet 90: 649, 1950.
64. Karim, M.: Isoxsuprine and the human parturient uterus. J Obstet Gynaecol Br Commonw 70: 992, 1963.
65. Karim, S. M. M.: Identification of prostaglandins in human amniotic fluid. J Obstet Gynaecol Br Commonw 73: 903, 1966.
66. Karim, S. M. M.: Appearance of prostaglandin $F_{2\alpha}$ in human blood during labour. Br Med J 4: 618, 1968.
67. Karim, S. M. M., Devlin, J.: Prostaglandin content of amniotic fluid during pregnancy and labor. J Obstet Gynaecol Br Commonw 74: 230, 1967.
68. Keirse, M. M. N. C., Turnbull, A. C.: Metabolism of prostaglandins within the pregnant uterus. Br J Obstet Gynaecol 82: 887, 1975.
69. Kloeck, F. K., Jung, H.: In vitro release of prostaglandins from the human myometrium under the influence of stretching. Am J Obstet Gynecol 15: 1066, 1973.
70. Korda, A. R., Lyneham, R. C., Jones, W. R.: The treatment of premature labour with intravenously administered salbutamol. Med J Austr 1: 744, 1974.
71. Kumar, D., Goodno, J. A., Barnes, A. C.: Isolation of progesterone from human pregnant myometrium. Nature (London) 195: 1204, 1962.
72. Kumar, D., Zourlas, P. A., Barnes, A. C.: In vitro and in vivo effects of magnesium sulfate on human uterine contractility. Am J Obstet Gynecol 86: 036, 1963.
73. Kumar, D., Zourlas, P. A., Barnes, A. C.: In vivo effect of amyl nitrite on human pregnant uterine contractility. Am J Obstet Gynecol 91: 1066, 1965.
74. Kumaresan, P., Han, G. S., Anandarangam, P. B., Vasicka, A.: Oxytocin in maternal and fetal blood. Obstet Gynecol 46: 272, 1975.
75. Landesman, R., De Sonza, F., J. A., Coutinho, E. A., Wilson, K. H., de Sousa, F. M. B.: The inhibitory effect of diazoxide in normal term labor. Am J Obstet Gynecol 103: 430, 1969.
76. Landesman, R., Wilson, K. H.: The relaxant effect of diazoxide on isolated gravid and nongravid human myometrium. Am J Obstet Gynecol 101: 120, 1968.
77. Landesman, R., Wilson, K. H., Coutinho, E. M., Klima, I. M., Marcus, R. S.: The relaxant action of ritodrine, a sympathomimetic amine, on the uterus during term labor. Am J Obstet Gynecol 110: 111, 1971.
78. Lanman, J. T., Than, R., Brinson, A.: Monkey uterine vein and fetal progesterone level. Abstract 113, Program, Eighth Annual Meeting, Society for the Study of Reproduction, 1975.
79. Lauersen, N. H., Wilson, K. H., Fuchs, F.: The effect of berotec (Th1165a) on spontaneous and induced uterine activity in the pregnant baboon. Am J Obstet Gynecol 121: 597, 1975.
80. Lewis, R. B., Schulman, J. D.: Influence of acetylsalicylic acid, an inhibitor of prostaglandin synthesis, on duration of human gestation and labor. Lancet 2 (7839): 1159, 1973.
81. Liggins, G. C.: Premature delivery of foetal lambs infused with glucocorticoids. J Endocrinol 45: 515, 1969.
82. Liggins, G. C., Fairclough, R. J., Grieves, S. A., Kendall, J. Z., Knox, B. S.: The mechanism of initiation of parturition in the ewe. Recent Progr Hormone Res 29: 111, 1973.
83. Liggins, G. C., Howie, M. B.: A controlled trial of antepartum glucocorticoid treatment for prevention of the respiratory distress syndrome in premature infants. Pediatrics 50: 515, 1972.
84. Liggins, G. C., Kennedy, P. C., Holm, L. W.: Failure of initiation of parturition after electrocoagulation of the pituitary of the fetal lamb. Am J Obstet Gynecol 98: 1080, 1967.
85. Lish, P. M., Hillyard, I. W., Dungan, K. W.: The uterine relaxant properties of isoxsuprine. J Pharmacol Exp Ther 129: 438, 1960.
86. MacDonald, P. C., Schultz, F. M., Duenhoelter, J. H., Gant, N. F., Jimenez, J. M., Pritchard, J. A., Porter, J. C., Johnston, J. M.: Initiation of human parturition. I. Mechanism of action of arachidonic acid. Obstet Gynecol 44: 629, 1974.
87. Majewski, J. T., Jennings, T.: Further experiences with a uterine relaxing hormone in premature labor. Obstet Gynecol 9: 322, 1957.
88. Mann, L. I., Bhakthavathsalan, A., Liu, M., Makowski, P.: Placental transport of alcohol and its effect on maternal and fetal acid-base balance. Am J Obstet Gynecol 122: 837, 1975.
89. Mathews, D. D., Friend, J. B., Michael, C. A.: A double-blind trial of oral isoxsuprine in the prevention of premature labor. J Obstet Gynaecol Br Commonw 74: 68, 1967.
90. Mati, J. K. G., Horrobin, D. F., Bramley, P. S.: Induction of labour in sheep and humans by single doses of corticosteroids. Br Med J 2: 149, 1973.
91. Merkatz, I. R., Mann, L. I., Lauersen, N. H., Fuchs, F.: Comparison of ritodrine and ethanol in premature labor. Abstr Gynecol Invest 7: 21, 1976.
92. Miller, F. C., Nochimson, D. J., Paul, R. H., Hon, E. H.: Effects of ritodrine hydrochloride on uterine activity and the cardiovascular system in toxemic patients. Obstet Gynecol 47: 50, 1976.
93. Mueller-Heubach, E., Myers, R. D., Adam-

sons, K.: Effects of adrenalectomy on pregnancy length in the rhesus monkey. Am J Obstet Gynecol 112: 221, 1972.

94. Murphy, B. E. P.: Does the human fetal adrenal play a role in parturition? Am J Obstet Gynecol 115: 521, 1973.
95. Nochimson, D. J., Riffel, H. D., Yeh, S., Kreitzer, M. S., Paul, R. H., Hon, E. H.: The effects of ritodrine hydrochloride on uterine activity and the cardiovascular system. Am J Obstet Gynecol 118: 523, 1974.
96. Novy, M. J., Cook, M. J., Manaugh, L.: Indomethacin block of normal onset of parturition in primates. Am J Obstet Gynecol 118: 412, 1974.
97. Nwosu, U. C., Wallach, E. E., Boggs, T. R., Bongiovanni, A. M.: Possible adrenocorticol insufficiency in postmature neonates. Am J Obstet Gynecol 112: 969, 1976 (b).
98. Nwosu, U. C., Wallach, E. E., Boggs, T. R., Nemiroff, R. L., Bongiovanni, A. M.: Possible role of the fetal adrenal glands in the etiology of postmaturity. Am J Obstet Gynecol 121: 366, 1975.
99. Nwosu, U. C., Wallach, E. E., Bolognese, R. J.: Initiation of labor by intra-amniotic cortisol instillation in prolonged human pregnancy. Obstet Gynecol 47: 137, 1976.
100. Nwosu, U. C., Wallach, E. E., Feldman, J. D., Bongiovanni, A. M.: Parturition-induced changes in maternal plasma cortisol levels. Obstet Gynecol 46: 263, 1975.
101. Pinto, R. M., Lerner, U., Mazzocco, N., Glauberman, M.: The oxytocic action of intra-amniotic estradiol-17_B on the pregnant human uterus. Am J Obstet Gynecol 94: 876, 1966.
102. Pinto, R. M., Votta, R. A., Montuori, E., Baleiron, H.: Action of estradiol 17_B on the activity of the pregnant human uterus. Am J Obstet Gynecol 88: 759, 1964.
103. Pose, S. V., Fielitz, C.: The effects of progesterone on the response of the pregnant human uterus to oxytocin. *Oxytocin*. Edited by R. Caldeyro-Barcia, H. Heller, Oxford, Pergamon Press, Inc. 1961, p 229.
104. Raja, R. L., Anderson, A. B. M., Turnbull, A. C.: Endocrine changes in premature labor. Br Med J 4: 67, 1974.
105. Rezek, G. H.: Lutrexin the treatment of premature labor. Ann NY Acad Sci 75: 995, 1959.
106. Rizzolo, E. A.: A uterine relaxant for premature uterine contractions. Clin Med 74: 53, 1967.
107. Robison, G. A., Butcher, R. W., Sutherland, E. W.: Cyclic AMP. Am Rev Biochem 37: 149, 1968.
108. Rudolph, A. M.: The effect of prostaglandins on fetal circulation. Presented at Symposium on Perinatal Medicine, Las Vegas, Nevada, April 1976.
109. Schultz, F. M., Schwarz, B. E., MacDonald, P. C., Johnston, J. M.: Initiation of human parturition. II. Identification of phospholipase A_2 in fetal chorioamnion and uterine decidua. Am J Obstet Gynecol 123: 650, 1975.
110. Schwarz, B. E., Schultz, F. M., MacDonald, P. C., Johnston, J. M.: Initiation of human parturition. III. Fetal membrane content of prostaglandin E_2 and F_2 and precursor. Obstet Gynecol 46: 564, 1975.
111. Scommegna, A., Burd, L., Goodman, C., Bieniarz, J., Seals, C.: The effect of pregnenolone sulfate on uterine contractility. Am J Obstet Gynecol 108: 1023, 1970.
112. Seppala, M., Aho, I.: Physiological role of meconium during delivery. Acta Obstet Gynecol Scand 54: 209, 1975.
113. Seppala, M., Aho, I., Tissari, A., Ruoslahti, E.: Radioimmunoassay of oxytocin in amniotic fluid, fetal urine, and meconium during late pregnancy and delivery. Am J Obstet Gynecol 114: 788, 1972.
114. Simmer, H. H., Tulchinsky, D., Gold, E. M., Frankland, M., Greipel, M., Gold, A. S.: On the regulation of estrogen production by cortisol and ACTH in human pregnancy at term. Am J Obstet Gynecol 119: 283, 1974.
115. Siiteri, P. K., MacDonald, P. C.: Placental estrogen biosynthesis during human pregnancy. J Clin Endocrinol 26: 751, 1966.
116. Stander, R. W., Barden, T. P., Thompson, J. F., Pugh, W. R., Werts, C. E.: Fetal cardiac effects of maternal isoxsuprine infusion. Am J Obstet Gynecol 89: 792, 1964.
117. Steele, P. A., Flint, A. P., Turnbull, A. C.: Proceedings: Evidence of steroid $C_{17,20}$ lyase activity in ovine foeto-placental tissue. J Endocrinol 64: 41P, 1975.
118. Sutherland, E. W., Rall, T. W.: The relation of adenosine-3′,5′-phosphate and phosphorylase to the actions of catecholamines and other hormones. Pharmacol Rev 12: 265, 1960.
119. Sybulski, S., Goldsmith, W. J., Maughan, G. B.: Cortisol levels in fetal scalp, maternal, and umbilical cord plasma. Obstet Gynecol 46: 268, 1975.
120. Sybulski, S., Maughan, G. B.: Cortisol levels in umbilical cord plasma in relation to labor and delivery. Am J Obstet Gynecol 125: 236, 1976.
121. Tuimala, R. J., Kauppila, A. J. I., Haapalahti, J.: Response of pituitary-adrenal axis on partal stress. Obstet Gynecol 46: 275, 1975.
122. Turnbull, A. C., Patten, P. T., Flint, A. P. F., Jeremy, J. Y., Keirse, M. J. N. C., Anderson, A. B. M.: Significant fall in progesterone and rise in oestradiol levels in human peripheral plasma before onset of labour. Lancet 1: 101, 1974.
123. Vane, J. R.: Inhibition of prostaglandin synthesis as a mechanism of action for aspirin-like drugs. Nature New Biol 231: 232, 1971.
124. Wagner, L., Wagner, G., Guerrero, J.: Effect of alcohol on premature newborn infants. Am J Obstet Gynecol 108: 308, 1970.
125. Wansbrough, H., Nakanishi, H., Wood, C.: Effect of epinephrine on human uterine activity in vitro and in vivo. Obstet Gynecol 30: 779, 1967.
126. Wesselius-de Casparis, A., Thiery, M., Yo Le Sian, A., Baumgarten, K., Brosens, I., Gamisans, O., Stolk, J. G., Vivier, W.: Results of

double-blind, multicentre study with ritodrine in premature labour. Br Med J 3: 144, 1971.
127. Wood, C., Elstein, M., Pinkerton, J. H. M.: The effect of progesterogens upon uterine activity. J Obstet Gynaecol Br Commonw 70: 839, 1963.
128. Zilianti, M., Aller, J.: Action of orciprenaline on uterine contractility during labour, maternal cardiovascular system, fetal heart rate, and acid-base balance. Am J Obstet Gynecol 109: 1073, 1971.
129. Zlatnik, F. J.: The applicability of labor inhibition to the problem of prematurity. Am J Obstet Gynecol 113: 704, 1972.
130. Zlatnik, F. J., Fuchs, F.: A controlled study of ethanol in threatened premature labor. Am J Obstet Gynecol 112: 610, 1972.
131. Zuckerman, H., Reiss, U., Rubinstein, I.: Inhibition of human premature labor by indomethacin. Obstet Gynecol 44: 787, 1974.
132. Zuspan, F. P., Coordinator, Progestational therapy during pregnancy; an invitational symposium. J Repr Med 3: 225, 1969.
133. Zuspan, F. P., Barden, T. P., Bieniarz, J., Cibils, L. A., Fuchs, F., Landesman, R., Mercer, J. P., Moawad, A. H., Pauerstein, C. J.: Premature labor: Its management and therapy. J Repr Med 9: 93, 1972.
134. Zuspan, F. P., Cibils, L. A., Pose, S. V.: Myometrial and cardiovascular responses to alterations in plasma epinephrine and norepinephrine. Am J Obstet Gynecol 84: 841, 1962.

JOHN L. SEVER, M.D., Ph.D.
DAVID A. FUCCILLO, Ph.D.

12

Perinatal Infections

Many viruses, protozoa and bacteria can cause birth defects, fetal disease or death. Recent data from the Collaborative Perinatal Project demonstrated that approximately 5% of all pregnancies are complicated by one or more reported clinical viral infections. Excluding the common cold, the most frequent infections were influenza or flulike illness, cold sores, herpes infections, viral gastroenteritis and viral pharyngeal pharyngitis tonsillitis. In addition, specific infections occurred at the rate of 1 to 18 per 10,000 pregnancies each for rubella, chickenpox, herpes zoster, viral bronchitis, measles, mumps, viral pneumonitis and infectious mononucleosis, warts and hepatitis.

The viruses which appear most important for man include cytomegalovirus, herpesvirus hominis, rubella, varicella, enteroviruses, Venezuelan equine encephalitis, dengue and possibly influenza and parainfluenza viruses. The bacterial infections of importance include syphilis, group B streptococcal infections, gram-negative sepsis and meningitis, pneumonia and gonorrhea. The sporozoan toxoplasmosis can also be an important cause of fetal infection and damage.

It is the purpose of this report to summarize the clinical and laboratory findings associated with perinatal infections and to indicate approaches to the management of these infectious diseases.

Virus Infections which Cause Malformations

Congenital infections which cause malformations in man include cytomegaloviruses, herpes simplex viruses, rubella, varicella and Venezuelan equine encephalitis viruses. Coxsackie B viruses have also been associated with congenital and neonatal infections.

CYTOMEGALOVIRUS

Cytomegaloviruses (CMV) are the most common cause of recognized congenital infections. Several serologic surveys in the United States have shown that approximately one-third to two-thirds of adult women have antibody to this group of closely related viruses.[26] In addition, CMV can be isolated from the cervix or urine of from 3 to 5% of pregnant women.[12] An increased number of infections are detected late in pregnancy. The great majority of infected women are asymptomatic. Occasionally, cervicitis and illness resembling infectious mononucleosis are caused by infection with these viruses. Infection can be documented by isolation of the virus from the urine or cervical area or by the development of antibody. The indirect hemagglutination test appears to be the most practical and reliable method for detecting antibody and seroconversions.[9]

Congenital infection occurs in 0.5 to 1.5% of births.[1] About 10% of these children exhibit permanent damage in the form of mental-motor retardation occasionally accompanied by microcephaly. Children with normal neurologic findings at 2 years of age generally have a good prognosis. The severe form of cytomegalic inclusion disease is relatively rare, occurring in 1 in 5,000 to 1 in 20,000 live births. Congenital infection can be documented by isolation of the virus from the nasopharynx and urine. Large, inclusion-containing cells may be present in the urine in approximately one-third of infected children. Elevated immunoglobulin M (IgM) levels (equal to or greater than 22 mg per 100 ml) are found in most infected newborns. Specific IgM cytomegalovirus antibody is present in the great majority of infected newborns.

Fetal infection apparently results from hematogenous spread from the mother. Damage to the brain includes direct tissue destruction with the formation of calcified areas. Similarly, chorioretinitis is associated with direct infection by the virus. Infected children shed the virus for many months and spread of infection from the baby to other members of the family has been well documented.

HERPES SIMPLEX

Two strains of herpes simplex virus (HSV) infect man. Type I generally infects the oral area and causes the common cold sore or fever blister.[21] Type II produces cervicitis and vaginitis and is though to be venerally transmitted. These strains differ in their antigenic and biologic properties. In a series of 28 cases of neonatal herpetic infection, 25 were found to be due to type II herpesvirus.[22]

Congenital infection with HSV may produce a syndrome which includes microcephaly, cerebral calcification, chorioretinitis and mental retardation.[29] If transplacental or transamniotic infection occurs near delivery, a spectrum of clinical disease in the newborn may range from a few cutaneous vesicles to a fatal generalized disease with jaundice, fever, hepatosplenomegaly, encephalitis, circulatory coagulation and death.[30]

The child with neonatal infection usually appears normal at birth, but symptoms of the disease develop during the first 3 weeks of age. This infection is usually acquired at birth by contact with the infection in the birth canal. The disease is manifested in three general forms: (*a*) vesicular lesions of the skin or throat with or without conjunctivitis (50% of cases exhibit these); (*b*) central nervous system involvement characterized by spinal fluid pleocytosis, elevated pressure and increased protein content (convulsions may also occur); (*c*) systemic disease manifested by hepatitis, jaundice, pulmonary disease, hemolytic anemia, petechiae, hepatomegaly and thrombocytopenia. The prognosis in children with localized vesicular lesions (and conjunctivitis) is good, although about 50% of them progress to more extensive disseminated infection. Systemic infection is fatal in over 90% of cases. Laboratory tests useful in the diagnosis of HSV infection are an elevation of IgM levels (equal to or greater than 22 mg per 100 ml) in the neonatal period or the presence of specific IgM HSV antibody. Virus can also be isolated from the lesions.

Chemotherapy for congenital infection using adenine arabinoside is under study. Preliminary reports suggest that some benefit may be achieved if the drug is started within the first few days after infection. Vaccines are not presently available but are being investigated. Delivery by cesarean section is recommended in order to avoid contact of the child with infected vaginal lesions, if these are found in a woman near term.

RUBELLA

Rubella is associated primarily with infections during the first trimester of pregnancy.[29] Infection during the second trimester, however, can result in infected and damaged infants. Severe congenital malformations and fetal damage occur in approximately 22% of babies following first trimester rubella and 6 to 10% following rubella in the 4th or 5th month of gestation.

The clinical findings for 14 children with congenital rubella who have been followed for 5 to 8 years are shown in Table 12.1. Deafness was the most frequent finding in these children. Other major damage due to the infection included congenital heart disease, microcephaly, hepatosplenomegaly, mental retardation and death. The high frequency of deafness and mental retardation in this group of patients was probably a reflection of the fact that these children have been kept under close observation for a number of years. Studies conducted only through the newborn period or the first

Table 12.1. Congenital rubella – clinical findings

	No. of cases
First trimester (11 cases)	
Deafness	9
Congenital heart disease	5
Microcephaly	4
Hepatosplenomegaly	3
Petechiae	3
Died	3
Mute	2
Low IQ	2
1 each: acute splenic tumor, conjunctivitis, spastic, cleft gum, cataract, inguinal hernia, retinopathy, high palate, abnormal facies, abnormal ears, jaundice	
Second trimester (3 cases)	
Deafness	2
Low IQ	2
1 each: delayed motor development, hernia, nystagmus, died, microcephaly	

few years of life have often failed to document the total damage due to rubella.

In the United States, approximately 10 to 15% of the women of child-bearing age are at risk for rubella infection. In the past, epidemics generally occurred at 7- to 10-year intervals. No major epidemic has occurred, however, since 1964. Local outbreaks are reported every spring.

The most useful laboratory test for the diagnosis of rubella is the hemagglutination inhibition method for antibody determination. With this method, susceptible individuals can be identified on the basis of absence of antibody and infection can be documented by the development of a seroconversion. Complement fixation tests are useful when the woman first consults a physician after the rash has appeared. In this case, the level of late appearing complement fixation antibody may still be increasing and thus a serioconversion can be documented by using the complement fixation method.

Most infected newborns have elevated IgM levels (equal to or greater than 22 mg per 100 ml) and rubella-specific IgM antibody.[28] In many cases rubella virus can be isolated from throat swabs for several months. The children are infectious and contact with pregnant women should be avoided.

Rubella virus is spread by the hematogenous route from the mother through the placenta to the fetus.[27] Maternal infection in the first trimester of pregnancy almost always results in placental infection. Only about one-third of the fetuses, however, show evidence of the virus. The virus in the fetus may be localized in one or a few organs, or it may be widely disseminated. Chronic infection of the fetus and child persists even in the presence of high titers of specific antibody. The shedding of virus, however, ceases in almost all infants at approximately 6 months to 1 year of age, suggesting that the immune status of the child is changed at this time. The nature of the immune deficiency which permits the chronic congenital infection is not known, but it may be related to absence of specific cellular immune responses.

Progressive rubella panencephalitis has been recognized as a rare late effect of congenital rubella. These children, in their second decade of life, show mental and motor deterioration, ataxia, sometimes myoclones and death. High rubella antibody titers are present in the serum and spinal fluid and the virus has been isolated from the brain of at least one child.

Rubella vaccines have now been administered to approximately 60,000,000 individuals in the United States. All of the vaccines produce a low incidence of side reactions, primarily arthritis and arthralgia, most marked in women of child-bearing age. All children and susceptible women of child-bearing age should be immunized. For adult women, special care must be taken to assure that the woman is not pregnant at the time of immunization and will not become pregnant within 2 months after immunization. This precaution is necessary because of the possible risk of infection of the fetus if the woman is pregnant. In many cases, it is most convenient to administer the vaccine in the immediate postpartum period.

VARICELLA

Varicella (chickenpox) infection in the first 16 weeks of pregnancy may result in damage to the central nervous system, encephalitis, hypoplasia of extremities, atrophic digits, chorioretinitis, microphthalmia, cataracts and scarring of the skin. Further studies are needed, however, to determine the frequency with which these defects occur.

Varicella in the last 4 days of pregnancy can also produce serious fetal damage including disseminated infection and death. Because of the severe nature of infection near term, varicella immune globulin (VIG) should be obtained and administered to the newborn as soon after birth as possible (0.3 to 0.6 ml per pound). VIG is available from the Center for Disease Control, Atlanta, Georgia.

Antibody tests are now available for varicella using the immune adherence method. This permits the rapid determination of immunity or documentation of infection by seroconversion. This test should be used whenever the diagnosis is in doubt.

VENEZUELAN EQUINE ENCEPHALITIS VIRUS

Studies from our laboratory have demonstrated that Venezuelan equine encephalitis virus is teratogenic for the rhesus monkey.[19] Infection of the fetus at 100 days of gestation routinely results in hydrocephalus and cataracts. These findings are consistent with clinical reports from Latin America which indicates similar findings in infants born to women who experience this disease.[33] This virus then appears to be capable of producing congenital infection and malformations in man and experimental animals.

COXSACKIE VIRUS

Group B Coxsackie viruses have been reported to be associated with both congenital and neonatal infection. These viruses have been isolated from stillbirths and aborted fetuses. In one study of 50 stillborn infants and neonatal deaths, Coxsackie B antigen was present in the myocardium of 5.[4] Myocarditis is the clinical finding most frequently associated with Coxsackie virus infection.[2] However, disseminated infection involving multiple organ systems has been reported. In a prospective study of 630 mothers of anomalous infants and control subjects, maternal seroconversion to Coxsackie viruses appeared to be increased during pregnancy with a variety of congenital defects.[3] Coxsackie B2 and B4 were associated with urogenital anomalies and type A9 with defects of the digestive system. Cardiovascular anomalies were associated with Coxsackie B3 and B4 infection during pregnancy, and the likelihood of congenital heart disease was increased by maternal infection with two or more Coxsackie B viruses rather than with one. Anomalous infants weighed less than their controls and were more often male. Further studies are in progress.

Virus Infections Which Cause Fetal Disease

RUBEOLA

Congenital infection with rubeola (measles) has been reported to be associated with a high incidence of stillbirths and abortions.[5] Fetal infection occurring before term may produce newborns with the clinical disease or development of disease soon after birth. Giant cell pneumonia has also been noted in newborns with this disease.[23] It has also been reported that mothers who had measles during the first trimester have increased rates of premature infants when compared to normal pregnancies.

ECHO VIRUSES

Several recent reports describe congenital infection with ECHO viruses. One study involved three infants congenitally infected with ECHO virus 19.[22] Pathologic findings closely resemble those found with herpes simplex virus; i.e., a generalized infection with massive terminal hemorrhage involving most organs of the body.

ECHO virus 14 was reported to be isolated from the liver of a newborn infant with fatal hepatic necrosis.[14] High immunoglobulin M titers were present at 6 days of age, indicating that possible infection was acquired in utero.

WESTERN EQUINE ENCEPHALITIS VIRUS

Transplacental passage of Western equine encephalitis virus with serologic confirmation has been demonstrated by a number of investigators.[6] Congenital encephalitis has been found in the newborn infant at the time of or shortly after delivery. No congenital abnormalities have been described.

MUMPS

Maternal mumps infection during the first trimester has been reported to be associated with increased fetal mortality. In one study, 60% of the abortions occurred within 2 weeks of onset of maternal disease. However, fetal infection was not demonstrated by viral isolation.[7]

Endocardial fibroelastosis in infants may be associated with congenital mumps in some cases. This association was based on data showing that infants with this disease have a high incidence of positive skin tests to mumps antigen. Other workers, however, have not been able to confirm this association or demonstrate hemagglutination antibodies to mumps virus in the sera of patients with this disease. In the Collaborative Perinatal Study, there were 10 cases of endocardial fibroelastosis, and in one, there was evidence of maternal mumps.

VARIOLA VIRUS (SMALLPOX)

This virus can be transmitted to the fetus as a result of maternal infection.[6] The infection may result in abortion or congenital disease with skin lesions and pneumonia in the neonatal infant. No congenital malformations have been associated with this virus.

HEPATITIS

Hepatitis type B-associated antigen can cross the placenta and appear in the cord blood.[17, 25] Type B hepatitis may also be transmitted by close contact from mother to infant after birth in the neonatal period. Most of these infants have no abnormal findings, but carry the antigen in their blood for at least several years. Some have laboratory evidence of liver damage.

Congenital hepatitis may result in stillbirth or abortion of the fetus. Newborn infants can appear with jaundice, hepatosplenomegaly or hemolytic anemia with a liver function test indicating an obstructive type of jaundice. About 80% of the infants survive for at least one year; 50% of these exhibit a chronic, persistent liver disease. There have been examples of mothers giving birth in successive pregnancies to infants with hepatitis, thus indicating a chronic maternal infection.

The availability of a serologic test helps to differentiate this hepatitis from other clinical hepatitis (produced by other viruses such as rubella, Coxsackie, CMV, herpes and varicella) in the newborn infant. Immune serum globulin (ISG) manufactured after 1972 should be offered to individuals who clearly have had an oral or percutaneous exposure to known HB_sAg-positive blood or fluids. This type of exposure would include accidental needle punctures or accidental injection. A single 5-ml intramuscular injection may be of benefit. When ISG of high anti-HB_s titer becomes available (HBIG), this will be used in preference to the present ISG.

INFLUENZA

The reports on congenital infection and damage with influenza are quite contradictory. There are many publications showing correlation between the disease and congenital malformations[10] but there are a number of negative reports.[30] The reasons for these contradictory reports can be explained in part by the methods employed for collecting data. Many studies have depended upon the self-diagnosis of the disease and self-reporting to correlate infection with pregnancy. Often there is little or no serologic data. This method can be very inaccurate and misleading. Other studies have depended upon the evaluation of clinical symptoms and signs. With this type of the approach the inapparent or subclinical infections were overlooked. Most investigations have been made with small numbers of patients and control subjects.

Some of the findings reported for influenza infections during pregnancy include increased incidence of fetal death, anencephaly, abortions, stillbirths, prematurity and congenital malformations. Most of the data available on these associations are at a low level of statistical significance.

VACCINIA VIRUS

Congenital infection with vaccinia rarely occurs as a result of reimmunization of pregnant women.[7] Primary maternal vaccination, however, in the first or second trimesters may lead to fetal infection and possibly stillbirth, abortion or prematurity and death.[13] Fetal infection develops as a disseminated type of disease with focal lesions on the skin, lungs, liver and other organs of the body. Lesions may be confused with those produced by herpes or varicella virus. Complications associated with vaccination are eczema vaccinatum, vaccinia necrosium and postvaccinial encephalitis. Infants or adults with exfoliative dermatitis, especially eczema, should not be vaccinated or exposed to recently vaccinated individuals. The low incidence of smallpox in the United States plus the complications associated with vaccination has influenced the Public Health Service to recommend discontinuing of routine smallpox vaccinations in the United States as of September 1971.

Bacterial and Protozoal Infections which May Affect Fetus

The most common bacterial infections in pregnant women are gram-negative infections of the urinary tract. Acute pyelonephritis has been associated with an increased incidence of premature labor and asymptomatic bacteriuria is reported to result in higher rates of small babies. Our own studies of symptomatic treated bacteriuria have shown high frequencies of abortions, stillbirths, prematurity and neonatal deaths. Because of the high frequency of these infections, considerable study is needed in this important area.

STREPTOCOCCI

A serious problem in some nurseries is group B streptococcal infections.[11] Infants dying of group B streptococcal sepsis in the immediate newborn period manifest a course of fulminating respiratory failure and have pathologic findings of pneumonia, whereas those who develop the disease in the late neonatal period have predominately leptomeningeal infection. In a recent study of this problem in Denver, Franciosi et al[8] found between 5 and 8% of mothers have positive vaginal or anal cultures for group B streptococcus, and 1 to 2% of babies are colonized. Group B neonatal sepsis occurs at rates of 2 to 3 per 1000 live births, or about 1 out of 10 babies colonized. The absence of placental inflammation and the high correlation of positive cultures from the maternal vagina suggest the infection is acquired by the newborn via contact at the time of birth or immediately prior to delivery. The mortality when group B sepsis occurs is 20 to 40%. In most cases, small infants are more likely to be affected. Franciosi et al[8] found 45% of husbands of women with positive cultures to have group B streptococci in prostatic or urethral secretions.

The epidemiology of group B streptococcal infections in the neonate suggests that prenatal screening and treatment of mothers will eliminate this problem in the nursery. However, this supposition needs to be tested in a prospective study. Other possible approaches include the immunization of women or the development of new, very rapid methods for the diagnosis of infection in infants.

SYPHILIS

The bacterial disease, syphilis, may result in severe fetal damage. The diagnosis of syphilis in the mother is extremely important. To assist in this effort, routine serologic tests for syphilis should be performed before marriage, early in pregnancy and again in the third trimester. Congenital clinical syphilis is rarely detected in the first year of life. Stillbirths occur in about one-fourth of the affected pregnancies. Clinically, many of the children have no abnormal findings for the first weeks to months of life. Early symptoms include failure to gain weight, fever, anemia, rashes, rhinitis, moist lesions about the mouth, genitalia and anus, and lymphadenopathy. In addition, there may be hepatosplenomegaly and pseudoparalysis of one or more extremities with osteochondritis and periositis. The central nervous system may be affected and the spinal fluid should be examined for cells and protein content. Radiologic examination is often useful in making the diagnosis. Osteochondritis at the major joints and periostitis of the long bones and skull are typical findings. Widened epiphysial lines are also observed frequently. Serologic tests of children should include quantitative serial determinations whenever the diagnosis is in doubt. IgM antibody is elevated in the newborn, and specific syphilis IgM in the child is diagnostic of infection.

SEPSIS NEONATORUM

This bacterial disease of infants occurs during the first 30 days of life and involves the blood stream and frequently the meninges. The frequency of occurrence of sepsis neonatorum differs among various hospitals. However, the average rate is found to be approximately 1 per 1000 live births. The risk to preterm infants increases to 1 case per 230. The predisposing factors include premature rupture of amniotic membranes, amniocentesis, toxemia, cesarean section and various other obstetric complications. The organisms most frequently involved are gram negative. *Escherichia coli* account for approximately two-thirds of the cases while Pseudomonas and Klebsiella cause the bulk of the remaining gram-negative infection. Occasionally, Hemophilus, Salmonella or Proteus may be isolated. Recently, there has been an increase in infections due to the gram-positive group B beta-hemolytic streptococci. The reasons for this shift remain obscure. Other gram-positive organisms occasionally involved include *Staphylococcus aureus, Staphylococcus epidermidis,* hemolytic and nonhemolytic streptococci and less familiar organisms such as *Vibrio fetus,* Mima and Listeria.

TOXOPLASMOSIS

Toxoplasma gondii is an intracellular sporozoan obligate parasite. It is a ubiquitous organism and infects many animals and birds in addition to man. Although it can be maintained in tissue culture, isolation is best accomplished by intraperitoneal inoculation of mice.

Toxoplasmosis can be transmitted by the ingestion of infected raw meat. For this reason, the eating of raw meat by pregnant women should be discouraged. In addition, droppings from cats may contain viable Toxoplasma organisms which can be transmitted either directly or indirectly by flies and other vectors. Because of this, it would seem wise to recommend good personal hygiene in handling cat excreta.

Malformations occur in approximately 20% of the cases of recognized congenital toxoplasmosis. These include microcephaly and frequently micro-opthalmia and hydrocephaly. Congenitally infected infants may also have chorioretinitis (65 to 90%), anemia (55 to 77%), convulsions, cerebral calcifications, jaundice, fever, splenomegaly, lymphadenopathy, hepatomegaly, vomiting, diarrhea, pneumonitis and rash. Severe neonatal illness is usually followed by neurologic sequelae, including mental retardation and seizures.

The prognosis in congenital toxoplasmosis is extremely poor. Approximately 12% of the patients die, and of those children who survive, 85% are mentally retarded, 80% have convulsions, over 60% are spastic, 50% have severely damaged vision and approximately 20% have hydrocephalus or microcephalus.

MYCOPLASMA INFECTIONS

Mycoplasmas are an enigmatic group of micro-organisms that are receiving increasing attention as a source of fetal and neonatal loss.[18] The evidence of an etiologic role of mycoplasma in infertility, premature labor and fetal or neonatal death is still largely circumstantial. The micro-organisms are relatively common in the vaginal flora of women in the reproductive age (29%), with the incidence increasing in proportion to sexual activity.[20] Kundsin and Driscoll[18] showed that the organism could be cultured from a greater proportion of high risk prenatal patients than normal patients, and that there was more likely to be an unfavorable outcome of pregnancy when the organism was present in either a high risk or the normal group. A prospective study of 100 pregnant women infected with *mycoplasma hominis* type I showed a significantly lower mean infant birth weight when compared with control subjects, but no differences in abortions, premature labor or premature rupture of membranes.[18]

Mycoplasma infections respond to broad spectrum antibiotic therapy, but well controlled prospective studies are needed to confirm the specific role these organisms play in prenatal mortality and to establish the benefits, if any, of treating culture-positive patients.

CONGENITAL PNEUMONIA

This condition is found in 25% of infants dying in the first 12 hr of life. Associated conditions include meningitis, splenitis, sepsis, otitis media and necrotizing enterocolitis. Several studies have shown significant correlation between the pathogenic bacteria in the lungs of the infants and the reproductive-urinary tract of the mother. The bacteria most frequently associated with disease in the newborn are *E. coli, S. aureus* (coagulase positive), hemolytic and nonhemolytic streptococci, *Aerobacte aerogenes, Proteus vulgaris* and *Pseudomonas aeruginosa*.

OPHTHALMIA NEONATORUM

A variety of bacteria can cause this condition. Routine ophthalmic prophylaxis has reduced the incidence of *Neisseria gonococcus* infection; however, because of the increase of this infection in women in the past few years, this disease continues to occur. Other bacteria which can cause this disease include streptococci, staphylococci, Pneumococcus, Hemophilus, *P. aeruginosa* and various other gram-negative organisms. Most of these infections are readily treatable. Gonococcal and Pseudomonas opthalmia, however, may progress rapidly to a panophthalmitis. TRIC agents also cause eye infections in newborns. These usually respond rapidly to antibiotics.

LISTERIA

Listeria monocytogenes, a gram-positive, nonacid fast/mobile bacillus plays a significant role in fetal wastage. Current knowledge about listeria has recently been reviewed.[16] The disease in the mother is usually manifested by a mild febrile illness with diarrhea, back or flank pain and pruritis. After the fever subsides, fetal death often occurs. If born alive, the infant is usually premature and critically ill and dies of circulatory collapse or meningitis. The infection appears to be spread across the placenta to the fetus. A study by Jansson et al[15] showed that there was serologic evidence of recent Listeria infection in 13% of 1462 pregnancies ending in abortion, stillbirth or diseased newborns. Listeria infections are sensitive to most antibiotics, and erythromycin appears to be the most effective agent. A prospective study similar to that of Franciosi et al[8] with group B streptococcus is needed to determine the role of *L. monocytogenes* in perinatal loss.

REFERENCES

1. Birnbaum, G., Lynch, J. I., Margileth, A. M., Longergan, W. M., Sever, J. L.: Cytomegalovirus infections in newborn infants. J Pediat 75: 789, 1969.
2. Brown, G. C., Evans, T. N.: Serologic evidence of Coxsackie virus etiology of congenital heart disease. J Am Med Assoc 199: 183, 1967.
3. Brown, G. C., Karunas, R. S.: Relationship of congenital anomalies and maternal infections with selected enteroviruses. Am J Epidemiol 95: 207, 1972.
4. Burch, G. E., Sun, S., Chu, K., Sobal, R. S., Colcolough, H. L.: Interstitial and coxsackie virus B myocarditis in infants and children. JAMA 203: 55, 1968.
5. Dyer, I.: Measles complicating pregnancy. S Med J 33: 601, 1940.
6. Eichenwald, H. F., McCracken, G. H., Kindberg, S. J.: Viral infections of the newborn. Progr Med Virol 9: 35, 1967.
7. Eichenwald, H. F., Shinefield, H. R.: Viral infections of the fetus and of the premature and newborn infant. Adv Pediat 12: 249, 1962.
8. Franciosi, R. A., Knostman, J. D., Zimmerman, R. A.: Group B streptococcal neonatal and infant infections. J Pediatr 82: 707, 1973.
9. Fuccillo, D. A., Moder. F. L., Traub, R. G., Henson, S., Sever, J. L.: Micro indirect hemagglutination test for cytomegalovirus. Appl Microbiol 21: 104, 1971.
10. Hakosalo, J., Saxen, L.: Influenza epidemic and congenital defects. Lancet 2: 1346, 1971.
11. Hey, D. J., Hall, R. T., Burry, V. F., Thurn, A. N.: Neonatal infections cuased by group B streptococci. Am J Obstet Gynec 116: 43, 1973.
12. Hildebrant, J. R., Sever, J. L., Margileth, A. M., Gallagan, D. A.: Cytomegalovirus in the normal pregnant female. Am J Obstet Gynecol 98: 1125, 1967.
13. Horstmann, D. M.: Viral infections in pregnancy. Yale J Biol Med 42: 99, 1969.
14. Hughes, J. R., Wilfert, C. M., Moore, M., Benirsche, K., Guevara, E. H.: Echovirus 14 infection associated with fatal neonatal hepatic ne-

crosis. Am J Dis Child 123: 61, 1972.
15. Jansson, E. O., Widholm, O., Tuuri, S.: Serologic studies on perinatal *Listeria monocytogenes* infection. Ann Cir Gynaecol Finn 60: 66, 1972.
16. Kelly, C. A., Gibson, J. L.: Listeriosis as a cause of fetal wastage. Obstet Gynecol 40: 91, 1972.
17. Keys, T. F., Sever, J. L., Hewitt, W. L., Gitnick, G. L.: Hepatitis associated antigen in selected mothers and newborn infants. J Pediatr 80: 650, 1972.
18. Kundsin, R. B., Driscoll, S. G.: Mycoplasmas and human reproductive failure. Surg Gynecol Obstet 131: 89, 1970.
19. London, W. T., Levitt, N. H., Kent, S. G., Sever, J. L.: The teratogenic effects of Venezuelan equine encephalitis virus in rhesus monkeys [Abstr]. American Society of Microbiology, Miami, 1973.
20. McCormack, W. M., Almeida, P. C., Bailey, P. E., Grady, E. M., Lee Y. H.: Sexual activity and vaginal colonization with genital mycoplasmas. JAMA 221: 1375, 1972.
21. Nahmias, A. J., Dowdle, W. R.: Antigenic and biologic differences in *Herpes virus hominis*. Progr Med Virol 10: 110, 1968.
22. Nahmias, A. J., Dowdle, W. R., Josey, W. E., Naib, Z. M., Painter, L. M., Luce, C: Newborn infection with *Herpesvirus hominis types* 1 and 2 J Pediatr 75: 1194, 1964.
23. Packer, A. D.: The influence of maternal measles (morbilli) on the newborn child. Med J Austr 1: 835, 1950.
24. Philip, G. S., Larson, E. J.: Congenital infection with Echo 19 virus. Am J Pathol 66: 23a, 1972.
25. Purcell, R. H., Holland, P. V., Walsh, J. H., Wong, D. C., Morrow, A. G., Chanock, R. M.: A complement fixation test for measuring Australian antigen and antibody. J Infect Dis 120: 383, 1969.
26. Sever, J. L.: Perinatal infections affecting the developing fetus and newborn. National Institute of Child Health and Human Development Conference on the Prevention of Mental Retardation through the Control of Infectious Diseases: Public Health Service Publication, 1962, pp 1692–1712.
27. Sever, J. L.: Rubella as a teratogen. Adv Teratol 2: 217, 1967.
28. Sever, J. L.: Immunoglobulin determination for the detection of perinatal infection infection. J Pediat 75: 1111, 1969.
29. Sever, J. L., Hardy, J. B., Nelson, R. B., Gilkeson, M. R.: Rubella in the Collaborative Perinatal Research Study, II. Clinical and laboratory findings in children through 3 years of age. Am J Dis Child 118: 123, 1929.
30. Sieber, O. F., Jr., Fulginiti, V. A., Brazie, J., Umlouf, J. H., Jr.: In utero infection of the fetus by Herpes simplex virus. J Pediatr 69: 30, 1966.
31. South, M. A., Tompkins, W. A. F., Morris, R., Rawls, W. E.: Congenital malformations of the central nervous system associated with genital (type 2) herpes virus. J Pediatr 75: 13, 1969.
32. Walker, W. M., McKee, A. P.: Asian influenza in pregnancy, relationship to fetal anomalies. Obstet Gynecol 13: 394, 1959.
33. Wenger, F.: Necrosis cerebral masiva del feta en caseo de encefalitis equina venezuelana. Invest Clin 21: 13, 1967.

RICHARD H. SCHWARZ, M.D.

13

Diabetes Mellitus

Of the metabolic and endocrine disorders seen concurrently with pregnancy, diabetes mellitus is by far the most frequent, and is indeed one of the most common medical complications of pregnancy. It is important to recognize that generally, the endocrinopathies, if blatant and uncontrolled, are incompatible with ovulatory cycles and conception. Concurrence with pregnancy is then most often the result of controlled pre-existent disease, or disease which exacerbates or first appears after conception. It is also important that only in the normal endocrine milieu does pregnancy proceed normally, and consequently there are a series of concerns for both the fetus and the mother when an endocrinopathy is present.

With the discovery of insulin, diabetes, which was rarely compatible with survival to childbearing, or if so, to the completion of pregnancy, has now become a leading medical complication of pregnancy. Prepregnancy and gestational diabetes together occur in 0.2 to 0.3% of pregnancies. Along with the opportunity for detection, one of the important reasons for this high incidence is the diabetogenic nature of pregnancy.

Mechanisms involved in this diabetogenic process include placental degradation of insulin, reduced insulin synthesis, and decreased peripheral utilization. In addition, fetal demands bring about a pseudostarvation state with increased lipolysis, which in turn, further increases insulin resistance as well as the tendency to ketoacidosis. Regardless of the mechanisms involved, the result in a normal gravida is islet cell hyperplasia; in the genetically predisposed, uncovering of diabetes; and in the established diabetic, an increase in insulin requirements. If we measure severity by insulin requirements, diabetes is worsened during pregnancy; however, this is a transient effect, with the insulin requirement returning quickly to prepregnant values after delivery, provided residual weight gain is not excessive. A permanent impact which might be life shortening, e.g., on the microvasculature, has not been demonstrated. Nonmetabolic risks to the diabetic in pregnancy include an increase in frequency of pyelonephritis, pre-eclampsia and hydramnios. Pyelonephritis clearly might be a threat to already damaged kidneys, as might preeclampsia. Most authorities feel that proliferative retinopathy and diabetic nephropathy with nitrogen retention are contraindications to the establishment of a pregnancy, and should lead to recommendations for termination in cases of established early pregnancy.

The impact of diabetes on pregnancy is equally dramatic since the fetus is subject to the mother's metabolic derangements, and also because diabetes is prone to attack small vessels, accelerating the decline of placental function. Perinatal mortality is increased, with rates of approximately 10% reported from most centers with a representative patient population. Mortality increases with the severity of diabetes, with rates in the White class A being only slightly higher than the population at large, while the class F patient has perhaps a 50% chance of having a surviving child. Recent series report even lower perinatal mortality; however, patient populations are weighted away from the classes of diabetics with significant vascular disease. The occurrence of hydramnios, pre-eclampsia or ketoacidosis significantly increases perinatal mortality.

To provide optimal care for the diabetic pregnancy, counseling should be provided preconceptionally in order to maintain all options, including adoption or a marriage without children. First, the patient should understand the implications for her health, and be aware that her diabetes will be at least transiently worsened. It is difficult to discuss the potential of a reduced life expectancy, since denial may be the patient's most secure emotional defense. Nevertheless, the juvenile diabetic with an already shorter life expectancy could have it further reduced, e.g., by an episode of pyelonephritis in pregnancy, and this information should be made available to the family if not the patient. In addition to the physical threat to the patient, there are the emotional and economic burdens as well. Prolonged hospitalization, separation from the family, multiple physician's visits, and costly laboratory studies are all considerations, and in the end there may be no baby to show for all of this.

Counseling must also inform the diabetic of the impact on her child. If the fetus survives its uterine environment, it has a 3-fold increased risk of having a birth defect and a 6-fold increase in the chance of a lethal malformation. Ventricular septal defects and sacrococcygeal deformities are especially increased, but there is no pathognomonic malformation for diabetes. Since the genetics of diabetes is unclear, it is not possible to predict accurately the risk of diabetes in the offspring. Consideration of autosomal recessive inheritance has been discredited by twin studies, with far less than 100% concordance, as well as diabetic-diabetic matings, also with lesser rates, which cannot be accounted for on the basis of lack of expression of the disease. It seems increasingly apparent that there are multiple genetic mechanisms involved and therefore there can be no rigid rules for risk counseling. Pedigrees of both parents must be obtained, and if the involved parent appears to be an isolated case, the risk is obviously lower than if both families are liberally represented with diabetes.

In addition to the long range concerns of malformations and diabetes, the newborn and his neonatologist face a number of more immediate concerns. Two of these concerns, hypoglycemia and macrosomia, are related to hyperglycemia in the mother. Since glucose crosses the placenta readily and is a function of maternal levels, whereas insulin does not cross, there results fetal islet cell hyperplasia and hyperinsulinism. With delivery and the withdrawal of the maternal source of glucose, neonatal hypoglycemia ensues. The severity of this hypoglycemia is a function of control of maternal blood sugar throughout the pregnancy. It is often most pronounced in the gestational diabetic who was not found to be hyperglycemic until late pregnancy, although much less pronounced in the insulin-dependent diabetic who was well controlled throughout pregnancy.

This same correlation applies to fetal macrosomia, which is the result of hyperglycemia and hyperinsulinism, and also, perhaps, increased concentrations of human chorionic somatomammotropin. Infants are large, not simply edematous, and have increased glycogen deposition. Macrosomic infants are generally born to class A, B and C diabetics, with small gestational age infants being born to those patients with vascular disease. As is the case with hypoglycemia, macrosomia can be significantly reduced by careful control of maternal blood sugar levels throughout the gestation. Macrosomia can result in mechanical problems at delivery, most of which can be eliminated by the appropriate application of cesarean section. Shoulder dystocia, however, cannot necessarily be predicted by the course of labor or pelvic measurement. Despite the easy descent of the head of the diabetic infant, its broad shoulders and short neck may present considerable problems in extraction, resulting in fractures or neural injuries. This is a sufficient concern for consideration of abdominal delivery if the baby is felt to be extremely large even if the pelvis seems adequate.

Finally, the diabetic offspring is subject to other metabolic problems, including hypocalcemia and hyperbilirubinemia. The subject of the propensity of the diabetic offspring to the respiratory distress syndrome (RDS) has been debated for some time, but it now seems clear that there is an association. There is an increase in RDS of as much as 7-fold, even when corrected for factors such as gestational age and route of delivery. Maturation of surfactant synthesis is delayed in the diabetic fetus and even with lecithin to sphingomyelin (L/S) ratios considered to be mature (2.0:1 to 2.5:1), there is a significant incidence of RDS, indicating that factors (acidosis, etc.) other than surfactant are important in the genesis of RDS.

The diagnosis of diabetes during pregnancy, of course, applies only to the gestational diabetic. Gestational diabetes should be suspected in patients with a family history of diabetes, glucosuria, large babies, unexplained reproductive failure and obesity. Screening ideally should be done by a full 3-hr glucose tolerance test; however, this presents logistic problems in most situations, and therefore the 2-hr sugar is selected as the most sensitive single indicator. Negative tests in early pregnancy should be repeated in the second and third trimesters because of the progression of diabetogenicity and abnormal 2-hr values should be pursued with full glucose tolerance tests. Some have proposed the use of the intravenous glucose tolerance test on the basis that the oral test overdiagnoses diabetes, especially with the delayed absorption of pregnancy. It has been our experience that borderline oral tests result, at most, in the introduction of an appropriate diet, a step not ill advised in these patients, most of whom are obese. To avoid the intolerance of the patient for the glucose solution, commercially available "cola" preparations are used, and are best tolerated when adequately iced. An adequate carbohydrate diet for at least 3 days prior to the test is imperative. A test is considered abnormal if any two values exceed the normal. The fasting level is least likely to be abnormal since it is lowered by the pseudostarvation state of pregnancy. A diagnosis of gestational diabetes, even though made in late pregnancy when little impact will be made on that gestation, is nonetheless important since it has likely identified an individual who is potentially an adult onset diabetic later in life, under appropriately stressful circumstances.

Management

The combination of pregnancy and diabetes, more than any other situation in obstetric practice, brings about the need for a collaborative effort, not only on the part of physicians but other professionals as well, including nurses, nutritionists and social workers. In addition, the treatment facility must provide appropriate laboratories, monitoring, ultrasound and a neonatal care unit capable of dealing with the high risk newborn. The internist involved in the care of the diabetic must have a special appreciation for the effects of pregnancy and the need for exceptionally tight control while the obstetrician must understand the basics of diet and insulin therapy and feel confident in participating in the diabetic as well as obstetric care. Finally, the neonatologist and anesthesiologist should be aware of the patient and her problems antenatally and participate in the decision making.

The first step in the medical management of the pregnant diabetic, if it has not been done recently, is a careful evaluation and classification of the diabetes. Although it was often recommended in the past that such an evaluation required hospitalization, it can be readily accomplished on an outpatient basis, given a cooperative patient and diabetes which is reasonably well controlled. In addition to the routine history and physical examination, it is necessary to focus particular attention on vascular and renal disease. The retina should be examined early in pregnancy, and repeatedly if there is any indication of progressive retinopathy. Although the internist as well as the obstetrician should examine the eyes, it is often necessary to dilate the pupils and it frequently requires an experienced ophthalmologist to evaluate the subtle and progressive changes. Renal function (glomerular filtration) is evaluated by a 24-hr creatinine clearance, and if there is proteinuria, a 24-hr quantitation should be done. The urine should be cultured even in the absence of symptoms, since there is with asymptomatic bacteriuria in pregnancy, a 15 to 20% incidence of subsequent pyelonephritis, for which the diabetic is already prone. If a significant bacteriuria exists, it should be treated with appropriate antimicrobials and clearance confirmed by repeat cultures.

Diet is the first consideration in the management of newly diagnosed gestational diabetic and, in addition, must be modified to accommodate pregnancy requirements in the prepregnant diabetic. The basic dietary assumptions are: (a) caloric requirements for the average sized pregnant woman are 2200 per day; (b) protein requirements are 1.0 to 1.5 g per kg of ideal body weight; (c) 60 to 70 g of fat are necessary to construct a palatable diet. Calories can be restricted in the overweight patient; however, 1500 calories is probably the minimum which will allow adequate protein intake. Since many overweight patients are accustomed to very large caloric intakes, there is the risk that the patient may not comply with a diet which is too restrictive. For the nonobese juvenile diabetic, more total calories may be necessary to compensate for fetal needs, plus urinary glucose loss. Failure to meet these needs will result in lipolysis and ketosis, with an increased propensity to ketoacidosis. In establishing the dietary program, the nutritionist must also consider the patient's economic status, likes and dislikes, work and sleep habits, who prepares the food and the ability of the patient to understand and comply with the diet. In the case of the gestational diabetic, a 2- to 3-week trial of diet therapy is indicated before insulin is added. A careful diet diary is helpful before initiating a program as well as periodically, to evaluate compliance.

Oral hypoglycemics are not approved for use in pregnancy. Hazards include refractory neonatal hypoglycemia and competition for bilirubin binding sites. Teratogenesis has been reported in animal studies with some preparations. Despite these contraindications, the agents have been used by some clinical investigators without problems. Nonetheless, routine clinical use is not recommended.

Diuretic therapy is indicated in the pregnant diabetic only for symptomatic edema, or as a component of antihypertensive therapy. Thiazides, specifically, have a hyperglycemic effect, and may increase insulin requirements. Potassium depletion must be guarded against if long term therapy is utilized.

When diet fails to lower the 2-hr postprandial blood sugar to 150 mg per 100 ml or less in the gestational diabetic, insulin therapy should be started. The obese gestational diabetic is one of the most insulin-resistant patients one deals with, and consequently it is safe to initiate insulin therapy on an outpatient basis when diet control fails. A single morning dose of from 10 to 20 units of intermediate acting (NPH) insulin will usually suffice, and follow-up should be based on postabsorptive blood sugars. The value of urine sugars is lessened by the reduced threshold; however, fractional urines should not be abandoned since they have a relative value in determining that time of day at which sugars are highest. It must be stressed, however, that it is only in the obese patient that insulin may be begun on an outpatient basis. The nonobese patient must be hospitalized for initial control. Insulin requirements in the established diabetic will generally increase progressively throughout pregnancy, and the total increase is not infrequently as great as 3- or 4-fold over prepregnancy needs. A sudden fall in insulin requirements is considered ominous, especially in late pregnancy. The single most important factor in successful pregnancy management is meeting the increased insulin requirements and maintenance of a euglycemic state. Some investigators have suggested that the mean blood sugar is to be maintained at 100 g per 100 ml or below; however, this approach is impractical and risky without extraordinary laboratory and clinical control. It is our preference to seek to maintain the 2-hr postabsorptive sugar at 150 mg per 100 ml or below, thereby reducing the risk of hypoglycemia associated with more rigid control. Even this level of control will seem too stringent to some nonpregnancy-oriented internists who find less tight control easier to deal with. Unfortunately, however, looser control results in more complications and a less favorable outcome. As insulin requirements increase, it becomes more difficult to achieve level blood sugar control with a single morning dose of intermediate acting insulin. When the total requirement reaches 40 to 50 units per day, it may be advisable to split the dose, giving a mixture of NPH and regular insulin before breakfast, and again before the evening meal. This often results in a smaller total dose, or at the least, a more level control with the same total dose since the blood sugar may climb during the night, resulting in the need to "chase" a higher fasting level each day. In addition to more level control, the split dose system provides a relatively simple system for establishing control and adjusting doses, as follows:

Morning regular controls prelunch sugar
Morning NPH controls predinner sugar
Evening regular controls bedtime sugar
Evening NPH controls fasting sugar

When the insulin-dependent patient is to be admitted for elective induction or cesarean section, no long acting insulin should be utilized on the day of delivery. Instead, a glucose infusion should be started in the morning and the patient should receive regular insulin in a total of one-half to two-thirds of the previous total dose divided into four subcutaneous doses every 6 hr. Supplemental insulin may be given if blood sugars warrant; however, the combination of low caloric intake (200 calories in 1000 ml of 5% glucose solution) and the increased demands of labor or surgery generally result in smaller requirements for insulin. In the case of a cesarean section, it is important to maintain a glucose infusion until a normal diet is tolerated to avoid problems in diabetic control. After delivery, insulin requirements fall dramatically, sometimes falling below prepregnancy levels for a day or two. If the total dose is less than 30 units prior to delivery, it is wise to withhold insulin completely on the first day and simply cover blood sugar levels as determined. In the case of the gestational diabetic, approximately 30% will have a residual insulin requirement postpartum, and the remainder will revert to a normal glucose tolerance curve. The latter group should be followed at least on an annual basis routinely and be checked at the time of stress, such as a serious infection.

The obstetric management of the diabetic is essentially limited to three areas: fetal evaluation, timing of delivery and the method of delivery. In addition to these purely obstetric functions, the obstetrician should serve as the coordinator of the perinatal care team.

The evaluation of fetal well-being is critical to the management of the diabetic pregnancy. Of those studies currently available, estriol determinations and oxytocin challenge tests (OCT) find most use. Estriol determinations have the most appeal since it is apparent that the fetopathy in diabetes is not simply a matter of uteroplacental vascular insufficiency (better evaluated by the OCT). This is particularly the case in classes A, B and C, where there is minimal vascular involvement. Although the 24-hr urinary estriol (or total estrogen) determinations have the disadvantage of the collection period and the possibility of incomplete collection, serum determinations have counterbalancing disadvantages. Because of the microgram rather than milligram quantities, assays are technically more of a problem and there is significant variation in serum levels throughout the day, which does not seem, as once thought, to follow a consistent diurnal pattern. The choice between urine and serum studies is probably best based on availability and consistency of reporting as well as the establishment of standard curves for a given laboratory. In our hands, 24 hr urinary estrogen determinations have proven to be reliable and the most useful. Determinations should be initiated at 30 to 32 weeks if the patient is stable. Studies should subsequently be done at least twice, or preferably, three times weekly after that, since diabetes is not a static condition. It is our practice to perform daily estriols on those patients hospitalized near term because of instability or the development of complications. A fall of 30% or more from the previous determination should be considered significant if the total volume and creatinine content indicate a complete collection.

In our hands, the OCT is utilized as an adjunct to estriol determinations and is most helpful in the more advanced classes of diabetics with significant vascular disease. Although a negative test generally is felt to offer reassurance of well-being for the ensuing 7 days, this presumption can apply only if the diabetes is stable and there are no complications such as preeclampsia, which can result in a fluctuating fetal environment. When the timing of delivery is dependent upon fetal maturation, amniocentesis should be performed (after placental localization by ultrasound), and the fluid assayed for L/S ratio, creatinine, ΔOD_{450} and fat cells. Although the L/S ratio (or shake test) is the most critical value, the other studies may be useful in borderline cases. Since the development of surfactant synthetic pathways is commonly delayed in the diabetic, and also because RDS does occur in diabetic offspring with L/S ratios above 2:1, it is important to await clearly mature values (>2.5 to 3.0:1). This merely confirms that factors other than surfactant deficiency are operative in the pathogenesis of RDS. The measurement of the biparietal diameter of the fetal head by ultrasound loses some value in estimating fetal maturity in the case of macrosomic fetuses, but should be used nonetheless. Serial measurements made between 20 and 30 weeks are critical in assessing fetal growth in diabetics with vascular disease suspected of having fetuses with intrauterine growth retardation. A minimum of 3 weeks between measurements is necessary to assess growth because of the small increments.

In the modern obstetric era, early delivery of all diabetics commonly had been practiced with a view toward preventing those stillbirths which might occur as the result of uteroplacental insufficiency. Unfortunately, in a number of cases, this results in exposing newborns to the risk of RDS as well as mothers to increased hazards of abdominal delivery. This practice of uniform early delivery can be avoided by individualized care with careful fetal and maternal evaluation to select those patients in whom early delivery is mandatory. Three groups of patients can be defined with regard to the timing of delivery. The first consists of the gestational diabetics and the stable prepregnancy diabetics (largely classes B and C). Provided that these patients remain well controlled, without complications such as pre-eclampsia or acute hydramnios, and if the parameters of fetal well-being indicate no jeopardy, early delivery is unnecessary. These patients can then safely be carried to term. However, if at any time after 38 weeks conditions become favorable for induction, it should be carried out since there is nothing further to be gained by the fetus with further intrauterine life. Should postmaturity supervene, however, it is difficult to justify further prolongation of the pregnancy with the possibility of additive deterioration of placental function. Finally, with this group, one must recognize the possiblity of fetal macrosomia and fetopelvic disproportion. Although this is usually easily recognized and dealt with, there is the more treacherous problem of shoulder dystocia. This is often difficult to anticipate since the pelvis may be large and labor may progress efficiently with dilatation and descent. Only after the birth of the head is the broad shouldered, short necked infant a problem. One can probably justify cesarean section even with an adequately sized pelvis if a very large baby (>10 pounds) is anticipated.

The second group to be considered might be termed the unstable diabetic group. Included in this category are the patients whose diabetes has been difficult to control, those with previous perinatal losses and those in whom the indices of fetal well-being are acceptable but fail to show progressive improvement (chronically low normal stable estriols). These patients should be delivered as soon as maturity can be established. Often, this is not clear-cut until 37 weeks because of the retardation of surfactant synthesis and the need to await a clearly mature L/S ratio (>2.5:1).

Finally, there is a group of patients who must be delivered promptly regardless of gestational age or fetal maturity. This category includes those who develop significant pre-eclampsia or acute hydramnios, and obviously, those patients in whom there is a deterioration in the parameters of fetal well-being. Unsettled at this time is the question as to whether corticosteriod therapy is of value when such a premature delivery is indicated. It seems, clinically, that there is value, especially in gestations of less than 32 weeks; however, the effect is not seen for 24 to 48 hr after administration, and the potential value must be balanced against the risks of delay.

The route of delivery is generally a simple decision once the timing has been determined. By and large, delivery should be by the most expeditious means, based upon a clincial evaluation of the suitability for induction of labor. In marginal situations, a limited trial with careful monitoring is justified in an effort to avoid the additional risks of cesarean section; however, there does not seem to be a place for prolonged and repeated attempts at induction. Analgesia and anesthesia should be dictated by the obstetric situation.

Summary

The management of the pregnant diabetic is a team venture which should be organized and coordinated by the obstetrician. An internist, knowledgeable about diabetes and pregnancy, a neonatologist, nutritionist, anesthesiologist, along with nurses and social workers, complete the team, and should provide care in a setting with complete laboratory and other essential clinical facilities. Because pregnancy is a diabetogenic event, it is critical in the management that the patient be maintained as nearly euglycemic as possible to secure the best outcome and the fewest neonatal problems. Risks to the mother include a transient decrease in carbohydrate tolerance, and an increased risk of pyelonephritis, pre-eclampsia and hydramnios. The offspring is subject to an increase in perinatal mortality, with a higher rate of RDS, congenital malformation, hypoglycemia, macrosomia, hypocalcemia and ultimate diabetes. Obstetric management entails careful evaluation of fetal well-being and maturity, with the timing and method of delivery being dependent upon the stability of the diabetes, the occurrence of complications, prior obstetric problems and the evaluation of the fetus. Despite the best efforts of all concerned, the outcome is not always favorable, with the perinatal mortality remaining at a level which seems irreducibly higher than that for the population at large; the patient herself assumes a risk which may not be large but assumes greater proportion in the more sever, long standing diabetic. The insulin era has created the concurrence of pregnancy and diabetes. Now, with modern perinatal medicine, the results are encouraging, but we would be remiss to suggest that the diabetic woman establish a pregnancy without a clear awareness of the ramifications of that disease.

SELECTED BIBLIOGRAPHY

1. Adam, P. A. L., Schwartz, R.: Diagnosis and treatment: Should oral hypoglycemic agents be used in pediatric and pregnant patients? Pediatrics 42: 819, 1968.
2. Beethan, W. P.: Diabetic retinopathy in pregnancy. Trans Am Ophthalmol Soc 48: 205, 1951.
3. Benjamin, F., Casper, D. J.: Comparative validity of oral and intravenous glucose tolerance tests in pregnancy. Am J Obstet Gynecol 97: 488, 1967.
4. Burt, R. L., Leake, N. H.: Oral glucose tolerance test during pregnancy and the early puerperium. Obstet Gynecol 33: 48, 1969.
5. Cruz, A. C., Buhi, W. C., Burk, S. A., Spellacy, W. N.: Respiratory distress syndrome with mature lecithin/sphingomyelin ratios: Diabetes mellitus and low Apgar score. Am J Obstet Gynecol 126: 78, 1976.
6. Dandrow, R. V., O'Sullivan, J. B.: Obstetrics hazards of gestational diabetes. Am J Obstet Gynecol 96: 1144, 1966.
7. Delaney, J. J., Ptacek, J.: Three decades of experience with diabetic pregnancies. Am J Obstet Gynecol 106: 550, 1970.
8. Driscoll, J. J., Gillespie, L.: Obstetrical considerations in diabetes and pregnancy. Med Clin North Am 49: 1025, 1965.
9. Gluck, L., Kulovich, M. V.: Lecithin/sphingomyelin ratios in amniotic fluid in normal and abnormal pregnancies. Am J Obstet Gynecol 115: 539, 1973.
10. Goebelsmann, E., Freeman, R. J., Mestman, J. H., Nakamura, R. M., Woodling, B. A.: Estriol in pregnancy. II. Daily urinary estriol assays in the management of the pregnant diabetic

woman. Am J Obstet Gynecol 115: 795, 1973.
11. Gugliucci, C. L., O'Sullivan, M. J., Opperman, W., Gordon, M., Stone, M. L.: Intensive care of the diabetic patient. Am J Obstet Gynecol 125: 435, 1976.
12. Hallman, N., Kulovich, M., Kirkpatrick, E., Sugarman, R. G., Gluck, L.: Phosphatidylinositol and phosphatidylglycerol in amniotic fluid: Indices of lung maturity. Am J Obstet Gynecol 125: 613, 1976.
13. Horger, E. O., III, Kellet, W. W., III, Williamson, H. O.: Diabetes in pregnancy. Obstet Gynecol 30: 46, 1967.
14. Kalin, C. B., Soelduer, J. S., Gleason, R. E., Rojas, L., Cavierini-Davalos, R. A., Marble, A.: Clinical and chemical diabetes in offspring of diabetic couples. N Engl J Med 281: 343, 1969.
15. Kass, E. H.: Pyelonephritis and bacteriuria. Ann Int Med 56: 46, 1962.
16. Khojandi, M., Tsai, A. Y.-M., Tyson, J. E.: Gestational diabetes: The dilemma of delivery. Obstet Gynecol 43: 1, 1974.
17. Kyle, G. C.: Diabetes and pregnancy. Ann Int Med 59 (Suppl 3): 1, 1963.
18. Lewis, S. B., Murray, W. K., Wallin, J. D., Coustan, D. R., Daane, T. A., Tredway, D. R., Navins, J. P.: Improved glucose control in nonhospitalized pregnancy diabetic patients. Obstet Gynecol 48: 260, 1976.
19. Lindback, T., Skaeraasen, J.: Phospholipid concentration in amniotic fluid from diabetic pregnant women. Pediatr Res 9: 858, 1975.
20. O'Sullivan, J. B., Charles, D., Malian, C. M., Dandrow, R. V.: Gestational diabetes and perinatal mortality. Am J Obstet Gynecol 116: 901, 1973.
21. Pedersen, L. M., Tygstrup, I., Pedersen, J.: Congenital malformations in newborn infants of diabetic women: Correlation with maternal vascular diabetic complications. Lancet 1: 1124, 1964.
22. Peel, J.: A historical review of diabetes and pregnancy. J Obstet Gynecol Br Commonw 79: 385, 1972.
23. Posner, N. A., Silverstone, F. A., Pomerance, W., Weiss, H., Weinstein, H.: The outcome of pregnancy in Class A diabetes. Am J Obstet Gynecol 111: 886, 1971.
24. Schwarz, R. H., Fields, G. A., Kyle, G. C.: Timing of delivery in the pregnant diabetic patient. Obstet Gynecol 34: 787, 1969.
25. Smith, S. G., Scragg, W. H., Jr.: Gestational diabetes. Obstet Gynecol 31: 228, 1968.
26. Warner, R. A., Cornblath, M.: Infants of gestational diabetic mothers. Am J Dis Child 117: 678, 1969.
27. White, P.: Pregnancy and diabetes: Medical aspects. Med Clin North Am 49: 1015, 1965.
28. Zucker, P., Simon, G.: Prolonged symptomatic neonatal hypoglycemia associated with maternal chlorpropamide therapy. Pediatrics 42: 824, 1968.

NORMAN F. GANT, M.D.
RICHARD J. WORLEY, M.D.

14

Pregnancy-induced Hypertension—A Chronic Disease Process*

This chapter is devoted to a discussion of the hypertensive disorders of pregnancy and is designed (*a*) to provide a working clinical classification of hypertensive disorders of pregnancy, (*b*) to present recently acquired pathophysiologic data which suggest that pre-eclampsia and/or eclampsia are chronic disease processes which affect both maternal and fetal patients many weeks before the onset of hypertension and (*c*) to present a clinical plan of management based upon laboratory and clinical data acquired at Parkland Memorial Hospital during the past 20 years. Utilizing the clinical approaches to therapy outlined in this chapter, significant reductions in perinatal mortality and maternal morbidity have been achieved at Parkland Memorial Hospital. Although the principles presented are based upon numerous clinical and often sophisticated laboratory studies, the practices suggested by these studies are not dependent upon expensive or time-consuming procedures. Instead, methods of management rely on clinical observations and commonly available laboratory studies. Additionally, the methods of management presented here rely heavily upon an understanding that this pregnancy-induced disease process is chronic in development and, if recognized as such, may be modified significantly by sound clinical judgment.

Before any classification of hypertensive diseases of pregnancy is presented, it is important to realize that the term "toxemia of pregnancy" has fallen into disrepute because no "toxin" has been identified even in the most fulminant cases. Because the etiology of hypertension occurring during pregnancy remains unknown, it seems more logical not to use the etiologic term "toxemia" but instead to utilize a descriptive expression. We have chosen the expression "pregnancy-induced hypertension" to designate those episodes of hypertension which are unique to pregnancy. Therefore, the following outline and terminology are proposed until true etiologic terms are available.

Classification

HYPERTENSION OF PREGNANCY

A. Pregnancy-induced hypertension
    1. Pre-eclampsia
        a. Mild
        b. Severe
    2. Eclampsia
B. Chronic hypertension preceding pregnancy (any etiology)

* This research was supported in part by United States Public Health Service Grant HD 08360.

C. Chronic hypertension (any etiology) with superimposed pregnancy-induced hypertension
   1. Superimposed pre-eclampsia and/or
   2. Superimposed eclampsia

D. Late or transient hypertension

Utilizing this outline as a rough clinical classification, it is apparent that virtually all of the hypertensive diseases occurring during pregnancy are included in these four major categories, which Chesley outlined in the 14th edition of *Williams' Obstetrics*.[5] The original outline has been modified here by the use of the term pregnancy-induced hypertension. This classification is self-explanatory with the exception of the late or transient hypertension category. This category includes only those patients with transient elevations in blood pressure which are observed during labor or in the early puerperium, and thus may encompass a wide spectrum of patients whose illnesses range from mild pregnancy-induced hypertension to those patients with latent or early symptoms of essential vascular hypertension.

Recent Studies of Pregnancy-induced Hypertension

MATERNAL PATIENT

Although the etiology of pregnancy-induced hypertension remains an enigma, recent studies have shown that the disease is chronic in development, and thus can be recognized early in gestation. In fact, those women who are destined to develop pregnancy-induced hypertension can be identified many weeks before the onset of clinical signs by utilizing two recently reported screening techniques.

The first of these screening procedures takes advantage of the increased vascular sensitivity to the pressor effect of infused angiotensin II which has been observed in women with pregnancy-induced hypertension.[4, 9, 34] Conversely, women who are normotensive late in pregnancy are relatively resistant to the pressor effects of angiotensin II.[1, 2, 9, 10] For example, in a nonpregnant individual approximately 7.4 ng per kg per min of angiotensin II is required to elevate baseline diastolic blood pressure 20 mm Hg, whereas in a normal term pregnant woman 12 to 14 ng per kg per min is required to elicit the same pressor response.[9, 22] In women acutely ill with pregnancy-induced hypertension, less than 8 ng per kg per min is required to elicit a similar pressor response. Significantly, this increased sensitivity to exogenously administered angiotensin II can be detected as early as the 22nd week of gestation in those women who are destined to develop pregnancy-induced hypertension, or as early as 18 weeks before the appearance of hypertension in some cases.[9]

Figure 14.1 illustrates a comparison of the response to angiotensin II infusions in normal and future hypertensive pregnant women. The 192 primigravid women in this prospective study were 16 years old or younger and were studied sequentially throughout their pregnancy, beginning as early in gestation as possible. At each

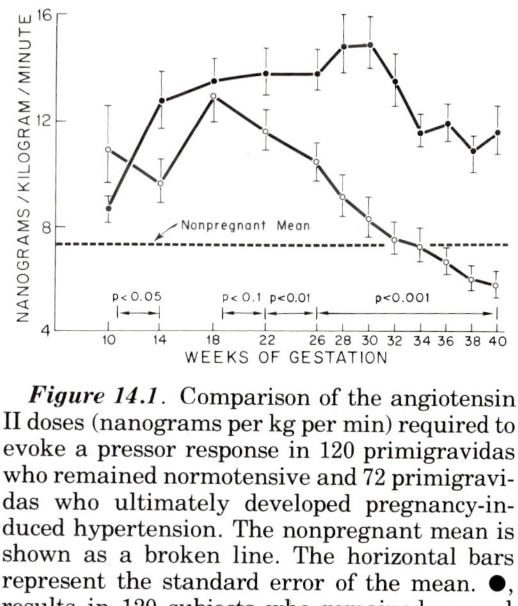

Figure 14.1. Comparison of the angiotensin II doses (nanograms per kg per min) required to evoke a pressor response in 120 primigravidas who remained normotensive and 72 primigravidas who ultimately developed pregnancy-induced hypertension. The nonpregnant mean is shown as a broken line. The horizontal bars represent the standard error of the mean. ●, results in 120 subjects who remained normal (769 infusions). ○, results obtained in 72 women who developed pregnancy-induced hypertension (421 infusions). The difference between the two groups became significant after week 23 ($P < 0.01$) and the two groups continued to diverge widely after the 26th week ($P < 0.001$). (Reprinted with permission from Gant, N. F., Daley, G. L., Chand, S.: A study of angiotensin II pressor response throughout primigravid pregnancy. J Clin Invest 52: 2684, 1973.)

clinic visit the patients received angiotensin II infusions sufficient to elicit an increase in diastolic blood pressure of 20 mm Hg higher than baseline. The dose required to elevate diastolic blood pressure 20 mm Hg was recorded as the pressor dose (nanograms per kg per min). In Figure 14.1 the pressor dose is shown on the vertical axis and is plotted as a function of weeks of gestation. The results obtained in women who remained normotensive throughout pregnancy are illustrated by the solid dots. Open circles represent the results obtained in those women who were destined to develop pre-eclampsia, but who were normal at the beginning of the study. It is evident that women destined to develop pregnancy-induced hypertension became progressively more and more sensitive to the pressor effects of infused angiotensin II after the 18th week of gestation. In fact, analysis of the data obtained between the 28th and 32nd week of gestation revealed that if less than 8 ng per kg per min was needed to elicit a pressor response during this 4-week period that the patient had a 90% chance of developing pregnancy-induced hypertension 10 to 12 weeks later. Conversely, if greater than 8 ng per kg per min was needed to elicit a pressor response during the same time period, the patient had a 90% chance of remaining normotensive throughout the remainder of pregnancy.

A similar study of angiotensin II pressor responsiveness in pregnancies complicated by chronic essential hypertension also was conducted. This study was designed (*a*) to outline prospectively vascular responsiveness to angiotensin II in gravidas with chronic essential hypertension, and (*b*) to ascertain whether increased sensitivity to infused angiotensin II could be detected before worsening of hypertension developed in those women who were destined to develop superimposed pregnancy-induced hypertension.[15]

Sixty-three women with chronic essential hypertension were studied prospectively throughout pregnancy. Two groups of patients were identified on the basis of clinical outcome and serial measurements of vascular reactivity to exogenously administered angiotensin II. The first group

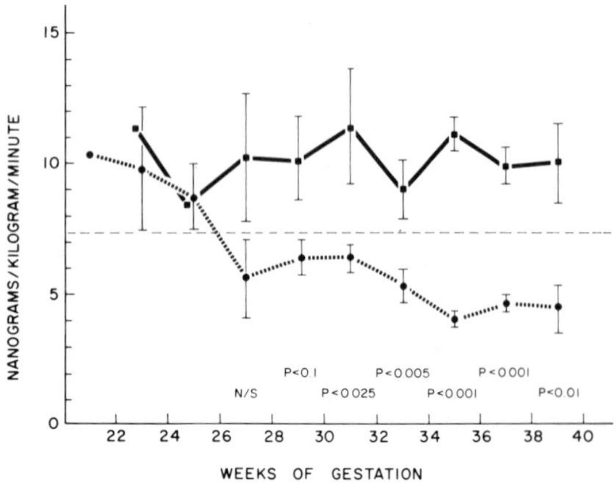

Figure 14.2. Comparison of angiotensin II responsiveness in 29 patients with essential hypertension and 34 patients with essential hypertension destined to develop superimposed pregnancy-induced hypertension. The dose of angiotensin II required to elevate resting diastolic blood pressure 20 mm Hg is shown in nanograms per kg per min on the vertical axis and is plotted as a function of weeks of gestation. The results obtained in gravidas with chronic hypertension alone are indicated by ■——■. The results obtained in gravidas with chronic hypertension destined to develop superimposed pregnancy-induced hypertension are shown as ●---●. The vertical bars represent the standard error of the mean. (Reprinted with permission from Gant, N. F., Whalley, P. J., Chand, S., MacDonald, P. C.: A prospective study of angiotensin II pressor responsiveness in pregnancies complicated by chronic essential hypertension. Am J Obstet Gynecol 127: 369, 1977.

consisted of 29 gravidas with chronic hypertension alone, and the second group was composed of 34 patients with chronic hypertension who were destined to develop superimposed pregnancy-induced hypertension. Shown in Figure 14.2 are the sequential pressor response values to angiotensin II for both of these groups of patients with chronic hypertension. In Figure 14.2 the dose of angiotensin II required to elicit a pressor response is shown on the vertical axis and is plotted as a function of weeks of gestation. Both groups of patients were resistant to the pressor effects of infused angiotensin between the 21st and 27th week of pregnancy. A clear separation between the two groups of patients developed after the 27th week of gestation, however, and the differences between the means became significant after the 30th week.

The pattern of angiotensin II responsiveness observed in these two groups of women with chronic essential hypertension is similar to that seen in both normal and future pre-eclamptic primigravid women. Indeed, the data obtained between the 28th and 32nd week of pregnancy suggest that pressor responsiveness to angiotensin II may also be used as a screening technique to identify those women with chronic hypertension who are destined to develop superimposed pregnancy-induced hypertension, as is the case in primigravid patients destined to develop pre-eclampsia/eclampsia. However, caution must be exercised in interpreting these data from the chronic hypertensive subjects in a manner analogous to that of the younger primigravid women. First, the number of patients and the number of infusions conducted in the study of chronic hypertensive gravidas are much smaller than those reported in the earlier study. Furthermore, superimposed pregnancy-induced hypertension is sometimes a difficult clinical diagnosis to make and as such is not nearly so "clean" a model as is the development of hypertension in a primigravid patient who was previously normotensive. Additionally, even when restricting the diagnosis of pregnancy-induced hypertension to primigravidas, any grouping of such patients will include a mixture of women with underlying hypertensive disease or chronic renal disease as was pointed out by McCartney[27] in his classic study of renal biopsies obtained in primigravid pregnancies with the clinical diagnosis of pre-eclampsia. Therefore, although individual determinations obtained between the 28th and 32nd week of gestation suggest that pressor responsiveness measured during this time might be used as a screening technique to identify those women destined to develop superimposed pregnancy-induced hypertension, additional studies conducted during this critical time period, 28 to 32 weeks, will be required before the reliability of such a screening technique is clearly established for gravidas with chronic hypertension.

Recently, a clinical test was described which correlates well with angiotensin II sensitivity or resistance. This test, which is noninvasive and can be done as an office procedure, is referred to as the "roll-over test."[8] The test is done by placing the 28- to 32-week pregnant patient in the lateral recumbent position and recording diastolic blood pressures for a minimum of 15 min or until diastolic blood pressure has become stable. At this point, the patient is "rolled over" onto her back and the blood pressure is taken again at 1 and 5 min. An increase in diastolic blood pressure of 20 mm Hg or more is regarded as a positive roll-over test (Figure 14.3). A positive roll-over test correlates well with increased sensitivity to angiotensin II and also with the ultimate development of pregnancy-induced hypertension. In prospective clinical studies of more than 700 women, those patients who exhibited a positive roll-over response ultimately developed pregnancy-induced hypertension in 76% of cases (Figure 14.4).[2, 16, 18, 23, 26, 37] Conversely, 92% of patients with a negative roll-over test re-

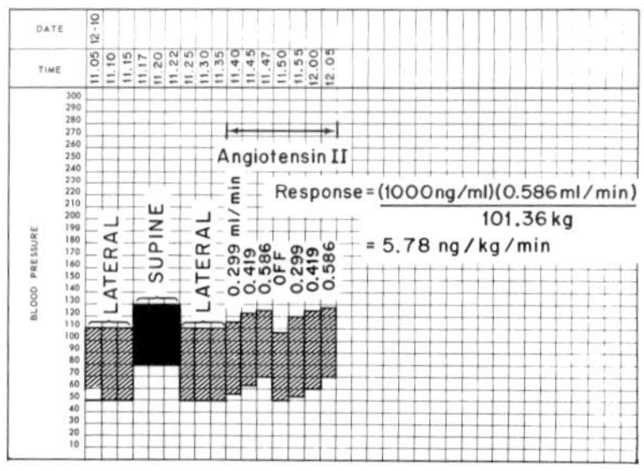

Figure 14.3. Illustration of a positive supine pressor test (roll-over test) followed by an angiotensin II infusion. After 15 min of lateral recumbency the patient was moved to the supine position and an immediate increase in diastolic blood pressure of 30 mm Hg was noted. After the patient was returned to the lateral position, diastolic blood pressure returned rapidly to baseline levels. An angiotensin II infusion was then begun. In this instance the patient required 5.7 ng per kg per min to elicit a pressor response on two occasions. (Reprinted with permission from Gant, N. F., Chand, S., Worley, R. J., Whalley, P. J., Crosby, U. D., MacDonald, P. C.: A clinical test useful for predicting the development of acute hypertension in pregnancy. Am J Obstet Gynecol 120: 1, 1974.)

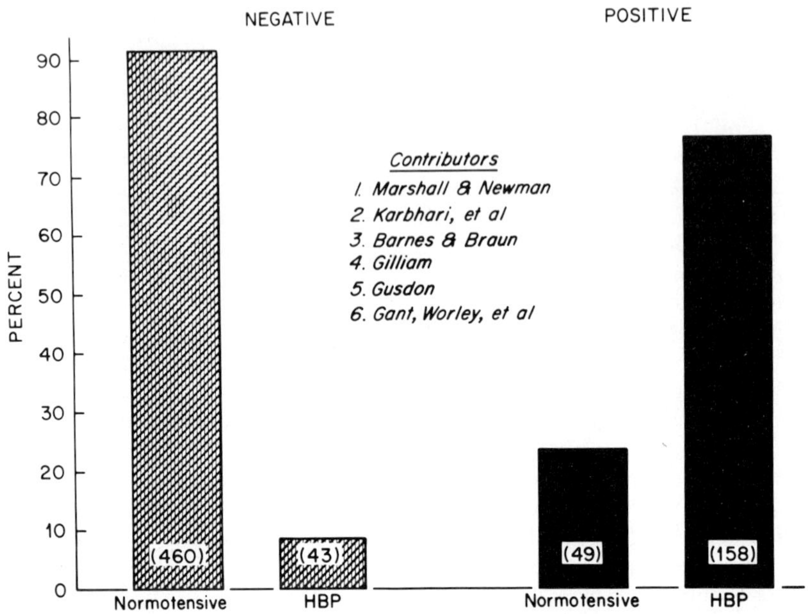

Figure 14.4. The clinical outcome in 710 patients with either a negative or positive roll-over test. Results obtained in patients with a negative test are shown in hatched bars and labeled "Normotensive" if they remained so throughout pregnancy and "HBP" if they ultimately developed hypertension. Solid bars with the same labeling are used to illustrate the results obtained in patients with a positive test. (The results shown in this illustration summarize the studies of Marshall and Newman,[26] Karbhari et al[23] and Gusdon et al.[18] The work of Barnes and Braun[2] has been submitted to the *Southern Medical Journal*. The series from Gillam[16] was presented as a personal communication as was the expanded series from Gant and Worley.)

mained normotensive throughout pregnancy.

With these two screening techniques, the physician now can identify a future pre-eclamptic patient as early as 3 months before the appearance of pregnancy-induced hypertension. This early identification of the gravida at high risk of developing pregnancy-induced hypertension will allow action to be taken that may delay the onset of the disease and/or modify its severity.

FETAL PATIENT

Thus far the discussion has centered primarily on the physician's first patient, the mother. From this point forward, however, let us consider the second patient, the fetus. Most investigators concur that pregnancy-induced hypertension jeopardizes the fetus by compromising uteroplacental blood flow. In fact, measurements of uteroplacental perfusion in pre-eclamptic women by a variety of techniques have uniformly detected 50 to 65% decrements either in flow[21, 28] or diameter of the spiral arterioles supplying the intervillous space.[3] Unfortunately, most of these attempts have either been too indirect to allow a true assessment of uteroplacental blood flow, too invasive for use in the human or have relied upon static measurements that cannot be expected to reflect uteroplacental perfusion accurately. Nevertheless, the need for a relatively noninvasive, accurate method of assessing blood flow through the intervillous space is clear, since availability of such a technique would allow one to study the uteroplacental dynamics of both normal and hypertensive pregnancies, and to assess responses of the latter to therapeutic regimens.

During the past 10 years our laboratory has addressed this problem. In so doing we have exploited the unique method by which estrogen is produced by the placenta. Measurements of the rate of placental clearance of maternal plasma prehormones for estrogen production have yielded a dynamic test of placental function. The placental clearance technique is based upon the fact that the placenta has little or no capability for de novo estrogen synthesis, but instead relies upon the delivery to it of ^{19}C steroids, primarily dehydroisoandrosterone sulfate (DS) and 16α-OH-dehydroisoandrosterone sulfate (16OHDS), for the synthesis of estradiol (E2) and estriol (E3), respectively.[32] Quantitatively, about half of placental estradiol production derives from DS of maternal adrenal origin and the other half from DS of fetal adrenal origin, whereas about 90% of estriol synthesis, especially in late pregnancy, derives principally from precursors supplied by the fetal adrenal.[32] This large fractional contribution of fetal precursors to estriol formation, however, reflects the relatively enormous production of 16OHDS in the fetal compartment, not greater efficiency in placental utilization of fetal rather than maternal precursors.[33]

In the nonpregnant women less than 0.1% of plasma DS is aromatized.[31] As early as the sixth week of human gestation, however, utilization of maternal plasma DS by the placenta for estradiol formation is readily demonstrable, and during the last weeks of pregnancy, 30 to 50% of maternal plasma DS is irreversibly converted to estradiol by the human placenta. All studies performed to date indicate that the amount of placental conversion of DS to E2 depends directly upon substrate availability, that plasma DS reaches its site of aromatization in the trophoblast by simple diffusion and that the trophoblastic supply of the aromatizing enzyme system is in excess.[25] Thus, since the production rate of DS by the maternal adrenal is relatively constant throughout pregnancy, the amount of DS aromatized by the placenta is a reflection of the amount of DS delivered to the intervillous space, or uteroplacental blood flow.

Although one can measure the extent of placental conversion of DS to E2 (the transfer constant), this measurement is a nonkinetic dimension and thus does not directly reflect the dynamics of flow which are in question. A kinetic dimension can be achieved, however, by measuring either the half-life or the metabolic clearance rate (MCR) of the prehormone. The metabolic clearance rate of a compound is that volume of blood or plasma completely and irreversibly cleared of hormone per unit of time. Since this computation identifies a volume of blood cleared as a function of time, it is much more readily applied to considerations of blood flow than is the half-life computation.

The MCR is usually measured by one of two practical methods. Hormones with a short half-life (high MCR) are best measured by the continuous infusion of isotope-labeled prehormone in tracer amounts until a steady state is achieved between the rate of its infusion and the rate of its disappearance from plasma. The metabolic clearance rate is then calculated from the known rate of infusion and the concentration of isotope-labeled hormone in plasma at steady state. The metabolic clearance rate of hormones with a relatively longer half-life (lower MCR) is best measured by computing the rate of disappearance of the isotope-labeled steroid from plasma after a single bolus injection. Either of these approaches is suitable for measuring the total metabolic clearance rate of maternal plasma ^{19}C prehormones, a portion of which is due to irreversible placental metabolism to estrogens.

As previously mentioned, aromatization of plasma DS in nonpregnant individuals is insignificant in amount. Moreover, the extent of conversion of plasma testosterone to estradiol in the nonpregnant subject is only 0.1 to 0.3%, and only about 1.5% of plasma androstenedione is converted to estrone.[24] Thus, even though extraglandular aromatization of plasma prehormones does occur in the nonpregnant individual, these conversions are insignificant when compared to the extensive placental aromatization of these compounds during pregnancy.

Because plasma dehydroisoandrosterone sulfate is the principle precursor of placental estrogen synthesis, the kinetics of dehydroisoandrosterone sulfate metabolism was first measured in pregnant subjects.[10] These studies showed that the metabolic clearance rate of dehydroisoandrosterone sulfate (MCR_{DS}) from maternal plasma is markedly increased during the course of human pregnancy. In fact, values 8-fold greater than those observed in the nonpregnant subject were found in normal pregnant women at or near term (Figure 14.5). Thus, not only is there a qualitative alteration in the metabolism of dehydroisoandrosterone sulfate during human pregnancy, but there is also a marked increase in the *rate* of its metabolism during pregnancy. Of the metabolic clearance rates of various steroidal hormones studied to date, DS is the only one whose metabolic clearance rate is so drastically altered during the course of human pregnancy. Therefore, an effort was made to ascertain the effect on the MCR_{DS} of pathologic aberrations as well as pharmacologic manipulations during pregnancy.

Among the first of these studies was a prospective assessment of serial MCR_{DS}

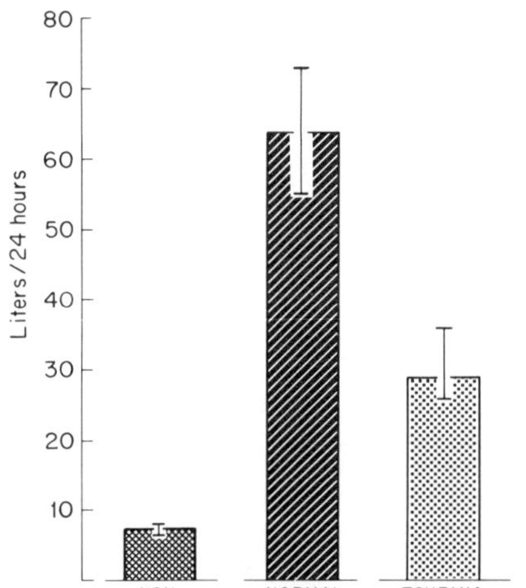

Figure 14.5. Metabolic clearance rate of DS (MCR_{DS}). The values for the nonpregnant group represent the MCR_{DS} determined in two normal men and two normal young women. The value for the MCR_{DS} in normal term pregnancy is the mean of 15 measurements in both primiparous and multiparous women. Values for MCR_{DS} in the "toxemia" group were obtained from six primigravid women with advanced pre-eclampsia characterized by hypertension, edema and proteinuria. (Reprinted with permission from Gant, N. F., Hutchinson, H. T., Siiteri, P. K., et al: Study of the metabolic clearance rate of dehydroisoandrosterone sulfate in pregnancy. Am J Obstet Gynecol 111: 555, 1971.)

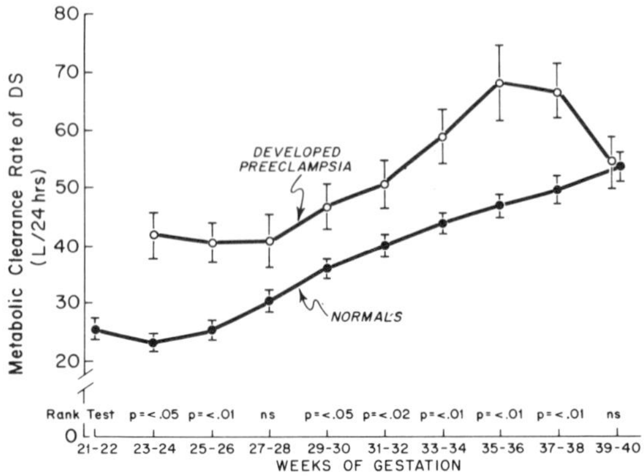

Figure 14.6.. The metabolic clearance rate of DS (MCR_{DS}) in normal primigravidas compared to primigravidas in whom pre-eclampsia ultimately developed. Note that the MCR_{DS} increased progressively throughout pregnancy in the 38 women who remained normal. In the 14 women who ultimately developed pre-eclampsia, initial values were higher and remained higher until 35 to 36 weeks' gestation (patients still clinically normal), at which time the values began to decrease. (Reprinted with permission from Gant, N. F., Madden, J. D., Siiteri, P. K., et al: A sequential study of the metabolism of dehydroisoandrosterone sulfate in primigravid women. Exerpta Medica International Congress Series No. 273, Endocrinology: Proceedings of the Fourth International Congress of Endocrinology, Washington, D. C., 1972, p 1026.)

determinations in young, primigravid women. These young subjects were chosen because of their high risk for ultimately developing pregnancy-induced hypertension. Results from this study showed that the MCR_{DS} in maternal plasma increased continually throughout normal pregnancy until the time of delivery (Figure 14.6).[14] Surprisingly, in those primigravidas who ultimately developed pregnancy-induced hypertension the MCR_{DS} initially was higher than in women who remained normotensive. The higher MCR_{DS} values observed in future pre-eclamptic patients persisted until approximately 4 to 6 weeks before the onset of hypertension, but then began to decline. This decrease in the MCR_{DS} continued until the appearance of hypertension, when the MCR_{DS} was similar to that observed in normal primigravid subjects at a comparable stage of gestation

(Figure 14.6). Furthermore, if these patients were not treated by bed rest or delivery, the metabolic clearance rate continued to decline and in some subjects reached nonpregnant values.[14]

In a similar study in gravidas with chronic hypertension who were destined to develop superimposed pre-eclampsia, the MCR_{DS} was higher than that of ambulatory chronic hypertensive subjects who did not develop superimposed pregnancy-induced hypertension (Figure 14.7).[11] In the patients who later developed superimposed pre-eclampsia the metabolic clearance rate began to decline before the appearance of superimposed pre-eclampsia (Figure 14.7), just as it did in primigravid women who later developed pre-eclampsia. Interestingly, in normotensive, chronic hypertensive and pre-eclamptic patients salt restriction or the administration of diuretics uniformly was followed by a decrease in the MCR_{DS} as well as a decrease in glomerular filtration rate (Table 14.1; Figure 14.8).[13, 30] Similarly, in gravidas with chronic hypertension, blood pres-

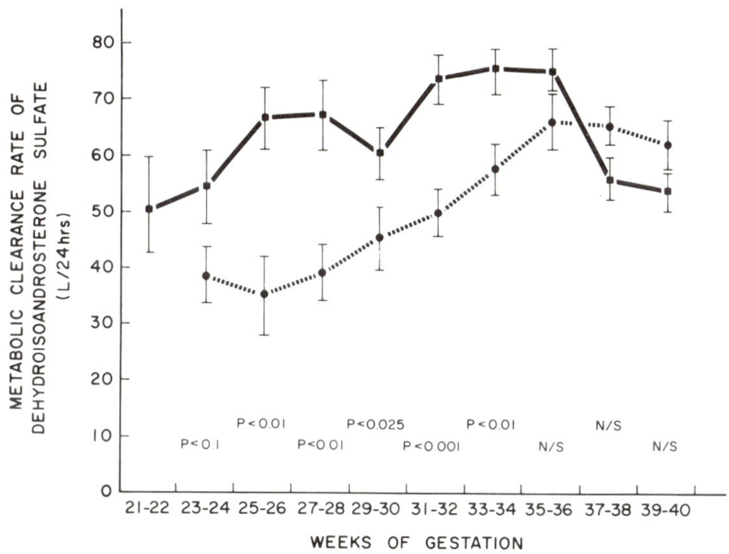

Figure 14.7. Comparison of the metabolic clearance rate of dehydroisoandrosterone sulfate (MCR_{DS}) in patients with chronic hypertension (●---●) and patients with chronic hypertension destined to develop superimposed pregnancy-induced hypertension (■——■). Vertical bars represent the standard error of the mean. The MCR_{DS} is plotted as a function of weeks of gestation. (Reprinted with permission from Gant, N. F., Madden, J. D., Chand, S., Worley, R. J., Strong, J. D., MacDonald, P. C.: The metabolic clearance rate of dehyroisoandrosterone sulfate. V. Prospective studies of essential hypertension complicating pregnancy. Obstet Gynecol 47: 319, 1976.)

Table 14.1. Individual patient values for metabolic clearance rate of dehydroisoandrosterone sulfate (MCR_{DS}) and the apparent volume of distribution of DA (AVD_{DS}) before and during therapy with furosemide in gravidas with chronic hypertension

Patient	MCR_{DS} (liters/24 hr)		Change (%)	AVD_{DS}		Change (%)	Change in diastolic blood pressure (mm Hg)
	Before therapy	During therapy		Before therapy	During therapy		
A. F.	86.0	74.0	↓ 13.9	12,500	11,111	↓ 11.1	0
C. B.	63.0	50.0	↓ 20.6	8,474	12,048	↑ 42.2	0
M. B.	64.0	51.0	↓ 20.3	6,097	6,666	↑ 9.3	0
O. I.	55.5	43.3	↓ 22.0	8,620	10,416	↑ 20.8	0
J. B.	58.5	47.0	↓ 19.6	7,042	8,474	↑ 20.3	0
Mean	65.4	53.1	↓ 18.8	8,546	9,743	↑ 14.0%	

sure reduction accomplished by treatment with intravenous hydralazine hydrochloride also resulted in a decrease in the MCR_{DS} (Table 14.2).[12] These studies suggested, but did not prove, that severe pregnancy-induced hypertension, salt restriction, diuretics and antihypertensive drugs decrease uteroplacental perfusion.

Since the MCR_{DS} measures the extent of removal of maternal plasma DS via all routes of metabolism and not specifically that fraction singularly and uniquely accounted for by placental removal to form estradiol, a technique has been developed that more specifically measures the placental kinetics of removal of DS from the maternal circulation. This technique combines the two concepts previously discussed regarding the metabolism of maternal dehydroisoandrosterone sulfate, i.e., measurement of the transfer constant of DS to placental estradiol and calculation of the metabolic clearance rate of dehydroisoandrosterone sulfate from maternal plasma. As indicated in Figure 14.9 these two measurements can be made in a single study that will allow one to compute specifically the rate of placental clearance of DS from maternal plasma. Thus, the total metabolic clearance rate of DS by all routes of removal can be measured as described above and as illustrated in Figure 14.9. In the same study the fraction of this total metabolism accounted for by the irreversible placental removal and conversion of dehydroisoandrosterone sulfate to the product hormone, estradiol, is also calculated. The product of these two, i.e., MCR_{DS} and percentage of DS converted to E2, equals the volume of maternal plasma cleared specifically by placental conversion of dehydroisoandrosterone sulfate to estradiol per unit time, or the placental clearance of DS to E2 (PC_{DSE2}).

Utilizing this technique definitive assessments can be made of the impact on uteroplacental function of various pathophysiologic aberrations of pregnancy, and of pharmacologic or nutritional manipulations of the gravida whose fetus is at risk.

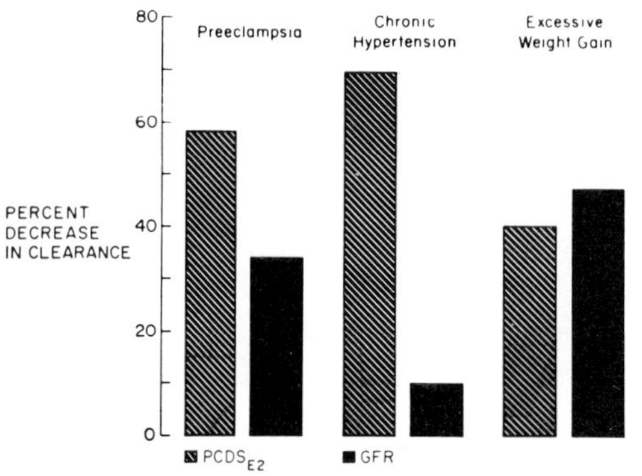

Figure 14.8. The percentage of decrease in the placental clearance of dehydroisoandrosterone sulfate ($PCDS_{E2}$) and glomerular filtration rate (*GFR*) following sodium restriction and diuretic therapy are shown for patients with pre-eclampsia, chronic hypertension and excessive weight gain. $PCDS_{E2}$ is represented by the striped bars and GFR is represented by the solid bars. (Reprinted with permission from Shoemaker, E. S., Gant, N. F., Madden, J. D., and MacDonald, P. C.: The effect of thiazide diuretics on placental function. Tex Med 69: 1, 1973.)

Table 14.2. Individual patient values for metabolic clearance rate of dehydroisoandrosterone sulfate (MCR_{DS}) and apparent volume of distribution of DS (AVD_{DS}) before and during therapy with hydralazine hydrochloride in gravidas with chronic hypertension

Patient	MCR_{DS} (liters/24 hr)		Change (%)	AVD_{DS} (ml)		Change (%)	Change in diastolic blood pressure (mm Hg)
	Before therapy	During therapy		Before therapy	During therapy		
A. S.	68	60	↓ 11.8	8,130	9,347	↑ 15.0	↓ 44
C. F.	66	59	↓ 10.6	9,615	12,980	↑ 35.0	↓ 44
J. C.	63	32	↓ 49.2	9,434	14,084	↑ 49.3	↓ 26
O. W.	46	19	↓ 58.7	6,060	9,700	↑ 60.1	↓ 30
F. D.	36	34	↓ 5.6	10,752	7,810	↓ 27.4	↓ 40
C. R.	50	35	↓ 30.0	8,333	6,896	↓ 17.2	↓ 40
J. A.	41	37	↓ 9.8	9,090	7,570	↓ 16.7	↓ 35
B. W.	69	60	↓ 13.0	13,510	12,650	↓ 6.4	↓ 40
Mean	54.9	42.0	↓ 23.5	9,365	10,129	↑ 8.1	↓ 37.4

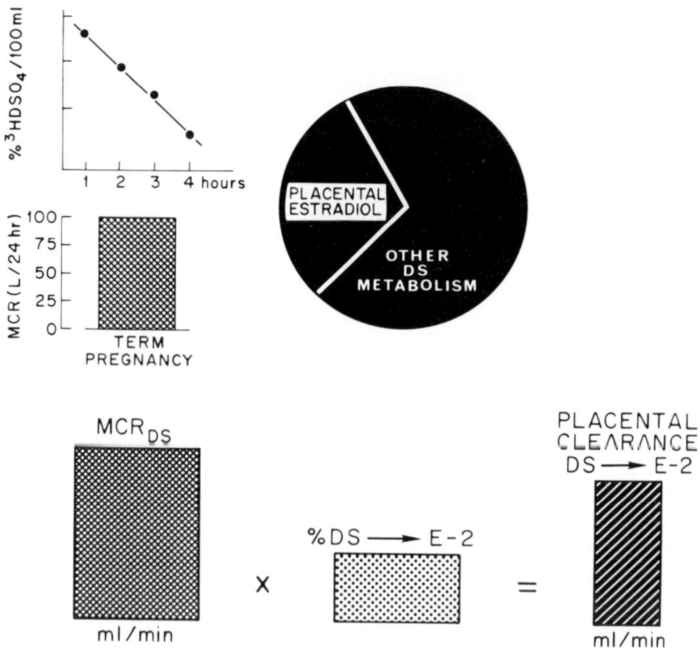

Figure 14.9. The placental clearance of dehydroisoandrosterone sulfate is computed as the product of the MCR_{DS} and the $[\rho]_{BU}^{DSE2}$ and expressed as the milliliters of maternal plasma DS cleared per unit time by the placenta for estradiol synthesis. (Reproduced with permission from Gant, N. F., Worley, R. J., MacDonald, P. C.: *Hypertension In Pregnancy*. Edited by M. Lindheimer, A. Katz, F. P. Zuspan, New York, John Wiley and Sons, 1976, pp 309–314.)

Furthermore, these results can be correlated with pregnancy outcome. At present such studies are in progress in our laboratory.

Treatment

For the past several years at Parkland Memorial Hospital the clinical management of pregnancies complicated by pregnancy-induced hypertension, chronic hypertension or a combination of both has been based upon the clinical and laboratory observations just presented. However, the clinical management of pregnancy-induced hypertension does not require the measurement of placental clearances or other complex laboratory procedures. In fact, therapy for both pregnancy-induced and/or chronic hypertension is based on clinical assessment of both the mother and fetus. Table 14.3 is an outline of the clinical management of such patients.

The outline of therapy in Table 14.3, which is based upon the clinical condition of both the maternal and fetal patients, has proven effective at Parkland Memorial Hospital. It is presented to serve as a guide for therapy. Each condition will be considered briefly and specific items of therapy discussed in detail.

The easiest clinical conditions to manage are those listed in category A. In these situations with a mature infant (greater than 37 weeks gestation) the most efficacious therapy for both mother and fetus has been to prevent convulsions by the administration of parenteral magnesium sulfate and to effect delivery. This approach is based upon the premise that the infant is sufficiently mature to survive ex utero and delivery is preferable to continued exposure to a compromised intrauterine environment. The mother is also best served by this approach since the only definitive treatment for pregnancy-induced hypertension remains delivery of the fetus.

A more difficult situation is presented when there is pregnancy-induced hypertension or chronic hypertension, the infant

Table 14.3. Clinical management of patients with pregnancy-induced and/or chronic hypertension

Clinical condition	Therapy
A. Pregnancy-induced hypertension (or chronic hypertension) when the fetus is mature	Definitive 1. Prevention of convulsions 2. Control of blood pressure 3. Delivery
B. Pregnancy-induced hypertension (or chronic hypertension) when the fetus is immature and there are signs of 1. Severe pre-eclampsia (or superimposed preeclampsia) 2. Fetal growth retardation 3. Fetal jeopardy	Definitive 1. Prevention of convulsions 2. Control of blood pressure 3. Delivery
C. Future or mild pregnancy-induced hypertension when the fetus is immature	Expectant 1. Ambulatory 2. Hospitalization

is immature and severe pre-eclampsia, fetal growth retardation or fetal jeopardy occur. Under these circumstances the intrauterine environment is no longer the best possible incubator for the fetus, so the infant is better delivered and placed in the care of a competent neonatologist. Therefore, in these clinical situations convulsions are either treated or prevented by the use of parenteral magnesium sulfate and the pregnancy is terminated.

It is important at this juncture to define the phrases severe pre-eclampsia, severe fetal growth retardation and fetal jeopardy. Severe pre-eclampsia is defined as the presence of any one of the following: (*a*) blood pressure greater than 160/120 mm Hg; (*b*) oliguria (24 hr urine output of less than 600 ml); (*c*) cyanosis or pulmonary edema; (*d*) visual symptoms and/or epigastric pain; (*e*) the presence of proteinuria greater than 3 to 4+ on a random catheterized urine specimen or proteinuria greater than 5 g per 24 hr urine specimen. Any one of these signs or symptoms identifies the pregnancy as being complicated by severe pre-eclampsia.

Severe fetal growth retardation is suggested when no fetal growth is observed on sequential physical examinations by the same physician combined with a failure of maternal weight gain, or even weight loss, after the 34th week of gestation. Actual documentation of fetal growth retardation is based upon serial ultrasound examinations of fetal thoracic and biparietal diameters.

The final indication for delivery regardless of gestational age is fetal jeopardy. At present two of the most widely accepted indicators of fetal jeopardy are the presence of meconium-stained amniotic fluid (obtained at the time of amniocentesis) and a positive oxytocin challenge test. However, it is important to emphasize that a positive oxytocin challenge test is not diagnostic of impending fetal death and at present can only be considered as suggestive of fetal distress. Although the same can be said about the significance of meconium-stained amniotic fluid, there are few who will not accept this finding as a sign of considerable fetal jeopardy. Regardless, if any of the clinical conditions listed under categories A or B in Table 3 are present, experience at Parkland Memorial Hospital has documented that fetal survival can be enhanced only by delivery of the infant.[20]

For those women in categories A and B an antihypertensive agent is utilized if diastolic blood pressure is greater than 110 mm Hg. For over 20 years at Parkland Memorial Hospital the drug of choice for this purpose has been hydralazine hydrochloride (Apresoline). Hydralazine is administered in intermittent intravenous doses of 5 to 10 mg to maintain diastolic blood pressure near 100 mm Hg. No attempts are made to lower blood pressure to normotensive readings since this represents a potential hazard for the fetus.[12] The use of antihypertensive medications in women classified in these two categories is limited strictly to the control of blood pressure during the intrapartum and postpartum periods. These agents are not utilized in ill advised, desperate attempts to prolong such gestations.

Infants born to mothers with these hypertensive disorders have been shown to have accelerated pulmonary maturation.[17] The evidence presented earlier that pregnancy-induced hypertension is a chronic disease which affects both mother and fetus many weeks prior to the development of hypertension suggests that the initiating factor responsible for the early lung maturation may be chronic stress or some other as yet undefined process. Thus one may anticipate that lung maturation is more advanced for gestational age in the infant of a woman with pregnancy-induced hypertension when compared to the infant of a normotensive gravida.[17] Therefore attempts to prolong pregnancies in which there are signs of severe pre-eclampsia, severe fetal growth retardation, or fetal jeopardy with the use of antihypertensive medications are ill advised because a significant reduction in blood pressure in these gravidas represents a distinct hazard to a fetus who quite likely would not only survive but thrive in an extrauterine environment.

Because lung maturation is frequently accelerated in infants of women with pregnancy-induced hypertension, the question naturally occurs as to whether or not amniocentesis should be performed in these pregnancies to document lung maturation. At Parkland Memorial Hospital we do not obtain amniotic fluid when delivery is absolutely indicated for maternal reasons. However, when indications for delivery are less urgent, amniotic fluid is obtained for L/S ratio determinations after the placenta is localized by sonography. With this precaution of placental localization, the risk of fetal injury from amniocentesis is significantly lowered. However, it must be kept in mind that even if the L/S ratio is less than 2:1 the fetal lung may still be mature. Even in normotensive pregnancies when the L/S ratio is less than 2:1 but above 1.5:1 only 40% of infants develop respiratory distress, and only 2% will succumb.[19] Therefore, it may be anticipated in pregnancies complicated by pregnancy-induced hypertension that a satisfactory fetal outcome can usually be expected when the L/S ratio is greater than 1.5:1 but less than 2:1.

Expectant therapy (clinical condition C) is used for patients who are destined to develop or who have already developed early or mild pregnancy-induced hypertension and have immature fetuses. This form of management is also utilized for all patients with chronic hypertension. In these instances treatment consists of either hospitalization or ambulatory care.

AMBULATORY CARE

Ambulatory care is limited to those patients with mild chronic hypertension who are less than 32 weeks pregnant and normotensive patients who have been identified by the roll-over test or angiotensin II sensitivity as destined to develop pregnancy-induced hypertension. The ambulatory, normotensive patients at high risk to develop pregnancy-induced hypertension are seen at weekly intervals and advised to remain at decreased physical activity at home. Preliminary results[35] indicate that the incidence of overt hypertension may thereby be decreased and the onset of hypertension delayed in these women. In no instances are these patients treated with salt restriction, antihypertensives or diuretics.

HOSPITALIZATION

At the first sign of hypertension in primigravid women or rising blood pressure in those with chronic hypertension, the patient is admitted to the hospital. Any blood pressure reading over 140/90 mm Hg in a previously normotensive woman is considered an indication for immediate hospitalization. There is in fact *no* place in modern obstetrics for ambulatory care of the patient with pregnancy-induced hypertension or chronic hypertension with superimposed pre-eclampsia. Therefore, in the Parkland Memorial Hospital Obstetric Clinics special attention is given to any elevation in blood pressure. If diastolic blood pressure exceeds 90 mm Hg the patient is promptly hospitalized and placed

LNMP: 8-21-73 Quickening: 12-30-73 EDC: 5-29-74 FHT 1st: 1-3-74

Complications: 15 year old Black Para 0-0-0-0 with PREGNANCY INDUCED HYPERTENSION

	Dates	3-16	3-19	3-22	4-2	4-8	4-15	4-22	4-29	5-1	5-2
	Weeks of Gestation	30	30	31	32	33	34	35	36	36	36
	Weight	136	129	129	130	130	130	131	132	134	136
	Blood Pressure	150/110	130/90	136/84	130/80	124/84	126/85	130/80	140/90	146/90	170/110
Renal Function	Plasma creatinine / urea	0.8 / 9				0.6 / 6			1.0 / 12		
Renal Function	Urine Creatinine total mgs.	1000				1200			1000		
Renal Function	Creatinine Clearance	123				124			69		
Renal Function	Urine Protein	Trace	0	0	0	0	0	0	0	1+	2+
Ultrasound	Biparietal (mm)		73			82				89	
Ultrasound	Growth Rate (mm/wk)					3.2				2.1	
Ultrasound	Gestation (weeks)		28			32				36	
Ultrasound	Placental Location		post								
Other	Plasma Estrogen (µg%)	2.8	3.0	3.5	4.4	6.1	6.4	9.5	10.7	11.3	11.2
Other	L/S Ratio									<2	
Other	Estimated Fetal Weight (Pounds)		3		4.0			4.5			

DELIVERY 5/2/74 C-Section BIRTH WEIGHT 2320 gm Apgar 9/9

Figure 14.10. Example of a good response to management on the high risk pregnancy unit at Parkland Memorial Hospital. All pregnancies followed on this unit have this form placed in their charts so that temporal changes are immediately apparent to the obstetrician. (Reproduced with permission from Hauth, J. C., Cunningham, F. G., Whalley, P. J.: Management of pregnancy-induced hypertension in the nullipara. Obstet Gynecol 48: 253, 1976.)

at decreased physical activity in the high risk pregnancy unit. Within 1 week the majority of women with pregnancy-induced hypertension become *normotensive* (Figure 14.10).[20] Furthermore, there is usually prompt clearing of edema and lesser degrees of proteinuria in the majority of cases. Most importantly, the patients are maintained in this high risk pregnancy unit until delivery because the return to outpatient management of such women will result in a return of hypertension in most instances.[20] In fact, the vasospastic process usually rapidly intensifies when the gravida is again managed as an outpatient and the hypertension then frequently becomes so severe that both mother and fetus may be compromised, necessitating early delivery which most likely could have been avoided had the patient maintained a sedentary existence.

The high risk pregnancy unit at Parkland Memorial Hospital is under the supervision of Dr. Peggy Whalley, who has recently reported outstanding clinical results based upon the management briefly outlined above.[20] Her high risk pregnancy unit has markedly lowered perinatal morbidity and mortality and has shown beyond doubt that early hospitalization of women with pregnancy-induced hypertension remote from term results in remarkable clinical outcomes for both the maternal and fetal patients. These results were achieved by merely restricting the patients to a sedentary form of existence and managing them without sodium restriction, without antihypertensive medications and without diuretics. Utilizing this simple clinical approach the status of the mother and her fetus has, in the majority of cases, been improved to such a degree that the development of severe preeclampsia and/or eclampsia largely has been prevented or delayed until after fetal lung maturation has occurred.

Further observations in patients with pregnancy-induced hypertension admitted to this high risk unit have shown that despite the consequent lowering or normalization of blood pressure, the underlying pregnancy-induced disease process is not cured and remains unrelieved except by delivery. Specifically, Worley et al[36] reported that, despite a return of blood pressure to normotensive ranges in the same patients reported by Hauth et al,[20] the placental clearance of dehydroisoandrosterone sulfate remained approximately one-half of that expected for the same period of gestation in normotensive gravidas. In fact, placental clearances of DS remained abnormally low throughout the remainder of pregnancy even though maternal blood pressure had fallen to normotensive ranges.

Since intense vasospasm or worsening of hypertension may develop suddenly or recur at any time before delivery (and even until a few days postpartum), each case is followed daily and clinically monitored as follows. (*a*) Blood pressure is recorded four times a day. If diastolic blood pressure increases to greater than 100 mm Hg a physician is notified immediately to reassess the patient. (*b*) A physician is summoned to the ward immediately if a patient complains of headache, visual disturbances, epigastric pain, lower abdominal pain (which might indicate abruption) or a decrease in fetal movement. (*c*) Weight is measured on alternate days and a sudden increase in weight, even in the absence of proteinuria and hypertension, is regarded as a grave prognostic sign which frequently heralds the rapid development of hypertension and proteinuria. (*d*) Fetal growth is evaluated by serial sonographic studies of both biparietal and thoracic diameters. If fetal growth retardation is documented the fetus is delivered. (*e*) Clean-voided urine specimens are checked three times a week for proteinuria. If overt proteinuria develops and persists delivery is indicated as outlined earlier. (*f*) Renal function is evaluated by plasma urea nitrogen levels and plasma creatinine values as well as 24-hr creatinine clearances obtained biweekly. If abnormally low creatinine clearances are obtained and confirmed in subsequent examinations, delivery is most often effected.

The goal of management on the High Risk Antepartum Unit is maintenance of maternal well-being and delivery of an infant who will survive and develop normally. Therefore, delivery is delayed until, but not past term unless hypertension persists or recurs after initial improvement following hospitalization. Factors other than hypertension alone also contribute to the decision to deliver the fetus as mentioned above, and include (*a*) rapid weight gain; (*b*) a decrease in creatinine clearance; (*c*) significant proteinuria; (*d*) fetal growth retardation; (*e*) headache, scotomata or epigastric pain; and (*f*) any indication of fetal jeopardy.

In summary, the regimen reported by Hauth, Cunningham and Whalley[20] allows the physician to observe nulliparous women with pregnancy-induced hypertension safely until fetal viability is assured. The regimen of modified bed rest combined with attention to fetal growth, maternal blood pressure changes, sudden weight gain and renal function results in a good clinical outcome in the majority of women so managed. Furthermore, although serial ultrasonography is helpful in assessing fetal growth, it is not absolutely necessary. Immunoreactive plasma estrogen measurements were performed twice weekly but in the final analysis did not influence the decision for delivery in any case.[6] Moreover, these tests sometimes indicated fetal well-being in a mother with obvious clinical deterioration, such as the case illustrated in Figure 14.10.

In their initial report of the results obtained on this high risk pregnancy unit, Dr. Whalley and her colleagues reported on 372 nulliparous women, usually black teenagers, who were admitted because of pregnancy-induced hypertension remote from term.[20] Of the 372 nulliparous women, 346 remained on the unit for care until the pregnancy was terminated. Perinatal mortality in this group of women who remained hospitalized was 9 per 1000. Furthermore, only five infants developed respiratory distress and all survived. The mean birth weight of the infants in this group was 2974 g, 83% of the infants weighing 2500 or more at the time of birth. The pregnancy outcomes of 26 women who left the high risk unit against medical advice, however, were dismal compared to those who remained. The perinatal mortality rate in this group was 154 per 1000!

The actual cost of providing care on this high risk antepartum ward has been approximately $15 per patient day. The cost can be kept at this level because the majority of services provided for these patients in this predominantly domiciliary care unit are janitorial, meal service and minimal nursing care which can be provided by specially trained LVN's. Although the charge to the patient may be approximately $70 to $100 per day, this represents a significant savings when compared to the cost of a neonatal intensive care stay for a grossly premature, seriously ill newborn infant. Such stays cost as much as $600 per day in the Dallas, Texas area, where the average stay is 10 days. It is apparent that the mother is not only the best incubator for the infant but is certainly the most cost-effective one as well.

DEFINITIVE THERAPY

The definitive treatment of pregnancy-induced hypertension is terminaton of the pregnancy. However, effective control of hypertension and the prevention or treatment of convulsions has made definitive treatment easier for the physician and certainly safer for both the mother and fetus. For the past 20 years, prevention or control of convulsions at Parkland Memorial Hospital has been effected by the use of parenteral magnesium sulfate ($MgSO_4 \cdot 7H_2O$). This agent has been used because it (*a*) definitely controls and/or prevents seizures due to pregnancy-induced hypertension; (*b*) the patient is alert and awake, in marked contrast to the use of barbiturates, tranquilizers or narcotics; (*c*) because the patient is awake, airway problems and aspiration of stomach contents are less likely; (*d*) the already compromised, frequently depressed fetus is not further depressed by narcotics, etc.; and (*e*) magnesium sulfate therapy is easily managed with a minimum of demands on nursing and physician time. (In those rare instances in which convulsions have not been controlled or prevented by the use of this agent alone, the addition of one or two doses of sodium amobarbital, 250 mg intravenously, has been successful.)

As with all drugs magnesium sulfate has certain disadvantages, which include the pain of the intramuscular injection and the danger of sciatic nerve damage. Both of these disadvantages can, of course, be overcome with the use of continuous intravenous administration via infusion pumps. However, this mode of therapy demands that physicians or trained nursing personnel always be in attendance so that overdoses can be prevented. Because of the inherent risk of continuous intravenous infusions and because of the demands on nursing and physician time, parenteral magnesium sulfate therapy at Parkland Memorial Hospital has been limited primarily to intramuscular administration, the only exception being the use of low dose intravenous loading doses to achieve rapid blood levels.

The use of parenteral magnesium sulfate at Parkland Memorial Hospital follows those guidelines established by Pritchard.[29] Specifically, a loading dose of 10 g of magnesium sulfate is administered as a 50% solution in divided doses, one-half of the dose deep intramuscularly in the upper outer quadrant of each buttock. Thereafter, a maintenance dose of 5 g of 50% magnesium sulfate is administered every 4 hr. If seizures have begun or appear imminent a rapid blood level of magnesium sulfate may be achieved by the intravenous administration of a 4-g dose of 20% magnesium sulfate given over a timed 5-min period.

The pharmacology of magnesium sulfate may be summarized by stating that the agent is a central nervous system depressant in toxic levels and also in toxic levels exerts a curare-like, neuromuscular blocking effect. Magnesium sulfate itself has no sustained hypotensive effects, but a transient and mild hypotensive response is often observed when magnesium sulfate is administered as an intravenous bolus. The normal physiologic blood levels of magnesium are approximately 1.5 to 2.5 mEq per liter. Therapeutic anticonvulsant blood levels are achieved when the concentration of magnesium reaches 4 to 7.5 mEq per liter. Signs of magnesium toxicity are reached at approximately 10 mEq per liter, at which point the patellar reflex is lost. Respiratory arrest usually occurs at plasma levels above 15 mEq per liter and total body paralysis at levels of approximately 25 mEq per liter. Therefore, any order for the administration of magnesium sulfate *must* specify that the drug is not to be given in the absence of patellar reflexes. The duration of action of the drug is, of course, dependent upon its route of administration, absorption from injection sites, and rate of clearance from blood. The intravenous administration of 4 g of magnesium sulfate as a 20% solution results in almost instantaneous blood levels in the therapeutic range, but when renal function is normal the serum magnesium concentration will return to normal within 30 to 60 min. It is important to emphasize that magnesium sulfate is almost exclusively cleared from the circulation by the kidneys, so the patient's renal status has great bearing on the duration of action of the drug. Therefore, following a loading dose of magnesium sulfate, a maintenance dose should not be given unless urine output has been greater than 100 ml during the past 4 hr and patellar reflexes are present.

In summary, magnesium sulfate orders for a patient with pre-eclampsia should include:

1. A 10-g loading dose (administered as 10 ml of 50% $MgSO_4 \cdot 7H_2O$ deep intramuscularly in each buttock.)
2. A 5-g maintenance dose (administered as 10 ml of 50% $MgSO_4 \cdot 7H_2O$ deep intramuscularly in alternating buttocks) every 4 hr (*a*) if patella reflexes are present and (*b*) if urine output is greater than 100 ml per 4 hr
3. Urine output every 4 hr
4. Vital signs with blood pressure every hr

Magnesium sulfate orders in a patient with eclampsia should include all the above plus the intravenous administration of 4 g of magnesium sulfate as a 20% solution to achieve immediate blood levels.

Control of hypertension in the preeclamptic or eclamptic patient is aimed at lowering maternal blood pressure to safer levels for the mother without compromising the fetus. Lowering the diastolic blood pressure to less than 100 mm Hg in chronic hypertensive patients results in significant decreases in the metabolic clearance rate of dehydroisoandrosterone sulfate, implying a significant decrease in uteroplacental perfusion.[12] Because of the significant risk of maternal cerebral vascular accidents, however, it is frequently imperative that maternal blood pressure be reduced to more acceptable levels. Thus, if diastolic blood pressure is above 110 mm Hg the use of antihypertensive medications is mandated for maternal indications. However, the goal of therapy is not to reduce blood pressure to normal levels, rather the goal is to lower and maintain diastolic blood pressure near 100 mm Hg. As previously mentioned hydralazine hydrochloride (Apresoline) has been used with notable success at Parkland Memorial Hospital for the past 20 years and is administered in intermittent small intravenous doses which produce a predictable and graded lowering of maternal blood pressure. Specific therapy with hydralazine hydrochloride consists of the intravenous administration of a 5-mg test dose and monitoring of blood pressure every 5 min. If the diastolic pressure is not lowered to about 100 mm Hg within 20 min, a 10-mg dose is similarly administered, and its effects are monitored as described. This dose is repeated until the diastolic blood pressure is lowered to approximately 100 mm Hg. The desired effect is usually achieved with 5 to 20 mg of hydralazine hydrochloride and the drug is repeated whenever diastolic blood pressure exceeds 110 mm Hg.

It is important to re-emphasize that this form of antihypertensive therapy is confined to the intrapartum and postpartum periods of time and is not used in ill advised attempts to prolong pregnancy. In fact, the experience at Parkland Memorial Hospital has shown that with rare exceptions even women with chronic hypertension should *not* be maintained on antihypertensive medications throughout pregnancy. Therefore, with the exception of women with high renin forms of hypertension who are successfully medically treated and normotensive at the beginning of pregnancy, the rule has been to stop all antihypertensive medications and follow these patients at weekly intervals until the 30th to 32nd week of pregnancy, when they are admitted to the high risk maternity ward. On this ward they are managed in the same fashion as women with pregnancy-induced hypertension until the 37th to 38th week of gestation, when delivery is effected.

The method of delivery for women with pregnancy-induced hypertension or chronic hypertension is based upon obstetric indications. If there are no obstetric contraindications to vaginal delivery, labor is induced by the intravenous administration of dilute oxytocin. All such inductions are monitored closely for frequency, duration and intensity of uterine contractions and fetal heart rate patterns.

Analgesia during labor is restricted to intermittent intramuscular or intravenous doses of 50 mg of meperidine with or without 25 mg of promethazine. If the fetus is premature attempts are made to minimize these doses and to avoid their administration during the 2 hr preceding delivery.

Anesthesia for spontaneous vaginal deliveries usually consists of pudenal block or local perineal and vaginal infiltration supplemented with self-administered nitrous oxide by mask. Spinal, epidural or caudal anesthesia is not used in hypertensive patients, who most often have constricted blood volumes. Endotrachael general anesthesia is used for more difficult forceps deliveries and cesarean sections. This anesthesia consists of a small intravenous dose of sodium thiopental, followed by succinylcholine, endotrachael intubation and nitrous oxide and oxygen. Because succinylcholine and magnesium sulfate may act synergistically to produce muscle paralysis, less succinylcholine is needed to maintain adequate muscle relaxation throughout the delivery.

Using the clinical approaches outlined in this chapter, perinatal mortality among pre-eclamptic primigravidas at Parkland Memorial Hospital in 1974 was 20 per 1000. By comparison, the overall Parkland perinatal mortality rate for the same year was 26 per 1000 and the national average 23 per 1000. Although this is an encouraging overall perinatal mortality rate for women with pregnancy-induced hypertension, the most impressive results are those previously cited from the high risk antepartum unit, where the perinatal mortality rate for infants of mothers who remained on the unit until delivery was 9 per 1000, but for infants of those who left against medical advice was 154 per 1000.

It should be apparent from the data presented in this chapter that pregnancy-induced hypertension is a chronic, insidious progressive disease of pregnancy. Furthermore, this disease is one which can be detected before the appearance of overt hypertension, and with its early detection or the early recognition of hypertension, significant modification of the disease process is possible utilizing the therapy outlined. In most instances the pregnancy can be prolonged until fetal maturity without the use of diuretics, antihypertensives or sodium restriction, all of which have been shown to affect the fetus adversely. Finally, the principles and practices outlined in this chapter are readily adaptable to any community hospital and competent practitioner of obstetrics.

REFERENCES

1. Abdul-Karim, R., Assali, N. S.: Pressor response to angiotonin in pregnant and nonpregnant women. Am J Obstet Gynecol 82: 246, 1961.
2. Barnes, A. B., Braun, R. D.: An evaluation of the roll-over test. South Med J (Submitted for publication.)
3. Brosens, I. A., Robertson, W. B., Dickson, H. G.: The role of the spiral arteries in the pathogenesis of preeclampsia. Obstet Gynecol Ann 172, 1972.
4. Chesley, L. C.: Vascular reactivity in normal and toxemic pregnancy. Clin Obstet Gynecol 9: 871, 1966.
5. Chesley, L. C.: Hypertensive disorders in pregnancy. *Williams' Obstetrics*. Edited by L. M. Hellman, J. A. Pritchard, Appleton-Century-Crofts, New York, 1971, p 685.
6. Duenhoelter, J. H., Whalley, P. J., MacDonald, P. C.: An analysis of the utility of plasma immunoreactive estrogen measurements in determining delivery time of gravidas with a fetus considered at high risk. Am J Obstet Gynecol 125: 889, 1976.
7. Gant, N. F., Chand, S., Whalley, P. J., MacDonald, P. C.: The nature of pressor responsiveness to angiotensin II in human pregnancy. Obstet Gynecol 43: 854, 1974.
8. Gant, N. F., Chand, S., Worley, R. J., Whalley, P. J., Crosby, U. D., MacDonald, P. C.: A clinical test useful for predicting the development of acute hypertension in pregnancy. Am J Obstet Gynecol 120: 1, 1974.

9. Gant, N. F., Daley, G. L., Chand, S., et al: A study of angiotensin II pressor response throughout primigravid pregnancy. J Clin Invest 52: 2682, 1973.
10. Gant, N. F., Hutchinson, H. T., Siiteri, P. K., et al: Study of the metabolic clearance rate of dehydroisoandrosterone sulfate in pregnancy. Am J Obstet Gynecol 111: 555, 1971.
11. Gant, N. F., Madden, J. D., Chand, S., Worley, R. J., Strong, J. D., MacDonald, P. C.: The metabolic clearance rate of dehydroisoandrosterone sulfate. V. Prospective studies of essential hypertension complicating pregnancy. Obstet Gynecol 47: 319, 1976.
12. Gant, N. F., Madden, J. D., Danniels, J. F., Siiteri, P. K., MacDonald, P. C.: The metabolic clearance rate of dehydroisoandrosterone sulfate. IV. Acute effects of induced hypertension, hypotension, and naturesis in normal and hypertensive pregnancies. Am J Obstet Gynecol 124: 143, 1976.
13. Gant, N. F., Madden, J. D., Siiteri, P. K., MacDonald, P. C.: The metabolic clearance rate of dehydroisoandrosterone sulfate. III. The effect of thiazide diuretics in normal and future preeclamptic pregnancies. Am J Obstet Gynecol 123: 159, 1975.
14. Gant, N. F., Madden, J. D., Siiteri, P. K., et al: A sequential study of the metabolism of dehydroisoandrosterone sulfate in primigravid women. Excerpta Medica International Congress Series No. 273, Endocrinology: Proceedings of the Fourth International Congress of Endocrinology, Washington, D. C., 1972, p. 1026.
15. Gant, N. F., Whalley, P. J., Chand, S., MacDonald, P. C.: A prospective study of angiotensin II pressor responsiveness in pregnancies complicated by chronic essential hypertension. Am J Obstet Gynecol 127: 369, 1977.
16. Gillam, J. S.: A clinical evaluation of a test of changes in postural diastolic blood pressures to predict the development of hypertension in primigravid pregnancies. (Personal communication.)
17. Gluck, L., Kulovich, M. V.: Lecithin/sphingomyelin ratios in amniotic fluid in normal and abnormal pregnancies. Am J Obstet Gynecol 115: 539, 1973.
18. Gusdon, Jr., J. P., Anderson, S. G., May, W. J.: A clinical evaluation of the "roll-over test" for pregnancy-induced hypertension. Am J Obstet Gynecol 127: 1, 1977.
19. Harvey, D., Parkinson, C. E., Campbell, S.: Risk of respiratory distress syndrome. Lancet 1: 42, 1975.
20. Hauth, J. C., Cunningham, F. G., Whalley, P. J.: Management of pregnancy-induced hypertension in the nullipara. Obstet Gynecol 48: 253, 1976.
21. Johnson, T., Clayton, C. G.: Diffusion of radioactive sodium in normotensive and preeclamptic pregnancies. Br Med J 1: 312, 1957.
22. Kaplan, N. M., Silah, J. G.: The effect of angiotensin II on the blood pressure in humans with hypertensive disease. J Clin Invest 43: 659, 1964.
23. Karbhari, D., Harrigan, J. S., LaMagra, R.: The supine hypertensive test as a predictor of incipient preeclampsia. Am J Obstet Gynecol 127: 620, 1977.
24. MacDonald, P. C., Rombaut, R. P., Siiteri, P. K.: The *in vivo* mechanism of origin of estrogen in subjects with trophoblastic tumors. Steroids 8: 589, 1966.
25. MacDonald, P. C., Siiteri, P. K.: Origin of estrogen in women pregnant with an ancephalic fetus. J Clin Invest 44: 465, 1965.
26. Marshall, G. W., Newman, R. L.: The roll-over test. Am J Obstet Gynecol 127: 623, 1977.
27. McCartney, C. P.: Pathological anatomy of acute hypertension of pregnancy. Circ Suppl 29–30: 37, 1964.
28. McClure Browne, J. C.: The uterine circulation in toxemia. Clin Obstet Gynecol 1: 341, 1958.
29. Pritchard, J. A., Pritchard, S. A.: Standardized treatment of 154 consecutive cases of eclampsia. Am J Obstet Gynecol 123: 543, 1975.
30. Shoemaker, E. S., Gant, N. F., Madden, J. D., MacDonald, P. C.: The effect of thiazide diuretics on placental function. Tex Med 69: 109, 1973.
31. Siiteri, P. K., MacDonald, P. C.: The utilization of circulating dehydroisoandrosterone sulfate for estrogen synthesis during human pregnancy. Steroids 2: 713, 1963.
32. Siiteri, P. K., MacDonald, P. C.: Placental estrogen biosynthesis during human pregnancy. J Clin Endocrinol Metab 26: 751, 1966.
33. Siiteri, P. K., MacDonald, P. C.: The origin of placental estrogen precursors during human pregnancy. Excerpta Medica International Congress Series No. 132. Proceedings of Second International Congress on Hormonal Steroids, Milan, 1966, p 726.
34. Talledo, O. E., Chesley, L. C., Zuspan, F. P.: Renin, angiotensin system in normal and toxemic pregnancies. III. Differential sensitivity to angiotensin II and norepinephrine in toxemia of pregnancy. Am J Obstet Gynecol 100: 218, 1968.
35. Worley, R. J., Cox, K., Gant, N. F.: Ambulatory care versus modified bedrest for the gravida identified as destined to develop pregnancy-induced hypertension. (In preparation.)
36. Worley, R. J., Everett, R. B., MacDonald, P. C., Gant, N. F.: Placental clearance of dehydroisoandrosterone sulfate and pregnancy outcome in three categories of hospitalized patients with pregnancy-induced hypertension. Proceedings of 22nd Annual Meeting of the Society for Gynecological Investigation, March 1975.
37. Worley, R. J., Gant, N. F., Cox, K.: An additional look at the roll-over test. (In preparation.)

F. GARY CUNNINGHAM, M.D., FACOG
JACK A. PRITCHARD, M.D., FACOG

15

Hematologic Disorders in Pregnancy

Hematologic abnormalities in the form of anemia and of acquired coagulopathies are more common among pregnant than nonpregnant women. Several of the anemias pose serious threats to the mother and fetus as do coagulopathies induced by pregnancy accidents. Hopefully, the description provided below of most of the anemias that are likely to be encountered during pregnancy and of several of the pregnancy accidents that commonly lead to consumptive coagulopathy will prove helpful in prevention, diagnosis and treatment.

Hematologic Disorders in Pregnancy

I. Anemias
   A. Definition of anemia
   B. Acquired anemias
      1. Iron deficiency
      2. Blood loss
      3. Chronic disorders
      4. Megaloblastic from folate deficiency
      5. Acquired hemolytic
      6. Aplastic (hypoplastic)
      7. Pernicious (B_{12} deficiency)
   C. Hereditary anemias
      1. Sickle hemoglobinopathies
         A. SS
         B. SC
         C. S-beta thalassemia
      2. Hemoglobin CC, C-beta thalassemia
      3. Beta thalassemia
         A. Minor
         B. Major
      4. Hereditary spherocytosis
II. Coagulopathies
   A. Thrombocytopenia
      1. Idiopathic thrombocytopenic purpura
      2. Thrombocytopenia from transfusions
   B. Placental abruption
   C. Pre-eclampsia/eclampsia
   D. Dead fetus
   E. Amniotic fluid embolism
III. Leukemia

Anemias

DEFINITION OF ANEMIA

The definition of anemia is complicated by differences in the hemoglobin concentrations between women and men, as well as between pregnant and nonpregnant women. On the basis of observations summarized in Table 15.1, and for reasons that follow, it can be said that a woman is anemic if the hemoglobin concentration is less than 12.0 g per 100 ml when nonpregnant, or is less than 10.0 g per 100 ml during pregnancy or the puerperium.[43]

The normal decrease in hemoglobin levels that accompanies pregnancy in healthy iron-sufficient women is the result of a relatively greater expansion of the plasma volume compared with the increase in red cell volume. This disparity is most apparent during midpregnancy. The plasma volume plateaus early in the third trimester while red cell production continues beyond that time, provided that iron is available. Therefore, the hemoglobin concentration of healthy pregnant women most often is 11.0 g per 100 ml or higher. Following normal delivery the hemoglobin concentration is not significantly lower than before delivery unless there has been appreciable hemorrhage. The hemoglobin level postpartum commonly fluctuates moderately for a few days before rising toward the nonpregnant level. This fluctuation is apparently due to relative hemoconcentration the consequence of labor, and subsequently to the mobilization and excretion of extracellular fluid that accumulates during normal gestation.

The differences between the hemoglobin concentrations in pregnant and nonpregnant women, coupled with the well recognized phenomenon of pregnancy hypervolemia, have led to the use by some of the term *physiologic anemia*. This is a poor and confusing term for describing a normal process, and should be discarded. Since the hemoglobin concentration is responsive to the oxygen level, the maternal hyperoxia which exists during most of normal pregnancy provides a logical explanation of the somewhat lower hemoglobin concentration during that period.

The frequency of anemia during pregnancy depends primarily on whether or not supplemental iron is taken during pregnancy. For example, in an earlier study at Parkland Memorial Hospital, the results of which are quite similar to several others, the hemoglobin concentration at the time of delivery averaged 12.4 g per 100 ml in women who took iron supplements, but was only 11.3 g per 100 ml in those women who received no iron.[41] In the women who took iron supplements the hemoglobin was only rarely less than 10.0 g per 100 ml, however, it was below this level in 16% of the women taking no iron. Furthermore, with iron supplementation the hemoglobin concentration was 11.0 g per 100 ml or more in 94% of women, whereas without supplementation it was 11.0 g per 100 ml or more in only 53%.

Classification of Anemias

Anemias during pregnancy can be classified as those that are *acquired* and those that are *inherited*. A limited classification of the more commonly encountered anemias is presented in Table 15.2. By far, the

Table 15.1. Hemoglobin concentration in healthy nonpregnant and pregnant women with proven iron stores*

	Hemoglobin concentration (g/100 ml)				
	Mean	<12 (%)	<11 (%)	<10 (%)	Lowest
Nonpregnant (n = 85)	13.7	1	0	0	11.7
Midpregnancy (n = 81)	11.5	72	29	4	9.7
Late pregnancy (n = 95)	12.3	36	6	1	9.8

* From Pritchard and Scott.[43]

Table 15.2. Causes of anemia during pregnancy

Acquired	Hereditary
Iron deficiency anemia	Sickle hemoglobinopathies
Acute blood loss anemia	Hemoglobin SS Disease
Anemia of chronic disorders	Hemoglobin SC Disease
Folate deficiency anemia	Sickle-beta thalassemia
Acquired hemolytic anemias	Thalassemia
Aplastic or hypoplastic anemia	Other hemolytic anemias
Vitamin B_{12} deficiency anemia	

two most common causes of anemia during pregnancy and the puerperium are iron deficiency and acute blood loss.

IRON DEFICIENCY ANEMIA

In a typical gestation with a single fetus the need for iron averages close to 800 mg, of which approximately 300 mg is required by the fetus and placenta, while the remainder is used to expand the maternal hemoglobin mass.[17, 48] Thus the iron requirements of pregnancy usually exceed considerably the iron stores even of healthy women. For example, in the United States, as well as in Sweden, iron stores in nonpregnant women have been demonstrated to be most often less than 500 mg, and not uncommonly, there is no storage iron demonstrable.[22, 43] Unless the difference between the amount of maternal storage iron and the iron requirements of normal pregnancy is made up by dietary or medicinal iron during pregnancy, iron-deficiency anemia will develop. Since the amount of iron transported to the fetus from the iron-deficient mother does not differ significantly from the amount normally transferred, at birth the infant of even a severely anemic mother does not have iron deficiency anemia.

The initial evaluation of a pregnant woman with a hemoglobin concentration of 9 to 10 g per 100 ml should include measurements of hemoglobin and red cell indices, reticulocyte count, careful examination of a stained smear of peripheral blood, a sickle cell preparation if the patient is black and perhaps measurement of serum iron concentration. Bone marrow examination is seldom performed at this point, although the demonstration of hemosiderin in marrow particles excludes iron deficiency as the cause of anemia. In severe iron deficiency anemia during pregnancy the erythrocytes exhibit the classic morphologic changes of hypochromasia, microcytosis and poikilocytosis. These changes are less likely to be as prominent in the pregnant woman as in the nonpregnant woman with a hemoglobin concentration of 9 to 10 g per 100 ml. In the moderately anemic pregnant woman the diagnosis of iron deficiency is usually presumptive, and is based largely on the exclusion of other causes of anemia.

If the pregnant woman with iron deficiency anemia receives therapeutic doses of iron, a hematologic response is first evident upon examination of the peripheral smear. New red cells, which are usually larger than normal and are polychromatophilic or basophilic, will be apparent 5 to 7 days after therapy is begun. The reticulocyte count also becomes elevated and usually reaches a maximum 5 to 10 days following iron therapy. Unless the anemia is severe, however, the degree of reticulocytosis most likely will be modest.

The rate of increase of hemoglobin concentration with iron therapy varies, but is usually somewhat slower than in nonpregnant women. This is related largely to blood volume differences. During the latter half of gestation the newly formed hemoglobin is added to the characteristically larger blood volume. Furthermore, since the blood volume commonly continues to expand during the period of therapy, the production of a given amount of hemoglobin by the pregnant woman usually does not result in a rapid increase in hemoglobin concentration. There is little evidence, however, that pregnancy itself depresses erythropoiesis in the iron-deficient woman who is being adequately treated.

There has been some divergence of opinion regarding optimal treatment of iron-deficiency anemia during pregnancy and the puerperium. Although the use of an effective parenteral iron medication guarantees that the mother receives the iron, oral preparations are preferred if the woman understands the importance of taking the medication regularly. If she will not, or much less likely, cannot take oral iron, parenteral therapy is the alternative. Whichever treatment is given, the objectives are reasonably prompt correction of the anemia and eventual restitution of iron stores. Both of these objectives can be accomplished with adequate doses of oral iron compounds that supply a daily dose of about 200 mg of elemental iron. To establish marrow iron stores oral therapy should be continued for 3 to 6 months after the anemia is corrected.[42]

Whenever parenteral iron therapy is

judged advisable during pregnancy, a satisfactory dose in most instances is one 5-ml ampule of iron-dextran providing 250 mg of iron to be given for each 1.0-g deficit in maternal hemoglobin concentration. Accordingly, if the hemoglobin level is 8.0 g per 100 ml, the number of ampules to be injected is 13 minus 8, or 5 ampules, plus 1 more ampule for the fetus and placenta. To provide sufficient iron for effective erythropoiesis, 250 mg of iron should be injected every 4 to 7 days. If after the first few injections there is no evidence of hematologic response as measured by increased reticulocytosis, it is important that the injections be stopped and the cause of anemia re-evaluated.

Folic acid may be given in combination with iron as a safeguard against folate deficiency, although in our experience the response of pregnant women with iron-deficiency anemia treated with iron and folic acid is no better than when iron alone is given.

Blood transfusions are seldom indicated for the treatment of iron deficiency anemia unless hypovolemia from blood loss coexists, or if an operative procedure must be performed on the severly anemic woman. The administration of whole blood to a woman with severe anemia and compromised cardiac function can lead to severe circulatory overloading with pulmonary edema and death. Exchange transfusion is an effective way to raise circulating hemoglobin of the severely anemic woman without inducing or intensifying circulatory overloading. A technique for exchange transfusion is outlined under "Sickle Cell Anemia."

ACUTE BLOOD LOSS ANEMIA

Severe hemorrhage demands immediate volume replacement, ideally with whole blood in amounts that restore and maintain adequate vital organ perfusion. In order to accomplish this seldom is it necessary to give blood to raise the hemoglobin concentration to normal values. In general, once dangerous hypovolemia has been treated and hemostasis achieved, the residual anemia should be treated with iron. Therapy should be continued long enough to repair hemoglobin mass and to allow for storage iron to be deposited.

ANEMIA OF CHRONIC DISORDERS

A number of subacute and chronic infections, chronic inflammatory states, neoplastic diseases, as well as mild to moderate renal insufficiency, is likely to produce moderate, and occasionally severe anemia. In these instances, the red cells are usually normocytic or very slightly microcytic, and both the serum iron concentration and iron binding capacity are typically decreased. The bone marrow differs from that of iron deficiency in that stainable iron is usually evident and erythroid hyperplasia is lacking. Reticulocytopenia is present. The anemia appears to result, at least in part, from alterations in reticuloendothelial function and iron metabolism, as well as a slightly shortened lifespan of the erythrocytes.[18] Iron released from the patient's senescent red blood cells is retained in the reticuloendothelial cells and not properly released to transferrin to be reutilized for production of new hemoglobin. The fate of iron administered in therapeutic doses is similar. There is currently no effective treatment except red cell transfusions should the patient become symptomatic from anemia.

Although some have found a higher incidence of anemia in women with *asymptomatic bacteriuria* during pregnancy, this has not been our experience at Parkland Memorial Hospital.[15, 60] Women who develop severe pyelonephritis during pregnancy, however, are likely to be overtly anemic once dehydration has been corrected. The exact incidence and severity of the anemia varies but seems to be related to the severity of the infection, and possibly to the presence or absence of septicemia or endotoxemia. Brumfitt[8] reported that 45% of pregnant women with acute pyelonephritis had anemia. It is also our experience that antepartum pyelonephritis is commonly complicated by anemia. The mean hemoglobin concentration in 40 women with antepartum pyelonephritis was 9.7 g per 100 ml, and in two-thirds of these women the hemoglobin level was less than 10 g per 100 ml. The anemia associated with pyelonephritis appears to be due to somewhat increased red cell destruction as well as impaired production.[13] Reticulocytopenia is common and red cell lifespan, as measured by ^{51}Cr labeling, is usually somewhat reduced.

Repair of the circulating hemoglobin mass following successful treatment for pyelonephritis appears to be delayed because of suppressed erythropoiesis as indicated by reticulocytopenia which persists for several weeks. Women who demonstrate anemia following pyelonephritis in midpregnancy will frequently have a hemoglobin concentration of less than 11 g per 100 ml at the time of delivery.

At least some cases of so-called *refractory anemia of pregnancy* probably are the consequence of one of these diseases that has gone unrecognized. The anemia of infection, chronic renal disease and malignancy is refractory in the sense that it is not corrected by treatment with iron, folic acid, vitamin B_{12} or any other known hematinic agent. Nonetheless, prophylaxis with iron and folic acid is recommended to offset any deficiency induced by pregnancy.

ANEMIA FROM FOLATE DEFICIENCY

The prevalence of megaloblastic anemia from folate deficiency during pregnancy varies considerably throughout the world. In the United States, overt anemia with frankly megaloblastic erythropoiesis is a most uncommon complication of pregnancy. When it occurs it is usually found late in pregnancy or in the puerperium. The woman with this disorder typically is one who consumes neither fresh vegetables, especially of the uncooked green leafy variety, nor foods with a high animal protein content. In our experience the earliest morphologic change in the peripheral blood smear that indicates folate deficiency is hypersegmentation of some of the neutrophils. As anemia develops, newly formed erythrocytes are produced in reduced numbers and are macrocytic. As maternal folate deficiency and, in turn, anemia become profound, then thrombocytopenia, leukopenia or both are likely to develop. The placenta and fetus extract folate from maternal sources so effectively that the infant is not born anemic, even though the mother is severely anemic from folate deficiency.[45]

In folate-deficient pregnant women with overt megaloblastic bone marrow changes, as little as 1 mg of folic acid administered orally once daily will produce a striking hematologic response. Within 3 to 6 days after treatment is started, the reticulocyte count is appreciably increased, and leukopenia and thrombocytopenia are corrected. Although the ineffective erythropoiesis from folate deficiency typically results in a considerable elevation of the plasma iron, pregnant women who develop megaloblastic anemia commonly become deficient in iron when treated with folic acid because any available iron stores are rapidly utilized for hemoglobin synthesis to fill newly produced red cells. Thus it is necessary to administer oral iron compounds in addition to folic acid.

Megaloblastic anemia tends to recur in subsequent pregnancies, very likely because of repeated dietary inadequacies, but also perhaps in part because of diminished absorption or utilization of folic acid. The use of estrogen plus progestin oral contraceptives is considered by some to predispose to folate deficiency. Several investigations, however, have not established any relationship between the use of oral contraceptives and folate deficiency.

FOLATE DEFICIENCY WITHOUT OVERT ANEMIA

A great deal of investigation in the past 15 years has been devoted to the possible role of folate deficiency in various forms of reproductive failure and, in turn, the value of prophylactic administration of folic acid throughout pregnancy. Hibbard, Hibbard and coworkers[24, 25] in England have maintained that folate deficiency is an important cause of placental abruption, abortion and fetal malformation. However, most investigations, including those from our laboratory, have found maternal folate deficiency to be no more common among women who experience these obstetric problems than those of the general obstetric population.[55, 62] From the foregoing, it appears most unlikely that intensive public health measures to provide folic acid supplementation to eradicate all possible maternal folate deficiency would have a marked effect on reducing these complications.

ACQUIRED HEMOLYTIC ANEMIA

Women with an acquired hemolytic anemia and a positive direct Coombs test sometimes demonstrate marked acceleration of hemolysis during pregnancy. Prednisone and other glucocorticoids are apparently as effective as when used in the nonpregnant state. Thrombocytopenia associated with this condition may also be favorably affected by such therapy.

Drug-induced hemolytic anemia occasionally is encountered during pregnancy. The red cell destruction is one of immunohemolysis which is mediated by one of several mechanisms and involves destruction of an intrinsically normal red cell. For example, anemia may result from an antibody that, in the presence of drugs such as quinine or penicillin, may cause lysis of red blood cells.

Especially in black women, hemolysis may more often be related to an inherited specific erythrocyte enzymatic deficiency, especially glucose-6-phosphate dehydrogenase (G-6-PD). Several oxidant drugs may induce hemolysis in these susceptible women. The more common agents with the potential for inducing hemolysis in G-6-PD-deficient women are sulfonamides, nitrofurantoin and analgesics and antipyretics, including aspirin. Infection and acidosis intensify drug-induced hemolysis. Young red blood cells contain higher levels of G-6-PD than do older erythrocytes, and are resistant to destruction; thus the anemia ultimately stabilizes. Unless there is coexisting bone marrow depression, the anemia is rather promptly corrected once the drug is discontinued.

The most fulminant acquired hemolytic anemia encountered in obstetrics is caused by the exotoxin of *Clostridium perfringens*. Although more common with septic abortion, clostridial septicemia and hemolysis have been encountered in puerperal infections. When hemolysis is overt, the mortality rate is high, and *acute tubular necrosis* is inevitable. Treatment is controversial; however, in our experience, intensive antibiotic therapy with usually limited but prompt surgical intervention to remove all infected products of conception, results in a maternal salvage rate equal to or better than after hysterectomy.[13, 47] Peritoneal or hemodialysis promptly instituted is necessary until renal failure resolves, which it usually does. Very infrequently irreversible *cortical necrosis* develops.

APLASTIC OR HYPOPLASTIC ANEMIA

Rarely encountered during pregnancy, *aplastic anemia* has a grave prognosis. None of the erythropoietic agents that produce remission of other anemias is effective, although corticosteroids may be of some value. When hypoplastic anemia antedates pregnancy, improvement is unlikely after pregnancy interruption. When the disease develops during pregnancy, however, termination occasionally results in remission.[53] Delivery should be accomplished vaginally whenever possible. If there are no large lacerations or incisions of the birth canal, and if the uterus is kept firmly contracted after delivery, intense thrombocytopenia is not likely to cause fatal hemorrhage. Moreover, the risk of sepsis is less likely with otherwise uncomplicated vaginal delivery than with cesarean section.

PERNICIOUS ANEMIA

Megaloblastic anemia caused by deficiency of vitamin B_{12} during pregnancy is rare. *Addisonian pernicious anemia,* in which there is failure to absorb vitamin B_{12} because of lack of intrinsic factor, is extremely uncommon in women of reproductive age. Moreover, unless women with this disease are treated with vitamin B_{12}, infertility may be a complication.[4] The two women with this condition that we have encountered were both over 35 years of age. Pernicious anemia had been diagnosed and treated prior to conception, and both did well with injections of 1 mg of vitamin B_{12} each month during pregnancy.

Hereditary Anemias

SICKLE HEMOGLOBINOPATHIES

Sickle cell anemia (SS disease), sickle cell-hemoglobin C disease (SC disease) and sickle cell beta thalassemia disease (S-beta thalassemia disease) are the three most important hemoglobinopathies which complicate pregnancy. Maternal and perinatal morbidity and mortality are variably but remarkably increased with each of these diseases.[19, 44]

Hemoglobin SS Disease (Sickle Cell Anemia)

In the United States 8 to 10% of black people have sickle cell trait, the result of inheritance of one gene for hemoglobin S and one for hemoglobin A. From this prevalence the frequency of sickle cell anemia among American blacks should be approximately 1 per 600. The disease is not nearly so common in pregnant blacks, however, with a frequency of only one-fourth to one-third the calculated prevalence. This disparity is undoubtedly due to childhood mortality from hemoglobin SS, and, in addition, the fertility, or at least the parity, of these women most often is reduced.

Pregnancy induces a serious burden on the woman with sickle cell anemia. Not only is the anemia likely to be intensified, but other forms of morbidity are increased. Severe episodic bone and joint pain, presumably due to red cell sludging in the microvasculature with infarction, occur more frequently and with greater intensity during pregnancy. Infections, especially pyelonephritis and pneumonitis, are more common. Pulmonary embolism and infarction are troublesome complications during pregnancy and the puerperium.

The reproductive performance of women with SS disease is notoriously poor. Pregnancy wastage from spontaneous abortion, stillbirths and neonatal deaths approaches 50% (Table 15.3).[19, 44]

Close monitoring, clinical as well as hematologic, of pregnant women with sickle cell anemia is mandatory for a favorable outcome. These women must be evaluated frequently and systematically throughout pregnancy and have access to emergency care at all hours, preferably provided by a physician who is well acquainted with the woman and her problems, and who appreciates the complexities of her disease and its interaction with pregnancy. Any complaint must be thoroughly investigated and often warrants hospitalization. To attribute pain simply to a so-called "sickle cell crisis," without ruling out other causes, is to invite disaster. Even though focal intravascular sickling seems to be a common cause of pain, this must be a diagnosis of exclusion. A vigorous examination for a source of infection, especially of the urinary tract, is mandatory, as well as a search for other obstetric complications which may give rise to severe pain, such as spontaneous abortion, ectopic pregnancy or placental abruption.

Table 15.3. Maternal deaths, abortions, perinatal deaths, and fetal salvage in women with sickle cell disease and sickle cell-hemoglobin C disease from Dallas* and Memphis†

Hemoglobinopathy	Dallas		Memphis	
	No.	%	No.	%
Hemoglobin SS disease				
Pregnancies	50		97	
Maternal deaths	0	0	6	6.2
Abortions	16	32	15	15.5
Perinatal deaths	9	17	32	33
Fetal salvage	27	52	50	52
Hemoglobin SC disease				
Pregnancies	78		34	
Maternal deaths	2	2.6	3	8.8
Abortions	5	6.4	8	23.5
Perinatal deaths	7	9.3	7	20.6
Fetal salvage	68	85	19	56

* Pritchard et al.[44]
† Fort et al.[19]

In the absence of infection or nutritional deficiency, especially folic acid, the hemoglobin concentration rarely falls below 7 g per 100 ml. Folic acid requirements, already increased by the increased erythropoiesis, are further increased by the demands for folate imposed by pregnancy. The dietary intake of folic acid by these women, especially at times of pain, is not likely to be optimal. Therefore, folic acid supplementation is recommended. A daily dose of 1 mg appears to be adequate.

With sickle cell anemia low birth weight from fetal growth retardation, prematurity or both, is common.[44] Because of the high incidence of stillbirths, the fetus is more likely better off ex utero if retarded growth is identified and the lungs are mature. When accurate dating of the gestation is not possible, and fetal growth retardation is suspected, measurement of the amniotic fluid lecithin to sphingomyelin ratio should be made, and if the results indicate that the lungs are mature, delivery is indicated.

The conduct of labor for the woman with SS disease is essentially the same as that of the woman with cardiac disease. She should be kept comfortable but not oversedated. In all cases, cross-matched blood should be immediately available, and if difficult vaginal delivery or cesarean section is anticipated, packed red cells should be given prior to delivery, or whole blood should be given during delivery. Aims of transfusion therapy are to maintain the hemoglobin concentration at 10 g per 100 ml or somewhat more. Likewise, at any time that cardiac work is significantly increased, such as with severe pregnancy-induced hypertension, it is recommended that the hemoglobin concentration be raised to about 10 g per 100 ml by the infusion of packed red blood cells but with care to prevent circulatory overload.

For the woman compromised by severe anemia, especially when associated with other factors predisposing to congestive heart failure, e.g., severe hypertension or infection, immediate partial exchange transfusion is warranted. We find the following method of exchange transfusion to be safe and effective. Two units of packed red blood cells are made ready for infusion utilizing a blood pump, a blood warming unit and a large bore indwelling venous catheter. Five hundred milliliters of blood are withdrawn rapidly from the opposite arm and the packed red cells are infused rapidly. The exchange transfusion may be repeated. The cardiac failure typically is characterized as "high output" and the benefits to be derived from digitalis glycosides therefore are questionable. Excessive blood loss at any time should immediately be replaced with *whole blood*.

Because of the chronic debility from sickle cell anemia, the increased complications caused by pregnancy, and the typically shortened lifespan of the woman, sterilization is indicated, even in women of low parity. As with other women with a serious incurable medical disorder, family size should be curtailed; at Parkland Memorial Hospital permanent sterilization is usually recommended after one pregnancy.

Hemoglobin SC Disease

The frequency of the gene for hemoglobin C in American blacks is approximately 1 in 50. It can be calculated, therefore, that 1 in 2400 black pregnant women will have SC disease. At Parkland Memorial Hospital the prevalence of SC disease among black pregnant women has been close to this figure.[44]

Unlike the woman with SS disease, the woman with SC disease, when not pregnant, seldom experiences severe morbidity. Pregnancy, however, increases morbidity and mortality.[16, 20, 44] Episodes of severe bone and joint pain, oftentimes never before a problem, frequently first appear during pregnancy. Likewise, episodes of "pneumonitis" may be encountered. The "pneumonitis" appears to be related to embolization of necrotic bone marrow which causes appreciable maternal morbidity and increased mortality.

Although spontaneous abortion in women with SC disease does not appear inordinately high, there is significantly increased perinatal mortality as emphasized by Pritchard et al,[44] as well as by Fort et al[19] (Table 15.3). The frequency of low birth weight infants is also appreciably increased.

Prenatal care given to the woman with SC disease is similar to that outlined for the women with SS disease. When pulmonary embolism, typically from necrotic bone marrow, is suspected heparin is recommended, although the benefits do not appear so great as with classic venous thromboembolism. The guidelines for blood transfusions in women with SC disease are similar to those for women with SS disease.

Careful clinical estimation, as well as ultrasonographic mensuration of fetal growth, as described for SS disease, is essential. Suspected fetal growth retardation with a lecithin to sphingomyelin ratio in amniotic fluid of 2 or more, warrants delivery. Although iron stores may be greater than in the general population, some women who have never been transfused may become iron depleted during pregnancy. It is recommended that in the absence of blood transfusion therapy an iron supplement be given in addition to folic acid.

Sickle Cell-Beta Thalassemia Disease

The inheritance of the gene for hemoglobin S from one parent and the allelic gene for beta thalassemia from the other parent results in sickle cell-beta thalassemia disease. When not pregnant these women may be asymptomatic and unaware of their disease. Although experience with this disease is not great due to its relative rarity, it has been the experience at Parkland Memorial Hospital that women with S-beta thalassemia behave during pregnancy like those with SC disease. They are prone to morbidity from bone marrow infarction accompanied by intense bone and joint pain, as well as pulmonary embolization. Likewise, the perinatal mortality rate for pregnancies complicated by S-beta thalassemia disease is similar to that for SC disease (Table 15.4). Again, the likelihood of low birth weight infants is increased. The general management of pregnancies complicated by S-beta thalassemia disease is the same as that outlined for SC disease.

Prophylactic Transfusion of Pregnant Women with Sickle Hemoglobinopathies

Transfusion of normal red cells not only to increase the hemoglobin concentration but to decrease the number of cells capable of sickling has been practiced sporadically. Ricks,[52] for example, reported a series of seven cases in which transfusion was employed with good maternal and fetal outcomes. More recently, Morrison and colleagues[32, 33] have reported their experiences with exchange transfusions used to try to decrease both maternal and fetal morbidity and mortality and their results are encouraging.

Table 15.4. Pregnancy outcome in 37 women with sickle cell-beta thalassemia disease*

	No.	%
Total pregnancies	37	
Maternal deaths	0	
Abortions	3	8.1
Fetuses	35	
Stillbirths	2	5.7
Neonatal deaths	1	2.9
Fetal salvage	32	84.2

* From Pritchard et al.[44]

Our previous extensive experiences indicated that pregnancy morbidity with sickle hemoglobinopathies is not limited to the third trimester of pregnancy.[44] Therefore a protocol was established that provided for red cell transfusion therapy to be initiated as soon as the diagnosis of pregnancy was established in any consenting woman who was demonstrated to have SS, SC or S-beta thalassemia disease.

At the outset red cells free of hemoglobin S were infused until the percentage of red cells that sickled was reduced to less than 50%, and the hematocrit was at least 32. With experience it became apparent that the beneficial effects of donor red cells were more the consequence of the ratio of normal to abnormal cells rather than the hematocrit. Therefore, the protocol has now been revised to maintain nonsickling red cells at 50% or higher, but without special concern for the hematocrit. In some cases of SC disease and S-beta thalassemia with nearly normal hematocrits, partial transfusion has been used to establish and maintain a population of red cells of which at least 50% did not sickle.

We have now treated 22 women during 23 pregnancies. Eleven of the pregnancies were complicated by SS disease, 9 by SC disease, and 3 by S-beta thalassemia disease. All of the women treated thus far have remained remarkably free of pain during pregnancy and the early puerperium. Very troublesome antibody formation as the consequence of multiple transfusions persists in one woman. Another woman with SS disease developed hepatitis with marked hyperbilirubinemia near the end of the second trimester, and late in pregnancy developed severe hypertension further complicated by congestive heart failure. Her fetus expired at this time, presumably from hypoxia. One woman with SS disease aborted spontaneously at 12 weeks, very soon after her initial transfusions. Twenty-one infants were liveborn and have subsequently done well.

Although Morrison and Wiser[33] claim a

remarkable decrease in the incidence of fetal growth retardation in infants born to mothers with transfusion therapy, our experiences are somewhat different. To date, we have commonly observed fetal growth retardation, although not severe, as well as fetal distress, manifested most often by meconium staining. Less often, abnormal fetal cardiac deceleration was observed during labor. The cesarean section rate to date has been high, and most often abdominal delivery was performed because of strong evidence of fetal growth retardation with an unfavorable cervix or because of fetal distress during labor.

Our observations, as well as those of Morrison et al,[32] indicate that the red cell transfusion therapy for the woman with the major sickle hemoglobinopathies is beneficial to her and her fetus. Nonetheless, there are risks involved which cannot be ignored, especially alloimmunization and hepatitis. Another difficult problem has been that women who are troubled by frequent attacks of pain when nonpregnant, and then go for many months free of pain, are likely to be less tolerant of pain when the protective effect of the transfusions dissipates. Morrison and Wiser[33] also rightfully point out that the expense of hospitalization and blood transfusion may be a deterrent to prophylactic transfusions.

Because of these problems associated with prophylactic transfusions, it is our belief currently that once a woman has given birth to an infant that most likely will survive, permanent sterilization should be urged.

SICKLE CELL TRAIT

The inheritance of one gene for hemoglobin S and another for hemoglobin A results in *sickle trait*. In the typical case hemoglobin S comprises only about one-third of the hemoglobin fraction. Although adverse pregnancy outcome has been attributed to women who have sickle trait, extensive experiences at Parkland Memorial Hospital indicate that the adverse effects of sickle trait on pregnancy are limited to a two-fold increase in the prevalence of bacteriuria.[7, 44, 61] When more than 1700 pregnancies in women with sickle trait were compared to a similar number of matched black women whose red cells did not sickle, no significant differences were found in perinatal mortality, frequency of low birth weight, Apgar scores, hematocrit or hypertension during pregnancy.[44] In addition, the mean birth weights for both groups of infants were the same (Table 15.5).

Ashcroft and associates[1] in Jamaica have similarly identified bacteriuria to be more common in women 35 to 64 years of age with sickle trait than in black women without hemoglobin S. They found no increase in the prevalence of renal disease, hypertension or cardiomegaly in women with sickle trait. Our observations on pregnancy performance, coupled with those of Ashcroft and associates in older

Table 15.5. Pregnancy experiences of black women at Parkland Memorial Hospital with sickle cell trait (AS hemoglobin) compared to black women without hemoglobin AS

	Birth weight (g)		Perinatal mortality (%)	Significant bacteriuria (%)	Pregnancy hypertension (%)	Mean hematocrit (vol/100 ml)
	Mean	<2501 (%)				
1972*						
Sickle trait (n = 350)	3041 (SEM = 34.8)	15.1	2.00	10.6	28.3	35.9
Sickle negative (n = 379)	3041 (SEM = 32.5)	15.8	2.11	5.1	33.3	36.7
1960–1963†						
Sickle trait (n = 1359)	3097 (SEM = 17.1)	13.2	3.31			36.6
Sickle negative (n = 1265)	3039 (SEM = 17.6)	15.3	3.32			37.1

* From Pritchard et al.[44]
† From Whalley et al.[61]

nonpregnant women with AS hemoglobin, do not support the concept that sickle cell trait is a disease.

Even though Brown and colleagues,[7] on the basis of observations made on a small number of pregnancies in women with sickle cell trait, suggest otherwise, the evidence seems clear that sickle trait is not overtly deleterious to the mother during pregnancy or subsequently, or to her fetus, except for the uncommon but unfortunate inheritance of a sickle cell hemoglobinopathy by the offspring.

HOMOZYGOUS HEMOGLOBIN C AND HEMOGLOBIN C-BETA THALASSEMIA DISEASES

Pregnancy and homozygous hemoglobin C disease or hemoglobin C-thalassemia disease appear to be rather benign associations. The anemia is usually, but not always mild.[13, 57] Severe anemia may be related to folic acid deficiency or other superimposed causes, such as infection. Serial measurements of hemoglobin concentrations and routine supplementation with folic acid and iron is recommended during pregnancy. Splenomegaly is common and, at times, may be marked. Infarction of the spleen can usually be treated symptomatically.

BETA THALASSEMIA

Beta Thalassemia Minor

Not all hypochromic microcytic anemia observed in pregnant women is a result of iron deficiency. Beta thalassemia minor is an inherited anemia characterized by slight to moderate reduction in hemoglobin concentration accompanied by red cell changes of hypochromasia and microcytosis. Wintrobe early described this condition in families of Mediterrean origin, and indeed, as many as 10% of the population in some areas of Italy have the gene for this disorder.[11] The incidence of thalassemia in white women in the United States without known Mediterrean ancestors, and in black women is much lower; however, for the latter it is estimated to be approximately 0.8%.[21]

The basic defect in thalassemia minor is impaired synthesis of the beta chain of globin. There is a compensatory increase in the synthesis of delta chains; therefore, the A_2 hemoglobin fraction is elevated. In normal adults hemoglobin A_2 rarely exceeds 2.5%, however, individuals with beta thalassemia minor usually have hemoglobin A_2 levels of 5% or more.[11] Pregnancy itself does not alter the percentage of A_2 hemoglobin.

During pregnancy, women with thalassemia minor are frequently anemic by previously defined standards (Table 15.1). Typically the hemoglobin concentration is 8 to 10 g per 100 ml late in the second trimester, with an increase to 9 to 11 g per 100 ml late in the third trimester, compared with 10 to 12 g per 100 ml when not pregnant. These values are significantly lower than those for normal iron sufficient pregnant women at comparable states of gestation. In normal women studied in late pregnancy the mean hemoglobin concentration was 12.3 g per 100 ml and in only 6% of these women was the hemoglobin concentration less than 11 g per 100 ml.[43] In contrast, the mean hemoglobin concentration for 34 women with beta thalassemia minor given supplemental iron was 10.9 g per 100 ml at term. In 56% the hemoglobin was less than 11 g per 100 ml, and in 21% it was less than 10 g per 100 ml (Table 15.6).

Although it is felt by some that iron supplementation during pregnancy for the woman with beta thalassemia minor should be withheld, data from Parkland Memorial Hospital indicate the opposite.[14] Scant to absent iron stores frequently coexisted with beta thalassemia minor during pregnancy as determined by histochemical studies of aspirated bone marrow. In 15 of 21 pregnant women storage iron was negligible, even though 12 of the women had been taking supplemental iron

Table 15.6. Hemoglobin concentration late in pregnancy in iron-supplemented normal and thalassemic women

	Hemoglobin (g/100 ml)				
	Mean	<12 (%)	<11 (%)	<10 (%)	Lowest
Normal (n = 95)	12.3	36	6	1	9.8
Beta thalassemia minor (n = 34)	10.9	85	56	21	8.4

for 1 to 4 months before the marrow was examined. Most likely in most of the pregnancies evaluated there would not have been enough storage iron to meet the requirements of pregnancy without iron supplementation.

Other than the mild anemia, thalassemia minor does not appear to lead to increased pregnancy complications. For example, 51 women with thalassemia minor were delivered of term infants whose mean birth weight was 3084 g. Four women were delivered of premature infants that included one set of twins. The mean birth weight of these infants was similar to that for all infants of black mothers who were delivered at Parkland Memorial Hospital while low birth weight (<2500 g) was not as common.[44]

Blood transfusions are rarely indicated for the pregnant woman with thalassemia minor except to treat hemorrhage. Iron and folic acid in prophylactic daily doses of 30 to 60 mg and 1 mg, respectively, is recommended. Any disease that depresses erythropoiesis or increases erythrocytic destruction will intensify the anemia; therefore, infection should be promptly identified and adequately treated.

Beta Thalassemia Major

The inheritance from both parents for the beta thalassemia gene results in *beta thalassemia major* or *Cooley's anemia*. The disease is severe and usually becomes apparent within the first year of life. Chronic severe anemia and hemochromatosis comprise the natural history of the disease. Fertility is impaired and pregnancy is uncommon. Survival beyond the third decade is unusual.

HEREDITARY SPHEROCYTOSIS

Hereditary spherocytosis is an autosomal dominant condition characterized by intermittent jaundice, splenomegaly and usually mild to moderate hemolytic anemia. Spherocytes are demonstrable in the peripheral smear and may approach 100%. The erythrocyte defect is *intrinsic*, and the abnormal red cells are destroyed prematurely by the spleen.[12] The tentative diagnosis is made by identifying the sperocytosis and the increased erythrocyte osmotic fragility associated with it. An acquired hemolytic anemia with spherocytosis must be excluded. Acceleration of hemolysis is rare in this hereditary hemolytic anemia but in certain circumstances erythropoiesis is remarkably impaired, leading to the so-called *aplastic crisis*. These events include folic acid deficiency and infection. The former may be even more common in pregnancy because of increased folate demands.

Troublesome anemia can be effectively relieved by splenectomy, which decreases the rate of hemolysis and thus the hemoglobin concentration is increased. Although Moore and associates[31] have recommended splenectomy during pregnancy, we have thus far found this unnecessary in the several cases managed at Parkland Memorial Hospital.

If iron stores determined by marrow examination are decreased or unknown, then iron supplementation is recommended, in addition to 1 mg of folic acid daily. Women with hereditary spherocytosis should be carefully monitored during pregnancy, and at any time there is indication of increased hemolysis or decreased erythropoiesis, hospitalization is warranted. Whenever possible splenectomy should be postponed until pregnancy is completed.

Coagulopathies

THROMBOCYTOPENIA

The platelet count has been reported by some, but not all, to decrease moderately during pregnancy.[26] In our experience the platelet count differs little from that of the normal nonpregnant state. A platelet count below 150,000 per mm^3 should be considered abnormal, although a count as low as 40,000 per mm^3 may be adequate for effective hemostasis. The critical level for effective hemostasis is determined to a considerable degree by the quality of the platelet function as well as by the magnitude of trauma to which the mother or fetus is subjected.

Thrombocytopenia during pregnancy may be the consequence of decreased production as found in cases of severe folate deficiency or of aplastic anemia, but more often is due to any of several mechanisms which lead to increased platelet destruction. These include thrombocytopenia associated with eclampsia or severe preeclampsia, systemic lupus erythematosus, other acquired hemolytic anemia, autoimmune thrombocytopenia and thrombocytopenia induced by drugs, infections or allergies.

Idiopathic Thrombocytopenic Purpura (ITP)

Idiopathic thrombocytopenic purpura (ITP) is a diagnosis reached by exclusion of other causes of thrombocytopenia. Since recent evidence indicates increased platelet destruction mediated by an immune mechanism, the adjective *idiopathic* may be inappropriate for this syndrome.[2] ITP rarely complicates pregnancy, but when it does, maternal and fetal mortality may be increased. Peterson and Larson[34] cite a maternal mortality rate of 2% and a perinatal mortality rate of 15%.

For the pregnant woman with ITP corticosteroids are recommended as initial treatment. Although they have a variable effect on the platelet count, reduction in capillary fragility and shortening of the bleeding time are often observed without an appreciable increase in platelet levels. As long as 2 weeks of treatment may be required before a substantial elevation of the platelet count is observed.[2] The majority of cases respond and the dose can be reduced after control of the acute episode. Splenectomy may be indicated if there is no improvement in 2 to 3 weeks, or if sufficient hemostatic function can be maintained only with massive doses of steroids or if after delivery spontaneous remission is not demonstrated in 2 to 6 months. Of patients who undergo splenectomy, 70 to 90% improve following the operation, and in two-thirds of these, platelet levels are permanently restored to normal. Some degree of shortened survival of platelets may persist, however, with normalization of the platelet count as the consequence of increased production. Splenectomy after the uterus enters the upper abdomen but remote from term may be technically difficult and, if possible, is best postponed. During periods of uncontrollable hemorrhage, or when major surgery is to be performed in the face of dangerous thrombocytopenia, transient improvement in platelet function may sometimes be achieved by transfusion with donor platelets.

Antiplatelet antibodies can cross the placenta and cause destruction of fetal platelets. In general, the severity of thrombocytopenia in the neonate is proportional to that of the mother at the time of delivery. For example, 80% of infants born to mothers with platelet counts of <100,000 per mm^3 will have some degree of thrombocytopenia.[58, 59] Territo and associates[59] recommend elective cesarean section at term to prevent possible fetal intracranial hemorrhage from labor if the maternal platelet count is less than 100,000 per mm^3. It remains to be established that otherwise uncomplicated, orderly labor and minimally traumatic delivery lead to greater morbidity in the infant than that associated with prophylactic cesarean section. Almost certainly, maternal hemorrhage and attendant complications from such will be greater in the severely thrombocytopenic woman who is delivered by cesarean section.

Thrombocytopenia from Transfusions

Consumptive coagulopathy, such as with severe abruptio placentae, and any severe obstetric hemorrhage which has been vigorously treated with stored blood, are, in our experience, the most common situations in which thrombocytopenia occurs in pregnant women. Management includes whole blood to correct volume deficits and avoidance of any surgical procedure which disrupts vessel integrity and thereby initiates uncontrollable hemorrhage. Platelets harvested from very recently drawn blood and promptly administered may on occasion be necessary to improve hemostasis. Such therapy is usually reserved for thrombocytopenic patients in whom intraoperative hemostasis cannot be adequately achieved and in those with continued postoperative bleeding.

Although donor platelets stored at 4°C have by decree a usable shelf life of 72 hr, *fresh donor* platelets, collected at room temperature and infused promptly survive and function better in the recipient. When platelet transfusions are necessary 8 to 10 platelet packs are given within 30 min. Occasionally the patient complains of mild chest discomfort and dyspnea, presumably due to platelet aggregates that reach the pulmonary microcirculation. It should be kept in mind that although each pack contains only 20 to 30 cc of platelet-rich plasma, each unit carries the same risk as a unit of whole blood in transmitting the hepatitis B antigen.[5]

Spontaneous repair of platelet levels usually takes 3 to 4 days from the time of the inciting insult. It is not unusual in these circumstances for thrombocytosis to then develop with the potential for thrombosis.

HEMATOLOGIC CHANGES ASSOCIATED WITH PLACENTAL ABRUPTION

Placental abruption so extensive as to kill the fetus is more likely in women who are hypertensive, who are of high parity or who previously suffered a placental abruption.[36] Blood loss generally is proportionate to both the extent and the duration of the placental abruption. Typically with total abruption, large volumes of blood are concealed within the uterus until delivery. Concealed hemorrhage commonly amounts to 2500 ml and may exceed 5000 ml. These observations of blood loss effectively refute the concept previously held by some that placental abruption often is associated with shock (hypotension) out of proportion to blood loss. Indeed the reverse is more often true.

Changes in the maternal coagulation mechanism indicative of consumptive coagulopathy are rather common with more extensive separation of the placenta. In our experience, if the degree of separation has been great enough to have killed the fetus, the plasma fibrinogen concentration will be 100 mg per 100 ml or less in approximately one third of the cases.[37, 38] With lesser degrees of separation gross deterioration of the coagulation mechanism with hypofibrinogenemia, thrombocytopenia and high levels of fibrin degradation products develop much less often.

Mechanisms operative in the genesis of coagulation defects associated with placental abruption include deposition of fibrin and other coagulants within the retroplacental clot. Although such "exsanguination coagulopathy" plays a role in the production of thrombocytopenia and hypofibrinogenemia, it is not the major mechanism involved in disruption of the coagulation system. The major mechanism in abruptio placenta most likely is the escape of thromboplastin from the placenta and decidua, and perhaps activated coagulation factor(s) in serum from the retroplacental clot which gains access into the maternal uterine venous outflow to cause disseminated intravascular coagulation.

In our experience, even in cases with severe hypofibrinogenemia due to placental abruption, red cells from the maternal circulation are rarely markedly distorted nor has hemoglobinemia or hyperbilirubinemia been evident until after extensive transfusion therapy.

Treatment of placental abruption, most often, has been remarkably simple. Reestablishment and maintenance of the maternal circulation was accomplished promptly following two general guidelines for fluid replacement. (1) Lactated Ringer's solution and whole blood are given in such amounts and in such proportions that (*a*) urine flow is at least 30 ml per hr and ideally approaches 60 ml per hr, and (*b*) the hematocrit is maintained at 30 or slightly higher. (2) If initial vigorous therapy with aqueous fluid and whole blood does not restore urine flow, then the central venous pressure is monitored and more fluids are given.

With this simplistic, but effective method of management, marked impairment of renal function has been rare and when it did occur, it was so transient that dialysis has not been necessary. In those instances in which transient renal failure has been observed, there was either considerable delay between the onset of symptoms of abruption and the initiation of appropriate fluid replacement therapy as outlined above, or there was pre-existing renal disease or both. In nearly 300 cases of placental abruption severe enough to kill the fetus that have been so managed during the past 20 years at Parkland Memorial Hospital, there have been no maternal mortalities.

If the fetus is alive and the estimated gestational age predicts that the fetus most likely will survive if delivered, cesarean section is immediately performed whenever fetal distress is evident or vaginal delivery is likely to be delayed. If the fetus is grossly immature or is dead, vaginal delivery is preferred. Occasionally, however, when other obstetric problems coexist, when progress in labor is unsatisfactory or when the rate of bleeding exceeds the capacity for blood replacement, cesaran section is necessary. In the past, an arbitrary time limit was established beyond which it was felt that further deterioration of the woman warranted operative intervention. Our experiences, as well as those of Brame and associates,[6] indicate that the time from the onset of abruption to delivery is not critical for a successful outcome provided adequate organ pefusion is maintained.

The administration of fibrinogen is limited to the unusual case in which severe disruption of the coagulation mechanism is apparent and cesarean section is necessary. If gross impairment of hemostasis is evident at sites of incision, 4 g of fibrinogen may be infused rapidly, or fibrinogen may be withheld and cryoprecipitate and fresh frozen plasma substituted. Usually a generalized ooze from abdominal incisions can be managed with appropriately placed drains after maximal hemostasis has been obtained through ligatures placed in the presence of a blood pressure adequate for perfusion. Vaginal delivery in the presence of gross disruption of the coagulation mechanism, irrespective of the cause is, in general, appreciably less morbid than is cesarean section. Moreover, any surgical dissection should be kept at a minimum, and cesarean section is less morbid than cesarean hysterectomy.

HEMATOLOGIC CHANGES IN PRE-ECLAMPSIA/ECLAMPSIA

Twenty-five years ago, evidence of intravascular coagulation in eclampsia was provided by McKay and associates,[29] who described intravascular deposition of fibrin in women with eclampsia studied at autopsy. Soon thereafter, Pritchard and coworkers[46, 49] documented a variety of coagulation changes in some women with pre-eclampsia and especially eclampsia. Subsequently other investigators substantiated this earlier work, and *disseminated intravascular coagulation* has been considered by some to not only be a common feature, but indeed essential to the development of pre-eclampsia and eclampsia. Since this time, extensive experiences from Parkland Memorial Hospital indicate that although there are a variety of coagulation changes in some instances of pre-eclampsia and eclampsia, these changes most likely are the consequence of the vasospasm rather than the cause.[39, 40]

Table 15.7. Measurements of some coagulation factors in women with eclampsia that might suggest disseminated intravascular coagulation*

	Term healthy nulligravidas	Women with eclampsia†
Platelets (per mm³)		
Mean	278,000	202,000
−2 SD	150,000	
<150,000	0/20	28/96
<100,000	0/20	16/96
<50,000	0/20	3/96
Fibrin split products		
8 μg/ml or less	17/20	58/66
16 μg/ml	3/20	6/66
>16 μg/ml	0/20	2/66
Plasma fibrinogen (mg/100 ml)		
Mean	415	412
−2 SD	285	
<285	0/20	7/93
Fibrin monomer, positive	1/20	1/21
Plasma thrombin time (sec)		
Mean	8.9	11.3
>2 sec longer than control	0	20/39

* Adapted from Pritchard, Cunningham and Mason.[39]

† Most abnormal of several determinations cited.

As shown in Table 15.7, the two most common hematologic derangements in women with eclampsia are thrombocytopenia and a prolonged thrombin time. The genesis of the prolonged thrombin time is not known. In 29% of 95 cases studied by us the platelet count was less than 150,000 per mm³ but less than 50,000 per mm³ in only 3%. Fibrinogen-fibrin degradation products that imply disseminated intravascular coaglation were occasionally found. Fibrin monomer was seldom identified and, unless associated with placental abruption, the plasma fibrinogen levels were the same as in healthy intrapartum nulligravidas. Overt *hemoglobinemia* was rarely identified; although indirect evidence of hemolysis, including elevated indirect bilirubin, reticulocytosis, nucleated red blood cells in the peripheral blood and distortion of red cells, was more common.

Although disseminated intravascular coagulation induced by thromboplastin released from the decidua or placenta has been suggested as the cause of hematologic changes in pre-eclampsia/eclampsia, the genesis of the thrombocytopenia may well be platelet adherence at sites of disrupted vascular endothelium. The experimental model produced by infusion of angiotensin II and other pressor amines results in disruption of the endothelial lining of arteries, especially in dilated segments that alternate with vasoconstricted segments.[9] Platelets and fibrin adhere to the denuded sites and when the process is intense, red cell damage, that is, microangiopathic hemolysis may result.[3, 10] The bulk of evidence indicates that hematologic changes associated with pregnancy hypertension are the *effect* of, rather than the *cause* of hypertension.

Appropriate management of pre-eclampsia/eclampsia complicated by severe thrombocytopenia or intravascular hemolysis is prevention of convulsions, control of severe hypertension and prompt delivery. These hematologic derangements indicate severe disease best treated by delivery. Although a few writers have advocated heparin therapy, there is no published evidence that heparin has a favorable effect on the disease. More important, giving heparin to a severely hypertensive woman, possibly with thrombocytopenia, is certain to increase the risk of intracranial hemorrhage as well as hemorrhage from other sites.

COAGULATION CHANGES WITH RETENTION OF A DEAD FETUS

In 1950, Weiner and associates[63] reported that some women who carry a dead fetus for a long time developed coagulation defects. Subsequent studies indicated that gross disruption of the maternal coagulation mechanism was most unlikely if the fetus had been dead for less than 1 month, but if the fetus was retained for longer periods, about 25% of women demonstrated significant coagulation changes.[35, 50]

In those women who develop a coagulopathy, the plasma fibrinogen usually falls gradually from levels normal for pregnancy to nonpregnant levels, but in some cases the decrease continues until clinically significant hypofibrinogenemia develops. Concomitant with the decrease in plasma fibrinogen, fibrin degradation products are somewhat elevated. Thrombocytopenia is common but is usually not severe.

Mechanisms which have been proposed to explain the development of the coagulopathy in women with a dead fetus are the same as those proposed for placental abruption. The major difference between the two conditions is the rate at which the coagulopathy develops, being much slower with a retained dead fetus. Consumptive coagulopathy is presumably mediated by the release of thromboplastin from the dead products of conception.[28, 56] Heparin infusion, but not epsilon amniocaproic acid, can correct the coagulation defects, and, although these observations serve to establish the cause of consumptive coagulopathy, they do not precisely identify the site where fibrinogen is converted to fibrin.[27]

Because of the changing attitudes for treatment of the woman with a dead fetus, consumptive coagulopathy is seldom observed. Most physicians will induce labor as soon as the clinical impression of fetal demise is substantiated either by x-ray or sonography. In general, in those cases in which fetal demise would be not quite as apparent, that is, early gestation, consumptive coagulopathy is less likely to develop. We have recently cared for a woman with severe hypofibrinogenemia at 18 weeks of gestation by menstrual dates, although her uterus was only 12 weeks' size. Massive hemorrhage occurred at the time of suction curettage and hematologic studies upon arrival at Parkland Memorial Hospital documented consumptive coagulopathy.

Cure is effected by delivery of the products of conception. In the unusual case in which hypofibrinogenemia is detected in the woman with an intact circulation, heparin may be carefully administered. Heparin blocks the pathologic consumption of fibrinogen and other clotting factors, thus allowing the coagulation mechanism to repair spontaneously. Once this has been accomplished the heparin is discontinued and promptly steps are taken to evacuate the dead products of conception.[27] It must be emphasized that this should be used only if the maternal circulatory system is intact.

If active hemorrhage is encountered at the time of vaginal delivery or surgical removal of the fetus, and overt consumptive coagulopathy is present, the administration of heparin almost certainly will enhance the bleeding. Under these circumstances we recommend whole blood and fluid replacement according to the guidelines for treatment of hemorrhage associated with placental abruption. Indications for the use of fibrinogen are also similar to those for placental abruption.

AMNIOTIC FLUID EMBOLISM

In some circumstances, entry of amniotic fluid into the maternal circulation may be fatal. The typical case of amniotic fluid embolism is seen in the woman who is laboring vigorously, or having just done so, is in the process of being delivered when she develops varying degrees of respiratory distress and circulatory collapse. If death is not immediate, serious hemorrhage with severe coagulation defects is soon evident.

The lethality of intravenously infused amniotic fluid varies remarkably depending upon the particulate matter which it contains. Meconium defecated into the amniotic fluid, a common event with myometrial hyperactivity, greatly increases its toxicity. Severe pulmonary vascular obstruction from this particulate matter, and perhaps from fibrin accumulation, causes acute cor pulmonale.[54] Severe hypoxia accompanied by decreased cardiac output is the consequence, and if the woman does not die immediately, coagulation defects causing hemorrhage are soon evident. Typically the blood, if not incoagulable, demonstrates a small, mushy clot which undergoes prompt lysis. Thrombocytopenia is likely to be severe and very intense fibrinolytic activity may accompany the consumptive coagulopathy.

Although there are women who have survived a degree of amniotic fluid embolism, the diagnosis is questionable unless amniotic fluid debris is demonstrated in the buffy coat of blood obtained from the right side of the heart, or within blood vessels in sections of the lung when examined postmortem. Therapy for severe amniotic fluid embolism is notoriously unsuccessful. Successful treatment of hypoxia often necessitates mechanical ventilation. Equally essential is blood replacement therapy.[51] The woman with cor pulmonale tolerates neither deficit nor excess in blood volume. The use of fibrinogen, heparin, fibrinolytic agents and antifibrinolytic agents has been described in various case reports but it is very difficult to evaluate their efficacy.

LEUKEMIA

Leukemia rarely complicates pregnancy, with an estimated incidence of 1 in 75,000 pregnancies.[30] McLain's[30] summary of over 500 cases indicates that about half are of the acute variety and half chronic. Survival for these women was the same as in nonpregnant leukemic patients and the data further suggest that pregnancy does not exert a profoundly deleterious effect on the course of leukemia.

Premature labor is common in this condition, and in general perinatal mortality is high. Treatment with most antineoplastic drugs in current use need not be withheld during pregnancy since available evidence indicates that their administration, especially after the end of the first trimester, does not seriously harm the fetus. Methotrexate is a notorious exception.

Because of the almost 100% fatality rate associated with acute leukemia, and the short mean survival time, it seems prudent to recommend abortion if the condition is identified early in pregnancy. The same considerations should be entertained for women who are identified to have chronic leukemias early in gestation.

REFERENCES

1. Ashcroft, M. T., Miall, W. E., Milner, P. F.: A comparison between the characteristics of Jamaican adults with normal hemoglobin and those with sickle cell trait. Am J Epidemiol 90: 236–246,1969.
2. Aster, R. H.: Thrombocytopenia due to en-

hanced platelet destruction. *Hematology,* Chap. 139. Edited by W. J. Williams, E. Beutler, A. J. Erslev, R. W. Rundles, New York, McGraw-Hill Book Co., 1972.

3. Baker, L. R. I., Brain, M. C.: Heparin treatment of haemolytic anemia and thrombocytopenia in preeclampsia. Proc Roy Soc Med 60: 477–485, 1967.
4. Ball, E. W., Giles, C.: Folic acid and vitamin B_{12} levels in pregnancy and their relationship to megaloblastic anemia. J. Clin Pathol 17: 165–170, 1964.
5. *Blood Component Therapy. A Physician's Handbook*. Second edition. Washington, D. C., American Association of Blood Banks, 1975.
6. Brame, R. G., Harbert, G.M., Jr., McGaughey, H. S., Jr., Thornton, W. N., Jr.: Maternal risk in abruption. Obstet Gynecol 31: 224–227, 1968.
7. Brown, S., Merkow, A., Wiener, M., Khajezadeh, J.: Low birth weight in babies born to mothers with sickle cell trait. JAMA 221: 1404–1407, 1972.
8. Brumfitt, W.: The effects of bacteriuria in pregnancy on maternal and fetal health. Kidney Int (Suppl) 8: 113–119, 1975.
9. Brunner, H. R., Varos, H.: Vascular damage in hypertension. Hosp Pract 10: 97–103, 1975.
10. Bull, B. S., Rubenberg, M. D., Dacie, J. V., Brain, M. C.: Microangiopathic haemolytic anaemia: Mechanisms of red cell fragmentation: *in vitro* studies. Br J Haematol 14: 643–652, 1968.
11. Comings, E. E.: Thalassemia. *Hematology,* Chap. 31. Edited by W. J. Williams, E. Beutler, A. J. Erslev, R. W. Rundles, New York, McGraw-Hill Book Co., 1972.
12. Cooper, R. A., Jandl, J. H.: Hereditary spherocytosis. *Hematology,* Chap. 38. Edited by W. J. Williams, E. Beutler, A. J. Erslev, R. W. Rundles, New York, McGraw-Hill Book Co., 1972.
13. Cunningham, F. G., Pritchard, J. A.: Unpublished data.
14. Cunningham, F. G., Pritchard, J. A., Scott, D. E.: Iron stores in pregnant women with hemoglobinopathies [Abstr]. Gynecol Invest 5: 12, 1974.
15. Cunningham, F. G., Whalley, P. J.: Asymptomatic bacteriuria during pregnancy. *Gynecologic and Obstetric Urology,* Chap. 25. Edited by J. J. Buchsbaum, J. D. Schmidt, Philadelphia, W. B. Saunders Co. (In press.)
16. Curtis, E. M.: Pregnancy in sickle cell anemia, sickle cell-hemoglobin C disease and variants thereof. Am J Obstet Gynecol 77: 1312–1320, 1959.
17. DeLeeuw, N. K. W., Lowenstein, L., Shieh, Y.: Iron deficiency in hydremia in normal pregnancy. Medicine 45: 291–298, 1966.
18. Erslev, A. J.: Anemia of chronic disorders. *Hematology,* Chap. 36. Edited by W. J. Williams, E. Beutler, A. J. Erslev, R. W. Rundles, New York, McGraw-Hill Book Co., 1972.
19. Fort, A. T., Morrison, J. D., Berreras, L., Diggs, L. W., Fish, F. A.: Counseling the patient with sickle cell disease about reproduction: Pregnancy outcome does not justify the maternal risk! Am J Obstet Gynecol 111: 324–330, 1971.
20. Fullerton, W. T., Hendrickse, J. P. deV., Watson-Williams, E. J.: Haemoglobin SC disease in pregnancy. *Abnormal Haemoglobins in Africa, A Symposium*. Edited by J. H. P. Jonxis, Philadelphia, F. A. Davis Co., 1965.
21. Goldstein, M., Patpongpanij, A., Minnich, V.: The incidence of elevated hemoglobin A_2 levels in the American Negro. Ann Intern Med 60: 95–99, 1964.
22. Hallberg, L., Hallgren, J., Hollender, A., Hogdahl, A., Tibblin, G.: Occurrence, causes and prevention of nutritional anaemias. Symp Swedish Nutr Found 6: 19, 1968.
23. Heys, R. F.: Child bearing and idiopathic thrombocytopenic purpura. J Obstet Gynaecol Br Commonw 73: 205–209, 1966.
24. Hibbard, B. M., Hibbard, E. D., Hwa, T. S., Tan, P.: Abruptio placentae and defective folate metabolism in Singapore women. J Obstet Gynaecol Br Commw 76: 1003–1007, 1969.
25. Hibbard, E. D., Smithells, R. W.: Folic acid metabolism and human embryopathy. Lancet 2: 1146–1151, 1965.
26. Hytten, F. E., Leitch, I.: *The Physiology of Human Pregnancy*. Second edition. London, Blackwell Scientific Publications, 1971.
27. Jimenez, J. M., Pritchard, J. A.: Pathogenesis and treatment of coagulation defects resulting from fetal death. Obstet Gynecol 32: 449–459, 1968.
28. Lerner, R., Margolin, M., Slate, W. G.: Heparin in the treatment of hypofibrinogenemia complicating fetal death *in utero*. Am J Obstet Gynecol 97: 373–378, 1967.
29. McKay, D. G., Merril, S. J., Weiner, A. E., Hertig, A. T., Reid, D. E.: The pathologic anatomy of eclampsia, bilateral renal cortical necrosis, pituitary necrosis, and other acute fatal complications of pregnancy, and its possible relationship to the generalized Shwartzman phenomen. Am J Obstet Gynecol 66: 507–515, 1953.
30. McLain, D. R., Jr.: Leukemia in pregnancy. Clin Obstet Gynecol 17 (4): 185–194, 1974.
31. Moore, A., Sherman, M. M., Strongin, M. J.: Hereditary spherocytosis with hemolytic crisis during pregnancy: Treatment by splenectomy. Obstet Gynecol (Suppl) 47: 19s–21s, 1976.
32. Morrison, J. C., Fort, A. T., Wiser, W. L., Fish, S. A.: The modern management of pregnancy sickle cell patients; A preliminary report. South Med J 65: 533–536, 1972.
33. Morrison, J. C., Wiser, W. L.: The effect of maternal partial exchange transfusion on the infants of patients with sickle cell anemia. J Pediatr 89: 286–289, 1976.
34. Peterson, O. J., Jr., Larson, P.: Thrombocytopenic purpura in pregnancy. Obstet Gynecol 4: 454–458, 1954.
35. Pritchard, J. A.: Fetal death *in utero*. Obstet Gynecol 14: 573–580, 1959.
36. Pritchard, J. A.: Genesis of severe placental abruption. Am J Obstet Gynecol 108: 22–27, 1970.
37. Pritchard, J. A., Brekken, A. L.: Clinical and laboratory studies on severe abruptio placentae. Am J Obstet Gynecol 97: 681–695, 1967.
38. Pritchard, J. A., Cunningham, F. G.: Unpublished data.
39. Pritchard, J. A., Cunningham, F. G., Mason, R.: Coagulation changes in eclampsia: Their fre-

quency and pathogenesis. Am J Obstet Gynecol 124: 855–864, 1976.
40. Pritchard, J. A., Cunningham, F. G., Mason, R. A.: Does coagulation have a causative role in eclampsia? NIH Proceedings, Hypertension in Pregnancy, October 1975, Chicago. (To be published.)
41. Pritchard, J. A., Hunt C.: A comparison of the hematologic responses following the routine prenatal administration of intramuscular and oral iron. Surg Gynecol Obstet 106: 516–522, 1958.
42. Pritchard, J. A., Mason, R. A.: Iron stores of normal adults and replenishment with oral iron therapy. JAMA 190: 897–901, 1964.
43. Pritchard, J. A., Scott, D. E.: Iron demands in pregnancy. *Iron Deficiency Pathogenesis, Clinical Aspects, Therapy*. Edited by L. Hallberg, H. G. Harwerth, A. Vanottie, New York, Academic Press, 1970.
44. Pritchard, J. A., Scott, D. E., Whalley, P. J., Cunningham, F. G., Mason, R. A.: The effects of maternal sickle cell hemoglobinopathies and sickle cell trait on reproductive performance. Am J Obstet Gynecol 117: 662–670, 1973.
45. Pritchard, J. A., Scott, D. E., Whalley, P. J., Haling, R. F., Jr.: Infants of mothers with megaloblastic anemia due to folate deficiency. JAMA 211: 1982–1986, 1970.
46. Pritchard, J. A., Weisman, R. Jr., Ratnoff, O. D., Vosburgh, G.: Intravascular hemolysis, thrombocytopenia and other hematologic abnormalities associated with severe toxemia of pregnancy. N. Engl J Med 250: 87–91, 1954.
47. Pritchard, J. A., Whalley, P. J.: Abortion complicated by *Clostridium perfringens* infection. Am J Obstet Gynecol 111: 484–490, 1971.
48. Pritchard, J. A., Wiggins, A. M., Dickey, J. C.: Blood volume changes in pregnancy and the puerperium. I. Does sequestration of red blood cells accompany parturition? Am J Obstet Gynecol 80: 956–962, 1960.
49. Pritchard, J. A., Ratnoff, O. D., Weisman, R., Jr.: Hemostatic defects and increased red cell destruction in preeclampsia and eclampsia. Obstet Gynecol 4: 159–164, 1954.
50. Pritchard, J. A., Ratnoff, O. C.: Studies of fibrinogen and other hemostatic factors in women with intrauterine death and delayed delivery. Surg Gynecol Obstet 101: 467–477, 1955.
51. Resnik, R., Swartz, W. H., Plumer, M. H., Benirshke, K., Stratthaus, M. E.: Amniotic fluid embolism with survival. Obstet Gynecol 47: 295–298, 1976.
52. Ricks, P.: Further experience with exchange transfusion in sickle cell anemia and pregnancy. Am J Obstet Gynecol 100: 1087–1090, 1968.
53. Rovinsky, J. J.: Primary refractory anemia complicating pregnancy and delivery. Obstet Gynecol Surv 14: 149, 1959.
54. Schneider, C. L. Henry, M. M.: Meconium embolism *in vivo*. Am J Obstet Gynecol 101: 909–913, 1968.
55. Scott, D. E., Whalley, P. J., Pritchard, J. A.: Maternal folate deficiency and pregnancy wastage. II. Fetal malformation. Obstet Gynecol 36: 26–28, 1970.
56. Sherman, E., Middleton, E. H.: The management of missed abortion with hypofibrinogenemia. Maryland State Med J 7: 300–304, 1958.
57. Smith, E. W., Krevans, J. R.: Clinical manifestations of hemoglobin C disorders. Bull Johns Hopkins Hosp 104: 17–19, 1959.
58. Tancer, M. L.: Idiopathic thrombocytopenic purpura and pregnancy: Report of 5 new cases and review of the literature. Am J Obstet Gynecol 79: 148–152, 1960.
59. Territo, M., Finklestein, J., Oh, W., Hobel, C., Kattlove, H.: Management of autoimmune thrombocytopenia in pregnancy and in the neonate. Obstet Gynecol 41: 579–584, 1973.
60. Whalley, P. J.: Bacteriuria of pregnancy. Am J Obstet Gynecol 97: 723–738, 1967.
61. Whalley, P. J., Martin, F. G., Pritchard, J. A.: Sickle cell trait and urinary tract infection during pregnancy. JAMA 189: 903–907, 1964.
62. Whalley, P. J., Scott, D. E., Pritchard, J. A.: Maternal folate deficiency and pregnancy wastage. I. Placental Abruption. Am J Obstet Gynecol 105: 670–678, 1969.
63. Weiner, A. E., Reid, D. E., Roby, C. C., Diamond, L. K.: Coagulation defects with intrauterine death from Rh isosensitization. Am J Obstet Gynecol 60: 1015–1022, 1950.

JAMES F. CONNAUGHTON, JR., M.D.
DIAN REESER, B.A.
LORETTA P. FINNEGAN, M.D.

16

Pregnancy Complicated by Drug Addiction

Introduction

Reports over the past decade show that increasing numbers of pregnant addicts are presenting themselves to medical facilities. However, the exact magnitude of narcotic dependency in pregnancy is difficult to determine, since statistics are generally based on hospital deliveries, and it is suspected that a considerable number of addicts may be delivered at home without a physician in attendance. The clinical management of these patients is difficult because of their tendency to neglect general health and prenatal care. In most cases, they do not seek medical assistance until the onset of labor. Social and emotional problems such as poor housing, inadequate income, lack of education and feelings of worthlessness and depression add to the overall difficulties of the pregnant addict, who fears calling attention to her drug habit and does not wish to risk confrontations with legal authorities.

Heroin addiction has the inherent problems of repeated infections from foreign body reactions, continued illegal activity, fatal overdose and inadequate nutrition. The perinatal management of drug-dependent women is complicated by these factors, as well as by premature labor and the potential narcotic withdrawal of the neonate.

Numerous investigators have published data concerning drug dependency in pregnancy and methods used for recognition and management of the passively drug-dependent infant.[2, 8, 9, 11, 12, 16–18, 20, 25, 28, 33, 39, 42, 44] Unfortunately, most reports are based on clinical experiences and do not adhere to strict research designs with the inclusion of control populations. Because researchers do not use the same parameters in measuring maternal, fetal and neonatal outcome, many controversies have arisen. A variety of conclusions concerning the effects of drugs on the pregnant woman and the neonate have been reported. Furthermore, recommendations show marked disagreement concerning both the type of drugs to be used for neonatal withdrawal and the appropriate management of the neonate after discharge from the hospital.

The ensuing discussion will describe the effects of prenatal drug abuse on the maternal-fetal unit and the various methods of management and will provide recommendations for the care of pregnant addicts.

Effects of Prenatal Drug Abuse on Maternal-Fetal Unit

The addicted woman usually suffers from chronic anxiety and depression. She lacks confidence and has extreme difficulty with interpersonal experiences, especially heterosexual relationships. Despite her need for psychosocial and medical treatment, the addict does not easily accomodate her lifestyle to this type of care.

In order to maintain the high cost of maintaining a habit, the addict will often indulge in robbery and prostitution. Because most of her time is spent either obtaining or abusing drugs, she is unable to perform the usual activities of daily living. She does have intermittent periods of alertness and well-being, but, for most of the day, she is either "high" or "sick." The "high" or euphoric state keeps her sedated, absorbed in herself and lost to all responsibility. The "sick" state, experienced during abstinence, is generally characterized by a craving for narcotics along with malaise, nausea, lacrimation, perspiration, tremors, vomiting, diarrhea and cramps. Because of this daily struggle for survival and fear of calling attention to her drug habit, the addict does not seek prenatal care. Furthermore, she is convinced by past experience that her fears and mistrust are a realistic reflection of her worth to society.

Several observations will help the physician identify a drug-dependent pregnant woman. There may be no history of prenatal care in a hospital setting or in a private physician's office. The woman is usually unmarried and frequently has venereal disease. Tatoos or self-scarring of the forearm disguise her needle marks. Because of diminished pain perception experienced while "high," she may have cigarette burns of her fingertips and clothes. Because of poorly cleaned or shared needles, she may have developed serum hepatitis. Furthermore, the use of poorly cleaned needles may produce cellulitis and abscesses of the arms, hands, feet, interdigital spaces and under the nails. The pregnant addict may initially be drowsy and lethargic, with pinpoint pupils. If her addiction is not recognized, she will develop the usual symptoms of withdrawal and become anxious and diaphoretic, develop an increased respiratory and heart rate and elevated blood pressure, complain of nausea and have cramps in the upper and lower extremities. If untreated, she may vomit or have diarrhea, and display extreme agitation. If the cramps occur during labor, they may be confused with abruptio placenta or premature contractions; during the postpartum period they are difficult to differentiate from endometritis.

The addict is predisposed to a host of maternal complications, including preeclampsia, toxemia, venous thrombosis, thrombophlebitis, abruptio placenta, retained placenta and postpartum hemorrhage. Fetal complications include low birth weight and a high neonatal morbidity and mortality rate.[12, 25, 27, 42, 44] From 10 to 15% of addicted infants are born to mothers who have had toxemia of pregnancy.[12, 25, 42, 44] Nearly 50% of heroin addicts deliver prematurely.[27, 33, 44] The infant of the opiate drug-dependent mother is not only premature, but also weighs less than the neonate of similar gestational age.[37, 43, 48]

Table 16.1 describes the incidence of toxemia and low birth weight newborns in heroin-addicted women.[25, 47, 33, 42, 44] These retrospective studies were completed prior to published data on treated patients, and demonstrated a high incidence of preeclampsia and low birth weight neonates (19 to 57%).

Blinick and his associates[2] reported meconium in the amniotic fluid of 33% of heroin-addicted pregnant women. Apparently, all of the fetuses in this study did well, and the stillborn rate did not differ from that of the general population (stillborn rate of 12 to 16 per 1,000 live births).[50] Stone[44] and Sussman[47] do not mention stillbirths associated with pregnant drug addicts, but Stern's report[42] (5 stillbirths of 70 infants delivered) indicates that the incidence of stillbirth could be much higher (71 per 1,000 live births).

Rementeria and Nunag[36] postulate that when a pregnant heroin addict undergoes severe withdrawal, muscular activity increases and the rate of metabolism and

Table 16.1. Incidence of toxemia and low birth weight in heroin-addicted women

Investigator	Year reported	No. of patients	Toxemia (%)	Low birth weight incidence (%)
Krause et al[26]	1958	18	10	39
Sussman[48]	1963	22		50
Perlmutter[34]	1967	22		57
Stern[43]	1966	66	15	19
Stone et al[45]	1971	382	11	49

oxygen consumption is elevated. It has been noted that fetal activity during maternal withdrawal also increases; therefore, it can be assumed that the oxygen needs of the fetus grow. The oxygen reserve of the placenta may be insufficient to meet the requirements of the fetus. If blood flow through the intervillous space is totally arrested, this oxygen reserve is completely exhausted in 2.5 min. During labor, contractions compromise uterine blood flow and consequently affect the oxygen reserve of the placenta.[4, 10] If labor should coincide with maternal withdrawal, the increased oxygen needs of the withdrawing fetus may coincide with a period of variable uterine blood flow. When a fetus is exposed to an environment of insufficient oxygen for a prolonged length of time, hypoxia and eventual death may occur. The older the fetus, the greater the metabolic rate and oxygen consumption. It is likely, therefore, that a pregnant woman undergoing severe withdrawal symptoms during the latter part of pregnancy is less able to supply the fetus with its required needs than during the first trimester.

Naeye et al[27] studied other fetal complications of maternal heroin addiction. These investigators evaluated 82 heroin-addicted women and found that nearly 60% of the mothers or infants had evidence of acute infection. Most infected mothers delivered prematurely, whereas those not infected delivered at term. The placentas of the heroin-exposed infants commonly revealed meconium histiocytosis, suggesting that the infants had experienced episodes of distress during fetal life, perhaps related to episodes of heroin withdrawal. Although the infants were small for gestational age, undernutrition of the addicted mothers as an explanation for retarded fetal growth could not always be documented. The authors proposed that periodic episodes of heroin withdrawal during pregnancy restricts fetal growth by reducing uterine or placental blood flow. However, the organ and cellular growth pattern associated with fetal growth retardation in uterine placental disorders is quite different from that observed in the offspring of heroin addicts.[18, 27] The high incidence of meconium histiocytosis in the placentas of heroin-exposed neonates suggests that the infants experienced episodes of hypoxia or some other form of distress during fetal life. Undernutrition in nonaddicted women restricts both the size and number of cells in many organs during the last trimester; the adrenal glands, liver and adipose tissue are most affected.[18, 26] By contrast, reduced organ size in infants exposed to heroin during the third trimester is due mainly to a subnormal number of cells. This suggests that maternal undernutrition is not the only factor responsible for growth restriction. In 1976, we compared heroin-addicted and nonaddicted patients who delivered at Philadelphia General Hospital without prior prenatal care. The incidence of low birth weight was 47.6% in the former group and 20% in the latter group. The nutritional status of the groups appeared to be similar. Therefore, a direct effect of heroin addiction on antenatal growth can be postulated.

Glass et al[15] assessed the effects of heroin on fetal and maternal adrenocortical funtion. Serum cortisol levels were comparable in both study and control infants, but addicted gravidas had significantly lower concentrations than nonaddicted mothers. Heroin decreases cortisol production in adults by inhibiting secretion of ACTH. Decreased cortisol levels were found in pregnant addicts at the time of delivery, but values were similar in the infants of addicted and nonaddicted mothers. The reason for these differences has not been explained. The authors stated that the findings may reflect a decreased responsiveness of the fetal pituitary to heroin or a relative insensitivity of the fetal adrenal cortex to fluctuations in ACTH secretion.

Northrop et al[31] evaluated estriol excretion of narcotic-maintained pregnant women during the last trimester. The concentration of urinary estriol remained low. After withdrawal, however, the urinary estriol concentrations rapidly increased and, in some cases, exceeded average values. Neither ACTH nor metyropone stimulated estriol excretion, although a daily dose of 4 mg of dexamethasone decreased urinary estrol excretion. The authors concluded that careful consideration must be given when fetal well-being is monitored by urinary estriols in the opiate-dependent woman.

The lecithin to sphingomyelin (L/S) ratio of amniotic fluid in normal and abnormal pregnancies has been studied by Gluck and Kulovich.[16] Only in normal pregnancy does the L/S ratio correlate with gestational age. Abnormalities of pregnancy including maternal, fetal and placental conditions may markedly affect the maturation of the fetal lung. Moderate to severe pre-eclampsia, retroplacental bleeding and ruptured membranes accelerate the L/S ratio whereas diabetes and erythroblastosis fetalis may delay fetal lung maturation. In a group of 10 narcotic-addicted patients it was noted that all had accelerated L/S ratios.[16] The studies of these individuals suggest that an association exists between major fetal organ system maturation and the L/S ratio. In 1971, Glass et al[14] reported an apparent decrease in the incidence of the respiratory distress syndrome (RDS) among low birth weight infants who developed symptoms of acute heroin withdrawal. Thirty-three preterm addicted infants were compared with 123 nonaddicted neonates of similar gestational age. The rate of RDS in nonaddicted infants was 53.7% at 32 and 33 weeks, 20.6% at 34 and 35 weeks and 6.9% at 36 and 37 weeks of gestational age. No RDS was noted among the 33 addicted neonates delivered prior to 38 weeks of gestation. By contrast, at Philadelphia General Hospital, 61 of 278 infants born to drug-dependent women were between 26 and 36 weeks of gestation. Eight of these infants underwent heroin withdrawal and developed a typical clinical picture of respiratory distress syndrome. This represents a 13% incidence of RDS, which is lower than the rate of occurrence in our preterm population of nonaddicted infants. It does demonstrate, however, that RDS can occur in the neonate withdrawing from narcotics.

When the drug habit is supported by prostitution, other perinatal complications may exist. Syphilis, gonorrhea and urinary tract infections plague the addicted pregnant woman. Anemia secondary to iron and folic acid deficiency often develops. Nutritional deficiencies, largely due to the lack of proper food, result from inhibition of the central mechanism which controls appetite and hunger. Adaptive or toxic responses to alcohol, barbiturates or narcotics may contribute to malnutrition by interfering with the absorption of ingested nutrients. Absorption abnormalities are common in alcoholics and drug addicts because of the high incidence of lesions of the intestine, liver and pancreas.

Peripheral neuritis, frequent in the alcoholic, is occasionally seen in the chronic drug addict. This usually is due to thiamine depletion, although a deficiency of vitamin B_6, pantothenic acid or nicotinic acid may produce identical signs. Hypoglycemia and vitamin B_6, thiamine or magnesium deficiencies may cause seizures in both alcoholics and drug addicts. Hepatitis, a frequent complication of injectable drug abuse, is depleting nutritionally secondary to a loss of protein, vitamins, minerals and trace elements. Intensive diet therapy is desirable in drug and alcohol addiction, and parenteral therapy may be necessary to correct fluid, mineral and vitamin deficits in acutely ill patients.[25]

Management of Pregnancy Complicated by Drug Abuse

Pregnant drug-abusing women must be managed appropriately to decrease maternal and prenatal morbidity and mortality. It is essential, therefore, to establish a comprehensive approach which specifically will meet the needs of these women. Although multiple drug use is seen, the majority of gravidas abuse opiates as the primary drug.

Before in-depth psychosocial counseling or management of obstetric complications can begin, the addict's physical dependence to opiate drugs must be treated. In 1972, the AMA Council on Mental Health and the Committee on Alcoholism and Drug Dependence provided guidelines for the treatment of morphine-type dependence. They recommended that a pregnant drug-dependent woman should undergo withdrawal prior to delivery. If there is insufficient time to accomplish withdrawal, the woman should be maintained (i.e., methadone or Demerol) during labor and then gradually withdrawn after the delivery process. Chappel,[5] Stimmel,[43] and our group at Philadelphia General Hospital[7, 11] disagree strongly and advocate the referral of pregnant addicts to addiction treatment programs. Withdrawal from opiates is not indicated in the third trimester because of the dual threat of inducing fetal withdrawal with neonatal death due to a meconium aspiration and the risk of premature labor.[7, 11, 36]

It has been stated that chronic opiate addicts have frequent endocrine aberrations including amenorrhea, anovulation and infertility. The women themselves believe that amenorrhea and infertility always result from the use of substantial amounts of heroin. Under experimental conditions, morphine has been shown to depress adrenocorticotrophic hormone release and adrenal function. Observed pregnancies, however, among women with chronic addiction cast doubt on the concept that narcotic use totally suppresses reproductive function.[1, 5, 7, 9] Wallach et al[51] found that women who were oligomenorrheic while using heroin began having regular menstruation, ovulation and conception with apparently normal pregnancies when methadone maintenance was started.

Blinick[1] found methadone maintenance to be successful in 105 pregnancies of narcotic-addicted women. He observed no maternal mortality complications of pregnancy with fetal wastage; however, one-third of the infants were premature by weight. No serious effects attributable to methadone were observed in the neonatal period and follow-up of a small number of the newborn infants revealed normal growth and development. His patients had been maintained on 80 to 100 mg of methadone hydrochloride.

Table 16.2 presents some of the largest studies compiled since 1969 evaluating the various methadone treatment programs for pregnant drug-dependent women.[7] It is noteworthy that even with the use of methadone in various dosages, the incidence of low birth weight infants was not significantly reduced.

Although methadone maintenance has been beneficial in the management of pregnant addicts, several investigators caution that medication without psychosocial support is less effective.[7, 8, 11, 12] In 1972, Statzer and Wardell[41] recognized the need for additional psychologic support and developed a specialized program at the Hutzel Hospital Project of the Detroit Maternal and Infant Care Program. In addition to the usual prenatal care, each patient was seen by a nutritionist, a social worker and a public health nurse. Additional personnel with specialized training in the psychologic requirements of the heroin user also were utilized.

Table 16.2. Recent literature statistics

Authors	Type of treatment		Total No. of patients	LBW* incidence		Incidence of infant withdrawal (%)
	No.	Dose		LBW/Total	%	
Harper[21]	11	60 mg	37	15/37	40	95
	26	60 mg				
Newman[28]	100	40 mg	120	N.R.†		79
	20	40 mg				
Scott and Ryan[39]	22	Mean dose	24	11/24	46	58
Blinick et al[2]	100	Detox. or maintenance dosage‡	100	34/100	34	N.R.†
Davis[8]	108	Various methadone maintenance	108	29/108	27	
Strauss et al[45]	72	Maintenance up to 100 mg	72	16/72	22.2	91.7
Newman et al[30]	70%	80 mg	313	110/313	35	80
	30%	80 mg				
Harper et al[20]	75%	60 mg	51	17/51	33.33	94
	25%	60 mg				

* LBW: low birth weight.

† Not reported.

‡ Patients were detoxified or maintained on methadone but no dosages were given in this report.

Newman[29, 30] has reported findings from the New York City Methadone Maintenance Treatment Program which support the successful use of methadone in pregnancy. A high incidence of neonatal withdrawal symptoms was noted which did not relate to the methadone dose. Newman also reported an extraordinarily high retention rate in the program after delivery with over 95% of the women remaining in treatment.

Harper et al[20] organized a family and maternity care program at the State University of New York, Downstate Medical Center for pregnant addicts, their spouses and the newborn infants. Methadone maintenance coupled with intense psychosocial support appeared to alleviate many of the common problems associated with addiction in pregnancy, although this regimen failed to prevent withdrawal in the newborn. Infant withdrawal, however, was not associated with increased mortality or known prolonged morbidity.

In Philadelphia, we recommend a comprehensive approach which has been used for over 300 pregnant addicts.[7, 11, 12] Patient management in the Family Center Program includes consultations with obstetricians, neonatologists and psychiatrists. Addictive care is arranged according to the patient's needs and her stage of pregnancy at enrollment. Some will choose to be managed drug free whereas others will elect methadone detoxification. In our experience, however, methadone maintenance has been the most successful approach, as we had only one successful detoxification during pregnancy. Eight other detoxified patients returned to heroin before delivery.

Generally, the addicted methadone patient is hospitalized for a detailed medical and drug history, complete physical evaluation and chest x-ray. Various laboratory tests (urinalysis, CBC, VDRL, blood type, Rh factor, SMA-12, and thin layer chromatography) are performed, and her opiate addiction is substantiated. During the 4-day admission she has the opportunity to meet and develop rapport with the professionals involved in the program.

The patient is started on 10 mg of methadone daily and increased only if a higher dosage is required to prevent withdrawal symptomatology. Methadone is kept, if possible, below 35 mg per day. Other drugs, such as tranquilizers and barbiturates, are strictly avoided unless the patient is addicted to these medications. In case of such addiction, the patient is transferred to a special detoxification ward where she can be weaned safely from drugs which are potentially more dangerous than opiates.

Psychosocial Counseling

Social rehabilitative processes in the Family Center Program involve three phases.[32] The initial phase introduces the patient to the program. A social worker helps the client to focus on her individual motivations for entering the program so that both the patient and the social worker can establish realistic goals and expectations. Honesty with the client in explaining the function and limits of the program and the facts of pregnancy and drug abuse is an absolute necessity. Often these realities serve as focal points for the patient, and she may become hesitant or ambivalent about the program. As a result, the social worker must be sensitive and show great understanding. The counselor will then try to assist the patient in achieving some sense of control over herself and her own life.

The second part of social rehabilitation generally is characterized by the patient's intensified internal struggle to give up the addict subculture which has become so familiar to her, and at times, comforting and protective. It is extremely important that the social worker reinforce and support the positive progress made by the client in the direction of autonomy from drugs.

During the last phase the counselor helps the patient initiate the lifetime process of developing independence to cope with her daily life. At this point, the patient usually is better able to assume at least some control of her life experiences and thus will assume a mothering role. She will accept more responsibility for her child's emotional development and will achieve a more positive mother-child relationship. Often, the patient has become drug free, and the formal rehabilitative process may be ended.

In order to strengthen the hospital or clinic-based psychosocial counseling, an outreach mechanism has been developed involving a public health nurse and a community worker. This program attempts to follow-up mothers and infants whose environment is impaired by the erratic lifestyle so common to the drug-dependent population. The fundamental role of the public health nurse is to develop and maintain the human relationship essential for encouraging these patients to return for obstetric, medical and psychosocial counseling. Homes are evaluated before and after infants are released. Since syphilis and gonorrhea are so common in this population, the nurse becomes involved in coordinating the activities of the patients with the social health clinic. The majority of the nurse's time is spent in the follow-up care of the mothers and in teaching necessary information about pregnancy. The nurse discusses nutrition, basic anatomy, signs of impending labor, danger signs of pregnancy, delivery and methods of contraception. After delivery of the infant, the nurse instructs patients in postpartum and infant care, child rearing practices and medical care for both mother and infant. In addition to these educational functions, the nurse identifies social or emotional problems and either institutes therapy immediately or refers patients to the social worker who will follow through with appropriate referral or counseling.

Labor and Delivery

On admission to the labor floor, a urine specimen is sent to the toxicology laboratory for verification of methadone use and to rule out the presence of other drugs. A record is made of the last dose of methadone taken, and, if necessary, methadone (10 to 20 mg intramuscularly) is given to the patient for prevention of withdrawal symptoms. During labor, the patient is managed with minimal regard to opiate addiction. Physicians in charge of the labor floor, however, are aware of her drug usage, and conduction anesthesia is initiated as early as possible to avoid the use of narcotic analgesics.

Early studies demonstrated that methadone administered in doses which produced satisfactory analgesia for labor contractions caused severe depression in newborns.[35] The drug also was noted to exert a variable effect on the interval and length of contractions.

Powell and Chen[34] studied the action of methadone on preparations of isolated uteruses from nonpregnant rabbits, rats, golden hamsters, cats and guinea pigs and uterine horns of rabbits and cats. Methadone inhibited uterine activity when rhythmic movements were present while stimulating a quiescent uterus. The authors concluded that methadone probably does not act on the uterine autonomic nervous system, but has a direct muscular action capable of relaxing an active and stimulating an inactive uterus. One might expect methadone to diminish the activity of the human uterus during labor and stimulate the uterus prior to active labor; however, clinical experience at Philadelphia General Hospital has not verified this concept.

Analysis of Methadone Program

To more completely evaluate the effectiveness of a comprehensive approach in the care of pregnant drug-dependent women and their newborns, data have been analyzed regarding the frequency of major obstetric complications and the morbidity and mortality in the passively dependent newborn infant. This data includes Family Center patients delivered at Philadelphia General Hospital from 1969 through 1975. Results are presented in relationship to the five groups of patients defined in Table 16.3.

The percentage of obstetric complications in these five groups are listed in Table 16.4. The data show a downward trend in the methadone-treated gravidas, but the differences are not significant when compared with the control groups. The incidence of low birth weight neonates (<2500 g) is significantly different between heroin-dependent women with no prenatal care (group A; 47.6%) and methadone maintenance patients with good prenatal care (group C; 17.1%) ($P < 0.001$). Infants born to nondrug-dependent mothers with no prenatal care (group D) had a 18.8% incidence of low birth weight in contrast to the 47.6% incidence in group A ($P < 0.001$). This difference is important since opiate dependency for the first time can be isolated as contributing to this serious perinatal problem. Those infants whose moters received comprehensive care in the Family Center (group C) had an incidence of low birth weight similar to control group E, (nondrug-dependent with prenatal care).

Infants of drug-dependent mothers were evaluated regarding morbidity, Apgar score, growth status at delivery and length of stay in the hospital (Table 16.5). Neonatal problems, such as infection, asphyxia neonatorum, transient tachypnea, aspiration pneumonia, intrauterine growth retardation, congenital syphilis and jaundice were seen most commonly in group A (74.6%) and group B (81.1%). The incidence of intrauterine growth retardation (IUGR) was 12.7% in group A compared to 2.4% in group D ($P < 0.001$). This finding again suggests that opiate use is a cause of IUGR. The incidence of IUGR was reduced to 7.0% and 7.2% in groups B and C with prenatal care and methadone treatment. These percentages are similar to control group E (7.0%).

Infants of group A gravidas remained in the hospital 19 days longer than the neonates from control groups D and E. The average hospital stay for infants of methadone-dependent mothers with or without prenatal care was 17 days versus 25.9 days for newborns of heroin-dependent women. Apgar scores at 1 min were similar in all groups; however, at 5 min, infants in the nondrug-dependent groups showed a slightly improved score.

Table 16.3. Comparative groups of 492 pregnant women delivered at Philadelphia General Hospital, 1969–1975

Group	Description
A (n = 63)	Heroin-dependent women; no prenatal care
B (n = 90)	Methadone maintenance; minimal prenatal care (1–3 visits; average 1.9)
C (n = 154)	Methadone maintenance; adequate prenatal care (4–21 visits; average 8.3) psychosocial counseling
D (n = 85)	Nondrug-dependent women; no prenatal care
E (n = 100)	Nondrug-dependent women; prenatal care 2–21 visits; average 9.1)

Table 16.4. Obstetric complications in 317 drug-dependent women and 185 control subjects, Philadelphia General Hospital, 1969–1975

Groups	No. of patients	Average No. of prenatal visits	Major* obstetrical complications (%)	LBW† (<2500 g) incidence (%)
A	63	0	28.1	47.6
B	90	1.9	24.7	36.4
C	154	8.3	26.6	17.1
D‡	85	0	22.4	18.8
E§	100	8.9	21.8	13.0

* Major: pre-eclampsia, abruptio placenta, premature labor, chorioamnionitis, fetal distress, rupture of membranes >24 hr.

† LBW = low birth weight.

‡ Control group: nondrug dependent; no prenatal care.

§ Control group: nondrug dependent; prenatal care.

Neonates of drug-dependent gravidas were evaluated for withdrawal symptomatology (Table 16.6). Group A infants were those with heroin withdrawal, and B and C were infants with combined methadone and heroin withdrawal or methadone alone. Toxicology studies revealed that nearly 50% of methadone-treated patients in the program had cheated at least once during pregnancy. The greatest incidence of cheating occurred among the group B patients. The most common neonatal symptoms were tremors, high pitched cries, sneezing, tachypnea, poor feeding, hyperactive Moro reflex, loose stools and sweating. Symptoms noted with less frequency included excoriation, mottling, nasal stuffiness, yawning, fever, projectile vomiting, watery stools, dehydration and generalized convulsions. There was no significant difference in the overall incidence of neonatal withdrawal in the three groups; however, marked differences were evident when the symptomatology was separated according to severity: mild, withdrawal requiring no drug therapy; moderate, withdrawal requiring drug therapy for 14 days or less; severe, withdrawal requiring drug therapy for longer than 14 days.

Severe neonatal withdrawal was most pronounced in group A, whereas infants in groups B and C generally had mild to mod-

Table 16.5. Incidence of morbidity in 307 infants of drug-dependent women in comparison to 185 control subjects, Philadelphia General Hospital, 1969–1975

Groups	Average prenatal visits	Baby days in hospital	Incidence of neonatal morbidity* (%)	Intrauterine growth retardation (%)	Apgar scores	
					1 min	5 min
A (n = 63)	0	25.9	74.6	12.7	7.0	8.3
B (n = 90)	1.9	18.1	81.1	7.0	7.3	8.4
C (n = 154)	8.3	16.6	66.2	7.2	7.6	8.9
D (n = 85)	0	7.1	43.0	2.4	7.9	9.2
E (n = 100)	8.9	6.7	45.0	7.0	8.2	9.4

* Most frequently occurring infant diagnosis: (1) asphyxia neonatorum; (2) aspiration pneumonia; (3) congenital syphilis; (4) intrauterine growth retardation; (5) prematurity; (6) hyperbilirubinemia; (7) sepsis; (8) hemolytic disease due to ABO incompatibility; (9) transient tachypnea; (10) hypocalcemia; (11) hypoglycemia; (12) hyaline membrane disease.

Table 16.6. Incidence of withdrawal symptomatology in 287 infants of drug-dependent mothers, Philadelphia General Hospital, 1969–1975

Groups	No withdrawal (%)	Mild withdrawal (%)	Moderate withdrawal (%)	Severe withdrawal (%)	Total withdrawal (%)
A n = 60	5.0	36.6	33.3	25.0	94.9
B n = 79	3.8	45.6	39.2	11.4	96.2
C n = 148	8.1	27.7	53.4	10.8	91.9

Table 16.7. Duration and dosage of methadone as related to withdrawal severity

Withdrawal severity	Daily methadone dosage (NS)*	Duration (weeks), $P < 0.05$
None	45.0 (n = 13)	45 (n = 7)
Mild†	26.5 (n = 52)	17 (n = 49)
Moderate‡	35.0 (n = 93)	25 (n = 88)
Severe§	44.0 (n = 24)	28 (n = 23)

* NS: not significant.
† Mild symptoms, no drug therapy necessary.
‡ Moderate symptoms necessitating drug therapy for ≤2 weeks.
§ Severe symptoms necessitating drug therapy for >2 weeks.

erate withdrawal. Thirteen percent of newborns whose mothers were taking very low doses of methadone experienced no withdrawal symptomatology. Table 16.7 describes the duration and dosage of methadone related to withdrawal severity in groups B and C. The effect of methadone dosage on withdrawal severity is not significant; however, the effect of duration in weeks is significant ($P < 0.05$). The most important aspect of this evaluation is that good prenatal care and methadone maintenance significantly reduces the incidence of severe neonatal withdrawal.

Longitudinal data have been collected at Philadelphia General Hospital concerning the long term disposition of infants born to drug-dependent patients. Information for group A mothers is not available since these patients generally went back to heroin usage after delivery and were lost to follow-up. Data is available for 59 patients in group B and 124 patients in group C. The average number of months between intake into the program and delivery was 2.0 months in group B and 4.9 months in group C. Approximately 1% of the patients in both groups decided to be drug free while the others chose methadone maintenance for thier addictive care.

Forty percent of the 59 patients in group B left the program against medical advice while only 20% of the 124 women in group C discontinued under similar conditions. The most frequent reason for termination in group C (27%) was voluntary detoxification post delivery. Table 16.8 describes status of patients in each group.

Those patients who remain in the Family Center for the longest period of time (group C) appear to be able to attain a drug-free status more often than those who seek sporadic Family Center services (group B). The success of group C is certainly an expression of individual motivation facilitated by counseling.

Comments and Recommendations

Previous reports have condemned methadone use in pregnancy suggesting that the severity of neonatal withdrawal was greater from methadone than heroin. Zel-

Table 16.8. Status of patients leaving program

Group	Total	Intake to delivery, average mos.	Intake to termination, average mos.	Reason for termination		
				Against medical advice (%)	Voluntary detoxification (%)	Transferred to another methadone program (after delivery) (%)
B	59	2.0	8.2	40.1	13.9	23.2
C	124	4.9	12.5	20.0	27.0	21.5

son[52] studied 42 infants whose mothers had used methadone alone or in combination with heroin compared to 34 neonates of heroin-addicted gravidas. His data demonstrated a higher incidence of severe withdrawal in infants of mothers taking methadone versus newborns of women on street heroin. The study however, failed to compare doses of methadone, heroin and/or heroin plus methadone. In our investigations, methadone maintenance (74% low dose) combined with prenatal care (group C) demonstrated a significant effect in decreasing severe neonatal withdrawal compared to infants of mothers on street heroin (group A).

We have had minimal success with drug detoxification. Only one of nine patients detoxified before delivery remained drug free while eight returned to opiates or were lost to follow-up. Recently, Zuspan et al[53] reported increased norephinephrine levels in the amniotic fluid of a patient being detoxified in the third trimester of pregnancy. He interpreted this finding as an indication of fetal stress, and, therefore, does not recommend detoxification until after delivery. Consequently, we do not attempt detoxification, especially during the last 8 weeks of gestation, when meconium aspiration is likely to occur.

From a review of the literature and our own experience with a large group of patients, it is clear that addicted pregnant women warrant specialized care with the use of the following parameters.

1. Any woman who requests help during pregnancy and admits to an opiate habit should be designated "high risk" and evaluated in a hospital setting.
2. If a program for drug rehabilitation is accessible, the personnel should be utilized as soon as possible for addictive management during pregnancy.
3. Detoxification of the pregnant addict is possible, but extremely difficult, and fraught with the possible hazards of abortion (first trimester patients) and possible fetal distress (third trimester patients). Our recommendation is that a low dose methadone maintenance program be instituted with qualified medical and paramedical support. If detoxification is requested or necessary (in areas where maintenance programs are unavailable), it should take place preferably between the 14th to 28th week of gestation and should be accomplished slowly (i.e., 5-mg reduction every 2 weeks).
4. Any mother who is addicted to barbiturates and tranquilizers as well as opiates should be detoxified during the second trimester in a very specialized detoxification center.
5. Infants born to mothers addicted to opiates should be considered high risk and admitted to an intensive care nursery where the personnel make use of an abstinence scoring system and treat the infants appropriately.

REFERENCES

1. Blinick, G., Jerez, E., Wallach, R. C.: Methadone maintenance, pregnancy and progeny. JAMA 225: 477–479, 1973.
2. Blinick, G., Wallach, R. C., Jerez, E.: Pregnancy in narcotic addicts treated by medical withdrawal. Am J Obstet Gynecol Vol 105: 997–1003, 1969.
3. Bracey, D.: Recommend new legislation to force pregnant addicts into prenatal treatment. Addictions 1: 13, 1972.
4. Caldeyro-Barcia, R.: Fetal malnutrition: The role of maternal blood flow. Hosp Pract 5: 33–43, 1970.
5. Chappel, J. N.: Treatment of morphine-type dependence. JAMA 221: 1516, 1972.
6. Cohen, S. N., Newmann, L. L.: Methadone maintenance during pregnancy. Am J Dis Child 126: 445–446, 1973.
7. Connaughton, J. F., Finnegan, L. P., Schut, J., Emich, J. P.: Current concepts in the management of the pregnant opiate addict. Addictive Dis 1: 21, 1975.
8. Davis, R.: The role of psychosocial support in methadone-maintained pregnancies. Presented at the NIDA Perinatal Research Conference, September 1974, Nashville, Tennessee. J Addictive Dis, 1975.

9. Davis, R. C., Chappel, J. N.: Pregnancy in the context of narcotic addiction and methadone maintenance. Proceedings of the Fifth National Conference on Methadone Treatment, March 17–19, 1973, Washington, D.C., 1973.
10. Dawes, G. S.: *Foetal and Neonatal Physiology*. Chicago, Year Book Medical Publishers, Inc., 1968, p 119.
11. Finnegan, L. P.: Narcotic dependence in pregnancy. J. Psychedel Drugs 7: 299, 1975
12. Finnegan, L. P., Connaughton, J. R., Emich, J. P., Wieland, W. F.: Comprehensive care of the pregnant addict and its effect on maternal and infant outcome. Contemp Drug Probl 1: 765–809, 1972.
13. Finnegan, L. P., MacNew, B.: Care of the addicted infant Am J Nursing 74: 685–693, 1974.
14. Glass, L., Rajegowda, B. K., Evans, H. E.: Absence of respiratory distress syndrome in premature infants of heroin-addicted mothers. Lancet 2: 685–686, 1971.
15. Glass, L., Rajegowda, B. K., Mukherjee, T. K., Roth, M. M., Evans, H. E.: Effect of heroin on cortisol production in pregnant addicts and their fetuses [Abstr]. Pediatr Res 7: 320, 1973.
16. Gluck, R., Kulovich, M. V.: Lecithin/sphingomyelin ratios in amniotic fluid in normal and abnormal pregnancy. Am J Obstet Gynecol 115: 539, 1973.
17. Goodfriend, M. J., Shey, I. A. Klein, M. D.: The effects of maternal narcotic addiction on the newborn. Am J Obstet 71: 29–36, 1956.
18. Gruenwald, P.: Chronic fetal distress and placental deficiency. Biol Neonate 5: 215, 1963.
19. Harper, R. G., Solish, G., Feingold, E., Sokal, M.: Heat stable alkaline phosphatase in methadone-maintained pregnancies. Addictive Dis 1: 89, 1975.
20. Harper, R. G., Solish, G. I., Purow, H. M., Sang, E., Panepinto, W. C.: The effect of a methadone treatment program upon pregnant heroin addicts and their newborn infants. Pediatrics 54: 300–305, 1974.
21. Harper, R. G., Solish, G. I., Sang, E., Purow, H.: The effect of a methadone treatment program upon pregnant addicts and their infants. Proceedings of the Fifth National Conference on Methadone Treatment, March 17–19, 1973, Washington, D.C., pp 1133–1137.
22. Hill, R. M., Desmond, M. M.: Management of the narcotic withdrawal syndrome in the neonate. Pediatr Clin North Am 10: 67–87, 1963.
23. Journal of the American Medical Association Editorial. Treatment of morphine-type dependence by withdrawal methods. JAMA 219: 1611–1615, 1972.
24. Jones, J.: Nutrition, drugs and their interrelations. Penn Med 35: p 3, 1974.
25. Krause, S. O., Murray, P. M., Holmes, J. B., Burch, R. E.: Heroin addiction among pregnant women and their newborn babies. Am J Obstet Gynecol 75: 754–758, 1958.
26. Naeye, R. L.: Malnutrition, a probable cause of fetal growth retardation. Arch Pathol 79: 284, 1965.
27. Naeye, R. L., Blanc, W., Leblanc, W., Khatamee, M. A.: Fetal complications of maternal heroin addiction: Abnormal growth, infections and episodes of stress. J Pediatr 83: 1055–1061, 1973.
28. Newman, R. G.: Results on 120 deliveries of patients in the New York City Methadone Maintenance Treatment Program. Proceedings of the Fifth National Conference on Methadone Treatment, March 17–19, 1973, Washington, D.C., pp 1114–1121.
29. Newman, R. G.: Pregnancies of methadone patients. N Y State J Med 1: 52–54, 1974.
30. Newman, R. G., Bashkow, S., Calko, D.: Results of 313 consecutive live births of infants delivered to parents in the New York City Methadone Maintenance Treatment Program. Am J Obstet Gynecol 121 (2): 233–237, 1975.
31. Northrop, G., Ditzler, J., Ryan, W. G, Wilbanks, G. O.: Estriol excretion profiles in narcotic-addicted women. Am J Obstet Gynecol 112: 704–712, 1972.
32. Oglesby, H.: Demographic characteristics and social work input in the social rehabilitative process of the pregnant opiate dependent mother in a comprehensive care program. Proceedings of the 36th Annual Meeting of the Committee on Problems of Drug Dependence of the National Research Council, March 11–14, 1974, Mexico City, Mexico.
33. Perlmutter, J. F.: Drug addiction in pregnant women. Am J Obstet Gynecol 99: 69–572, 1967.
34. Powell, C. E., Chen, K. K.: Action of dolophine on the animal uterus. J Am Pharm Assoc 37: 516–518, 1948.
35. Prescott, F., Ransom, S. G.: Amidone (Miadone) as an obstetric analgesia. Lancet 2: 501–503, 1947.
36. Rementeria, J. L., Nunag, N. N.: Narcotic withdrawal in pregnancy: Stillbirth incidence with a case report. Am J Obstet Gynecol 116: 1152–1156, 1973.
37. Rosenthal, T., Patrick, S. W., Krug, D. C.: Congenital neonatal narcotic addiction: A natural history. Am J Publ Health Nation's Health 54: 1252–1262, 1964.
38. Rothstein, P., Gould, J. B.: Born with a habit: Infants of drug-addicted mothers. Pediatr Clin North Am 21: 307–321, 1974.
39. Scott, N. R., Ryan, J. J.: Clinical evaluation of pregnant methadone maintenance patients and their newborn infants. Proceedings of the Fifth National Conference on Methadone Treatment. March 17–19, 1973, Washington, D. C., 1128–1132.
40. Singh, E. J., Zuspan, F. P.: Content of amniotic fluid prostaglandins in normal, diabetic and drug-abuse human pregnancy. Am J Obstet Gynecol 118: 358–361, 1974.
41. Statzer, D. E., Wardell, J. N.: Heroin addiction during pregnancy. Am J Obstet Gynecol 94: 253–257, 1966.
42. Stern, R.: The pregnant addict: A study of 66 case histories, 1950–1959. Am J Obstet Gynecol 94: 253–257, 1966.
43. Stimmel, B., Adamson, K.: Narcotic dependence in pregnancy. JAMA 235: 1121–1124, 1976.

44. Stone, M. L., Salerno, L. J., Green, M., Zelson, C.: Narcotic addiction in pregnancy. Am J Obstet Gynecol 109: 716–723, 1971.
45. Strauss, M. E., Andresko, M., Stryker, J. C., Wardell, N. N., Dunkel, L. D.: Methadone maintenance during pregnancy: Pregnancy, birth and neonate characteristics. Am J Obstet Gynecol 120: 895–890, 1974.
46. Sullivan, R. D., Fischbach, A. L., Hornick, F. W.: Treatment of a pregnant opiate addict with oral methadone. Arizona Med 29: 30, 1972.
47. Sussman, S.: Narcotic and methamphetamine use during pregnancy, effect on newborn infants. Am J Dis Child 106: 325–330, 1963.
48. Vandervort, W. J., Paulshock, B. Z.: Laboratory screening of heroin addicts. JAMA 220: 1014, 1972.
49. Waldeman, H.: Psychiatric emergencies during pregnancy and in the puerperium. Muench Med Wochenschr 115: 1039–1043, 1973.
50. Wallace, H. M.: Factors associated with perinatal mortality and morbidity. Clin Obstet Gynecol 13: 13–43, 1970.
51. Wallach, R. D., Jerez, E., Blinick, G.: Pregnancy and menstrual function in narcotic addicts treated with methadone. Am J Obstet Gynecol 105: 1226, 1969.
52. Zelson, C.: Infant of the addicted mother. N Engl J Med 288: 1393–1395, 1973.
53. Zuspan, F. P., Gumpel, J. A., Mejia-Zelaya, A., Madden, J., Davis, R.: Fetal abuse from methadone withdrawal. Am J Obstet Gynecol 122(1): 43–46, 1975.

Part IV

NEONATAL

MHAIRI G. MACDONALD, MBchB, MRCP(UK), FAAP
HERMAN M. RISEMBERG, M.D., FAAP

17

Neonatal Emergencies
FETAL NEONATAL TRANSITION ACUTE INTENSIVE CARE

Introduction

During labor and the first hours of neonatal life, important changes occur in the fetus and neonate. This chapter is concerned with the physiologic adaptation of the fetus to extrauterine life, as a basis for the pathophysiology of maladaptation.

Acute intensive care of the fetus and neonate may bring improvements in mortality rate, morbidity and perhaps quality of survival. The implementation of intensive care in the perinatal period will be the second priority of this review.

Physiologic and Pathologic Cardiorespiratory Adaptation

Section I

CARDIOVASCULAR SYSTEM

Throughout pregnancy blood is supplied to the intervillous space by the uterine and ovarian vessels. The normal maternal arterial pressure (Figure 17.1) is 85 mm Hg to 90 mm Hg, whereas intramyometrial and amniotic fluid pressure is in the range of 10 to 15 mm Hg.

During labor, the maternal arterial pressure remains unchanged, but with contractions, the myometrial pressure rises rapidly, impairing venous return. When the intramyometrial pressure reaches 120 mm Hg, the arterial supply to the intervillous space is interrupted, producing circulatory stasis.

Amniotic fluid pressure reaches levels of about 60 mm Hg at the peak of a contraction (Figure 17.2). Between contractions the circulatory changes rapidly revert to normal, and under ordinary circumstances there are no gross changes in the acid-base status of the fetus, apart from a mild combined respiratory and metabolic acidosis with pH values of 7.25 to 7.30 at the time of birth.[35] pH values return to normal spontaneously within the first few minutes of life.

In the normal neonate at birth, circulatory changes occur rapidly. The cardiac output and blood flow to the pulmonary artery increase, pulmonary vascular resistance decreases and the ductus arteriosus closes. The resulting increase in the return of blood to the left atrium is accompanied by an increase in left atrial pressure, closure of the foramen ovale and completion of the transition from fetal to neonatal circulation. The systemic pressure immediately rises and the umbilical vessels become constricted. This adaptation is mediated via the bradykinin system (Figure 17.3) as a response to the increased oxygen content of the pulmonary arterial blood.[37, 38]

Cardiovascular Maladaptation

If myometrial hypertonicity develops during labor (abruptio placentae, oxytocin induction, etc.) or if contractions become too frequent and the duration of relaxation

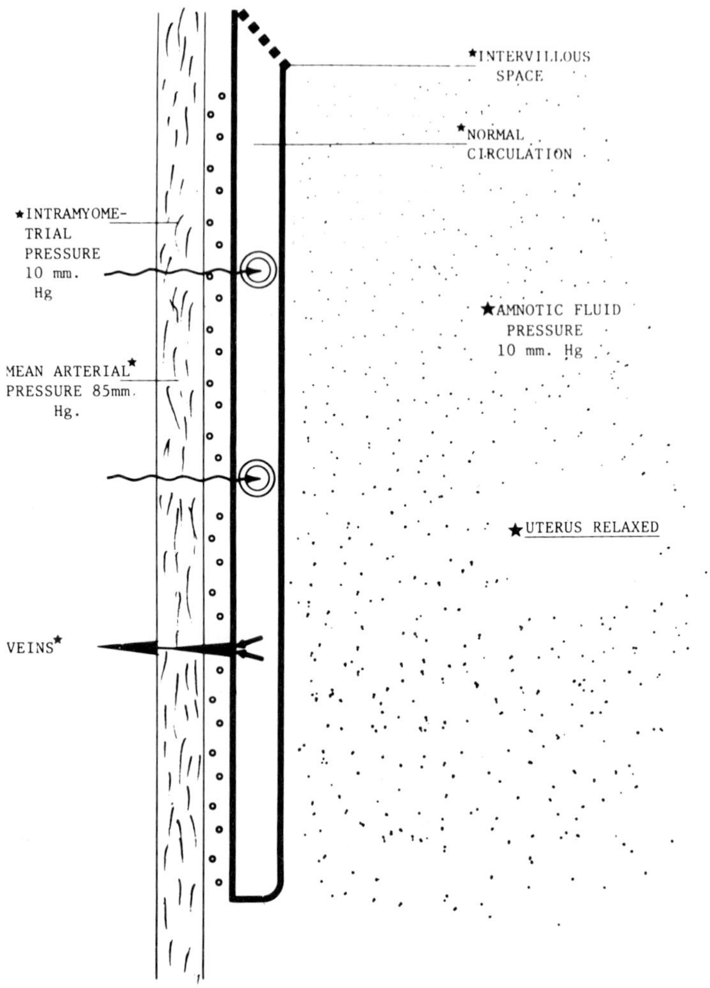

Figure 17.1. Placental perfusion during uterine relaxation.

decreases, circulatory maladaptation will occur, and the condition of the fetus will deteriorate rapidly, with the development of hypoxemia and acidosis. When the fetus is chronically stressed during pregnancy, as in intrauterine growth retardation, mild hypoxemia and acidosis will be present even before the initiation of labor. The condition of the fetus may then deteriorate rapidly, even during normal labor, and if not recognized, will result in severe neonatal asphyxia and fetal death.

The circulatory changes that ensue in utero during fetal stress may be irreversible, even after correction of the causative factors. During stress, the cardiovascular system of the fetus will respond by selectively increasing the blood flow to the brain and heart, and by decreasing the blood flow to the placenta and other organs.[7] This so-called "diving reflex" is comparable to circulatory changes observed in seals and dolphins during diving.

At birth the circulation of the distressed neonate may fail to adapt to the new environment, with persistance of fetal circulation and a large right to left shunt leading to hypoxemia and acidosis. The combination of hypoxemia and acidosis then causes constriction of the pulmonary vasculature, increasing the shunt.[34]

Respiratory System

From the 20th to the 22nd weeks of gestation, epithelial alveolar cells (pneumon-

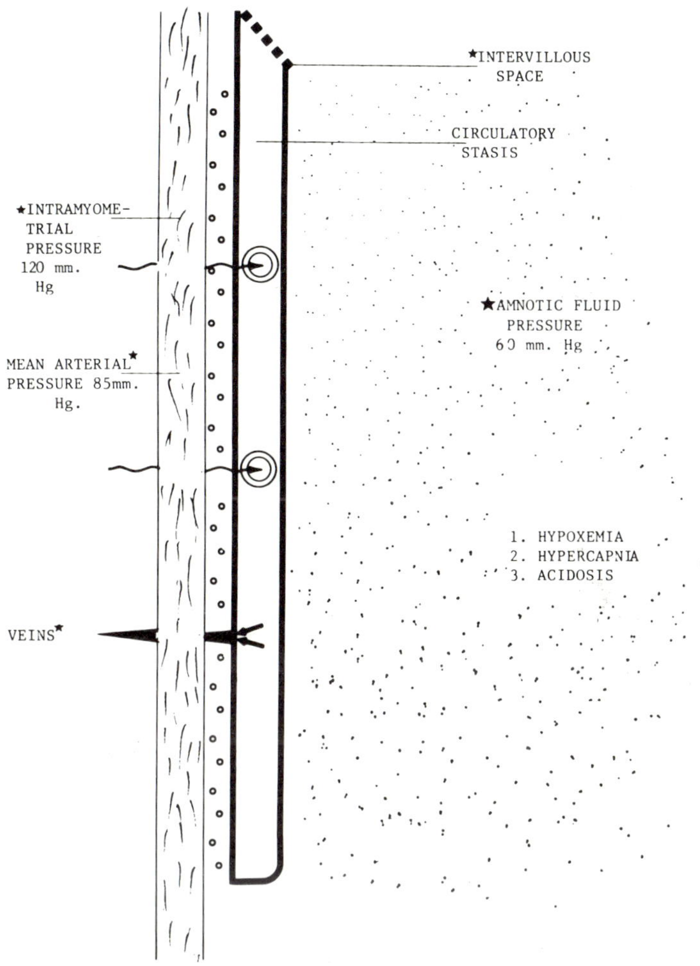

Figure 17.2. Placental perfusion during uterine contraction.

ocytes type II) are seen in the fetal lungs. By the 28th week of gestation, there is an increase in cell number, and the cells take on a granular appearance. The granules contain disaturated phospholipids (lecithin and sphingomyelin), which are secreted into the alveoli, forming an inner lining to the alveolar wall. The lung phospholipids are known collectively as pulmonary surfactant. Lecithin shows the greatest surface activity and increases in quantity during pregnancy, so that in the mature lung, the quantity of lecithin present is 4 to 5 times greater than the quantity of sphingomyelin. Because of the active excretion of pulmonary fluid into the amniotic cavity, it is possible to predict the degree of maturation of the fetal lungs by determining the lecithin to sphingomyelin ratio in the amniotic fluid.[9, 18] Chronic intrauterine stress (intrauterine growth retardation), prolonged rupture of membranes and heroin addiction may accelerate surfactant maturation, whereas maternal diabetes and severe erythroblastosis fetalis may delay maturation.[5]

At birth the lungs are airless and half-filled with fluid; hence, the first two or three respiratory efforts may require negative respiratory pressures as high as 70 cm of H_2O. The presence of pulmonary surfactant counteracts the retracting tissue forces that tend to collapse the alveoli. The lungs remain expanded, and a functional residual capacity is established. The remaining pulmonary fluid is excreted into the pulmonary and lymphatic capillaries and, after a few seconds, a normal respira-

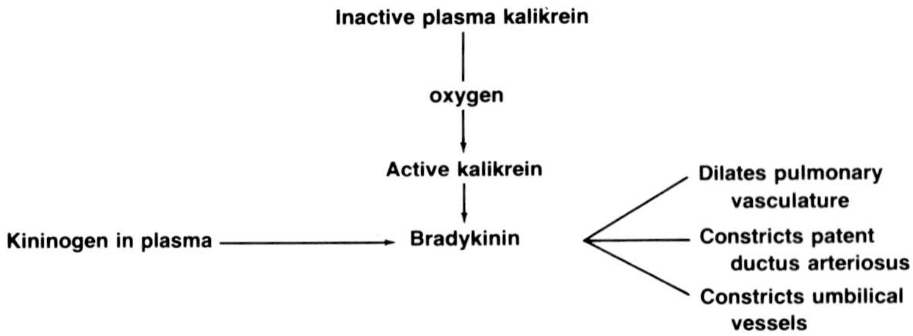

Figure 17.3. The bradykinin system.

tory pattern is established. The tidal volume necessary to maintain physiologic interchange of gases is approximately 5 cc per kg, and the pressures generated by the respiratory effort range from 5 to 10 cm H_2O.

The lungs of premature infants may contain an inadequate amount of pulmonary surfactant, producing labored respirations, progressive atelectasis and hypoxemia. Combined metabolic and respiratory acidosis develops, seriously embarrassing respiratory and circulatory adaptation.

Neonatal Asphyxia

After normal labor and delivery, the neonate will establish a normal respiratory pattern almost immediately. At 1 min of life, the infant will be pink, crying and active, with normal reflexes and muscle tone, a heart rate between 120 and 160 beats per min and an Apgar score of 8 to 10.[3] If the neonate is a product of intrauterine asphyxia, apnea will be present at birth, and the recognition of the degree of asphyxia becomes the first priority of the neonatal evaluation.

Animals respond to asphyxia with a rapid succession of gasping movements, increasing heart rate and elevation of blood pressure.[2, 13] Asphyxia prolonged over 1 to 2 min produces primary apnea, accompanied by mild bradycardia and hypotension. One or 2 min later gasping movements reappear, lasting from 4 to 6 min, with the last gasp occurring approximately 9 to 10 min after the onset of the asphyxia. The onset of secondary apnea is signaled by severe bradycardia and hypotension and, unless resuscitation is begun, death will follow. A similar sequence of events probably occurs in the human fetus, with the outcome for the patient determined by the speed with which asphyxia is recognized and treated.

Differential Diagnosis of Primary and Secondary Apnea

Primary Apnea. The newborn is cyanotic, and reflexes are diminished. The heart sounds and the pulse are usually normal, but bradycardia in the range of 60 to 100 per min may be present, and the Apgar score is from 3 to 5. After gentle suction and the administration of oxygen, gasping respirations appear, with rapid improvement in the infant's condition. At 5 min the Apgar score will be 8 to 10, and the immediate and long term prognosis is excellent.

Secondary Apnea. The neonate appears ashen, reflexes are absent, heart sounds are distant, the pulses are weak and bradycardia is usually severe, with a pulse rate between 20 and 60 per min. The Apgar score is between 1 and 3. Stimulation fails to evoke gasping movements, and unless immediate resuscitation is performed, the neonate will suffer irreversible asphyxia. Spontaneous respiration may not be achieved for 5 to 15 min after commencing resuscitation efforts. Long term disabilities may occur.

Resuscitation of Neonate

Anticipation of problems allows the team to take an orderly approach to resuscitation, using the following recommended steps: (*a*) evaluation of the degree of apnea; (*b*) suction; (*c*) administration of oxygen; (*d*) administration of buffers; (*e*) cardiac massage; (*f*) thermal regulation.

Rapid Evaluation. This preferably is performed by two individuals: the leader to evaluate the Apgar score, and the other to listen to the heart rate and tap out the rate on the resuscitation table.

Suction. If the infant is meconium stained, larynx and trachea must be suctioned immediately through an endotracheal tube. If the infant is not meconium stained, gentle but rapid nasal pharyngeal suction should be performed. The duration of this procedure should not exceed 30 sec, since prolonged suction may evoke a vasovagal reaction.[10]

Administration of Oxygen. This is the most important resuscitation procedure, and must not be delayed. If the patient has primary apnea, oxygen should be administered by facial mask; if secondary apnea is present, oxygen must be administered by positive pressure through an endotracheal tube. During intubation it is helpful to have the observer place a finger over the suprasternal notch to monitor the introduction of the tube into the trachea. Intubation may be facilitated by freezing the endotracheal tubes and keeping them in an ice bucket in the delivery room.

If, after 5 min, autonomous respiration is not established, a neonatal volume respirator should be used. This will free the team leader to proceed with further evaluation.

Administration of Buffers. Most patients with secondary apnea require a buffer such as sodium bicarbonate, which can be given via the umbilical vein, at the rate of 2 to 3 mEq per kg over a period of 5 to 10 min.[14] Sterile heparinized syringes should be kept available so that blood may be obtained for baseline pH estimation. Initial administration of buffer should not be delayed while awaiting the result of this estimation.

Cardiac Massage. When peripheral pulses are weak or absent, cardiac massage must be started immediately. Manual compression of the heart, via sternal massage, will improve the cardiac output satisfactorily. This maneuver is most easily carried out by embracing the back of the infant with the hands and using the thumbs to depress the sternum, using a ratio of one cardiac massage to three respirations.

Thermal Regulation. The asphyctic newborn cannot maintain his normal body temperature, and his survival may be jeopardized by cold stress. It is essential, therefore, to place the infant in a neutral thermal environment during resuscitation.

After 5 min of intensive care, the apneic infant must be re-evaluated, including blood pressure and hematocrit determination. If the infant is in shock or is anemic, plasma or blood transfusions must be administered. Once the infant has been successfully resuscitated, careful follow-up is essential, as hypoglycemia, hypocalcemia and unstable temperature regulation commonly occur. Furthermore a carefully planned long term follow-up may lead to the early detection of abnormalities in growth and development of prognostic significance.

Section II

DEVELOPMENTAL EVALUATION

Prompt evaluation of fetal growth and development must be made in order to anticipate potential emergencies. Used in conjunction with obstetric data, physical measurements, including weight, head circumference and length, and physical signs such as the degree of development of the ear cartilage, breast tissue, genitalia, sole creases and muscle tone and posture, help to determine physical and neurologic maturation and permit an accurate determination of gestational age.[16]

A full term infant has a gestational age of 37 to 41 completed weeks, a weight between 3000 and 3600 g, a head circumference of 33.5 to 35 cm, and a length between 49 and 51 cm. In the absence of fetal stress, these infants adapt themselves rapidly to extrauterine environment and have an excellent prognosis.

The difference between appropriate for gestational age (premature) and small for gestational age (dysmature) infants is important. *Premature infants* have an intrauterine life of less than 37 weeks and are appropriately developed for gestational age. The most serious complication to be expected is respiratory distress syndrome, and the incidence is related to gestational age. Hypoglycemia and hypothermia are also important complications of prematurity. These infants should be provided with a neutral thermal environment from birth because they have difficulty in maintaining normal body temperature.

Dysmature infants, in contrast, are small for gestational age. They are commonly associated with maternal toxemia, low socioeconomic environment, intrauterine infections and certain malformations associated with chromosomal abnormalities. Blood glucose should be monitored from birth since they tend to develop hypoglycemia. The presence of microcephaly is usually a poor prognostic sign, since it is most commonly observed in infants with intrauterine infections or chromosomal abnormalities.

Large for gestational age infants are often products of mothers with diabetes. Hypoglycemia, respiratory distress syndrome, hyperbilirubinemia and polycythemia are frequent findings. Nevertheless, the size of a number of large infants may be genetically determined or associated with excessive maternal weight gain during pregnancy.

Section III

RESPIRATORY DISTRESS IN NEWBORNS

The diagnosis of the cause of respiratory distress may be difficult, since it may be due to cardiac, vascular, pulmonary or surgical causes. Considerable progress has recently been made in the treatment of conditions manifested by cardiorespiratory difficulties, and prompt recognition of the etiology will permit early treatment and, if necessary, early referral to a regional intensive care center.

Respiratory Distress of Cardiovascular Origin

Because of the complex circulatory adaptation of the newborn, congenital heart disease may not manifest clinically in the first few hours of life, and respiratory distress seen immediately after birth is not usually of cardiac origin. There are two main groups of congenital heart disease seen in the neonatal period—cyanotic and acyanotic.

Heart murmurs are not always of diagnostic value. Thus, complex congenital heart disease may present without heart murmurs (e.g., transposition of the great vessels), whereas noncardiac conditions may present with murmurs (e.g., functional murmurs associated with respiratory diseases). The hyperoxia test (administration of 100% oxygen for 15 min) may help to differentiate between cardiac and noncardic causes of respiratory disease. Patients with congenital heart disease of the cyanotic type will have only minor changes in the partial oxygen pressures after the hyperoxia test, whereas the noncardiac patient will demonstrate a dramatic increase in the partial oxygen pressure.

Cyanotic Group

Transposition of the great vessels accounts for 90% of cyanotic congenital heart disease in the neonatal period. Tricuspid atresia, truncus arteriosus, tetralogy of Fallot with pulmonary atresia and pulmonary atresia with intact ventricular septum are less common. In the last few years progress in surgical and medical techniques has brought about a distinct increase in the survival of this group of patients, making early diagnosis and treatment essential.

Congestive Heart Failure Group (Figure 17.4)

Hypoplastic left heart syndrome acounts for 90% of infants who present with congestive heart failure in the early newborn period. It is important to rule out coarctation of the aorta and severe aortic stenosis by early cardiac catheterization, as these two conditions can be treated surgically.

Respiratory Distress of Vascular Origin

Persistent fetal circulation syndrome, associated with intrauterine asphyxia, may be the cause of circulatory maladaptation in the immediate neonatal period. Hypoxemia and acidosis are secondary to large right to left shunts. The syndrome is manifested clinically by low Apgar scores (1 to 3), early cyanosis and respiratory distress. The cyanosis may persist despite the administration of 100% oxygen. The pH and PCO_2 are initially within normal limits, but metabolic acidosis develops rap-

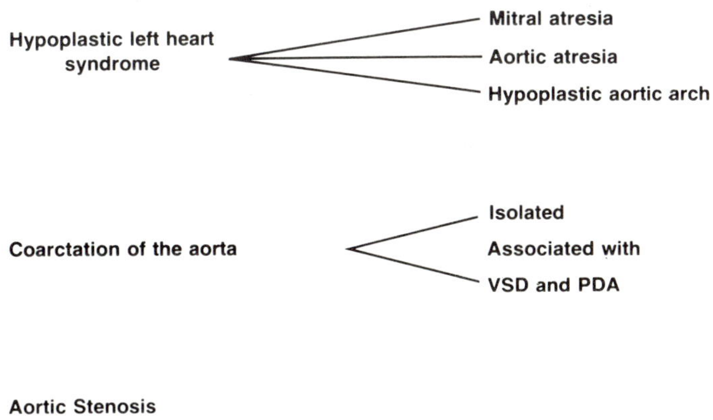

Figure 17.4. Congenital heart disease manifesting initially with congestive heart failure. VSD, ventricular septal defect; PDA, patent ductus arteriosus.

idly, with consequent clinical deterioration.

In some instances this syndrome presents with coronary insufficiency, associated with cardiac enlargement and congestive heart failure. One hundred percent oxygen should be administered, and the metabolic acidosis must be corrected.

Coarctation of Aorta

Early diagnosis of coarctation of the aorta is possible if the peripheral pulses are examined routinely in neonates. When the coarctation is associated with a ventricular septal defect and/or patent ductus arteriosis, congestive heart failure develops rapidly. Early medical and surgical treatment may permit survival in most patients.

Respiratory Distress of Pulmonary Origin

Respiratory Distress Syndrome (RDS). This is the most common cause of respiratory distress in the neonatal period. It is seen predominantly in premature babies, but RDS in infants near term is not a rarity, especially in those delivered by cesarean section prior to initiation of labor.[17] Maternal diabetes and severe erythroblastosis fetalis are conditions that often lead to RDS.

Deficiency of pulmonary surfactant is the most important factor in the pathogenesis of the syndrome, but pulmonary hypoperfusion, low total serum proteins, deficient fibrinolytic enzymes and renal hypoperfusion may also play an important role.

RDS is seen more commonly in boys than in girls and, in twin pregnancies, the second twin is usually more severely affected. Pulmonary atelectasis is more severe in prematures of low gestational age because they have very small respiratory units, a frail chest wall and decreased pulmonary surfactant. Infants present with tachypnea, retractions, grunting respirations and cyanosis. Symptoms and signs are usually present immediately or soon after birth. If untreated, hypoxemia and combined respiratory and metabolic acidosis are followed by respiratory insufficiency. X-ray of the chest characteristically shows a reticular granular pattern, with air bronchograms throughout both lung fields.

The treatment of respiratory distress syndrome consists of correcting hypoxemia and preventing respiratory failure. In infants larger than 1500 g, prompt oxygen therapy via hood or mask is advisable but, if arterial PO_2 fails to rise above 50 mm Hg in an oxygen environment of 60% or more, treatment with nasal constant positive airway pressure (CPAP) is recommended.[33] In premature infants under 1500 g, early utilization of nasal CPAP, as well as correction of base excess deficit with sodium bicarbonate (not exceeding 3 mEq per kg per dose), may dramatically change the outcome of RDS. CPAP therapy should be initiated with a starting positive pressure of 5 cm of water, and gradually increased, if necessary, until the grunting respirations disappear. Positive airway pressures above 10 cm H_2O are not advised.

A pH value below 7.25, in association with a PCO_2 value greater than 70 mm Hg and/or PO_2 below 50 mm Hg in 100% oxygen, is an indication for mechanical respiratory assistance. The patient should have endotracheal intubation and be placed on a neonatal ventilator that is capable of providing positive end expiratory pressure. Provision of a thermogenically neutral environment, as well as adequate circulatory support using blood or plasma, are important supporting measures. Any rapid change in the condition should alert the physician to the possibility of a developing pneumothorax. Early transfer of infants with respiratory distress syndrome to an intensive care center enhances the chance of intact survival.

Transient Tachypnea of Newborn. This is usually seen in full term infants, and is associated with transient retention of pulmonary fluid. It is manifested clinically by shallow and rapid breathing, but blood gases are usually normal. X-rays may reveal retention of lung fluid and, occasionally, cardiomegaly. The tachypnea may persist for 48 to 72 hr, during which time the child requires close observation. The prognosis is good.

Pneumothorax. This is commonly seen following resuscitation in patients born with neonatal asphyxia, and also as a complication of RDS. Tachypnea, with or without cyanosis, is the presenting symptom. The diagnosis may be made in an acute emergency by transilluminating the chest wall with a high intensity light source such as a Chun Gun (Radiation Measurement, Incorporated, Middleton, Wisconsin), but chest x-ray is the diagnostic procedure of choice when time allows. If the pneumothorax is under tension, or large enough to produce mediastinal shift, the air must be evacuated immediately, preferably by introducing a Teflon needle (Abbocath size 14 or 16). A small pneumothorax which is not under tension may be treated effectively by placing the full term infant in 100% oxygen for 2 to 3 hr.

Meconium Aspiration Pneumonia. This is associated with a clinical history of a meconium-stained newborn with or without symptoms of neonatal asphyxia. It is strongly recommended that endotracheal suction be carried out in these infants immediately after birth, since this may prevent the development of aspiration pneumonia. In affected infants, clinical manifestations usually appear immediately after birth, and commonly progress to respiratory failure. The chest x-ray is characterized by bilateral patchy infiltrates and areas of emphysema. Early referral of the symptomatic patient to a neonatal center should improve the prognosis for these infants.

Bacterial Pneumonia and Premature Rupture of Membranes. A history of infection in the mother, or premature rupture of membranes, is commonly associated with congenital bacterial pneumonia. The clinical picture consists of respiratory distress, associated with varying degrees of circulatory collapse and metabolic acidosis. Prompt administration of antibiotics (ampicillin and gentamycin), fluids (blood, plasma, Plasmanate (Cutter)), and the correction of metabolic acidosis will rapidly improve tissue perfusion and the clinical condition.

The association of prolonged rupture of membranes and neonatal pneumonia is frequent enough, when membranes have been ruptured longer than 24 hr, to warrant a special review of maternal and neonatal management. Asymptomatic infants who are products of mothers with prolonged rupture of the membranes should have a postnatal evaluation which includes the performance of blood, gastric aspirate, nasal pharyngeal and skin cultures. Patients should be placed in an observation nursery for the next 48 hr, and close observation is the treatment of choice. If the infants are born with symptoms (tachypnea, hypothermia, fever, gastrointestinal symptoms, etc.), cultures should be taken as in the preceding group, with the inclusion of a spinal tap. Treatment with antibiotics should be started immediately.

Miscellaneous Causes of Respiratory Distress. These include diaphragmatic hernia, hypoplastic lungs, congenital lobar emphysema, choanal atresia and congenital lymphangectasia. The immediate care of an infant with diaphragmatic hernia should include the insertion of an oral or nasal gastric tube which should be aspirated continuously. Positive pressure ventilation, if required, should be administered via an endotracheal tube, and never by face mask.

The majority of newborn infants breathe through the nose. Choanal atresia, therefore, usually causes considerable respiratory distress. The emergency treatment consists of the immediate insertion of an oral airway.

Metabolic Adaptation

Section IV

CARBOHYDRATE METABOLISM

In utero the fetus derives all of his energy requirements from the oxidation of carbohydrates. [20] In view of the fact that the fetal blood sugar is approximately 70 to 80% of the maternal value, it is apparent that sugars do not cross the placenta by simple diffusion. The fetal liver is unable to store glycogen and to regulate the glucose content of the blood until 12 to 14 weeks of gestation, and does not assume full capacity until 20 to 24 weeks. The majority of hepatic glycogen stores are formed during the last trimester of pregnancy, and the level steadily increases to approximately twice the adult concentration at term.

In utero, therefore, the fetus is continuously nourished via the placenta. At birth the supply of glucose ceases abruptly, and the infant becomes entirely dependent upon the external environment for all nutritional needs. For some hours after birth the infant is unlikely to receive a significant caloric intake, and the energy required for muscular activity, respiration and maintenance of body temperature must be derived from his own body stores. Initially, this is reflected by a rapid decrease in the glycogen content of most tissues. The liver glycogen concentration decreases rapidly, to approximately 10% of its original value, within 2 to 3 hr of birth.

Hypoglycemia

Clinical signs and symptoms associated with neonatal hypoglycemia were first reported by Hartman and Jaudon in 1937.[19] Neurologic complications, however, were not described until 1959, when two of eight neonates with severe symptomatic hypoglycemia became spastic and mentally retarded.[11] The importance of neonatal hypoglycemia as a potential cause of cerebral damage, and even death, has since been confirmed by many workers.

Based on primary pathophysiology, hypoglycemic newborn infants may be divided into four clinical categories. The first includes infants of mothers with frank diabetes and those with gestational diabetes, and infants with severe erythroblastosis fetalis. These infants suffer from hypoglycemia due to hyperinsulinism. Beta cell hyperplasia is present in the pancreas, and hypoglycemia tends to occur within the first hours of life.

The second group includes infants who have experienced intrauterine undernutrition. They are frequently the infants of toxemic mothers, infants with placental abnormalities or the smaller of twins. These infants have low levels of hepatic glycogen and a high ratio of brain weight to liver weight. Thus, they have decreased energy stores in the presence of an increased oxygen consumption and metabolic rate.

A third category includes the very immature infant who has been separated from the placenta early in the third trimester and therefore has not fully benefited from the period of maximum glycogen storage. The preterm infant, in the face of complications such as respiratory distress syndrome or anoxia, has metabolic needs increased out of proportion to his substrate stores.

The fourth group is the least common, and includes infants with genetic or developmental defects such as galactosemia, glycogen storage disease, maple syrup urine disease, insulinoma and leucine sensitivity.

The symptoms produced by hypoglycemia are nonspecific. They include episodes of apnea, cyanosis, bradycardia, tachypnea, jitteriness, tremors, convulsions, coma, sweating, hypothermia, limpness, weak or high pitched cry, refusal to feed and irregular respirations. Many of these manifestations are also seen in infants with other problems including infection, hypocalcemia, hypomagnesemia, meningitis, drug withdrawal and intracranial hemorrhage.

Because of the lack of specific symptoms, there has been some controversy over the definition of true hypoglycemia. It is now customary to regard as hypoglycemia a glucose level below 30 mg per 100 cc in the term infant, and a level less than 20 mg per 100 cc in the preterm infant. The question of whether these levels are as serious in the asymptomatic as in the symptomatic infant is still essentially unanswered. There is some suggestion, however, that the asymptomatic infant may fare better from the point of view of long term prognosis.[31]

Because studies are not totally conclusive, and because hypoglycemia has definitely been shown to shorten the survival time of newborn animals in nitrogen and to depress oxygen uptake of the human brain in insulin coma, it would certainly seem desirable to maintain normoglycemia in all newborn infants.

Infant of Diabetic Mother

The infant of the diabetic mother has many problems, one of which is a tendency to early hypoglycemia. It has now been fairly well documented that all of the signs and symptoms seen in these infants can be reduced by close control of maternal diabetes, especially during the last trimester of pregnancy.[30] The hypoglycemia appears to result from a state of hyperinsulinism produced by elevated maternal blood sugar levels. The resulting high fetal plasma glucose concentration stimulates the pancreatic beta cells to produce increased quantities of insulin. Approximately half of the infants born to insulin-dependent diabetics are hypoglycemic within 3 hr of birth, and about one-fifth of those born to gestational diabetics develop early hypoglycemia. There are no documented reasons for using oral hypoglycemic agents in obstetric patients. Not only may these drugs be teratogenic, but they also produce a particularly severe and prolonged hypoglycemia in the newborn.[1] They have been shown to stimulate pancreatic islet growth in newborn animals and to potentiate insulin activity.

A small number of the infants born to mothers with severe diabetes, usually those with evidence of vascular disease, appear undernourished at birth rather than overgrown and plethoric. The placenta is often small and infarcted. These infants are appropriately classed with neonates suffering from lack of nutritional reserves.

Hypoglycemia Due to Lack of Nutritional Reserves

Pre- and post-term infants and infants that are light weight for gestation (including twins) are born with limited reserves of glycogen and fat secondary to inadequate placental carbohydrate transfer. The majority of those who develop symptomatic hypoglycemia are light weight for gestation, and most are born to mothers with toxemia of pregnancy. Associated hypoxia and hypothermia may result in inefficient utilization of the limited glucose reserves, thereby increasing the probability of neuronal damage.

Management of Hypoglycemia

All infants at risk for hypoglycemia should have blood sugar levels monitored at birth, and thereafter every 4 hr, for at least the first 24 hr of life. Dextrostix (Ames) estimations on capillary blood, obtained from the heel of the infant, are satisfactory for screening purposes. If the Dextrostix reading is falling significantly despite adequate oral caloric intake, or is below 45 mg per 100 ml, an accurate blood sugar estimation should be obtained.

The only satisfactory methods for measuring blood sugar in neonates are those which are specific for glucose, and the method most commonly used is that based on the glucose oxidase reaction. Methods which determine total reducing substances in the blood do not reflect the true blood glucose level since, in the newborn infant, the concentration of nonglucose reducing substances in the blood tends to be far greater than in older children and adults.

There are also other sources of error. If blood is taken from the heel when skin circulation is impaired, misleadingly low levels of glucose may be obtained due to glycolysis in the stagnant peripheral blood. Red cell glycolysis may considerably reduce the glucose content of the sample if there is delay between collection and analysis.

If the Dextrostix reading is below 45 mg per 100 ml and the infant is symptomatic treatment should not be delayed until the laboratory blood sugar estimation is available. In the asymptomatic infant, treatment may await the laboratory result and, if the infant is then found to be suffering from hypoglycemia as previously defined, treatment is instituted immediately. Initially a bolus of 20% glucose (10% glucose if using the umbilical vein), 2 to 3 cc per kg, is administered as an intravenous push. A smaller volume of 50% glucose may be given, but we prefer to avoid this if possible because of the potentially damaging effect of this solution on the vascular linings. The initial bolus is followed by a continuous infusion of 10 to 15% glucose to provide a total fluid intake appropriate for age and weight. Treatment is discontinued once the blood sugar has remained within the normal range for 24 hr or more. The concentration of glucose solution is reduced gradually, since the sudden cessation of intravenous therapy commonly causes a return of hypoglycemic symptoms. Glucagon, 300 μg per kg by intramuscular injection, can be used in the treatment of hypoglycemia. However, although this treatment is usually effective in infants suffering from hyperinsulinism, it is unlikely to be effective in infants suffering from a lack of hepatic glycogen stores. Since glucagon has a marked stimulant effect on insulin production, it is advisable to start an intravenous infusion of 10 to 15% dextrose soon after the injection has been given.

Section V

CALCIUM METABOLISM AND HYPOCALCEMIA[26]

The incidence of neonatal hypocalcemia is not well defined, although in preterm infants it appears to range from 26 to 50%. Throughout pregnancy the fetus is supplied, via the placenta, with both calcium and maternal parathyroid hormone. Calcium is transported actively by the placenta and accumulated by the fetus at a progressively increasing rate towards term. The active transport of calcium maintains a fetal plasma level higher than the maternal level, and allows fetal calcification to proceed normally, despite poor maternal nutrition or placental insufficiency. Therefore, light weight for gestation infants usually have a normal calcium store at birth, whereas the truly preterm infant, who has missed the period of most rapid intrauterine calcium accumulation, is born relatively calcium deficient. All newborns exhibit a physiologic state of relative hypoparathyroidism at birth, along with inadequate renal phosphate excretion. This physiologic state is exaggerated in the preterm infant and in the infant of the diabetic mother. In addition to functional hypoparathyroidism and/or renal immaturity, there are several other factors associated with hypocalemia in the neonate. These include obstetric trauma, asphyxia, treatment of acidosis with bicarbonate and a diet consisting of modified cow's milk, which has a high phosphate content compared with breast milk. Early hypocalcemia occurring in the first 24 to 36 hr of life is seen in infants of diabetic mothers, premature infants, anoxic infants and those suffering cerebral trauma . A later form of hypocalcemia commonly occurs between the fifth and seventh days of life in infants fed on full strength modified cow's milk formula. As the disorder is virtually never seen in breast-fed infants, it seems likely that cow's milk, with its high phosphate content, stresses the suboptimal parathyroid status of the neonate. Neonatal hypocalcemia is also associated with a maternal hyperparathyroidism, exchange transfusion using citrated blood and maternal deficiency of vitamin D. The parathyroid glands may be congenitally absent, in association with an absent thymus and immunologic deficiency.[15]

Like the symptoms of hypoglycemia, the symptoms of hypocalcemia are nonspecfic in the newborn. Twitching, hypertonia, jitteriness and focal convulsions are most frequently described in the full term infant. Since these symptoms mimic those of cerebral trauma and anoxia, and since hypocalcemia is commonly associated with both of these conditions, it is essential to exclude coexistent hypocalcemia before drawing conclusions concerning the degree of brain damage in these infants. Symptoms in the preterm infant differ somewhat from those in the term infant. It is unusual for these infants to display the hypertonia and hyperactivity seen in the term infant. In contrast, these infants tend to be hypotonic. They have poor color, may become apneic, and show symptoms similar to those of hypoglycemia.

Whenever hypocalcemia is suspected on clinical grounds, serum calcium should be estimated. If the infant is symptomatic and hypoglycemia has been excluded, treatment should be instituted immediately. An electrocardiograph may show a prolongation of the Q-T interval; however, absence of this sign does not exclude hypocalcemia.

Management of Hypocalcemia

Although, unlike hypoglycemia, hypocalcemia does not appear to cause structural damage to the central nervous system, it seems appropriate, with the present state of knowledge, to actively treat these infants, particularly those with associated convulsions. In the presence of symptoms, a trial of therapy is indicated, while awaiting confirmation of hypocalcemia from the laboratory. It has become standard practice to treat all infants with a serum calcium level of 7 mg per 100 ml or less. Serum calcium, as routinely measured, includes protein-bound calcium in addition to the physiologically crucial free ionized calcium. Nomograms are available to allow estimation of the ionized fraction.[25] Immediate treatment consists of the intravenous infusion of calcium gluconate in a 10% solution, in a dose of 1 cc per kg body weight, at a rate no faster than 1 cc per min. If the symptoms are due to hypocalcemia, they should disappear with treatment. Occasionally, however, symptoms may cease because of the nonspecific sedative effect of the calcium solution, so that serum should be obtained before the calcium infusion to allow confirmation of hypocalcemia. It is advisable to monitor the infant electrocardiographically while administering the calcium and to stop the infusion temporarily if there is evidence of cardiac arrhythmia.

In the nonacute situation, calcium lactate solution may be given orally, up to a total dose of 1 g per kg birth weight per day. Milks such as breast milk and PM 60/40 (Similac) with relatively low phosphate content are a useful adjunct to therapy.

Since a rebound hypocalcemia may result from abrupt cessation, treatment should be tapered gradually when a normal serum calcium is achieved. Occasionally, associated hypomagnesemia may render the hypocalcemia resistant to treatment. The administration of magnesium sulfate, in a 50% solution, in two to three doses of 0.2 cc per kg body weight, 12 hr apart, will usually produce a satisfactory response in both serum calcium and serum magnesium levels.

Section VI

FURTHER ASPECTS OF CHEMICAL ADAPTATION

Renal function is relatively inefficient in all infants for the first 1 to 2 weeks of life. This problem is exaggerated in the preterm infant, and excessive loads of fluid or solute are inadequately excreted. Maternal overhydration has been reported to produce hyponatremia and seizures in the fetus.[6]

Hypernatremia may be produced either by administering excess solute or by dehydrating the infant, and may cause brain damage. In the first 24 to 48 hr of life, the infant does not require a significant intake of sodium. In the preterm infant glucose utilization is relatively sluggish, and hyperglycemic coma may result from the use of hypertonic intravenous glucose solutions. Many of these infants also exhibit a lowered renal threshold for glucose, and the resulting osmotic diuresis may cause severe dehydration.

Section VII

NEONATAL SEIZURES—METABOLIC AND OTHER CAUSES (TABLE 17.1)

Estimates of the frequency of seizures in the newborn period vary considerably. Reports from Britain indicate an incidence between 12 and 15 per 1000 live births.[8, 22] In general, the frequency of seizures in the first 48 hr of life has declined whereas frequency of seizures occurring later in the first week of life has increased. Seizures occurring early in the neonatal period are most likely to be associated with cerebral birth injury and show numerical response to improved obstetric care. These seizures carry the worst prognosis. In studies in Britain, between one-third and one-half of these infants died, and fewer than half of the survivors escaped neurologic or intellectual deficit. These studies also reconfirmed the coexistence of metabolic imbalance with cerebral birth injury, and emphasized the need to estimate calcium, glucose and electrolyte status in these infants.

Seizures initially occurring subsequent to the first 48 hr of life are, in the majority of cases, metabolic in origin, and, of these, most are due to hypocalcemia. The tendency for the frequency of these later occurring seizures to increase since the early 1950's is probably related to the decreasing popularity of breast feeding. Seizures due to inherited aminoacidopathies and galactosemia tend to occur after the first 48 hr of life, since an adequate intake of nutritional precursors must precede the production of toxic metabolic products.

Table 17.1. Some important causes of neonatal seizures*

A. First occurring within 48 hr of birth
Cerebral trauma and/or perinatal asphyxia
Intracranial hemorrhage
Metabolic—hypoglycemia, hypocalcemia, hyponatremia, hypernatremia, pyridoxine dependence
Developmental abnormalities of the brain
Bacterial sepsis and/or meningitis
Congenital viral (Torch) infection
B. First occurring subsequent to 48 hr of birth
Metabolic—hypocalcemia, hypomagnesemia, hyponatremia, hypernatremia
Intraventricular hemorrhage in preterm infants
Sepsis and/or meningitis
Drug withdrawal in infants of addicted mothers
Aminoacidopathies and galactosemia

* Groups A and B given in the approximate order of frequency.

Clinical Presentation of Seizures in Newborns

Recognition of seizures in the newborn can be very difficult because they are likely to be very subtle, especially in the preterm infant. The full grand mal type of episode is rare. The nervous system of the neonate functions primarily at the level of the brain stem, with little evidence of higher cortical function. A focal discharge in the cortex has difficulty recruiting sufficient response from surrounding cells to produce a seizure, whereas this is relatively easily accomplished at a subcortical level.

Seizures may take the form of brief extensor spasms, episodes of apnea and/or bradycardia, tonic-clonic movements of one area, eye rolling, facial twitching, paroxysmal blinking, continuous sucking or chewing movements or excessive swallowing and yawning.

Diagnosis of Seizures in Newborns

A careful history is essential for evidence of perinatal trauma or asphyxia, maternal drug or alcohol addiction or a history of previous infants with neonatal seizures. However, regardless of history, initially the infant should be assumed to be suffering from a potentially reversible problem. In this way damaging conditions such as hypoglycemia will not be neglected. Lumbar puncture should always be considered in the seizing infant to exclude meningeal infection and intracranial hemorrhage. Subdural tap may also be indicated in the infant with a full fontanel. EEG may help to confirm the cerebral origin of an abnormality if recorded during a seizure; however, it is unlikely to advance the diagnosis further, and treatment should not be delayed while awaiting this test.

Treatment of Neonatal Seizures

Immediately following any required acute resuscitation, a Dextrostix reading should be obtained, and glucose given as previously described should hypoglycemia be present. If the Dextrostix reading is greater than 45 mg per 100 ml, a trial of calcium therapy is indicated. In infants not responding to these measures, it is our practice to administer 50 mg of pyridoxine intravenously, since relative deficiency of this coenzyme is a rare cause of seizures in the immediate neonatal period. If therapy is appropriate, seizure activity should cease abruptly.

Once specific metabolic causes have been excluded, purely symptomatic therapy must be considered, particularly in status epilepticus. In cases where seizures are associated with significant cyanosis or status epilepticus, 10 to 15 mg per kg of phenobarbital may be given intravenously over several minutes. Diazepam is an effective alternative, although it should be avoided in icteric infants because it is prepared with *sodium benzoate* (see under "Hemolytic Anemia and Jaundice"). It is administered in aliquots, no faster than 0.1 mg per min, up to a maximum of 1.0 mg. Both of these drugs may produce significant respiratory depression, so that appropriate equipment for respiratory support must be available when they are used. Paraldehyde is not associated with significant respiratory depression when given slowly intravenously in a dose of 150 mg per kg, or per rectum in a dose of 300 mg per kg.

Continued suppression of seizures is usually achieved using oral phenobarbitone in a dose of 5 to 15 mg per kg per day or 4 to 6 mg per kg per day of oral diphenylhydantoin. These drugs may be used in combination in resistant cases.

Section VIII

HEMATOLOGIC ADAPTATION[21, 29]

Blood formation can first be detected in utero on about the 19th day of gestation, and may be divided into three distinct phases, namely, mesoblastic, hepatic and myeloid. By the 22nd day, blood islands may be observed throughout the mesodermal tissues of the fetus. During the sixth week of gestation, the activity of this stage declines, and from the third to sixth month, hematopoiesis takes place predominantly in the spleen and the liver. Extramedullary hematopoiesis is superseded by the myeloid phase from the sixth month onward, although blood cell formation can still be observed in the spleen during the first week of postnatal life.

The bulk of hemoglobin in utero is hemoglobin (Hb) F, with smaller quantities of hemoglobin A and hemoglobin A2. The quantity of HbF present in the red cells is inversely proportional to the gestational age, with the blood of the term infant containing approximately 50% HbF, falling to approximately 10% by the age of 4 to 5 months. HbF has a number of properties not shared by adult hemoglobin, which include resistance to acid elution and denaturization by alkali. Fetal blood also has a greater affinity for oxygen than adult blood. This appears to be due, in part, to the lower content of an organic phosphate, 2,3-diphosphoglycerate, in fetal red cells. 2,3-Diphosphoglycerate binds to reduced hemoglobin, decreasing its affinity for oxygen, but the effect upon HbA is more than 50% greater than it is on HbF. The greater capacity of adult red cells to release oxygen may have clinical application in the hypoxic newborn, since transfusion with adult cells should, hypothetically, improve tissue oxygenation.

From the sixth month of gestation onwards there is an increase in hematocrit. The normal value for newborn hemoglobin concentration is in the range of 14 to 20 g per 100 ml, and the normal value for hematocrit ranges between 45% and 60%. In the first few hours after birth there is an increase in hemoglobin and hematocrit values due to physiologic hemoconcentration. Then follows a slow decline by the end of the first week of life to very near the original values. Capillary hemoglobin values are 0.5 to 2 g per 100 ml higher than venous values. This difference can be minimized by warming the limb before capillary samples are obtained.

Polycythemia

Hemoglobin values in preterm infants may be 1 to 2 g per 100 cc lower than those in term infants, whereas values in infants that are light weight for gestational age tend to be higher by a similar amount. Many light weight for gestation and some post-term infants suffer relative hypoxia in utero, and tend to compensate for this by producing an excess of red blood cells.

Hemoglobin and hematocrit values at birth may be altered considerably as a result of placental transfusion. In normal pregnancies the infant is probably optimally delivered onto a surface which is level with the mother's perineum, with rapid cord clamping. If there is reason to suspect significant anemia in the newborn, there may be some benefit in allowing placental-fetal transfusion by delaying cord clamping. However, unnecessary transfusion from the placenta may result in a polycythemic infant. Polycythemia may also result from twin to twin transfusion in monozygotic twins, rarely from fetal-maternal transfusion, and is frequently seen in infants of diabetic mothers, in whom increased production of erythropoietin is one of many responses to hormonal imbalance.

Complications of polycythemia include congestive cardiac failure, vascular thrombosis, respiratory distress, exacerbation of physiologic jaundice, hypoglycemia and thrombocytopenia. A venous hematocrit greater than 65% or a capillary hematocrit greater than 70% is indication for therapy in the form of partial exchange transfusion with plasma, removing sufficient blood to lower the venous hematocrit below 60% while maintaining blood volume.

Anemia Due to Hemorrhage in Prenatal Period

Anemia may be present at birth as a result of intrauterine hemolysis or hemorrhage. The average blood volume for a term infant is approximately 80 cc per kg, so that a rapid bleed of as little as 50 cc can cause a shock state in the newborn. Bleeding may occur from the fetal to the maternal circulation, from one twin to another, from the rupture of abnormal placental vessels and from placenta previa.

When the site of bleeding is not obvious, a sample of maternal blood should be examined for fetal red cells. It is now recognized that, in as many as 50% of pregnancies, some fetal cells pass into the maternal circulation at some time during gestation or the birth process. In 10% of pregnancies these losses range from 0.5% to 40 cc of blood. In about 1% losses are even greater and may approximate 100 cc.

Fetal blood cells are demonstrated in the maternal circulation using the Kleihauer technique of acid elution.[23] This test is based on the increased resistance of HbF to acid elution, as compared with HbA. When fixed smears are immersed in a disodium hydrogen phosphate solution, buffered to an acid pH, HbA is eluted from the erythrocytes, but HbF is not.

The newborn with severe acute intrauterine hemorrhage is born in a collapsed state. In many ways he represents a clinical picture very similar to that seen in the asphyxiated infant; however, tachycardia is often associated with hemorrhage, whereas bradycardia is a more usual finding in the asphyxiated infant. The hemoglobin concentration may not fall immediately, but the central venous pressure is low, and the hematocrit will fall precipitately over the first few hours of life if treatment is not instituted. This fall is due to movement of fluid from the extravascular space into the intravascular space in an attempt to maintain blood volume. The state of the infant at birth should be judged on clinical grounds, and too much reliance should not be placed on the hemoglobin concentration.

Infants traumatized during the birth process, particularly during breech delivery, may bleed internally, and the site of hemorrhage may not be obvious immediately. Laceration of internal organs may cause serious blood loss, as may hemorrhage into the scalp after vacuum (ventouse) delivery.

Treatment of Intrauterine Hemorrhage

Treatment of acute blood loss should not await the results of investigation. A catheter should be placed in the umbilical vein, and blood withdrawn for hemoglobin and hematocrit values, platelet count, Coombs test, cross-matching and coagulation screen. Blood volume should be rapidly expanded, preferably with group O Rh-negative blood, in a volume of 10 to 20 cc per kg body weight. If blood is not available, plasma may be substituted initially, and, since there is often some delay while fresh frozen plasma is thawed, an artificial plasma substitute, 5% Plasmanate (Cutter), may be used. Plasma therapy should be replaced by blood transfusion as soon as possible. Overtransfusion can be avoided by frequently assessing the central venous pressure via the umbilical vein. Subsequent management depends upon the source of bleeding.

Hemorrhage in Neonatal Period

The diagnosis and rational treatment of the bleeding infant requires a thorough physical examination and a careful history, including maternal history. If the infant has swallowed maternal blood, he may present with hematemesis and/or melena for a period of up to 48 hr after birth. Diagnosis is made using the Apt test,[4] which depends upon the ability of fetal hemoglobin to protect red blood cells from denaturization with alkali. One part of stool or vomit is mixed with 5 parts of water. The specimen is shaken, and then centrifuged for 10 min at 3000 rpm. The pink supernatant solution is decanted, and to 5 cc is added 1 cc of 0.25 N (1%) NaOH. After 2 min, blood containing adult hemoglobin changes from a pink to a brown-yellow color, whereas blood containing predominantly fetal cells remains pink.

The majority of hemorrhagic episodes in the neonatal period are due to coagulation defects. In the normal term infant, factors 5 and 8 and fibrinogen show normal adult levels at birth, but all other factors are present in lower quantities than found in the normal adult. Bleeding results from accentuation of these physiologic deficiencies by vitamin K deficiency, intravascular coagulation, inherited permanent abnormalities of the coagulation system, quantitative or qualitative abnormalities of the platelets, vascular abnormalities and trauma alone or in association with any of the other factors.

Vitamin K Deficiency

Vitamin K is required for the hepatic synthesis of prothrombin, plus factors 7, 9 and 10. The quantity of vitamin K-dependent factors in the blood of all newborns begins to fall shortly after birth, and reaches nadir on the third or fourth day of life. This is often referred to as the "physiologic dip" and may be associated with hemorrhagic diathesis. The tendency to hemorrhage increases with increasing prematurity. A single dose of vitamin K, given soon after birth, usually prevents bleeding, and early feeding with formula derived from cow's milk may also lessen this tendency. Feedings based on cow's milk contain 4 times (6 μg per 100 cc) as much vitamin K as human breast milk (1.5 μg per 100 cc) No advantage is associated with the prenatal administration of vitamin K to the mother.

The term "hemorrhagic disease of the newborn" (HDN) was introduced in 1894 by Townsend.[36] Typically, infants developing this disease are full term and fed on breast milk. A bleeding tendency develops on the second to fourth day of life, i.e., at the nadir of the physiologic dip. Bleeding from the gastrointestinal tract is the most common manifestation, but bleeding from the umbilicus and nose and into the skin and internal organs also occurs. Vitamin K deficiency is characterized serologically by a prolonged clotting time and a very prolonged prothrombin time (see Table 17.2). It should be suspected as the major cause of hemorrhage in any newborn infant who has not received vitamin K at birth. The response to vitamin K is less predictable in the preterm infant, probably because of a combination of relative immaturity of the liver and the effect of anoxia on hepatic production of coagulation factors. Infants born to mothers receiving anticonvulsants and oral anticoagulants are also at risk for hemorrhage due to deficiency of the vitamin K-dependent factors. Information currently available indicates that vitamin K in the nonwater-soluble form, and in the dose recommended by the American Academy of Pediatrics (1 mg intramuscularly) is safe, and is the drug of choice for prophylaxis against HDN, even in infants suffering from glucose-6-phosphate dehydrogenase deficiency.[39] Intravenously administered vitamin K is effective within 3 to 4 hr, but in the case of acute severe hemorrhage, clotting factors should be administered in the form of fresh blood (less than 48 hr old), or fresh frozen plasma. (Plasmanate does not contain clotting factors, and should not be used for this purpose.) The estimated incidence of HDN, in infants not receiving vitamin K at birth, varies from 0.25 to 0.5%.

Disseminated Intravascular Coagulation (DIC)

Disseminated intravascular coagulation is now recognized as an important disorder, frequently seen in neonatal practice. It is not itself a primary disease, but is a response to deleterious stimuli. Sepsis, hypoxia, acidosis and maternal eclampsia are common initiating factors. Clinical manifestations include the appearance of purpura and bruising, oozing from puncture sites, gastrointestinal bleeding, pulmonary hemorrhage and bleeding into internal organs. Intraventricular hemorrhage is common in preterm infants with respiratory disease. The factor which initiates the coagulation cascade has not yet been defined, but results in the widespread deposition of fibrin clots throughout the body. There is consumption of coagulation factors in the process, in particular fibrinogen, factor 5 and factor 8, with a resulting bleeding diathesis. Platelets aggregate in the clots, producing thrombocytopenia. Physical trauma to red blood cells, as they attempt to pass through the fibrin strands, leads to a characteristic red cell fragmentation. Laboratory diagnosis of DIC in the neonate rests on the combined findings of a falling hematocrit, thrombocytopenia, decreased fibrinogen levels (below 200 mg per 100 ml), increased prothrombin time and partial thromboplastin time and red cell fragmentation (see Table 17.2). In the majority of infants with this disease, recovery results from treatment of the primary disease. Exchange transfusion with fresh heparinized blood may be used in severe cases. In milder cases, the "vicious circle" of the disease may be broken simply by transfusing with plasma or fresh blood, in a volume of 10 cc per kilo body weight, in addition to treating the underlying illness. Cessation of bleeding and a stable hematocrit and platelet count, indicate therapeutic success.

Neonatal Hemorrhage Due to Other Causes

A deficiency in number or quality of platelets is an important cause of hemorrhage in the newborn, and should be suspected when bleeding is characterized by cutaneous petechiae and purpuric spots. The number of platelets considered normal in the neonate tends to vary somewhat with the reporting authority. It generally is considered that thrombocytopenia is present when the platelet count is less than 150,000 mm^3 in the term infant, and less than 100,000 mm^3 in the preterm infant.

There are numerous causes of thrombocytopenia in the newborn including DIC, infection (particularly viral infection), isoimmune disorders and maternal drug therapy with thiazide diuretics, furosem-

Table 17.2. Major diagnostic features of vitamin K deficiency versus disseminated intravascular coagulation (DIC)

Feature	DIC	Vitamin K deficiency
History		
Mother receiving oral anticoagulants or anticonvulsants	Absent	May be present
Perinatal asphyxia	Frequently present	Occasionally present, particularly in preterm infants
Vitamin K administered at birth	Usually present	Absent in term infants; may be present in preterm infants
Infant otherwise well	Never present	Usually present
Hematologic parameter		
Prothrombin time	Prolonged	Prolonged
Partial thromboplastin time	Prolonged	Prolonged
Red cell fragmentation	Present	Absent
Fibrinogen level	Decreased	Normal
Fibrin split products	Often increased	Normal
Platelet count	Decreased	Normal

ide or tolbutamide. A short lived but profound thrombocytopenia may appear in infants born to mothers suffering from idiopathic thrombocytopenia or disseminated lupus erythematosis, and a low platelet count is frequently seen in infants with giant hemangiomatous malformations.

When the platelet count is sufficiently low to produce a bleeding tendency, usually at a level between 10,000 and 20,000 mm^3, immediate treatment is required. Fresh blood or a pure platelet transfusion (10 cc per kg) should effectively reverse the bleeding tendency, but the effect may not persist longer than 6 to 8 hr. Exchange transfusion is indicated for the isoimmune type of thrombocytopenia to remove maternal antibodies from the circulation. Washed platelets should be used, since most donor platelets carry common antigens against which maternal antibodies are active. This disorder may appear in isolation, or in association with rhesus isoimmunization. A significant increase in the number of large, immature platelets in the circulation is a clue to diagnosis. The majority of the remainder of the clotting disorders in the neonatal period is due to inherited factor deficiencies. More than 90% of these are cases of hemophilia (factor 8) or Christmas disease (factor 9). Only severely affected cases are likely to be diagnosed in infancy unless there is a family history of the disease. A number of cases will present after circumcision, which should never be performed in the delivery room. Bleeding can be controlled by maintaining deficient factor levels above 30%, using fresh frozen plasma or specific factor fractions.

Hemolytic Anemia and Jaundice

The bulk of bilirubin produced for excretion derives from red cell breakdown, 1 g of hemoglobin producing 35 mg of bilirubin. Detectable jaundice occurs when the serum bilirubin concentration rises above 2 mg per 100 ml. Before passage through the liver, bilirubin is soluble in fat, but is insoluble in water. Fat-soluble (indirect) bilirubin may cross the placenta and the so-called blood brain barrier. Water-soluble (direct) bilirubin is rapidly excreted in the stool and the urine. One molecule of albumin binds 2 molecules of bilirubin. The second of these binding sites binds the bilirubin less firmly than the first, so that displacement of bilirubin is relatively easy and may occur with asphyxia, acidosis and in the presence of substances which compete for albumin sites. The latter include sulfonamides, salicylates and *sodium benzoate,* which is a carrier substance used in the preparation of many drugs. Before delivery, excretion of bilirubin is handled largely by the placenta, but at birth, the infant liver is required to take over this function. The liver in most newborns is relatively deficient in glucuronyl transferase activity, and, in a situation of increased bilirubin production, may fail to cope with the increased load.

The differential diagnosis of jaundice in the newborn is shown in Table 17.3. All infants with more than the slightest icterus require the basic investigation of direct and total bilirubin estimation, Coombs testing, blood group, hemoglobin determination and blood films to show red cell morphology. Urinalysis for reducing substances should also be routine, since the test is simple and noninvasive, and these substances are found in excess in the rare case of galactosemia presenting with jaundice. A full sepsis workup is performed if clinically indicated.

Physiologic Jaundice

Hepatic immaturity is a major cause of jaundice in the neonatal period. This is related to a deficiency of glucuronyl trans-

Table 17.3. Differential diagnosis of jaundice in newborns

Significant jaundice in the first 48 hr of life
Blood group incompatibilities
Infection
Jaundice appearing after the first 48 hr of life, and resolving prior to the 14th day of life
Physiologic jaundice and jaundice of prematurity
Infection
Jaundice appearing after the first 48 hr of life, and not resolving by the 14th day of life
Infection, including neonatal hepatitis
"Breast milk" jaundice
Obstructive jaundice due to anatomic abnormality of the biliary system
Galactosemia
Hypothyroidism

ferase activity in the liver, and is exaggerated in the preterm infant. Jaundice usually appears on the third or fourth day of life, and is so rare in the first 24 hr of life that other causes always should be considered in an infant presenting with early jaundice. The jaundice does not usually persist beyond the age of 7 days in the term infant, or 14 days in the preterm infant. Persistence beyond 14 days indicates the need for further investigation to exclude hypothyroidism or surgical causes.

Hemolytic Disease

Until recent years, rhesus isoimmunization has been the major cause of perinatal hemolysis in the Western hemisphere. However, with the advent of RhO D-immune gammaglobulin (Rhogam), the incidence of this disease has fallen considerably, highlighting other forms of hemolytic problem, in particular ABO incompatibility.

Anemia results when erythropoiesis fails to compensate for hemolysis and, in the hydropic infant, the hemoglobin at birth is often less than 6 g per 100 ml. After birth, the hemoglobin continues to fall, since hemolysis will continue for as long as maternal antibodies are present in the infant's blood stream. Anemia is seldom seen in association with ABO incompatibility, possibly because of later onset of intrauterine hemolysis, combined with a slower rate of hemolysis than is seen with Rh isoimmunization. The disease differs from Rh incompatibility in that increased antibody titers, against incompatible blood group antigens, are not present prenatally in the mothers of ABO-incompatible infants. Jaundice is usually absent at birth in both diseases, but becomes evident during the first 24 to 48 hr after birth. The Coombs test is always positive in rhesus isoimmunization. In ABO disease, however, the Coombs test may be negative, although the frequency of negative results decreases as techniques for Coombs testing become more sensitive. Significant hyperbilirubinemia is less frequent in ABO disease than in rhesus isoimmunization, and bilirubin levels tend to rise more slowly.

Breast Milk Jaundice

Jaundice develops in a small proportion of breast-fed infants, and appears to be due to a substance secreted in the milk which depresses glucuronyl transferase activity in the liver. This compound may be the steroid, pregnane-3-alpha-20-beta-diol. Jaundice appears toward the end of the first week and persists for 3 to 6 weeks.

Obstructive Jaundice

Increase in the conjugated component of the total serum bilirubin, over 2 mg per 100 ml, arouses suspicion of obstructive jaundice. Approximately half of these cases have biliary atresia, and the majority of the remainder have neonatal hepatitis. Recently there have been suggestions that certain types of neonatal hepatitis may lead to eventual biliary atresia, making both diseases part of the spectrum of the same pathologic process.

Hypothyroidism

This problem may present with prolonged hyperbilirubinemia, in the absence of other clinical stigmata of cretinism. Thyroid function studies always should be obtained in cases where icterus persists for more than 14 days.

Bilirubin Toxicity

Bilirubin values are monitored every 4 to 6 hr in infants at risk for hyperbilirubinemia. Indirect, or conjugated, bilirubin is readily deposited in brain tissue once serum levels reach a significant level. In otherwise healthy term infants, neurotoxic effects do not usually appear unless the concentration of unconjugated bilirubin rises above 20 mg per 100 ml, but significantly lower levels may cause brain damage in the presence of prematurity, acidosis, asphyxia or hypoproteinemia. Substances which compete for bilirubin binding sites on the albumin molecule will have a similar effect. Symptoms of brain damage, or kernicterus, in the neonate include loss of primitive reflexes (including the suck reflex), hypotonia, high pitched cry and opisotonic posturing with or without seizures. Sequelae in surviving infants include choreoathetosis, high tone deafness and mental retardation.

Treatment of Jaundice

The type of therapy to be used is indicated by the serologic parameters measured. It is commonly accepted that in rhesus isoimmunization a cord hemoglobin level of below 10 g per 100 cc, in association with a cord bilirubin value greater than 4 mg per 100 cc, is indication for immediate exchange transfusion at birth. We have found that a cord bilirubin value of greater than 4 mg per 100 cc is also an indication for early therapy in ABO incompatibility.[40] In the latter disease phototherapy has been used with some success, although exchange transfusion may still be required in a small number of patients. A rate of rise of the serum bilirubin value of greater than 0.5 mg per hr requires immediate intervention and, in less severely affected infants, a bilirubin concentration greater than 20 mg per 100 cc. This latter figure may only be reliably used in full term infants who are otherwise clinically well. Most preterm infants weighing less than 2000 g receive exchange transfusion at a serum bilirubin concentration no greater than 15 mg per 100 ml.

Exchange transfusion is associated with some risk to the newborn, and should be performed only in a center with staff well practiced in the technique. Where prenatal tests have indicated a high risk infant, nursery staff should be informed in advance of delivery. Fresh O-negative blood should be cross-matched for the infant, using a sample of maternal serum. Packed cells are used in severely anemic infants, whereas whole blood exchange transfusion is employed to replace the infant's sensitized red blood cell population, and simultaneously to remove both bilirubin and circulating maternal antibodies.

In 1958, Cremer et al[12] showed that in some cases of neonatal jaundice the serum bilirubin concentration could be significantly reduced by the illumination of the infant with blue light. This form of treatment is effective in infants with physiologic jaundice, and probably also in some cases of hemolytic jaundice.[27, 32] Bilirubin breakdown is enhanced by light, producing photo-oxidation products, the exact nature of which is unknown. The site of breakdown appears to be in the skin, and excretion is enhanced by a stimulant effect of the light upon gastrointestinal motility. Since the quantity of unconjugated, rather than conjugated, bilirubin increases in the intestinal tract of infants receiving phototherapy, it has been postulated that phototherapy may change the stereoscopic orientation of the bilirubin molecule, with the resulting molecule so closely resembling the conjugated form of bilirubin that it is excreted without further hepatic processing.[28]

Since the possible side effects of the photo-oxidation products are not known, the treatment should be used only when, and for as long as, clinically indicated. Usual indications for phototherapy are a serum bilirubin value greater than 13 to 15 mg per 100 ml in a term infant, and above 10 mg per 100 ml in preterm infants. In the acidotic or asphyxiated infant, these levels are accordingly lower.

Known side effects of phototherapy are not severe, and include a transient generalized morbilliform rash and loose stools. A liberal fluid intake is essential, since treatment increases fluid losses from the skin and gut. Light therapy should be avoided in the infant with a direct bilirubin value greater than 2 mg per 100 ml.[24]

Phenobarbital has been advocated in the treatment of physiologic jaundice. It appears to be effective for this purpose when given to the mother prior to delivery, but has not been of proven benefit when administered directly to the neonate, particularly once icterus has developed. Phenobarbital probably produces an effect by enhancing the activity of hepatic glucuronyl transferase. Clearly, however, this approach involves the unnecessary treatment of a large number of normal infants, in order to achieve an as yet unknown degree of therapeutic success in the few infants who develop significant hyperbilirubinemia. Side effects of phenobarbital therapy in the newborn include transient skin rashes and undesirable sedation.

REFERENCES

1. Adam, P. A. J., Schwartz, R. Diagnosis and treatment: Should oral hypoglycaemic agents be used in pediatric and pregnant patients. Pediatrics 42: 819, 1968.

2. Adamsons, K., Jr., Behrman, R., Dawes, G., et al: Resuscitation by positive pressure ventilation of Rhesus monkey asphyxiated at birth. J Pediatr 65: 807, 1964.
3. Apgar, V.: A proposal for a new method of evaluation of the newborn infant. Current Res Anesthesiol Analges 32: 260, 1953.
4. Apt, L., Downey, W. S.: A simple test for the differentiation of adult and fetal hemoglobin in bloody stools. J Pediatr 47: 6, 1955.
5. Avery, M. E.: *The lung and Its Disorders in the Newborn Infant*. Second edition. Philadelphia, W. B. Saunders Company, 1968.
6. Battalgia, F., Prystowsky. H.: Fetal blood studies. XIII. The effect of the administration of fluids intravenously to mothers upon the concentration of water and electrolytes in plasma of human fetuses. Pediatrics 25: 2, 1960.
7. Behrman, R. E., Lees, M. H., Peterson, E. N., DeLamoy, C. W., Seeds, A. E.: Distribution of the circulation in the normal and asphyxiated fetal primate. Am J Obstet Gynecol 108: 956, 1970.
8. Brown, J. K., Cockburn, F., Forfar, J. O.: Clinical and chemical correlates in convulsions of the newborn. Lancet 1: 135, 1972.
9. Clements, J. A., Platzker, A. C. G., Tierney, D. F., Hobel, C. J., Creasy, R. K., Margolis, A. J., Thibeault, D. W., Tooley, W. H., Oh, W.: Assessment of the high risk of the respiratory-distress syndrome by a rapid test for surfactant in amniotic fluid. N Engl J Med 286: 1077, 1972.
10. Cordero, L., Jr., Hon, E. H.: Neonatal bradycardia following nasopharyngeal stimulation. J Pediatr 78: 441, 1971.
11. Cornblath, M., Odell, G. B., Levin, E. J.: Hypoglycaemia associated with the toxaemia of pregnancy. J Pediatr 55: 545, 1959.
12. Cremer, R. J., Perryman, P. W., Richards, D. H.: Influences of light on the hyperbilirubinaemia of infants. Lancet 1: 1094, 1958.
13. Dawes, G.: *Fetal and Neonatal Physiology*. Chicago, Year Book Medical Publishers, 1968.
14. Dawes, G. S., Hibbard, E., Windle, W. T.: The effect of alkali and glucose infusion on permanent brain damage in Rhesus monkeys asphyxiated at birth. J Pediatr 65: 801, 1964.
15. DiGeorge, A. M.: Congenital absence of the thymus and immunologic consequences. Birth Defects 4: 116, 1968.
16. Dubowitz, L. M. S., et al: Clinical assessment of gestational age in a newborn infant. J Pediatr 77: 1, 1970.
17. Fedrick, J., Butler, N. R.: Hyaline membrane disease. Lancet 2: 768, 1972.
18. Gluck, L., Mulovich, M. V., Borer, R. C., Brenner, P. H., Anderson, G. G., Spellacy, W. N.: Diagnosis of the respiratory distress syndrome by amniocentesis. Am J Obstet Gynecol 109: 440, 1971.
19. Hartman. A. F., Jaudon, J. C.: Hypoglycaemia. J Pediatr 11: 1, 1937.
20. Haworth, J. C.: Carbohydrate metabolism in the fetus and the newborn. Pediatr Clin North Am 12: 573, 1965.
21. *Hematology in the Perinatal Patient*. Mead Johnson Symposium on Perinatal and Developmental Medicine, No. 4, 1973.
22. Keen, J. H., Lee, D.: Sequelae of neonatal convulsions: Study of 112 infants. Arch Dis Child 48: 542, 1973.
23. Kleihauer, E., Braun, H., Betke, K.: Demonstration von fetalem hemoglobin in den erthyrocyten eines blutausstrichs. Klin Wochenschr 35: 637, 1957.
24. Kopelman, A. K., Brown, R. S., Odell, G. B.: The "bronze" baby syndrome: A complication of phototherapy. J Pediatr 81: 466, 1972.
25. McLean, F., Hastings, A.: The state of calcium in the fluids of the body. I. The conditions affecting the ionisation of calcium. J Biol Chem 108: 285, 1935.
26. Mizrahi, A., London, R. D., Gribetz, D.: Neonatal hypocalcemia—Its causes and its treatment. N Engl J Med 278: 1163, 1968.
27. Moller, J., Ebbesen, F.: Phototherapy in newborn infants with severe Rhesus hemolytic disease. J Pediatr 86: 135, 1975.
28. Odell, G. B.: Personal communication.
29. Oski, F. A., Naiman, J. L.: Hematologic problems in the newborn. *Major Problems in Clinical Pediatrics*, Vol. IV, Second edition. Philadelphia, W. B. Saunders Company, 1972.
30. Pedersen, J.: *The Pregnant Diabetic and Her Newborn: Problems and Management*. Baltimore, The Williams & Wilkins Co., 1967.
31. Pildes, R. S., Cornblath, M., Warren, I., Page-El, E., DiMenza, S., Merrit, D. M., Peeva, A. A.: Prospective controlled study of neonatal hypoglycaemia. Pediatrics 54: 5, 1974.
32. Reid, M. McC., Marks, E., McClure, G., Elwood, J. H.: Phototherapy in Rh hemolytic disease. Lancet 1: 874, 1972.
33. Risemberg, H. M., Fomufird, K., Hazelbaker, N., Nishida, H., Peralta, M. J.: Assisted ventilation with nasal continuous positive airway pressure and its effects on morbidity and mortality in respiratory distress syndrome. Johns Hopkins Med J 135: 171, 1974.
34. Rudolph, A. M., Yuan, S.: Response of the pulmonary vasculature to hypoxia and H^+ ion concentration changes. J Clin Invest 45: 399, 1966.
35. Seeds, A. E., Behrman, R. E.: Acid-base monitoring of the fetus during labor with blood obtained from the scalp. J Pediatr 74: 804, 1969.
36. Townsend, C. W.: The hemorrhagic disease of the newborn. Arch Pediatr 11: 559, 1894.
37. White, P.: Diabetes mellitus in pregnancy. Symposium on Management of the High-Risk Pregnancy, September 1974, p 343.
38. Whitfield, C. R., Sproule, W. B., Brudenell, M.: The amniotic fluid lecithin: Sphingomyelin area ratio (LSAR) in pregnancies complicated by diabetes. J Obstet Gynaecol Br Commonw 80: 918, 1973.
39. Zinkham, W. H.: Peripheral blood and bilirubin valves in normal full-term primaquine sensitive Negro infants: Effects of vitamin K. Pediatrics 31: 983, 1963.
40. Risemberg, H. M., Mazzi, E., MacDonald, M. G., Peralta, M., Heldrich, F.: The correlation of cord bilirubin levels with hyperbilirubinemia in ABO incompatibility. Arch Dis Childhood, 1977.

Index

Ed,

A small token to you for your personal generosity to me at a difficult time in my life. May our friendship grow in the future as it has in the past. It is truly an honor and privilege to know and work with a fully human as yourself.

Ron

(Oct 6, 1977)